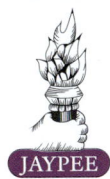
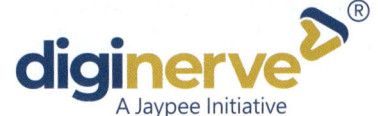

# DigiNEET

Master your MBBS studies and NEET PG preparation effortlessly with DigiNEET. Designed by India's top faculty, this all-in-one program covers all 19 subjects, helping you build a strong foundation and excel with confidence.

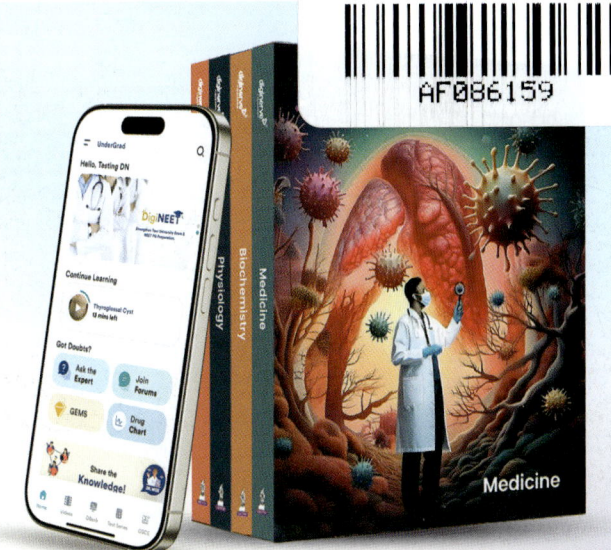

## Course Features

 1,400+ hrs of Video Lectures

 1,500+ Topics in Notes

 15,000+ Questions in QBank

 1,800+ GEMS

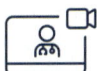 450+ OSCEs

 Test Series

 Drug Chart

 Dr. Wise AI Chatbot

 Regular Webinar

 Printed Notes*

*Printed notes are available at an additional cost.

**Unlock 5 Days of Full Access**

DOWNLOAD DIGINERVE APP

### Just 4 steps to unlock 5 days full access

1. Scan the QR code
2. Download the app
3. Sign up with your details
4. Start accessing premium content – free for 5 days!

*T&C Apply

+91-8800-418-418   marketing@diginerve.com

Download the App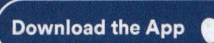

# Part-2
# An Insider's Guide to Cases in Clinical Medicine

## Second Edition

**Archith Boloor**
MBBS MD (Internal Medicine)
Additional Professor and HOU
Department of Medicine
Kasturba Medical College, Mangaluru
Manipal Academy of Higher Education
Karnataka, India
*archithb@gmail.com*

### Co-Editors

**Nikhil Kenny Thomas**
MBBS MD (Internal Medicine) DM DrNB (Medical Gastroenterology)
Consultant Gastroenterologist
Department of Gastroenterology and Hepatology
St. Luke Hospital, Pathanamthitta
Dr KM Cherian Institute of Medical Sciences, Chenganur, Kerala, India
*nikhilkennythomas@gmail.com*

**Mohamed Faizan Thouseef**
MBBS MD DNB (Internal Medicine)
Assistant Professor
Department of Medicine
Kasturba Medical College, Mangaluru
Manipal Academy of Higher Education
Karnataka, India
*mfaizan1709@gmail.com*

### Foreword
**Ashok Kumar Das**

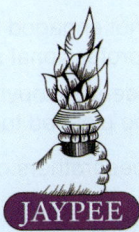

## JAYPEE BROTHERS MEDICAL PUBLISHERS
*The Health Sciences Publisher*
New Delhi | London

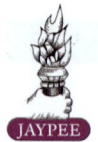 **Jaypee Brothers Medical Publishers (P) Ltd**

**Headquarters**
EMCA House
23/23-B, Ansari Road, Daryaganj
New Delhi 110 002, India
Landline: +91-11-23272143, +91-11-23272703
+91-11-23282021, +91-11-23245672
E-mail: jaypee@jaypeebrothers.com

**Overseas Office**
J.P. Medical Ltd
83 Victoria Street, London
SW1H 0HW (UK)
Phone: +44 20 3170 8910
E-mail: info@jpmedpub.com

**Corporate Office**
4838/24, Ansari Road, Daryaganj
New Delhi 110 002, India
Phone: +91-11-43574357
Fax: +91-11-43574314
E-mail: jaypee@jaypeebrothers.com

**EU GPSR** Authorised Representative
Logos Europe, 9 rue Nicolas Poussin
17000, La Rochelle, France
Phone: +33 (0) 6 67 93 73 78
E-mail: contact@logoseurope.eu

Website: www.jaypeebrothers.com
Website: www.jaypeedigital.com

© 2026, Jaypee Brothers Medical Publishers

The views and opinions expressed in this book are solely those of the original contributor(s)/author(s) and do not necessarily represent those of editor(s) and publisher of the book.

All rights reserved. No part of this publication may be reproduced, stored or transmitted in any form or by any means, electronic, mechanical, photocopying, recording or otherwise, without the prior permission in writing of the publishers.

All brand names and product names used in this book are trade names, service marks, trademarks or registered trademarks of their respective owners. The publisher is not associated with any product or vendor mentioned in this book.

Medical knowledge and practice change constantly. This book is designed to provide accurate, authoritative information about the subject matter in question. However, readers are advised to check the most current information available on procedures included and check information from the manufacturer of each product to be administered, to verify the recommended dose, formula, method and duration of administration, adverse effects and contraindications. It is the responsibility of the practitioner to take all appropriate safety precautions. Neither the publisher nor the author(s)/editor(s) assume any liability for any injury and/or damage to persons or property arising from or related to use of material in this book.

This book is sold on the understanding that the publisher is not engaged in providing professional medical services. If such advice or services are required, the services of a competent medical professional should be sought.

Every effort has been made where necessary to contact holders of copyright to obtain permission to reproduce copyright material. If any have been inadvertently overlooked, the publisher will be pleased to make the necessary arrangements at the first opportunity.

**Inquiries for bulk sales may be solicited at:** jaypee@jaypeebrothers.com

*An Insider's Guide to Cases in Clinical Medicine*

First Edition: 2023
Second Edition: **2026**
ISBN: 978-93-6616-219-5

*Printed in India*

**Dedicated to**

All the young budding doctors who shall be the future caretakers of our society

# Contributors

**Abu Thajudeen** MD
Department of Neurology
Father Muller Medical College
Mangaluru, Karnataka, India

**Ashwini** MV MD DM
Department of Cardiology
Kasturba Medical College, Manipal
Manipal Academy of Higher Education
Karnataka, India

**Madhav H Hande** MD DrNB
Associate Consultant
Department of Nephrology
Manipal Hospital, Whitefield
Bangaluru, Karnataka, India

**Manoj Kumar Devera** MD
Department of Internal Medicine
Sri Venkateswara Institute of Medical Sciences
Tirupati, Andhra Pradesh, India

**Mohammed Shaheen**
Department of Emergency Medicine
Hamad Medical Corporation
Doha, Qatar

**Prajwal Pai** MD
Department of Medical Gastroenterology
Kasturba Medical College, Manipal
Manipal Academy of Higher Education
Karnataka, India

**PS Gayathri Thampi** MD
Department of Internal Medicine
Kasturba Medical College, Mangaluru
Manipal Academy of Higher Education
Karnataka, India

**Sagi Pranathi** MD
Department of Neurology
Andhra Medical College
Visakhapatnam, Andhra Pradesh, India

**Saladi Sri Vijay Sasikanth**
Department of Internal Medicine
Kasturba Medical College, Mangaluru
Manipal Academy of Higher Education

**Sheetal Raj M** MD
Department of Internal Medicine and Program Director
Geriatric Medicine Fellowship
Kasturba Medical College, Mangaluru
Manipal Academy of Higher Education
Karnataka, India

**Siddharth Satish Bableshwar**
Department of Internal Medicine
Kasturba Medical College, Mangaluru
Manipal Academy of Higher Education
Karnataka, India

**Varun M Nair** MD
Department of Internal Medicine
Kasturba Medical College, Mangalore
Manipal Academy of Higher Education
Karnataka, India

**Vidarshan Mathavan**
Department of Internal Medicine
Kasturba Medical College, Mangaluru
Manipal Academy of Higher Education
Karnataka, India

**Vivek Hari** MD
Department of Nephrology
Madras Medical College
Chennai, Tamil Nadu, India

**Vivek K Koushik** MD DrNB
Consultant Nephrologist
Prashanth Hospitals, Kolathur
Chennai, Tamil Nadu, India

# Foreword

It is my proud privilege and an immense pleasure to write the foreword for the second edition of *An Insider's Guide to Cases in Clinical Medicine*, written by Professor Dr Archith Boloor.

Dr Boloor is a great teacher with astute clinical acumen with a flair for imparting knowledge and empowering undergraduate and postgraduate students with clinical knowledge, skill, and bedside diagnosis.

This second edition of *An Insider's Guide to Cases in Clinical Medicine* has many new case discussions, further enriching earlier discussions with latest facts.

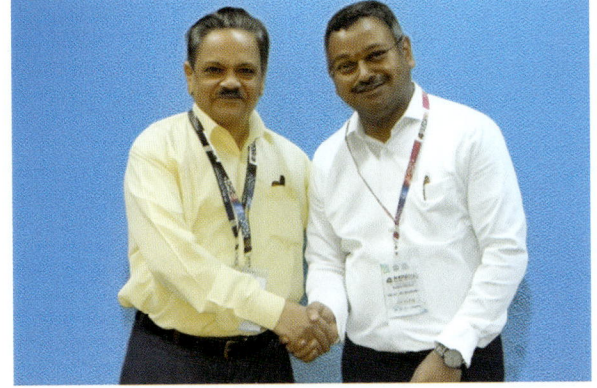

This case-based clinical medicine book is a well-structured, thoughtfully, and carefully curated compilation of long and short cases. This book is also focused on examination-oriented teaching and discussion of most of the cases that a student encounters in day-to-day practice, especially in the exit and admission qualifying examinations.

Dr Archith Boloor is a gifted medical teacher and well known all over India. His bedside clinics are superb, exemplary, and much sought after. I have found that the questions discussed in the book are the usual examination questions. It is a must "go to book" for the examination going undergraduates and postgraduates.

Each case follows a consistent pattern and structure. It underscores the prime importance of thorough history taking, appropriate physical examination, and relevant investigations, leading to a clinical diagnosis. The inclusion of laboratory investigations, treatment, preventive strategies, follow-up, and a reflective discussion ensures that readers not only grasp the core clinical concepts but also understand the reasoning behind each decision and the broader implications for patient care.

What truly distinguishes this book is its ability to empower the students, faculty, and clinicians to apply the knowledge bedside. Today, bedside clinical teaching has possibly got a beating, the resurgence of clinical empowerment is the need of the hour, and this book fulfils the unmet need of clinical teaching.

I am confident that *An Insider's Guide to Cases in Clinical Medicine* will serve as a practical and integral guide for medical students, interns, postgraduate trainees, and even practicing clinicians who wish to strengthen their clinical reasoning skills.

I wholeheartedly recommend this book for them.

**Ashok Kumar Das** MD PhD DNB FAMS FICP FRCP
Dean Academics and Emeritus Professor, Department of Medicine
Mahatma Gandhi Medical College and Research Institute, Sri Balaji Vidyapeeth, Puducherry, India
Current Chairman of the Academic Committee of National Academy of Medical Sciences, New Delhi, India
Former Professor and Head, Department of Endocrinology, JIPMER, Puducherry, India
Past National President, Association of Physicians of India, Research Society for the Study of Diabetes in India
*ashokdas82@gmail.com*

# Preface to the Second Edition

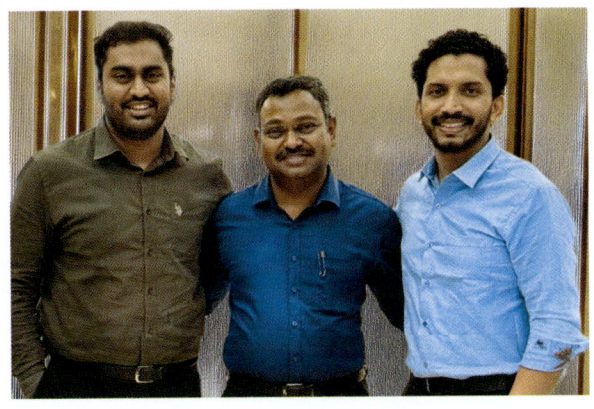

It is one of those days. A wet Mangalorean morning. The rain poured down last night, pitter-pattering against the window while he stayed awake to the words of numerous definitions and diagnoses pitter-pattering inside his very hollow cranium. He woke up in the morning, none the wiser. Annoyed, irritated, and almost an hour past his alarm. Nothing drives a medical student up the wall more than the potent cocktail of insomnia, a damp laboratory coat and a disappointed professor demanding you to pull out factoids from your brain that nobody bothered to put there. "Oscillating top of vertical column of blood that faithfully reflects the pressure changes in the right atrium during the cardiac cycle"—Who even remembers that? WHY even remember that? What is the point of all this? Thoughts raced through his head as the plopping sound of his shoes grabbed pace. The last thing he needs today is to be late.

Doctors are trained every day to make life-altering decisions in record time. With 6 minutes to reach the examination hall, he had to take a shortcut. With little regard for his own safety, he ran across a car that honked a couple times loudly. The future of health is tied in the hands of doctor students who run wantonly at red lights. He reached the hall with classical NYHA Grade 4 breathlessness, but he reached on time. A small win in a big list of losses that would adorn the rest of his day.

The internal examiner walked in with the external examiner, showing off the wards and the beds. Most of the patients finding solace in the rather twisted fact that they get paid for having a chronic medical condition, which is interesting enough to be quizzed upon, but not life-threatening enough to be treated immediately. The students all waited with their slot numbers, for what is a long case other than a stage performance where you are graded on your umm's and your ahaa's. He held his card which said "1". Either he would set the bar, or he would drown in it. Right next to the table where the examiners were sitting, now engaged in casual conversation like newlyweds: The patient which had 1 assigned on his bed looked intimidating enough. Breathless, barely conscious-looking, definitely something from the large chunk of medicine that he was not feeling confident about. Well, at this point, that was all of medicine. But there were 20 minutes to salvage this situation. 20 minutes to prepare for anything that the external or the internal examiner could combinedly throw at him.

As he approached the patient, he felt some energy surging through him. "I can do this." "I have studied for four and a half years. It is impossible that I will not know anything". "Surely, I can answer what is needed to make it through this." The positive reaffirmations reverbed through his head giving him all the confidence he desperately needed. But that is not the way life would have it, of course! From the white noise in his brain, he could hear distinctly the two newlyweds chatting...

"Oh, my day is absolutely ruined. I was on the way here and this absolute moron ran across the red light in front of my car. If I find him somewhere, I have some words he needs to hear."

"Ahaa, It is okay. Today is the first day of the examination, you can take it out on a couple of these kids." "That is the plan. Cannot wait for the first one..."

Now what you read above is an example of an unforeseen event. No amount of preparation or pre-emptive thinking can protect you from these. Of course, the more prepared you are, the less you will suffer from the consequences of these unforeseen events. But it is unforeseen nevertheless. Your practical examination, your long cases, and your short cases are the opposite of unforeseen events. Every teacher worth their money will prepare you carefully and consistently to do well in these foreseen cases! In creating this book, I chose to enlist the help of some of my best performing students, their experiences, and their opinions to curate a book of cases that will help you perform well. Not only is the book a haven for exam-oriented preparationists, it also has the important facts and figures that will help you get an extra edge on any sort of evaluation. The book doubles down on its usefulness, both as a guide for cases as well as a way to read up medicine in a capsulized form. We have done our absolute best to incorporate all of the details, which are pertinent to the undergraduate level, but we have also tried to keep it interesting and challenging for the postgraduate level. The deficit for such a book in the market, and also the enthusiastic contributions of my successful students all inspired me to compile this book. It is our utter delight to present this to you, our biggest readers and supporters. We hope we have done justice to the vastness of medicine while doing similar justice to the curiosity of the student.

The crux of medicine is always in the clutches of the patient. The rest of it is found in books like these, slowly coercing both knowledge and experience into swallowable, bite-sized pieces that will save you on one of those days. It would be a matter of great honor and pride for this book to receive that tag.

**Archith Boloor**
**Nikhil Kenny Thomas**
**Mohamed Faizan Thomas**

# Acknowledgments

We place on record our heartfelt gratitude for the appreciation the book *An Insiders Guide to Cases in Clinical Medicine* has received from students and teachers all over India. That book was a comprehensive description of clinical examination of all the systems important for the practical examination. We felt the need for a case-based approach to common cases kept for examination with emphasis on the descriptive discussion of each of the cases.

Firstly, we would like to thank our families—the unwavering pillars of strength that have supported us throughout every challenge of our life. Our friends, colleagues, and well-wishers who have always supported our work were not an exception this time too. Lastly, we want to thank all our students, each and every one, because without their unrelenting urge to learn, we would not have the drive to compile our teachings in the form of a book.

We remain profoundly grateful to Dr Ashok Kumar Das for his gracious foreword. To have his thoughtful words precede this work is both a privilege and an enduring honor. His endorsement lends this endeavor a depth of meaning that far exceeds the written page.

We are thankful to all our friends whose contributions and knowledge flowed seamlessly at a very short notice.

We thank Dr Mohammed Shaheen, Dr Madhav H Hande, Dr Ashwini MV, Dr Vivek K Koushik, Dr Abu Thajudeen, Dr Saladi Sri Vijay Sasikanth, Dr Manoj Kumar Devera, Dr Vidarshan Mathavan, Dr Prajwal Pai, Dr PS Gayathri Thampi, Dr Varun M Nair, Dr Vivek Hari, Dr Sagi Pranathi, and Dr Siddharth Satish Bableshwar for their contributions.

We are especially grateful for the ongoing encouragement from the management and administration of our university, the Manipal Academy of Higher Education (MAHE), Manipal, Karnataka, India.

We convey our sincere gratitude to Shri Jitendar P Vij (Group Chairman), Mr Ankit Vij (Managing Director), Mr MS Mani (Group President), Mr Rishi Sharma (Regional Business Developmental Manager-North), Dr Madhu Choudhary (Director-Educational Publishing), Ms Pooja Bhandari [Director-Production (Books and Journals)], Mr Ajay Kumar Sharma [Deputy General Manager (Books and Journals)], Ms Sunita Katla (Executive Assistant to Group Chairman and Publishing Manager), Ms Samina Khan (Executive Assistant to Director-Educational Publishing), Dr Aditya Tayal (Senior Editorial Manager-Content Strategy), Mr Vijay Kumar Bhatia (Manager-Production), Mr Bishan Singh (Production Manager), Ms Seema Dogra (Cover Visualizer), Ms Neha Verma (Graphic Designer-Cover), Mr Laxmidhar Padhiary (Team Lead-Production), Mr Kapil Dev Sharma (Typesetter), Mr Sumit Kumar (Team Lead-Graphic Designer), and their team members, for their help in the formatting and their well-received technical assistance and unwavering support during the process of developing this project.

A very special gratitude goes out to all our teachers, who are solely responsible for what we are today and for having ignited the passion of teaching and writing in us.

Lastly, we thank God Almighty, for what was, what is, and what will be.

**Archith Boloor**
**Nikhil Kenny Thomas**
**Mohamed Faizan Thomas**

# Contents

## SECTION 1: RESPIRATORY SYSTEM

**Case Sheet Format** .................................................................................................................................. 3

**Diagnosis Format** ..................................................................................................................................... 7
- Chronic Obstructive Pulmonary Disease   *8*

**Sample Case Sheet and Discussion** ........................................................................................................ 8
- Pleural Effusion   *15*
- Fibrosis   *29*
- Pneumothorax   *36*
- Suppurative Lung Disease   *41*

**Respiratory System: Summary of Findings in Common Respiratory Diseases** ................................... 49

**Schematic Approach to Clinical Diagnosis in Respiratory System** ..................................................... 50

## SECTION 2: CARDIOVASCULAR SYSTEM

**Case Sheet Format** ................................................................................................................................ 53

**Diagnosis Format** ................................................................................................................................... 56

**Sample Case Sheet and Discussion** ...................................................................................................... 57

*Valvular Heart Disease*   *57*
- Mitral Stenosis   *57*
- Mitral Regurgitation   *74*
- Aortic Stenosis   *87*
- Aortic Regurgitation   *97*

*Congenital Heart Disease*   *108*
- Atrial Septal Defect   *108*
- Ventricular Septal Defect   *116*
- Patent Ductus Arteriosus   *121*
- Eisenmenger's/Cyanotic Heart Disease   *123*

**Schematic Approach to Clinical Diagnosis in Cardiovascular System** ............................................... 133

**Summary of Findings in Common Cardiovascular Diseases** ............................................................. 134

## SECTION 3: GASTROINTESTINAL SYSTEM

**Case Sheet Format** .............................................................................................................................. 139

**Diagnosis Format** ................................................................................................................................. 142

**Sample Case Sheet and Discussion** .................................................................................................................. 143
- Cirrhosis  *143*
- Hepatomegaly  *168*
- Splenomegaly  *171*
- Ascites  *176*

## SECTION 4: NERVOUS SYSTEM

**Case Sheet Format** ............................................................................................................................................ 193

**Sample Case Sheet and Discussion** .................................................................................................................. 201
- Stroke  *201*
- Spinal Cord Diseases  *252*
- Peripheral Neuropathy  *275*
- Guillain-Barré Syndrome  *296*
- Ataxia  *305*
- Parkinson's Disease  *316*
- Muscle Disease  *322*
- Motor Neuron Disease  *328*

## SECTION 5: OTHERS

- Approach to Anemia  *337*
- Approach to Anemia  *338*
- Approach to Jaundice  *345*
- Approach to Lymphadenopathy  *350*
- Approach to Edema  *354*

**Comprehensive Geriatric Assessment** .............................................................................................................. 357
- Approach to Arthritis  *361*
- Approach to Arthritis  *361*

*Index*  *367*

# Abbreviations

| | | | | | |
|---|---|---|---|---|---|
| °C | : | Degree Celsius | AVNRT | : | AV nodal re-entrant tachycardia |
| °F | : | Degree Fahrenheit | APB | : | Atrial premature beat |
| ALL | : | Acute lymphoblastic leukemia | ALS | : | Amyotrophic lateral sclerosis |
| ABPA | : | Allergic bronchopulmonary aspergillosis | ADL | : | Activities of daily living |
| ACS | : | Acute coronary syndrome | ACPA | : | Anticitrullinated protein antibody |
| ACR | : | American College of Rheumatology | APLA | : | Antiphospholipid antibody syndrome |
| ARF | : | Acute renal failure | AP | : | Anteroposterior |
| ADHD | : | Attention deficit hyperactivity disorder | Bx | : | Biopsy |
| ADR | : | Adverse drug reaction | BAL | : | Bronchoalveolar concentration |
| ARDS | : | Acute respiratory distress syndrome | B/L | : | Bilateral |
| AGN | : | Acute glomerulonephritis | BIH | : | Benign intracranial hypertension |
| AION | : | Anterior ischemic optic neuritis | BAV | : | Bicuspid aortic valve |
| AKI | : | Acute kidney injury | BBB | : | Bundle branch block |
| ALL | : | Acute lymphoblastic leukemia | BC | : | Bone conduction/blood culture |
| ASCVD | : | Atherosclerotic cardiovascular disease | BCAT | : | Brief cognitive assessment tool |
| ACD | : | Anemia of chronic disease | BER | : | Benign early repolarization |
| ADC | : | Apparent diffusion coefficient | BLS | : | Basic life support |
| ACA | : | Anterior cerebral artery | BSA | : | Body surface area |
| ACE | : | Addenbrooke's cognitive examination | BP | : | Blood pressure |
| ACEI | : | Angiotensin converting enzyme inhibitor | BT | : | Bleeding time |
| ARB | : | Angiotensin receptor blocker | BUN | : | Blood urea nitrogen |
| ACTH | : | Adrenocorticotropic hormone | BM | : | Bone marrow |
| ADHF | : | Acute decompensated heart failure | BMI | : | Body mass index |
| AEM | : | Ambulatory electrocardiogram monitoring | BMV | : | Bag and mask ventilation/balloon mitral valvotomy |
| AI | : | Aortic insufficiency | BVP | : | Biventricular pacing |
| AIDP | : | Acute inflammatory demyelinating polyneuropathy | B-ALL | : | B-cell acute lymphoblastic leukemia |
| AF | : | Atrial fibrillation | BADL | : | Basic activities of daily living |
| AICA | : | Anterior inferior cerebellar artery | CRP | : | C-reactive protein |
| AICD | : | Automated implantable cardioverter defibrillator | CXR | : | Chest X-ray |
| AML | : | Acute myeloid leukemia | CCA | : | Common carotid artery |
| ANS | : | Autonomic nervous system | C/L | : | Contralateral |
| ARVD | : | Arrhythmogenic right ventricular dysplasia | CMT | : | Charcot-Marie tooth disease |
| ASD | : | Atrial septal defect | CN | : | Cranial nerve |
| AVF | : | Arteriovenous fistula | C/O | : | Complaints of |
| AVM | : | Arteriovenous malformation | CT | : | Computed tomography |
| AVR | : | Aortic valve replacement | CAMCOG | : | Cambridge cognitive examination |
| AVRT | : | Atrioventricular re-entrant tachycardia | COST | : | Cognitive state test |

# Abbreviations

| | | | | | |
|---|---|---|---|---|---|
| CPR | : | Cardiopulmonary resuscitation | DVT | : | Deep venous thrombosis |
| CCF | : | Congestive cardiac failure | DLE | : | Disseminated lupus erythematosus |
| CHF | : | Congestive heart failure | DAS | : | Disease activity score |
| CBC | : | Complete blood count | DWI | : | Diffusion weighted imaging |
| CBD | : | Common bile duct | ECA | : | External carotid artery |
| CHB | : | Complete heart block | EAT | : | Ectopic atrial tachycardia |
| CKD | : | Chronic kidney disease | ECG | : | Electrocardiogram |
| CIDP | : | Chronic inflammatory demyelinating polyneuropathy | ECF | : | Extracellular fluid |
| | | | ECHO | : | Echocardiogram |
| CLD | : | Chronic liver disease | ECMO | : | Extracorporeal membrane oxygenation |
| CLL | : | Chronic lymphoid leukemia | EPS | : | Extrapyramidal system |
| CML | : | Chronic myeloid leukemia | EF | : | Ejection fraction |
| CMV | : | Cytomegalovirus | EM | : | Erythema multiforme |
| CNS | : | Central nervous system | ECD | : | Endocardial cushion defects |
| CVA | : | Cerebrovascular accident | EDH | : | Extradural hematoma |
| CNS | : | Central nervous system | EOM | : | Extraocular muscles/movement |
| CABG | : | Coronary artery bypass graft | EPO | : | Erythropoietin |
| CAD | : | Coronary artery disease | EDM | : | Early diastolic murmur |
| CAUTI | : | Catheter associated UTI | ESM | : | Ejection systolic murmur |
| CBE | : | Clinical breast examination | ESRD | : | End-stage renal disease |
| CRF | : | Chronic renal failure | ET | : | Endotracheal tube |
| COPD | : | Chronic obstructive pulmonary disease | ESV | : | End-systolic volume |
| CCCU | : | Critical coronary care unit | EULAR | : | European League Against Rheumatism |
| CCS | : | Canadian Cardiovascular Society | FMS | : | Fibromyalgia syndrome |
| CVS | : | Cardiovascular system | FBS | : | Fasting blood sugar |
| CVP | : | Central venous pressure | FEV1 | : | Forced expiratory volume in first second |
| CP angle | : | Cerebellopontine angle | FTT | : | Failure to thrive |
| CPB | : | Cardiopulmonary bypass | FVC | : | Forced vital capacity |
| CDC | : | Centers for disease control and prevention | GI | : | Gastrointestinal |
| CDAI | : | Clinical disease activity index | GBS | : | Guillain–Barré syndrome |
| CGA | : | Comprehensive geriatric assessment | GCS | : | Glasgow Coma Scale |
| CSF | : | Cerebrospinal fluid | GERD | : | Gastroesophageal reflux disease |
| DDx or D/D | : | Differential diagnosis | GH | : | Growth hormone |
| DPI | : | Dry powder inhaler | Hb | : | Hemoglobin |
| DIC | : | Disseminated intravascular coagulation | HMF | : | Higher mental functions |
| DIP joint | : | Distal interphalangeal joint | HOCM | : | Hypertrophic obstructive cardiomyopathy |
| DKA | : | Diabetic ketoacidosis | HBV | : | Hepatitis B virus |
| DLCO | : | Diffusion lung capacity for carbon monoxide | HL | : | Hodgkin lymphoma |
| DM | : | Diabetes mellitus | HUS | : | Hemolytic uremic syndrome |
| DR | : | Diabetic retinopathy | HAI | : | Hospital acquired infection |
| DNR | : | Do not resuscitate | HE | : | Hepatic encephalopathy |
| DTR | : | Deep tendon reflex | HDS | : | Hemodynamically stable |
| DTA | : | Descending thoracic aorta | HIT | : | Heparin-induced thrombocytopenia |
| DSM | : | Diagnostic and statistical manual of mental disorders | HCC | : | Hepatocellular carcinoma |

| | | |
|---|---|---|
| HTN | : | Hypertension |
| HIV/AIDS | : | Human immunodeficiency virus/acquired immunodeficiency syndrome |
| HD | : | Huntington's disease |
| HDL-C | : | High density lipoprotein cholesterol |
| IADL | : | Instrumental activities of daily living |
| IP joint | : | Interphalangeal joint |
| IGF | : | Insulin-like growth factor 1 |
| ICA | : | Internal carotid artery |
| ICD | : | Intercostal drain |
| ICS | : | Intercostal space/inhaled corticosteroid |
| ICH | : | Intracerebral hemorrhage |
| IVH | : | Intraventricular hemorrhage |
| INO | : | Internuclear ophthalmoplegia |
| INR | : | International Normalized Ratio |
| ICP | : | Intracranial pressure |
| IBD | : | Inflammatory bowel disease |
| IBS | : | Irritable bowel syndrome |
| IDDM | : | Insulin-dependent diabetes mellitus—Type 1 diabetes |
| ICSOL | : | Intracranial space occupying lesion |
| IHD | : | Ischemic heart disease |
| IJV | : | Internal jugular vein |
| ILD | : | Interstitial lung disease |
| IMN | : | Infectious mononucleosis |
| IVC | : | Inferior vena cava |
| INH | : | Isoniazid |
| IPPV | : | Intermittent positive pressure ventilation |
| ITP | : | Immune thrombocytopenic purpura |
| IV | : | Intravenous |
| JME | : | Juvenile myoclonic epilepsy |
| JRA | : | Juvenile rheumatoid arthritis |
| JVP | : | Jugular venous pressure |
| KUB | : | Kidney, ureters, and bladder |
| KDIGO | : | Kidney disease improving global outcomes |
| KF Ring | : | Kayser-Fleischer ring |
| LSM | : | Late systolic murmur |
| LV | : | Left ventricle |
| LVH | : | Left ventricular hypertrophy |
| L\A | : | Local anesthetic |
| LDL-C | : | Low density lipoprotein cholesterol |
| LP | : | Lumbar puncture |
| LMN | : | Lower motor neuron |
| LVE | : | Left ventricular enlargement |
| LVF | : | Left ventricular failure |
| LOC | : | Loss of consciousness |
| LQTS | : | Long QT syndrome |
| LGIB | : | Upper gastrointestinal bleed |
| MAP | : | Mean arterial pressure |
| MAT | : | Multifocal atrial tachycardia |
| MCTD | : | Mixed connective tissue disease |
| MoCA | : | Montreal cognitive assessment |
| MMSE | : | Mini-mental state examination |
| MCA | : | Middle cerebral artery |
| MCP joint | : | Metacarpophalangeal joint |
| MDS | : | Myelodysplastic syndrome |
| MDM | : | Mid-diastolic murmur |
| MLF | : | Medial longitudinal fasciculus |
| MND | : | Motor neuron disease |
| MS | : | Mitral stenosis/multiple sclerosis |
| MVP | : | Mitral valve prolapse |
| MVR | : | Mitral valve replacement |
| MSA-C | : | Multisystem atrophy—cerebellar |
| MSA-P | : | Multisystem atrophy—Parkinson's |
| MCTD | : | Mixed connective tissue disease |
| MI | : | Myocardial infarction |
| MRC | : | Medical Research Council |
| mMRC | : | Modified Medical Research Council |
| MRI | : | Magnetic resonance imaging |
| MDI | : | Metered dose inhaler |
| MODS | : | Multiorgan dysfunction syndrome |
| NHL | : | Non-Hodgkin lymphoma |
| NASH | : | Non-alcoholic steatohepatitis |
| NCV | : | Nerve conduction velocity |
| NMJ | : | Neuromuscular junction |
| NPPV | : | Noninvasive positive pressure ventilation |
| NPH | : | Normal pressure hydrocephalus |
| NTS | : | Nucleus tractus solitarius |
| REM | : | Rapid eye movement |
| NREM | : | Non-rapid eye movement |
| NST | : | Non-stress test |
| NSTEMI | : | Non-ST-elevation myocardial infarction |
| NSAIDs | : | Nonsteroidal anti-inflammatory drugs |
| NYHA | : | New York Heart Association |
| NG Tube | : | Nasogastric tube |
| O/E | : | On examination |
| OSA | : | Obstructive sleep apnea |
| OA | : | Osteoarthritis |

| | | |
|---|---|---|
| OP | : | Organophosphorus |
| PA | : | Posteroanterior |
| PAN | : | Polyarteritis nodosa |
| PDA | : | Patent ductus arteriosus |
| PAH | : | Pulmonary artery hypertension |
| PCI | : | Percutaneous coronary intervention |
| PCA | : | Posterior cerebral artery |
| PCV | : | Packed cell volume |
| PCWP | : | Pulmonary capillary wedge pressure |
| PD | : | Parkinson's disease |
| PE | : | Pulmonary embolism |
| PEEP | : | Positive end expiratory pressure |
| PEFR | : | Peak expiratory flow rate |
| PAH | : | Pulmonary artery hypertension |
| PIP Joint | : | Proximal interphalangeal joint |
| PICA | : | Posterior inferior cerebellar artery |
| PLS | : | Progressive lateral sclerosis |
| PND | : | Paroxysmal nocturnal dyspnea |
| PUO/FUO | : | Pyrexia (fever) of unknown origin |
| PVC | : | Premature ventricular contractions |
| pO2/paO2: | | Partial pressure of oxygen |
| paCO2 | : | Partial pressure of carbon dioxide |
| PMI | : | Point of maximal impulse |
| PPBS | : | Post-prandial blood sugars |
| qSOFA | : | Quick sequential organ failure assessment |
| QSART | : | Quantitative sudomotor axon reflex test |
| RA | : | Rheumatoid arthritis |
| RF | : | Rheumatoid factor |
| RAI scan | : | Radioactive iodine scan |
| RAS | : | Reticular activating system |
| RAPD | : | Relative apparent pupillary defect |
| RCM | : | Restrictive cardiomyopathy |
| RCC | : | Renal cell carcinoma |
| RDW | : | Red cell distribution width |
| RS | : | Respiratory system |
| RSOV | : | Ruptured sinus of Valsalva |
| RS3PE | : | Remitting seronegative symmetrical synovitis with pitting edema |
| RHD | : | Rheumatic heart disease |
| RLN | : | Recurrent laryngeal nerve |
| RR | : | Respiratory rate |
| RV | : | Right ventricle |
| RVH | : | Right ventricular hypertrophy |
| RVF | : | Right ventricular failure |
| REMS | : | Regional examination of musculoskeletal system |
| SAAG | : | Serum–ascites albumin gradient |
| SAH | : | Subarachnoid hemorrhage |
| SACD | : | Subacute combined degeneration of cord |
| SANRT | : | Sinoatrial node re-entrant tachycardia |
| SLRT | : | Straight leg raise test |
| SOFA | : | Sequential organ failure assessment |
| SIRS | : | Systemic inflammatory response syndrome |
| SSPE | : | Subacute sclerosing pan-encephalitis |
| SDAI | : | Simplified disease activity index |
| STMS | : | Short test of mental status |
| SV | : | Stroke volume |
| SVT | : | Supraventricular tachycardia |
| SMA | : | Spinal muscular atrophy |
| SDH | : | Subdural hematoma |
| SCM | : | Sternocleidomastoid |
| SLE | : | Systemic lupus erythematosus |
| STEMI | : | ST-elevation myocardial infarction |
| SVC | : | Superior vena cava |
| SSR | : | Sympathetic skin response |
| SLICC | : | Systemic Lupus International Collaborating Clinics |
| TAPVC | : | Total anomalous pulmonary venous connection |
| TIA | : | Transient ischemic attack |
| TB | : | Tuberculosis |
| TBI | : | Traumatic brain injury |
| TIN | : | Tubulointerstitial nephritis |
| TG | : | Triglycerides |
| TST | : | Thermoregulatory sweat test |
| TMJ | : | Temporomandibular joint |
| TSH | : | Thyroid stimulating hormone |
| U/L | : | Unilateral |
| UA | : | Unstable angina |
| UMN | : | Upper motor neuron |
| UIP | : | Usual interstitial pneumonitis |
| UGI | : | Upper gastrointestinal |
| UGIB | : | Upper gastrointestinal bleed |
| URTI | : | Upper respiratory tract infection |
| UTI | : | Urinary tract infection |
| US/USG | : | Ultrasonogram |
| VA | : | Visual acuity |
| VAP | : | Ventilator acquired pneumonia |
| VC | : | Vital capacity |
| VDRL | : | Venereal Disease Research Laboratory |
| VPC | : | Ventricular premature contractions |
| VSD | : | Ventricular septal defect |
| VT | : | Ventricular tachycardia |
| V/Q | : | Ventilation/perfusion |
| VUR | : | Vesicoureteric reflux |
| WHO | : | World Health Organization |
| WPW | : | Wolff–Parkinson–White syndrome |
| ZES | : | Zollinger-Ellison syndrome |

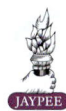 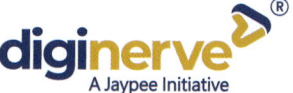

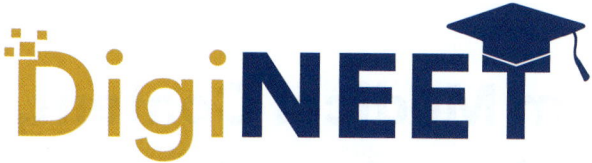

Simplify your undergraduate studies and NEET PG preparation with this comprehensive program covering all 19 subjects. Crafted by India's top faculty, it includes video lectures, printed notes, OSCEs, a QBank, test series, and the innovative Dr. Wise AI Chatbot.

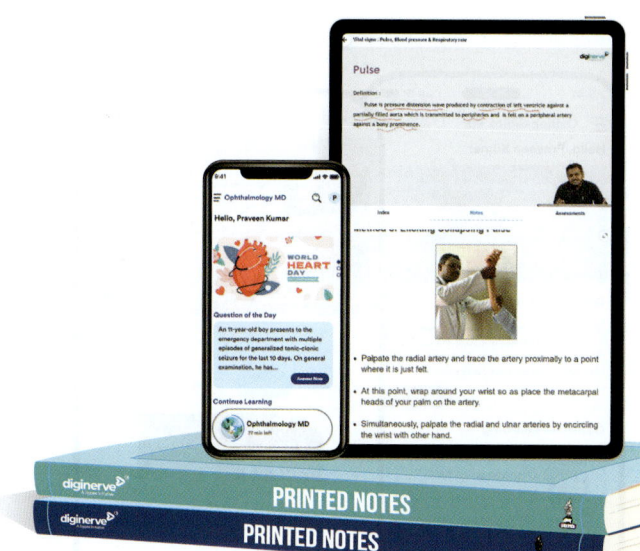

## Course Features

1400+ hrs Video Lectures

1500+ Topics in Notes

15000+ Questions in QBank

1800+ GEMS

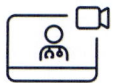
450+ OSCEs

Test Series

Dr. Wise AI Chatbot

Drug Chart

**Regular Webinars by Esteemed Faculty**

## Access Anytime, Anywhere

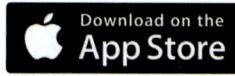 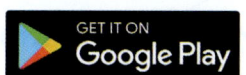 

Scan to Download

+91-8800-418-418     marketing@diginerve.com

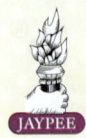
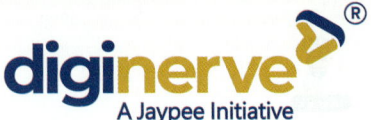

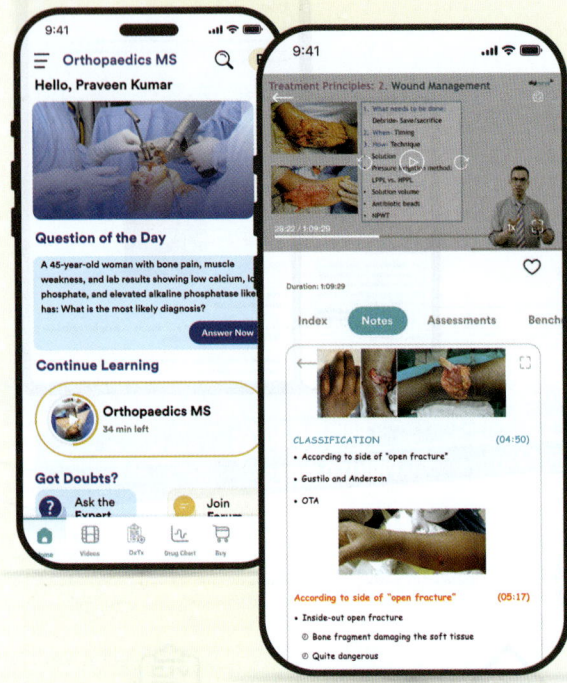

# Premium Medical Content, Anytime, Anywhere

**Trusted by 150K+ Users**

**20+** Courses    **3600+** Hrs of Video Content    **790+** Mentors

## A host of features for **UnderGrads, PostGrads** and **Professionals**

Available on 

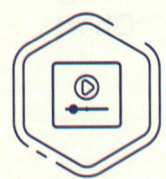 Video Lectures     Notes    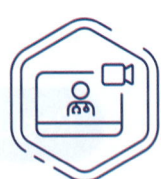 OSCEs

 Drug Chart     Question Bank     Dr. Wise AI Chatbot

📞 +91-8800-418-418    ✉ marketing@diginerve.com

# Respiratory System

## Section Outline

- Case Sheet Format
- Diagnosis Format
- Sample Case Sheet and Discussion
  - Chronic Obstructive Pulmonary Disease
  - Pleural Effusion
  - Fibrosis
  - Pneumothorax
  - Suppurative Lung Disease
- Schematic Approach to Clinical Diagnosis in Respiratory System

# Case Sheet Format

## HISTORY TAKING

Name:

Age:

Sex:

Residence:

Occupation:

Chief complaints:

1. _____ × days
2. _____ × days
3. _____ × days

**History of presenting illness:**
**Cough:**
- Duration
- Onset
- Progression
- Variation
  - Diurnal variation
  - Seasonal variation
  - Postural variation
- Aggravating factors
- Relieving factors

**Expectoration:**
- Duration
- Onset
- Progression
- Variation
  - Diurnal variation
  - Seasonal variation
  - Positional variation
- Aggravating and relieving factors
- Quantity of sputum
- Color
- Smell
- Blood tinged
  - How often
  - Quantity
  - Fresh or altered

**Dyspnea:**
- Duration
- Onset
- Grade
- Progression
- Aggravating factors
- Relieving factors
- Orthopnea
- Trepopnea
- Platypnea
- Paroxysmal nocturnal dyspnea (PND)
- Any respiratory system complaints
  - Wheeze
  - Cough with expectoration

**Chest pain:**
- Duration
- Onset
- Site
- Type of pain
- Radiation
- Diurnal variation (nocturnal angina)
- Variation with respiration
- Aggravating factors
- Relieving factors
- Associated symptoms
  - Nausea, vomiting, sweating
- Local tenderness

**Wheeze:**
- Duration
- Onset
- Progression
- Episodic or continuous
- Variation
- Allergy
- Skin rashes
- Aggravating and relieving factors

**Fever:**
- Episodic or continuous
- Grade
- Chill and rigors
- Aggravating factors
- Relieving factors
- Variation
  - Diurnal variation

**History of:**
- Nasal discharge
- Recurrent cold/epistaxis
- Recurrent headaches
- Weight loss
- Anorexia
- Evening rise of temperature
- Smoking
- Belching
- Regurgitation of food
- Hoarseness of voice

**Past history:**
- Asthma
- Chronic obstructive airway disease

- Tuberculosis
- History of contact with tuberculosis
- Diabetes mellitus (DM)
- Hypertension (HTN)
- Ischemic heart disease (IHD)
- Seizure disorder

**Family history:**
(Draw pedigree chart representing three generations)

**Personal history:**
- Bowel habits
- Bladder habits
- Appetite
- Loss of weight
- Occupational exposure
- Sleep
- Dietary habits and taboo
- Food allergies
- Smoking (in Smoking Index or Pack years)
- Alcohol history (_____ grams of alcohol/day or _____ units of alcohol/week)

**Menstrual and obstetric history:**
- G____P____L____A____
- Age of menarche ____
- Menopause at ____
- Flow—amenorrhea/oligomenorrhea/menorrhagia

**Summarize:**

**Differential diagnosis:**

1.

2.

3.

## GENERAL EXAMINATION

**Patient:**
- Conscious
- Cooperative
- Obeying commands

**Body mass index:**
Weight (kg)/$H_2$ (m)

**Vitals:**
- Pulse
  - Rate
  - Rhythm
  - Volume
  - Character
  - Vessel wall thickening
  - Radio-radial delay and radiofemoral delay
  - Peripheral pulses
- Blood pressure
- Respiratory rate
  - Regular
  - Abdominothoracic (male) or thoracoabdominal (female)
  - Usage of accessory muscles
- Jugular venous pulse
  - Waveform
- Jugular venous pressure
  - ____ cm of blood above sternal angle (+ 5 cm water)
- Pulse oximetry
- Pain

**On physical examination:**
- Pallor:
- Icterus:
- Cyanosis:
- Clubbing:
- Lymphadenopathy:
- Edema:

**Others:**
- Use of accessory muscles of respiration
- External markers of tuberculosis if any
- External markers of malignancy if any
- Features suggesting type of respiratory failure

## SYSTEMIC EXAMINATION

### Upper Respiratory Tract Examination
- Nostrils:
- Nasal septum:
- Nasal polyps:
- Sinus tenderness:
- Tonsils:
- Postpharyngeal wall:

### Lower Respiratory Tract Examination

#### Inspection
- Shape and symmetry:
- Spine:
- Subcostal angle:
- Trachea:
- Apex beat:
- Respiratory movements:

| Area | Right | Left |
|---|---|---|
| Infraclavicular area | | |
| Mammary area | | |
| Suprascapular area | | |
| Infrascapular area | | |

- Visible pulsations/sinus/scars:

## Palpation

(Warm the palms by rubbing against each other before palpation)
- Spine: Position and tenderness
- Trachea:
- Apex:

**Respiratory movements:**

| Area | Right | Left |
|---|---|---|
| Supraclavicular | | |
| Infraclavicular | | |
| Mammary | | |
| Suprascapular | | |
| Infrascapular | | |

**Dimensions/measurements:**

| | | |
|---|---|---|
| Transverse diameter | | |
| Anteroposterior diameter | | |
| Transverse/anteroposterior ratio | | |
| Chest circumference | Expiration | |
| | Inspiration | |
| Right hemithorax | Expiration | |
| | Inspiration | |
| Left hemithorax | Expiration | |
| | Inspiration | |
| Chest expansion | Right hemithorax | |
| | Left hemithorax | |
| | Total | |
| Spinoscapular distance | (Right side) and (left side) | |
| Spinoacromial distance | (Right side) and (left side) | |

**Vocal fremitus:**

| Areas | Right | Left |
|---|---|---|
| Supraclavicular | | |
| Infraclavicular | | |
| Mammary | | |
| Axillary | | |
| Infra-axillary | | |
| Suprascapular | | |
| Interscapular | | |
| Infrascapular | | |

- Tactile fremitus:
- Friction fremitus:
- Tenderness:
- Subcutaneous emphysema:
- Rib crowding:
- Bony tenderness:

## *Percussion*

| Areas | Right | Left |
|---|---|---|
| Supraclavicular | | |
| Clavicular | | |
| Infraclavicular | | |
| Mammary | | |
| Axillary | | |
| Infra-axillary | | |
| Suprascapular | | |
| Interscapular | | |
| Infrascapular | | |

- Shifting dullness:
- Tidal percussion:
- Traube's space:
- Kronig's isthmus:
- Liver dullness:

**Heart border:**
- Right heart border:
- Left heart border:

## *Auscultation*

**Breath sounds:**
- Vesicular/bronchovesicular/bronchial (tubular/cavernous/amphoric)
- Comment on intensity of breath sound—normal/increased/decreased

| Areas | Right | Left |
|---|---|---|
| Supraclavicular | | |
| Infraclavicular | | |
| Mammary | | |
| Axillary | | |
| Infra-axillary | | |
| Suprascapular | | |
| Interscapular | | |
| Infrascapular | | |

**Vocal resonance:**

| Areas | Right | Left |
|---|---|---|
| Supraclavicular | | |
| Infraclavicular | | |
| Mammary | | |
| Axillary | | |
| Infra-axillary | | |
| Suprascapular | | |
| Interscapular | | |
| Infrascapular | | |

**Adventitious sounds (mention in specific areas):**
- Crepitations
- Rhonchi/wheeze (inspiratory or expiratory/polyphonic or monophonic)
- Pleural rub

**Additional tests:**
- Coin test:
- Bronchophony:
- Egophony:
- Whispered pectoriloquy:
- Succussion splash:
- Post-tussive crepitations:
- Shifting dullness:

## Other Systems

**Cardiovascular system:**
- Inspection:
- Palpation:
- Percussion:
- Auscultation:

**Gastrointestinal system:**
- Inspection:
- Palpation:
- Percussion:
- Auscultation:

**Nervous system:**
- Higher mental functions:
- Cranial nerves:
- Sensory system:
- Motor system:
- Reflexes:
- Cerebellar system:
- Meningeal signs:

# Diagnosis Format

## ANATOMICAL DIAGNOSIS

- Lung (right/left/bilateral) disease with (upper/middle/lower) lobe
- Pleural disease

## PATHOLOGICAL DIAGNOSIS

Consolidation/fibrosis/collapse/obstructive lung disease/restrictive lung disease/effusion/pneumothorax.

## ETIOLOGICAL DIAGNOSIS

Tuberculosis/bronchogenic carcinoma/smoking/occupation/trauma.

## COMPLICATIONS

Respiratory failure (type I or type II)/cor pulmonale.

## EXAMPLES

**Example 1:** Right upper lobe fibrosis post-tubercular etiology, no evidence of respiratory failure or cor pulmonale.

**Example 2:** Bilateral obstructive lung disease—emphysema secondary to smoking with evidence of type 2 respiratory failure and cor pulmonale.

**Example 3:** Left-sided pleural effusion secondary to malignancy with no evidence of respiratory failure or cor pulmonale.

# Sample Case Sheet and Discussion

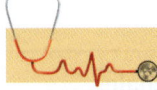

## Case 1: Chronic Obstructive Pulmonary Disease

*Brief History*

A 65-year-old farmer, beedi smoker for 25 years, came to the OPD with complaints of cough and breathlessness for 15 days. He has fever since last 15 days. Sputum is yellowish in color. No hemoptysis. Breathlessness is grade 4. Cough is more during night. No chest pain. No chills and rigors. No PND.

Patient gives history of similar complaints of breathlessness and cough since last 5 years. The symptoms are more during rainy season and winter season. He is also giving history of swelling of the lower limb since last 6 months. Not a known case of hypertension, diabetes, IHD, TB.

*General Examination*
- Elderly male
- Moderately built and nourished
- Conscious, co-operative
- Height: 177 cm
- Weight: 70 kg
- BMI: 22.36 kg/m²
- PR: 76/min, regular, normal volume and character, all peripheral pulses well felt.
- BP: 160/70 mm Hg, right arm supine, no postural drop
- RR: 28/min, abdominothoracic.
- JVP: Normal
- Bilateral pitting pedal edema present
- No pallor, icterus, cyanosis, clubbing or lymphadenopathy
- Fine tremors of the outstretched hands present
- No flapping tremors
- No thyroid swelling
- Surgical scar present over scalp.

*Systemic Examination*
Respiratory System Examination

*Inspection*
- Shape of the chest: Normal
- No kyphoscoliosis, no shoulder drooping, no supraclavicular hollowing or infraclavicular flattening.
- Accessory muscles of respiration are acting.
- Trachea appears central.
- Apex beat not visible.

*Palpation*
- Trachea central.
- Apex beat not palpable
- Chest movements normal in all areas.
- AP diameter: 18.5 cm, transverse diameter: 29 cm.
- AP-transverse ratio: 0.64
- Chest circumference: 88 cm.
- Right hemithorax: 44 cm, left hemithorax: 44 cm
- Chest expansion: 4 cm, 2 cm each on both sides.
- Vocal fremitus: Normal

*Percussion*
- Normal resonant note heard in all areas
- Liver dullness percussed in the 6th right intercostals space in the midclavicular line
- Cardiac dullness obliterated.

*Auscultation*
- Intensity of breath sounds reduced bilaterally
- Normal vesicular breath sounds bilaterally
- Bilateral inspiratory and expiratory wheeze heard.
- Fine early inspiratory crepitations heard in left interscapular area.
- Vocal resonance normal in all areas.

*Diagnosis*
Chronic obstructive airway disease, predominantly emphysema with cor pulmonale. Not in respiratory failure.

## DISCUSSION

**Q. What are the causes of pedal edema in COPD patients?**

- Right ventricular failure as a result of pulmonary artery hypertension.
- Changes in the salt and water balance in COPD patients due to hypoxia and hypercapnia.

    The most consistent change in renal function in patients with hypoxic COPD, particularly those with edema, is a reduction in renal blood flow.

    Hypoxia and hypercapnia may interact to reduce renal blood flow. Hypercapnia reduces renal blood flow through catecholamine release and via a neurally mediated action. In addition, arginine vasopressin (AVP) levels may be inappropriately high in them probably due to renin-angiotensin-aldosterone system activation.

- Activation of renin-angiotensin-aldosterone system and elevation in the levels of circulating catecholamines (as a result of reduced renal blood flow) also causes salt and water retention and peripheral edema in COPD patients.
- Subclinical autonomic dysfunction which is common in COPD patients also can lead to hormonal changes and salt and water retention.

    This is counter-regulated by a number of factors including the release of atrial natriuretic peptide (released due to the increased atrial stretch in the presence of PAH)

favoring natriuresis. When the protective mechanisms are overwhelmed by the edema promoting factors patients COPD patients develop edema.
*Reference:* Crofton and Douglas.

### Q. Definition of cor-pulmonale.

- Cor-pulmonale was classically defined as "hypertrophy of the right ventricle resulting from diseases affecting the function and/or structure of the lungs except when these pulmonary alterations are the result of diseases that primarily affect the left side of the heart (WHO expert committee report, 1963).
*Reference:* Crofton and Douglas
- Cor-pulmonale is defined as dilation and hypertrophy of the right ventricle with or without failure secondary to disease affecting the pulmonary vasculature, lung parenchyma and/or chest wall.

Since this definition does not indicate the presence of right heart failure, and since the presence of edema does not always imply underlying right heart failure in stable chronic obstructive pulmonary disease (COPD) patients, the terms cor-pulmonale and right heart failure are not synonymous. Pulmonary hypertension (PH), however, is always the underlying pathologic mechanism for right ventricular hypertrophy in cor-pulmonale.

Pulmonary hypertension associated with lung disease is defined as resting mean pulmonary artery pressure (mPAP) greater than 20 mm Hg which is different from the definition of primary pulmonary hypertension (mPAP >25 mm Hg).

### Q. Define COPD, chronic bronchitis and emphysema.

- COPD is a preventable and treatable pulmonary disease associated with some significant extrapulmonary effects that may contribute to the severity in individual patients.
- Pulmonary disease is characterized by airflow limitation, which is not fully reversible.
- The airflow limitation is usually progressive and associated with an abnormal inflammatory response of the lung to various noxious particles or gases.

New definition as per GOLD 2023—heterogeneous lung condition characterized by chronic respiratory symptoms (dyspnea, cough, expectoration, exacerbations) due to abnormalities of the airway (bronchitis, bronchiolitis) and/or alveoli (emphysema) that cause persistent, often progressive, airflow limitation.

- **Emphysema:** An anatomically defined condition characterized by abnormal and permanent enlargement of the airspaces distal to the terminal bronchioles. It is accompanied by destruction of the airspace walls, without obvious fibrosis (i.e., there is no fibrosis visible to the naked eye) **(Figs. 1.1 and 1.2).**
- **Chronic bronchitis:** It is defined as a chronic productive cough for 3 months in each of two successive years in a patient in whom other causes of chronic cough (e.g., bronchiectasis) have been excluded.
- **Small airways disease:** A condition in which small bronchioles are narrowed.

### Q. What are the types of chronic bronchitis?

- Simple chronic bronchitis
- Chronic mucopurulent bronchitis
- Chronic asthmatic bronchitis
- Chronic obstructive bronchitis.

### Q. What are the risk factors for COPD?
Refer **Box 1.1**.

### Q. What are the physical examination signs in COPD?

- Cyanosis
- Pedal edema and dilated neck veins
- Asterixis

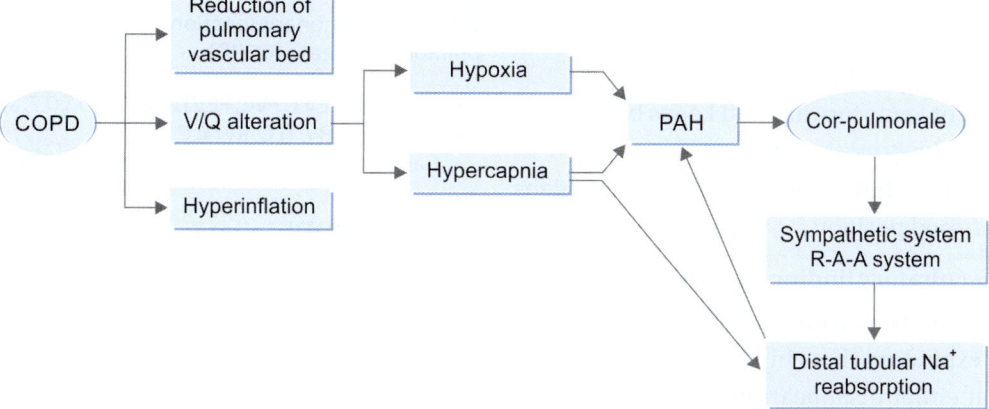

**Fig. 1.1:** Mechanism of pedal edema in respiratory diseases.
(COPD: chronic obstructive pulmonary disease; PAH: pulmonary arterial hypertension; R-A-A: renin-angiotensin-aldosterone)

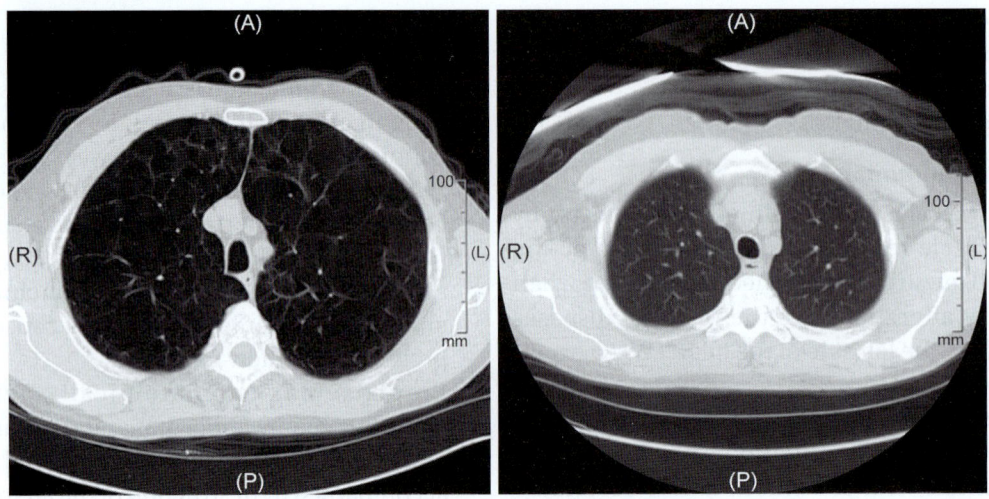

**Fig. 1.2:** COPD versus normal CT scan.

**Box 1.1:** Risk factor for chronic obstructive pulmonary disease (COPD).

**Environmental**
- Tobacco smoke
- Indoor air pollution. Cooking with biomass fuels
- Toxic industrial inhalants: Occupational dust exposure (e.g., coal dust, silica, and cadmium)
- Respiratory infections: Recurrent infection; HIV infection (associated with emphysema), previous tuberculosis
- Low-birth weight and bronchopulmonary dysplasia
- Lung growth: Childhood infections or maternal smoking may affect growth of lung during childhood
- Low socioeconomic status and antioxidant deficiency
- Cannabis smoking

**Host factors**
- Genetic factors: α1-antiproteinase deficiency TGF β-1 polymorphism, SERPINE2 gene expression
- Airway hyperreactivity

- **Hoover's sign:** Intercoastal indrawing
- **Pursed lip breathing:** Patient exhales with pursed lips to prevent alveolar collapse during expiration by increasing the expiratory pressure (PEEP).
- **Tripod sign:** Patient leans forward and keeps both hands on the knees or thighs
- **Dahl's sign/Thinker's sign:** Hyperpigmentation of thighs due to constant tripod position

**Q. What are the auscultatory finding you will get in COPD?**
- Vesicular breath sounds with prolonged expiration
- Inspiratory and expiratory rhonchi
- Crepitations that either disappear or change in location and intensity after coughing
- Forced expiratory time >4 seconds.

**Q. List the comorbidities in COPD.**

Refer **Box 1.2**.

**Box 1.2:** Common comorbidities in chronic obstructive pulmonary disease (COPD).

- Cardiovascular disorders:
  - Pulmonary hypertension
  - Right heart failure and cor-pulmonale
  - *Vascular disease:* Coronary artery disease, cerebrovascular disease, and peripheral vascular disease
  - Systemic hypertension
- Nutritional disorders:
  - Cachexia
- Musculoskeletal disorders:
  - Muscle dysfunction
  - Osteoporosis
- Cancer: Lung cancer
- *Other:* Sleep disorders, sexual dysfunction, diabetes, depression, anxiety, anemia, osteoporosis, peptic ulcer, and glaucoma

**Q. List the PFT abnormalities in COPD?**

Refer **Box 1.3**.

**Box 1.3:** Pulmonary function tests findings in chronic obstructive pulmonary disease (COPD).

- Reduced: FEV1, FVC, FEV1: FVC ratio <0.7, and PEF
- Increased: RV, TLC, RV/TLC
- Gas transfer factor for carbon monoxide (diffusion) is reduced

**Q. What is BODE index?**

Refer **Box 1.4**.

**Q. What are the complications of COPD?**

- **Mucopurulent relapses:** It may develop due to secondary bacterial infection *by Streptococcus pneumoniae, Haemophilus influenzae,* or *Moraxella catarrhalis.* It presents with fever and increased production of purulent sputum.

**Box 1.4:** BODE index.

- It is a multidimensional prognostic index. It takes into account several indicators of COPD prognosis [body mass index (BMI), obstructive ventilatory defect severity, dyspnea severity, and exercise capacity].
- The components are derived from measures of the body mass index (weight in kg/height m²), $FEV_1$ percent predicted, the modified Medical Research Council dyspnea, and 6-minutes walk test.
- A BODE score greater than 7 is associated with a 30% 2-year mortality.
- A score of 5 to 6 is associated with 15%, 2-year mortality.
- If score is less than 5, the 2-year mortality is less than 10%.

- **Carbon dioxide narcosis:** Persistent retention of $CO_2$ (hypercarbia: high $PaCO_2$) manifests as clouding of consciousness, altered behavior, drowsiness, headache, and papilledema.
- **Respiratory failure:**
  - *Type 1 respiratory failure (low $PaO_2$ normal $PaCO_2$):* In mild-to-moderate COPD
  - *Type II respiratory failure:* Acute or chronic in severe COPD
- **Secondary polycythemia:** Due to hypoxemia which stimulates erythropoiesis
- **Pulmonary hypertension and right ventricular failure (cor-pulmonale)**
- **Pneumonia**
- **Tuberculosis**
- **Lung cancer**
- **Pneumothorax (emphysema)**
- **Deep vein thrombosis**
- **Pulmonary embolism**

### Q. Define acute exacerbation of COPD.

- **Definition:** "An event in the natural course of COPD characterized by a change in patient's baseline dyspnea, cough, and/or sputum that is beyond normal day-to-day variations. It is acute in onset and may warrant a change in regular medication in a patient with underlying COPD."
- **Causes of exacerbation:** (1) Infection of the tracheobronchial tree and (2) air pollution. In about one-third of cases, no cause can be identified.
- **Trigging factors:** Infections by bacteria, viruses, or a change in air quality.

### Q. What are the criteria and classification of acute COPD exacerbation?

Refer **Box 1.5**.

## EMPHYSEMA

### Q. Define emphysema.

Emphysema (pulmonary) is a chronic lung disease characterized by abnormal irreversible (permanent) dilatation of the airspaces distal to the terminal bronchiole. This is associated with destruction of their walls but without obvious fibrosis.

**Box 1.5:** Criteria and classification of acute COPD exacerbation.

**Major criteria**
- Increase in sputum volume
- Change in sputum color (generally yellow and green)
- Worsening of baseline dyspnea

**Additional criteria**
- Upper respiratory infection in past 5 days
- Fever of no apparent cause
- Increase in wheezing and cough
- Increase in respiration rate or heart rate 20% above baseline
- Various nonspecific signs and symptoms may accompany these findings, such as fatigue, insomnia, depression, and confusion

**Degree of exacerbation**
- Mild exacerbation = 1 major criterion + 1 or more additional criteria
- Moderate exacerbation = 2 major criteria
- Severe exacerbation = all 3 major criteria

### Q. What are the types of emphysema?

Emphysema is classified according to its anatomic distribution (location of the lesions) within the lobule into four major types **(Figs. 1.3A and B)**:
1. Centriacinar
2. Panacinar
3. Paraseptal
4. Irregular.

#### Centriacinar (centrilobular) emphysema
- Dilatation involves the central or proximal parts of the acini (formed by respiratory bronchioles), whereas distal alveoli are spared.
- Common and severe in the upper lobes, especially in the apical segments.
- **Association:** It occurs in heavy smokers and in association with chronic bronchitis and coal workers' pneumoconiosis.

#### Panacinar (panlobular) emphysema
- All the airspaces beyond terminal bronchiole are more or less uniformly/equally dilated.
- **Site:** More common in the lower lobes, and is usually most severe at the bases.
- It is associated with α1-antitrypsin (α1-AT) deficiency.

#### Distal acinar (paraseptal) emphysema
- Dilatation affects the distal airspace at the periphery of the lobule and the proximal portion is normal.
- It is found near the pleura. Dilated spaces of more than 1 cm in size are known as bullae, which may rupture and cause spontaneous pneumothorax.

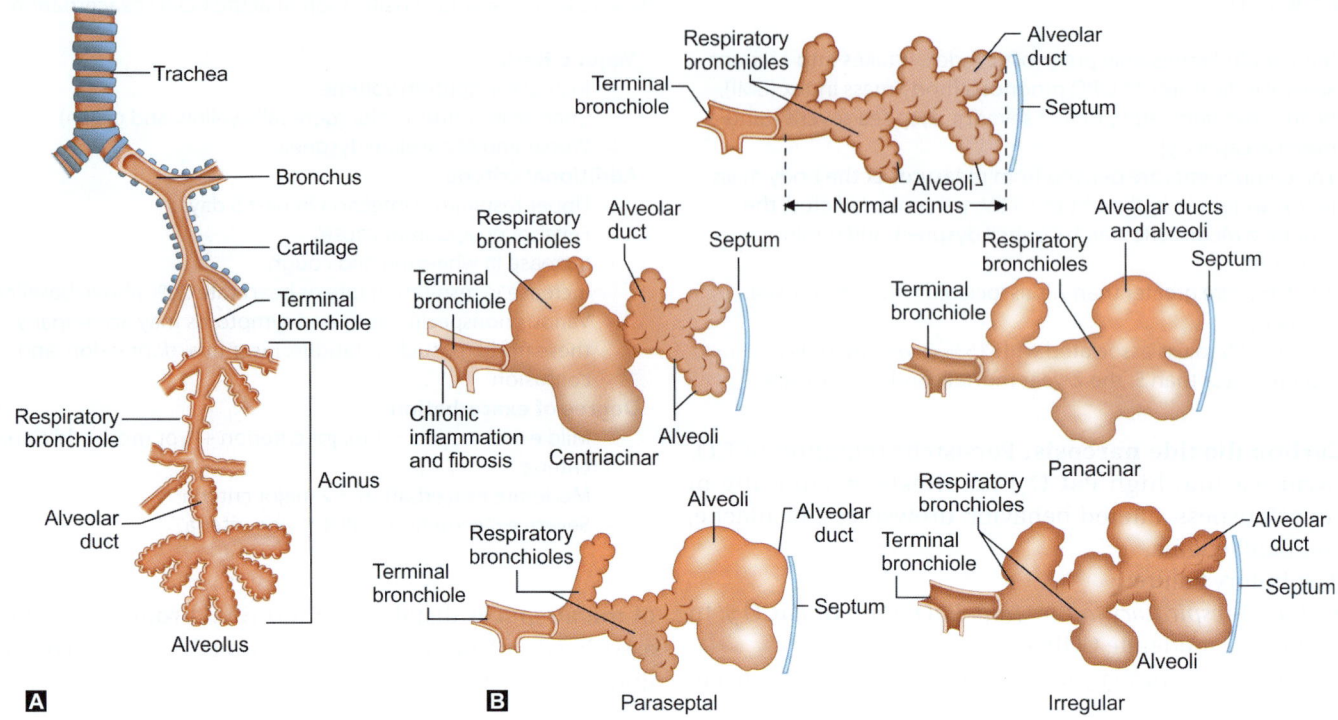

**Figs. 1.3A and B:** (A) Normal components of respiratory tree; (B) Types of emphysema.

- It occurs adjacent to areas of fibrosis, scarring, or atelectasis.

**Irregular (scar or cicatricial) emphysema**
- Acinus is irregularly involved and may be asymptomatic.
- It is most common form of emphysema.
- It occurs near the scar and is commonly found around old healed inflammatory process such as tuberculous scars.

**Q. What are blue bloaters?**

Refer **Figure 1.4A**.

It is a distinctive clinical pattern seen in chronic bronchitis, the characteristics of which are:
- Marked/heavy cyanosis ("blue") and peripheral edema ("bloated") and secondary polycythemia.

**Q. What are pink puffers?**

Refer **Figure 1.4B**.
- It is a distinctive clinical pattern seen in emphysema of lung.
- Patients are thin and noncyanotic at rest (hence "pink").
- They have marked dyspnea ("puffer") and have prominent use of accessory muscle. They develop steadily progressive dyspnea.

**Q. List the differences between emphysema and chronic bronchitis.**

Refer **Table 1.1**.

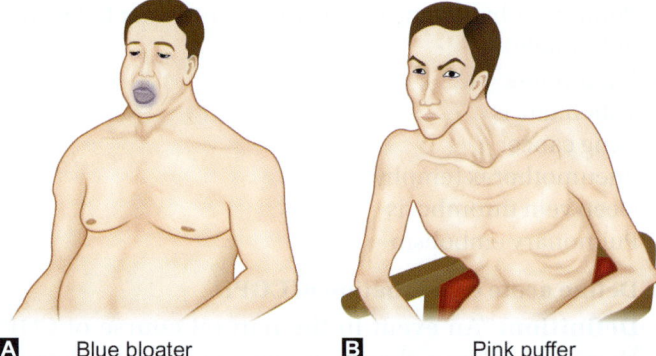

**Figs. 1.4A and B:** (A) Blue bloater (in chronic bronchitis); (B) Pink puffer (in emphysema).

**Table 1.1:** Differences between emphysema and chronic bronchitis.

| Feature | Emphysema | Chronic bronchitis |
|---|---|---|
| **Clinical features** | | |
| Dyspnea | Severe | Mild to moderate |
| Cough | Develops after dyspnea starts | Frequent, develops before dyspnea starts |
| Sputum—amount and nature | Scanty and mucoid | Copious and purulent |
| Frequency of mucopurulent relapses | Less | More |
| Cyanosis | Absent | Present |
| Pulmonary hypertension | Late and mild | Early and severe |

| Feature | Emphysema | Chronic bronchitis |
|---|---|---|
| Right ventricular failure and respiratory failure | Late and often terminal | Repeated episodes |
| Mechanism of airway obstruction | Loss of elastic recoil | Decreased airway lumen due to mucus and inflammation |
| **Investigations** | | |
| Hematocrit (PCV) | Normal | Increased |
| $PaO_2$ | Normal to low "pink puffer" | Low "blue bloater" |
| $PaCO_2$ | Normal mildly increased | High (>40) |
| $FEV_1$ | Decreased | Decreased |
| Diffusing capacity | Reduced | Normal |
| Chest X-ray | Features of hyperinflation, bullae, and tubular heart | Increased bronchovascular markings and cardiomegaly |
| Elastic recoil | Decreased | Normal |
| Airway resistance | Normal to slightly increased | Increased |
| Cor-pulmonale | Late and mild | Early and marked |
| Prognosis | Good | Poor |

($FEV_1$: forced expiratory volume in the first second; $PaCO_2$: partial pressure of carbon dioxide; $PaO_2$: partial pressure of oxygen)

### Q. What are the differences between asthma and chronic obstructive pulmonary disease?

Refer **Table 1.2**.

**Table 1.2:** Differentiating features of asthma and chronic obstructive pulmonary disease (COPD).

| Characteristics | Bronchial asthma | COPD |
|---|---|---|
| Age of onset | Usually children and young adults | Usually older individuals |
| Risk factors | Family history of allergy, exposure to allergens, and occupational sensitizers | Smoking, atmospheric pollution, occupational exposure, and α1-antitrypsin deficiency |
| **Respiratory symptoms** | | |
| Main symptoms | Wheezing, cough, and dyspnea | Chronic dyspnea and productive cough |
| Nature of symptoms | Vary from time to time and even over hours and days | Usually continuous symptoms |
| Triggers | Exercise, dust, or exposure to allergens | Unrelated to triggers |
| Recovery of symptoms | Symptoms improve spontaneously or with treatment | Slowly progressive despite therapy |
| Comorbidities | Generally absent | Often present (cardiovascular diseases, metabolic syndrome, depression, osteoporosis, and muscle wasting) |
| Chest X-ray | Normal | Hyperinflation |
| Spirometry | Reversibility of airway obstruction and normal between symptoms | $FEV_1/FVC<0.7$ and persistent airflow limitation |

($FEV_1$: forced expiratory volume in the first second; FVC: forced vital capacity)

### Q. What is cricosternal distance?

Cricosternal distance is the distance between the inferior border of the cricoid cartilage and the suprasternal notch:
- Measure the distance between the suprasternal notch and cricoid cartilage using your fingers.
- In healthy individuals, the distance should be 3–4 fingers. Cricosternal distance is actually based on the size of the patient's fingers so if their fingers are significantly different in size from your own, it may be worth using their fingers for the assessment.

### Q. What are the causes of abnormal cricosternal distance?

A distance of fewer than 3 fingers suggests underlying lung hyperinflation (e.g., asthma, COPD).

### Q. What is preserved ratio impaired spirometry (PRISm)?

PRISm is considered as a subtype that is more likely to progress to COPD. PRISm is defined as the ratio of forced expired volume in the first second to forced vital capacity ($FEV_1$:FVC) greater than or equal to 0.7 with an $FEV_1$ less than 80% predicted.

### Q. What are the clinical and molecular phenotypes of asthma?

Five predominant phenotypes in adult patients:
1. Mild-early-onset allergic disease
2. Moderate early-onset allergic disease
3. Late-onset eosinophilic non-allergic disease
4. Severe early-onset eosinophilic allergic disease
5. Late-onset non-allergic neutrophilic severe asthma with fixed airflow obstruction.

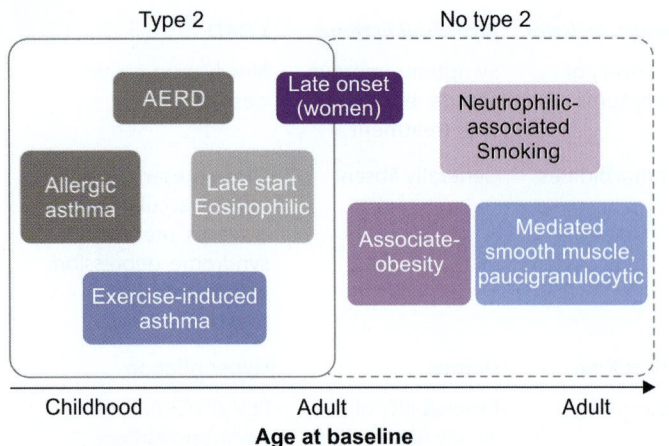

Biomarkers can help discriminate patients into the asthma phenotypes and endotypes that have been identified. Several biomarkers exist for T2 inflammation, including blood and sputum eosinophil counts, Feno values, IgE levels, and specific IgE test (skin prick test or ImmunoCAP) results.

For non-T2 asthma few potential biomarkers include IL-6, YKL-40, and serum and sputum IL-17.

## Targeted Therapy of Asthma

| Biologic | Target | Commonly used criteria | Benefit |
|---|---|---|---|
| Omalizumab | IgE | IgE ≥30 IU/mL, positive SPT response or specific IgE levels to perennial allergens | Significant improvement of asthma control and asthma control test scores |
| Mepolizumab | IL-5 | Blood eosinophil count ≥300 cells/μL | Decrease exacerbations by 39–52% |
| Reslizumab | IL-5 | Blood eosinophil count ≥400 cells/μL | Decrease exacerbations by 50–59% |
| Benralizumab | IL-5 receptor α | Blood eosinophil count ≥300 cells/μL | ✦ Decreased exacerbations by 45–51%<br>✦ Improvement in prebronchodilator FEV1 by 0.106–0.159 L<br>✦ Improvements in ACQ-5 scores |
| Dupilumab | IL-4Ra | ✦ Blood eosinophil count ≥150 cells/μL<br>✦ Feno >25 ppb | ✦ Decreased exacerbations by 46–48%<br>✦ Improvement in prebronchodilator FEV1 by 0.13–0.14 L<br>✦ Improvements in ACQ-5 scores<br>✦ Improved prebronchodilator $FEV_1$ |
| Tezepelumab | TSLP | **Trial criteria:** uncontrolled asthma on ICS/LABA; history of exacerbation FEV1: 40–80% of predicted value; post-BDR ≥12% | ✦ Phase 2 trials showed improvement in exacerbation rates by 62–71%<br>✦ Reduction in blood eosinophil counts, serum IgE levels, and Feno values |

## Case 2: Pleural Effusion

*Brief History*
Middle aged male, smoker with history of dry cough and breathlessness of 10 days duration.

*General Examination*
- Patient is conscious, oriented
- Moderately built. BMI: 18.5
- No pallor/icterus/pedal edema/lymphadenopathy. Grade 1 clubbing present **(Figs. 1.5A and B)**.
- Pulse: 72/min, regular, normal volume, no special character. All peripheral pulses well felt
- JVP: not raised
- BP: 110/70 mm Hg
- RR: 22/min
- Temperature: 99.4°F.

*Systemic Examination*
Respiratory System
- Upper respiratory tract: Nicotine stain of teeth present.
- Lower respiratory tract.

*Inspection*
- Shape is elliptical, bilateral symmetrical.
- Trachea appears central, apical impulse not visualized.
- Decreased chest movements in the left side in all areas. Right side movements are normal.
- No visible pulsations/dilated veins.
- Spine appears to be normal.

*Palpation*
- Chest is bilateral symmetrical.
- Trachea is central.
- Apical impulse could not be localized.
- Intercostals tenderness present in 5th, 6th, 7th spaces left side.
- Respiratory movements decreased in the left apical, mammary and infrascapular areas.
- Chest expansion is 4.5 cm. 3 cm by right hemithorax. 1.5 cm by left hemithorax. AP: Transverse diameter = 7:5.
- Vocal fremitus decreased in the left mammary infra-axillary and infrascapular areas.
- Right side of chest has no positive findings.

*Percussion*
- Stony dull note present in left infra-axillary, infrascapular, interscapular and mammary areas.
- Right side normal resonant note was present
- Liver dullness noted in the right 5th intercostals space in midclavicular line.

*Auscultation*
- Diminished breath sounds in the left infra-axillary, infrascapular and the mammary areas.
- Tubular bronchial breath sounds present in the left interscapular areas.
- Normal vesicular breath sounds present in the right side.
- Vocal resonance decreased in the left mammary, infra-axillary and infrascapular areas. VR increased in the left interscapular areas.

*Cardiovascular System*
Within normal limits.

*Central Nervous System*
No focal neurological deficits.

*Per Abdomen*
No organomegaly.
Diagnosis: Left-sided pleural effusion? Empyema secondary to pneumonia, not in respiratory failure.

## DISCUSSION

### Q. What is the normal amount of fluid in pleural space?

Normal pleural fluid is a clear, ultrafiltrate of plasma, present in small amounts within the pleural space, typically between 0.1 and 0.3 mL per kilogram of body weight. It acts as a lubricant, facilitating smooth lung movement during breathing. The fluid is characterized by low protein concentration, typically less than 2% (1–2 g/dL), and a low white blood cell count (less than 1,000/μL).

### Q. What are features that differentiate empyema from pleural effusion?

In empyema patient will be toxic with fever, clubbing and intercostal tenderness. All other features will be similar to pleural effusion **(Fig. 1.6)**.

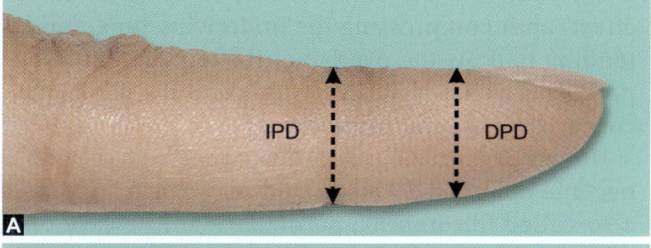
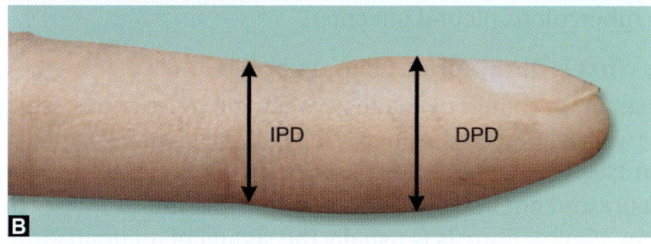

**Figs. 1.5A and B:** (A) Normal finger; (B) Clubbing of finger.
(IPD: interphalangeal distance; DPD: distal phalangeal distance)

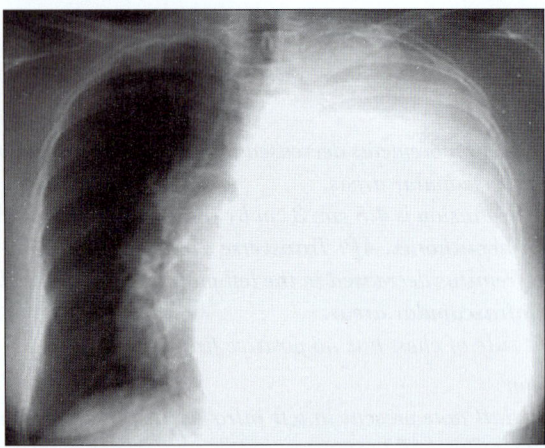

**Fig. 1.6:** Chest X-ray shows left-sided massive pleural effusion.

**Q. Name the clinical course of empyema.**
- **Early exudative stage:** Once infected by pathogenic organisms, the connective tissue layers within the pleural membranes become edematous and produce an exudation of proteinaceous fluid that starts to fill the pleural cavity. The pleural fluid is thin with a relatively low white cell count and the visceral pleura and underlying lung remain mobile.
- **Fibrin purulent stage:** As the inflammatory process continues, newly formed layers of fibrin become laid down on the epithelial surface within the pleural cavity, particularly on the parietal pleura. The empyema fluid becomes thicker and more turbid, containing a higher white cell count. With the deposition of fibrin on both pleural surfaces, lung movement may become increasingly restricted.
- **Organizational stage:** May begin within 2 weeks. Thickened fibrinous layers organize as collagen and become vascularized by an ingrowth of capillaries. The inner layers of the thickened empyema cortex continue to show a considerable inflammatory cell infiltrate and the fibrous outermost layers exert an increasingly restrictive effect, both compressing the underlying lung and also tending to draw the overlying ribs together, ultimately producing a chest deformity with a dorsal scoliosis that is concave towards the affected side.

Ultimately an inadequately treated empyema cavity may become obliterated and its rind may calcify, producing a so-called fibrothorax, particularly in the case of old tuberculous pleural infection.

**Q. What is fibrothorax/pleural fibrosis?**
Distinction should be made between pleural plaques, which are well-demarcated lesions of the parietal pleura, and pleural fibrosis, which is a diffuse process involving both layers of pleura and not infrequently extending into the surface of the lung. Pleural fibrosis is usually the sequel of an unabsorbed pleural effusion. The lesion may be unilateral or bilateral. The physiological effects of pleural fibrosis are decreased lung volumes, without reduction in transfer coefficient, and decreased compliance. The localized type mimics pleural effusion, with local reduction in movements, percussion note and breathe sounds. The generalized type may cause marked limitation of chest wall movements, retraction of intercostals spaces and flattening of the chest wall, mimicking the features of extensive pulmonary fibrosis.

**Q. What is therapeutic thoracocentesis—how much pleural fluid to remove?**
Large pleural effusions should be drained incrementally, draining a maximum of 1.5 L on the first occasion. Any remaining fluid should be drained 1.5 L at a time at 2-hour intervals, stopping if the patient develops chest discomfort, persistent cough or vasovagal symptoms. Re-expansion pulmonary edema is a well-described serious but rare complication following rapid expansion of a collapsed lung through evacuation of large amounts of pleural fluid on a single occasion and the use of early and excessive pleural suction. Putative pathophysiological mechanisms include reperfusion injury of the underlying hypoxic lung, increased capillary permeability and local production of neutrophil chemotactic factors such as interleukin-8.

**Q. How to palpate for scalene lymph nodes?**
Feel for the scalene nodes above the first rib next to the insertion of scalenus anterior muscle with patients head slightly tilted to that side. Place your index finger between the clavicle and sternocleidomastoid muscle and press down gently towards the first rib. A palpable scalene node is a soft mobile mass just above a hard first rib.

**Q. What is the lymphatic drainage of the lung and pleura?**
Parietal pleura to axillary lymph node whole of right lung and left lower lobe to right supraclavicular lymph node, left upper lobe to left supraclavicular lymph node.

**Q. Name the causes of loculated pleural effusion.**
It occurs in conditions that cause intense pleural inflammation such as tuberculosis, empyema, hemothorax produces characteristic D-shaped pattern on chest X-ray **(Fig. 1.7)**.

**Q. Where do you perform thoracocentesis?**
Thoracocentesis is performed preferably in sitting position with arms resting on a table or by lying on the affected side with ipsilateral arm over the head. It should be attempted one interspace below the spot where tactile fremitus is lost and the percussion note becomes dull, posteriorly several inches from the spine, where the ribs are easily palpated and just superior to a rib to avoid the neurovascular bundle.

**Q. What is D'Espine sign? How do you interpret it?**
- Normally, vesicular breath sounds from the right and left lung are louder than the sounds heard over the vertebral body at the same level.

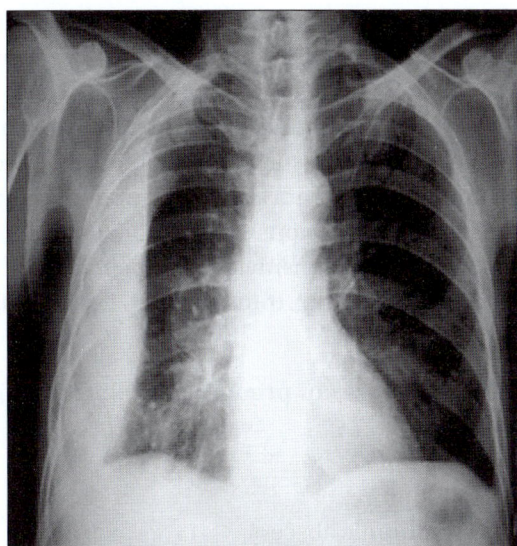

**Fig. 1.7:** Chest X-ray of loculated effusion.

- If the sounds over the vertebral body are louder, and actually tubular in quality, the D'Espine sign is positive.
- D' Espine considered the sign to be positive if heard over the seventh cervical vertebra or more caudal.
- In the infant, it is present at the C7 vertebral level, by the tenth year it reaches T3, and in the adult it is at the level of T4.
- So, in an adult one should listen for the sign around T4 region where the trachea bifurcates. **The further caudal, the more a positive sign is to be significant**.

### Interpretation

A positive D'Espine sign implies that the posterior mediastinum contains a solid lesion connecting the tracheobronchial system with the vertebral body. The commonest causes of solid lesions include, bronchogenic malignancies, lymph nodes (lymphomas, sarcoids, metastatic malignancies and tuberculosis).

### False-positive D'Espine sign can occur in:

- Kyphoscoliosis without posterior mediastinal tumor
- A unilateral false-positive sign can occur in patients with intrathoracic tracheal deviation.

### Q. What are the clinical features of PEM?

- Easily pluckable hair
- Flag sign (transverse depigmentation of hair)
- Sparse hair
- Cracking (flaky paint or crazy pavement dermatosis seen on the legs)
- Poor wound healing, decubitus ulcers
- Edema
- Hepatomegaly
- Parotid enlargement
- Dry cracked tongue.

### Q. What is the importance of skinfold thickness?

Measurement of skinfold thickness is useful for estimating body fat stores, because about 50% of body fat is normally in the subcutaneous region. Skinfold thickness can also permit discrimination of fat mass from muscle mass. The Triceps Skin Fold thickness (TSF) is a convenient site that is generally representative of the body's overall fat level. A thickness <3 mm suggests virtually complete exhaustion of fat stores. The mid-arm muscle circumference (MAMC) can be used to estimate skeletal muscle mass, calculated as follows:

MAMC (cm) = upper arm circumference (cm) – [0.314 × TSF (mm)]

Wasting of the temporalis muscle results in the gaunt appearance of the starved. The skeletal muscles of the extremities also serve as an indicator of malnutrition.

### Q. What are the causes of niacin deficiency?

- Isoniazid therapy
- Hartnup's disease
- Malabsorption
- Alcohol-dependent patients who do not eat.
- Very low protein diets given for renal disease.
- Carcinoid syndrome and pheochromocytomas.

### Q. How to differentiate hydropneumothorax and pleural effusion?

- Shifting dullness present in hydropneumothorax, absent in pleural effusion
- Straight line dullness present in hydropneumothorax.
- Succussion splash present in hydropneumothorax, absent in pleural effusion
- Coin test present in hydropneumothorax, absent in pleural effusion
- Amphoric bronchial breathing may be present in hydropneumothorax due to bronchopleural fistula.

### Q. What are the causes of pleural effusion with trachea shifted to the same side?

In collapse with obstruction of bronchus in bronchogenic carcinoma.

### Q. What are the causes of hypotension in a patient with pleural effusion?

- Addison's disease secondary to TB of adrenal glands.
- Sepsis (empyema thoracis).
- Pericardial effusion, constrictive pericarditis.

### Q. What are the features of malignant pleural effusion?

- History of cough, hemoptysis, emaciation. Elderly, chronic smoker.
- Presence of lymphadenopathy—supraclavicular, scalene and axillary groups (parietal pleura drains to axillary nodes).
- Clubbing, anemia or polycythemia.
- Associated with superior mediastinal syndrome or Horner's syndrome.

- Massive and rapidly progressive repeated accumulating pleural effusion with mediastinal shift or fixity of mediastinum.
- Causes—bronchogenic carcinoma, metastasis (from breast, thyroid), mesothelioma, lymphoma.

**Q. What are the features of bronchogenic carcinoma on general examination?**

In addition to the above:
- Superior sulcus tumors (Pancoast tumors), can compress the cervical sympathetic plexus, causing classic Horner syndrome (ipsilateral ptosis, miosis, enophthalmos, and anhidrosis).
- Superior vena cava syndrome (SVCS) results from obstruction of blood flow (dilated veins over neck, face and chest, edema of face)
- Supraclavicular and scalene lymph nodes.
- Clubbing—hypertrophic osteoarthropathy.
- Cushingoid habitus (obesity, moon like face)—paraneoplastic syndrome.

**Q. What is the significance of lymphadenopathy in pleural effusion?**
- Tuberculosis—cervical (posterior triangle), supraclavicular, axilla.
- Bronchogenic carcinoma—supraclavicular (especially right side), scalene.
- Lymphoma—generalized lymphadenopathy.
- Associated with splenomegaly in miliary TB, lymphoma, acute leukemias, cirrhosis of liver.

**Q. What is Light's criteria?**

To differentiate transudate and exudate effusions (**Box 1.6**).
- Pleural fluid protein/serum protein >0.5
- Pleural fluid LDH/serum LDH >0.6
- Pleural fluid LDH more than two-thirds normal upper limit for serum.

Exudative pleural effusions meet at least one of the following criteria, whereas transudative pleural effusions meet none.

**Box 1.6:** Modified Light's criteria for distinguishing pleural transudate from exudate.

> **Modified Light's criteria**
> *Pleural fluid is an exudate if one or more of the following criteria are met:*
> *Pleural fluid*
> - Serum protein ratio >0.5
> - Serum LDH ratio >0.6
> - LDH >2/3 upper limit of normal serum LDH
> - Protein >30 g/L
>
> If only one of the above criteria is met, then calculate the fluid to serum albumin gradient.
>
> If the albumin gradient >12 g/L, consider a transudate.

- **False positive:** If one or more of the exudative criteria are met and the patient is clinically thought to have a condition producing a transudative effusion.
- **Example:** Effusion in CHF on diuretic therapy. May have higher protein. In such case difference between the protein levels in the serum and the pleural fluid should be measured. If >3.1 g/dL considered transudative.

**Table 1.3** shows the sensitivity and specificity of tests to distinguish exudative from transudative effusions. **Box 1.7** shows the Roth's criteria.

**Q. What are the causes of predominant left sided pleural effusion?**
- Acute pancreatitis.
- Esophageal rupture.
- Left side subphrenic abscess.
- Dressler's syndrome.

**Q. What are the causes of predominant right sided pleural effusion?**
- Rupture of amoebic liver abscess.
- Meig's syndrome.
- Right side subphrenic abscess.

**Q. What are the causes of recurrent pleural effusion?**
- Bronchogenic carcinoma.
- Pulmonary TB.
- Mesothelioma.

**Table 1.3:** Sensitivity and specificity of tests to distinguish exudative from transudative effusions.

| | Sensitivity for exudates (%) | Specificity for exudates (%) |
|---|---|---|
| Light's criteria | 98 | 83 |
| Pleural fluid cholesterol level >60 mg/dL | 54 | 92 |
| Pleural fluid cholesterol level >43 mg/dL | 75 | 80 |
| Ratio of pleural fluid cholesterol/serum cholesterol >0.3 | 89 | 81 |
| Serum albumin level minus pleural fluid albumin level ≤12 g/L | 87 | 92 |

(LDH: lactate dehydrogenase)

**Box 1.7:** Roth's criteria.

> Clinically if a patient should have a transudative effusion, but meets Light's criteria for an exudative effusion, measure serum-pleural fluid albumin gradient, or measure the serum-pleural protein gradient (**Roth's criteria**).
> - Serum-effusion albumin gradient of >1.2 g/dL—transudative
> - Serum-effusion protein gradient >3.1 g/dL—transudative

- Lymphoma.
- Congestive cardiac failure.
- Collagen vascular diseases.

**Q. What are the causes of pleural fluid eosinophilia?**

Diseases associated with pleural fluid eosinophilia:
- Pneumothorax
- Hemothorax
- Benign asbestos
- Pulmonary embolism
- Parasitic disease—paragonimiasis, hydatid disease, amebiasis, ascariasis
- Fungal disease—histoplasmosis, coccidioidomycosis
- Drug-induced—dantrolene, bromocriptine, nitrofurantoin, valproic acid
- Lymphoma—Hodgkin disease and carcinoma
- Churg-Strauss syndrome.

**Q. What is the diagnostic algorithm of pleural effusion?**
Refer **Figure 1.8.**

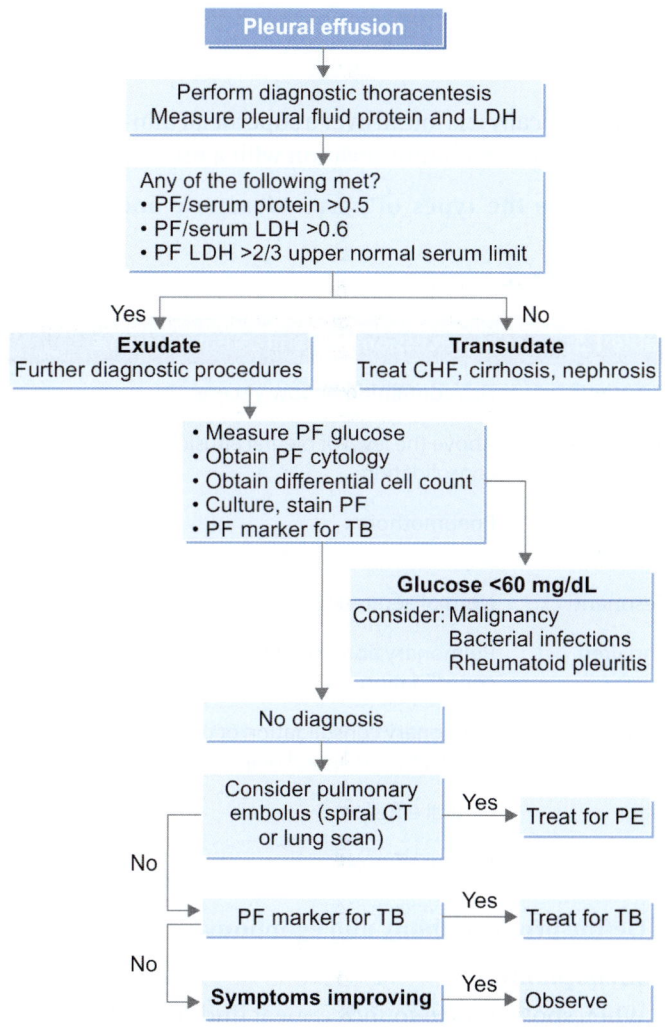

**Fig. 1.8:** Diagnostic algorithm of pleural effusion.

**Q. What is the lymphatic drainage of pleura?**
Refer **Figure 1.9.**

**Q. Name the lung diseases causing decreased vocal fremitus or resonance.**

**Decreased VR:** Usually due to defective production or transmission of sound vibrations.
- Partial obstruction of an air passage (as in partial laryngeal stenosis or glottis edema)
- Hypertrophic emphysema
- Thickened pleura
- Small pleural effusion
- Partial pneumothorax
- Edema of chest wall
- Malignant disease of pleura
- A feeble voice from a disease or debility may also result in decreased vocal resonance

**Absent vocal resonance:**
- Deaf mutism
- Vocal cord paralysis
- Large pleural effusion
- Severe emphysema
- Pneumothorax
- Acute pulmonary edema
- Absence of lung tissue (as in diaphragmatic hernia or after lobectomy).

**Q. Name the types of bronchial breathing.**
Refer **Table 1.4.**

| Table 1.4: Types of bronchial breathing. | | |
|---|---|---|
| Cavernous (low pitched) | Peculiar hollow character | ◆ Underlying cavity with irregular walls<br>◆ Open pneumothorax<br>◆ Pulled trachea syndrome |
| Tubular (high pitched) | Tubular or aspirate quality | ◆ Consolidation of lung tissue<br>◆ Pulmonary infarction<br>◆ Atelectasis or collapse (secondary to partial obstruction) |
| Medium pitched | ◆ Intermediate between cavernous and tubular<br>◆ Incomplete loss of elasticity | ◆ Incomplete loss of elasticity of diseased lung as in:<br>◆ Tuberculous infiltration<br>◆ Bronchial carcinoma<br>◆ Fibrosis<br>◆ Partial lung collapse |
| Amphoric (high pitched) | Echo or metallic quality | ◆ Large cavity with smooth walls<br>◆ Pneumothorax communicating with bronchus |

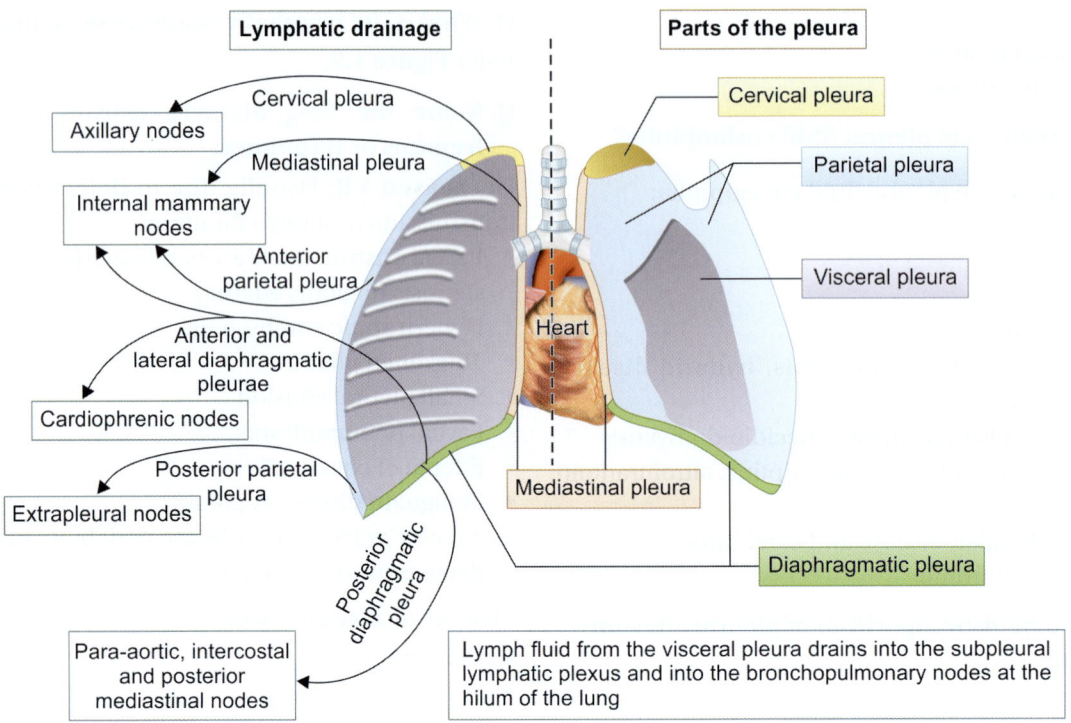

**Fig. 1.9:** Lymphatic drainage of pleura.

**Q. What are the different types of percussion notes?**

**Normal lung resonance:**
- Normal percussion note of the chest is due to the underlying lung tissue, containing a normal amount of air in the air vesicles, air sacs and air passages.
- It has a distinctive character with a low pitch.
- Normal lung resonance varies slightly from case to case and over the different areas of the chest in the same person, front wall of the chest yields a more resonant note compared to the back because of less musculature.
- Lesions that are more than 5 cm away from the chest wall or less than 2–3 cm in diameter does not alter the percussion note.

**Impaired resonance:**
- A percussion notes, completely devoid of resonance or displaying absolute or extreme dullness, is referred to as impaired resonance.
- Seen in cases of lung fibrosis with thickened pleura.

**Stony dullness:**
- Absolute dull percussion note associated with pain when percussing in the examiner's pleximeter as one would experience percussing over a stone.
- This can be seen with pleural effusion.

**Woody dullness:** Usually seen in consolidation.

**Cracked pot resonance:**
- This is a variety of tympanic note which can be elicited normally over the chest of an infant, or child during the act of crying.
- Pathologically it is found over a superficial thin-walled lung cavity that is in communication with a bronchus.

**Q. What are the types of percussion note and causative lesions?**

Refer **Table 1.5.**

**Table 1.5:** Types of percussion note and causative lesions.

| | |
|---|---|
| Tympanic | Gas containing hollow viscera |
| Subtympanic | Above the level of pleural effusion or consolidation |
| Hyper-resonant | Pneumothorax |
| Resonant | Normal aerated lung |
| Impaired | Pulmonary fibrosis sometimes collapse or consolidation |
| Dull | Pulmonary consolidation or collapse, thickened pleura, tumor, raised diaphragm |
| Flat | Pleural effusion |
| Stony dull | Pleural effusion |

**Q. Define bronchophony and egophony.**

**Bronchophony:**
- When spoken voice sounds appear unduly loud or intense and close to the ear. The individual words or syllables;

however, are indistinguishable. This condition is known as bronchophony.
- Normally heard over the larynx and trachea.
- Pathologically heard over lung consolidation as in lobar pneumonia, massive bronchopneumonia, caseous or tuberculous pneumonia.
- Compressed lung tissue as in pleural effusion (above the level of fluid) or intrathoracic tumor (causing lung compression).

### Egophony
- When spoken voice sounds during auscultation display peculiar quivering, nasal quality like the bleating of a goat, the sign can be imitated by saying ninety-nine while holding one's nose.
- Pleural effusion, along the border or just above the level of percussional dullness.

### Q. What is pulsus paradoxus and how do you elicit pulsus paradoxus?

In normal people blood pressure falls by 3–5 mm Hg during inspiration. In respiratory disorders there can be large pressure swings during the respiratory cycle.

When measuring blood pressure initially as the cuff pressure is reduced the systolic sound is heard initially only during expiration and but with further reduction in cuff pressure it is audible throughout expiration and inspiration. The pressure difference between initial systolic sound and the sound heard throughout the respiratory cycle gives the measurement of pulsus paradoxus.
- Pulsus paradoxus results from alterations in the mechanical forces imposed on the chambers of the heart and pulmonary vasculature often due to pericardial disease, particularly cardiac tamponade and to a lesser degree constrictive pericarditis.
- It is also seen in nonpericardial cardiac diseases such as right ventricular myocardial infarction and restrictive cardiomyopathy.
- Noncardiac disease states can occasionally lead to pulsus paradoxus including severe chronic obstructive pulmonary disease (COPD), severe asthma, tension pneumothorax, large bilateral pleural effusions, and pulmonary embolism.

### Q. What are the signs of hypercarbia?
- **Warm hands:** In carbon dioxide retention, the hands are strikingly warm and an irregular flapping tremor.
- **Pulse:** High volume bounding pulse.
- **Blood pressure:** In cases of acute exacerbation of COPD and acute severe asthma there is pulsus paradoxus.
- **JVP:** In cases of severe airway obstruction JVP gets elevated during expiration and falls during inspiration.
- **Edema:** Peripheral edema is often seen with hypercapnic with hypoxia, however, hypoxic normocapnic patients seldom have edema.
- Altered mental status.

### Q. How do you elicit succussion splash? What are the conditions causing succussion splash?
- Explain the procedure
- Percuss the chest of affected side
- Demarcate the fluid level
- At the junction of resonant and dull note place the stethoscope
- Sway the patient suddenly and observe the splashing sound produced

**Conditions causing succussion splash:**
- Hydropneumothorax
- Pyopneumothorax
- Herniation of stomach or colon into the thoracic cavity through diaphragm
- Large cavity with fluid and air in the lung.
- Succussion splash cannot be elicited in cases of hydropneumothorax if the fluid is thick as in empyema and loculated pleural effusion.

### Q. What is the normal amount of fluid present in the pleural cavity and pericardial cavity?

In pleural cavity the normal amount of fluid is about 15 mL (8 +/- 4 mL) and normal amount of fluid in pericardial cavity is about 30 mL (average 20–35 mL).

### Q. What is the rate of formation of pleural fluid?
- It is 0.01 mL/kg/hour
- It is produced and absorbed in parietal pleura.

### Q. What are the characteristic features of normal pleural fluid?

Normally, pleural fluid has the following characteristics:
- Clear ultrafiltrate of plasma that originates from the parietal pleura
- pH 7.60–7.64
- Protein contain less than 2% (1–2 g/dL)
- Fewer than 1,000 WBCs per cubic millimeter
- Glucose content similar to that of plasma
- Lactate dehydrogenase (LDH) less than 50% of plasma
- Sodium, potassium and calcium concentration similar to that of the interstitial fluid.

### Q. What are the causes of increased pleural fluid production?

The following processes play a role in the increased production of pleural fluid:
- Altered permeability of the pleural membranes (e.g., inflammation, malignancy, pulmonary embolus)
- Reduction in intravascular oncotic pressure (e.g., hypoalbuminemia, cirrhosis)

- Increase capillary permeability or vascular disruption (e.g., trauma, malignancy, inflammation, infection, pulmonary infarction, drug hypersensitivity, uremia, pancreatitis)
- Increase capillary hydrostatic pressure in the systemic and/or pulmonary circulation (e.g., CHF, superior vena cava syndrome)
- Reduction of pressure in the pleural space, preventing full lung expansion (e.g., extensive atelectasis, mesothelioma)
- Decrease lymphatic drainage or complete blockage, including thoracic duct obstruction or rupture (e.g., malignancy, trauma)
- Increase peritoneal fluid, with migration across the diaphragm via lymphatic or structural defect (e.g., cirrhosis, peritoneal dialysis)
- Movement of fluid from pulmonary edema across the visceral pleura
- Persistent increase in pleural fluid oncotic pressure from an existing pleural effusion, causing for the fluid accumulation

**Q. What are the differences between transudative and exudative effusions?**
Refer **Table 1.6**.

**Table 1.6:** Differentiation of transudative from exudative effusion.

| Characteristics | Transudative effusion | Exudative effusion |
|---|---|---|
| Cause and mechanism | Noninflammatory process: Ultrafiltrate of plasma, due to increased hydrostatic pressure or decreased serum oncotic pressure with normal vascular permeability | Inflammation process and is rich in proteins due to increased vascular permeability |
| Appearance | Clear, serous | Cloudy/purulent/ hemorrhagic/chylous |
| Color | Straw yellow | Yellow to red |
| Specific gravity | <1.018 | >1.018 |
| **Protein** | | |
| Absolute value | Low, <2 g/dL, mainly albumin | High, >2 g/dL |
| Pleural fluid: serum ratio | <0.5 | >0.5 |
| Clot | Absent | Clots spontaneously because of high fibrinogen |
| **Leukocytes** | | |
| Total leukocytes | <1,000/mm$^3$ | >1,000/mm$^3$ |
| Type of cells | >50% lymphocytes or mononuclear cells | >50% lymphocytes (tuberculosis, malignancy) |
| Differential leukocytes | Mesothelial cells | >50% polymorphs (acute inflammation) |
| **Erythrocytes** | <500/mm$^3$ | Variable |
| **Bacteria** | Absent | Usually present |
| **Lactate dehydrogenase (LDH)** | | |
| Absolute value | <200 IU/L | >200 IU/L |
| Pleural fluid LDH: serum LDH ratio | <0.6 | >0.6 |
| **Glucose** | >60 mg/dL (usually same as in blood) | <60 mg/dL (variable) |

**Q. What are the causes of effusion?**
Refer **Table 1.7**.

**Table 1.7:** Classification and causes of pleural effusion.

| Types of effusion | Causes | |
|---|---|---|
| Transudative effusion | - Cardiac failure<br>- Hypoproteinemia (e.g., nephrotic syndrome, cirrhosis of liver, severe malnutrition)<br>- Constrictive pericarditis | - Hypothyroidism<br>- Meigs' syndrome (benign ovarian tumors with ascites and pleural effusion)<br>- Peritoneal dialysis |

| Types of effusion | Causes | |
|---|---|---|
| Exudative effusion | • Tuberculosis<br>• Bacterial pneumonia<br>• Malignancy<br>• Pulmonary infarction<br>• Autoimmune diseases (e.g., rheumatoid arthritis, systemic lupus erythematosus)<br>• Acute pancreatitis<br>• Postmyocardial infarction syndrome (Dressler's syndrome) | • Drug-induced effusion<br>• Benign asbestos- related effusion<br>• Intra-abdominal abscess<br>• Meigs' syndrome (can be transudative as well)<br>• Ruptured amebic liver abscess, chylous pleural effusion<br>• Acute rheumatic fever |

**Note:** Pulmonary embolism: Can cause both transudative and exudative effusion.

### Q. What is the difference between hemorrhagic effusion and hemothorax?

Refer **Table 1.8**.

**Table 1.8:** Difference between hemorrhagic effusion and hemothorax.

| Hemorrhagic effusion | Hemothorax |
|---|---|
| RBC <100,000/microliter | RBC >100,000/microliter |
| PCV <50% of blood | PCV >50% of blood |
| Tumor, trauma, PTE, pancreatitis, TB | Tumor, trauma, PTE |

### Q. What is the differences between chylous and chyliform (pseudochylous effusion)?

Refer **Table 1.9**.

**Table 1.9:** Differences between pseudochylous thorax and chylothorax.

| Feature | Pseudo-chylothorax | Chylothorax |
|---|---|---|
| Triglycerides | <0.56 mol/L (50 mg/dL) | >1.24 mmol/L (110 mg/dL) |
| Cholesterol | >5.18 mmol/L (200 mg/dL) | <5.18 mmol/L (200 mg/dL) |
| Cholesterol crystals | Often present | Absent |
| Chylomicrons | Absent | Present |
| Etiology | Tuberculosis, rheumatoid arthritis, poorly treated empyema | Neoplasm (lymphoma, metastatic carcinoma), trauma (operative, penetrating injuries), miscellaneous (tuberculosis, sarcoidosis, cirrhosis, lymphangioleiomyomatosis, obstruction of central veins, amyloidosis) |

### Q. What are the differences between empyema and chylous/chyliform effusion?

On centrifugation—the milky appearance clears in empyema but not in the other two cases.

### Q. What is pleural fluid analysis?

Interpretation of pleural fluid parameters is shown in **Table 1.10**.

**Table 1.10:** Interpretation of pleural fluid parameters.

| Parameter | Interpretation |
|---|---|
| Appearance of pleural fluid | Putrid odor (anaerobic empyema), food particles (esophageal rupture), bile-stained (chylothorax/biliary fistula), milky (chylothorax/pseudochylothorax), anchovy sauce-like fluid (ruptured amebic abscess) |
| **Parameter** | **Interpretation** |
| Pleural fluid glucose concentration | |
| Low glucose concentration (<60 mg/dL) | Suggests empyema, malignancy or tuberculosis |
| Very low glucose concentration (<15 mg/dL) | Empyema, rheumatoid effusions |
| Pleural fluid eosinophilia (>10% of all cells) | May be observed in resolving infections, pneumothorax, hydropneumothorax, hemothorax and asbestos-related pleural effusion, dantrolene, bromocriptine, nitrofurantoin, paragonimiasis or Churg-Strauss syndrome |
| Pleural fluid erythrocyte counts >100,000/mm$^3$ | Most often in malignancy or pulmonary infarction/embolism, but may result from a traumatic tap |
| Low pH of pleural fluid <7.2 | Complicated parapneumonic effusion, esophageal rupture, rheumatoid pleuritis, tuberculous pleuritis, malignant pleural disease, hemothorax, systemic acidosis, paragonimiasis, lupus pleuritis, urinothorax |
| Raised pleural fluid amylase | Pancreatic diseases and esophageal rupture. However, routine amylase estimation is not recommended unless the clinical features suggest either of the two diseases |
| Pleural fluid antinuclear antibody titers or rheumatoid factor | No diagnostic significance and is not indicated in most cases |
| Mesothelial cells | Absent: Tuberculosis<br>Markedly increased: Pulmonary embolism |

## Q. What are the features of microscopic analysis of pleural fluid?

**The microscopic appearance of pleural fluid**

*Neutrophilic effusion*
- Neutrophils more than 50% of total cells
- Acute process affecting the pleura
  - Parapneumonic effusion
  - Pancreatitis
  - PTE

*Lymphocytic effusion*
- Lymphocytes more than 50% of total cells
- Chronic process affecting the pleura
- Tuberculosis/fungal infections
- Neoplasia

*Eosinophilic effusion*
- Eosinophils more than 10% of total cells
- Drug induced—amiodarone/nitrofurantoin
- Collagen vascular diseases
- Blood/air in the pleural space
- Repeated thoracentesis

*Neoplastic cells*
- Adenocarcinoma (70%)
- Lymphoma (50%)
- Squamous cell carcinoma (20%)

**Biochemical investigations in pleural fluid**

**LDH:** Indicator of the ongoing inflammation should be measured. Each time thoracentesis is done in the case of unknown effusion.

**Glucose:** Low glucose (<60 mg/dL) indicates:
- Complicated parapneumonic effusion
- Neoplastic effusion
- TB
- Rheumatoid pleuritis (very low)

*Amylase*
- Pancreatic effusion
- Esophageal rupture

*pH*

pH <7.2 indicates:
- Complicated parapneumonic effusion
- Malignant effusion (chemical pleurodesis not effective)
- TB
- Rheumatoid pleuritis

## Q. Describe the management of hemothorax.
- Tube thoracostomy to prevent empyema and
- To assess the rate of bleed
- Bleed >200 mL/hr mandates thoracotomy

## Q. What is the management of chylothorax?
- Investigate with CT thorax and lymphangiogram
- Treated with pleuroperitoneal shunt
- Tube thoracostomy contraindicated

## Q. What are the causes of effusion in AIDS?
- Infections—bacterial pneumonia/tuberculosis/fungal infections
- Lymphoma
- Kaposi sarcoma

## Q. Name some sclerosing agents used in pleurodesis.
Antibiotics (tetracycline, doxycycline, erythromycin, minocycline) as well as antiseptics (silver nitrate, iodopovidone), chemotherapeutic agents (mitomycin, bleomycin, cytarabine, doxorubicin, mitoxantrone), microorganisms (*Corynebacterium parvum*, *Streptococcus pyogenes* (OK432), and autologous blood have been used for performing chemical pleurodesis.

## Q. What are the causes of effusion with no mediastinal shift?
- Small effusion
- Bilateral effusion
- Loculated effusion
- Effusion with underlying collapse/fibrosis
- Effusion with fixed mediastinum (usually malignancy).

## Q. Differential diagnosis of encysted effusion.
- Pleural thickening
- Mass lesion

## Q. Describe about the imaging in pleural effusion.
Chest radiographs are useful to confirm the presence of effusion. The findings of effusion vary with the amount of effusion. On an upright posteroanterior (PA) view, a minimum of 200 mL of fluid is required to obliterate the costophrenic angle, called the meniscus sign of a pleural effusion. However, in a lateral view, 50 mL of fluid can be diagnosed with this sign. Ultrasound of the chest is more sensitive and useful for the diagnosis of pleural effusion and also helps in planning thoracentesis. All unilateral effusion in adults needs thoracentesis to determine the cause of pleural fluid.

## Q. What is the management of transudative effusion?
Refer **Figure 1.10**.

## Q. What is parapneumonic pleural effusion?
Parapneumonic pleural effusion (PPPE) is PE associated with lung infection, usually pneumonia, abscess, or infected bronchiectasis. When not associated with lung infection, it is called IPE (infectious PE). Up to 54% of pneumonias studied with chest ultrasound are associated with PPPE during their clinical course, and about 40% of these are complicated PPPE or empyema **(Table 1.10)**.

Categories of parapneumonic effusion **(Table 1.11)**

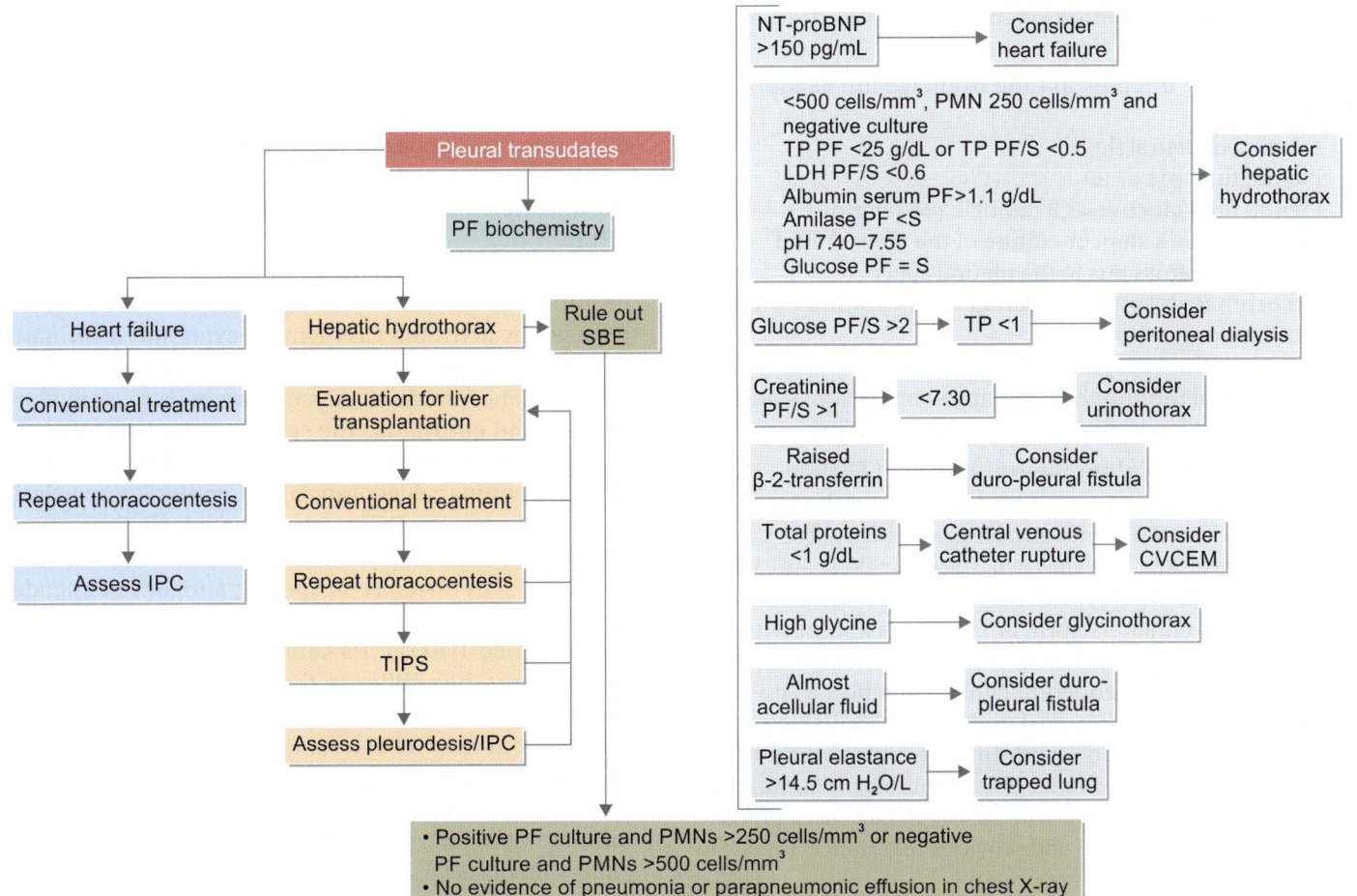

**Fig. 1.10:** Algorithm for the treatment of pleural transudate. (CVCEM: central venous catheter extravascular migration; IPC: indwelling pleural catheter; LDH: lactate dehydrogenase; NT-proBNP: n-terminal pro-brain natriuretic peptide; PF: pleural fluid; PF/S: pleural fluid/serum ratio; PMN: polymorphonuclear; SBE: spontaneous bacterial empyema; TIPS: transjugular intrahepatic portosystemic shunt; TP: total proteins)

**Table 1.11:** Parapneumonic pleural effusion and empyema: Light's classification and corresponding treatment.

| Category | Type | Characteristics | Treatment |
| --- | --- | --- | --- |
| 1. | Nonsignificant | <1 cm thick on an ipsilateral decubitus view. Thoracocentesis not required | Antibiotic |
| 2. | Typical parapneumonic | > 1 cm thick, glucose >40 mg/dL, pH >7.20, negative Gram's stain and culture | Antibiotic + consider therapeutic thoracentesis |
| 3. | Borderline complicated | pH 7–7.20 or LDH >1,000, negative Gram's stain and culture | Antibiotic + pleural drainage tube + consider fibrinolytics |
| 4. | Simple complicated | pH <7.0, positive Gram's stain or culture. Not loculated, no pus | Antibiotic + pleural drainage tube + fibrinolytics |
| 5. | Complex complicated | pH <7.0, positive Gram's stain or culture. Multiloculated | Antibiotics + pleural drainage tube + fibrinolytics + consider VAT |
| 6. | Simple empyema | Frank pus. Single loculation or free-flowing fluid\ | Antibiotics + pleural drainage tube + fibrinolytics + consider VAT |
| 7. | Complex empyema | Frank pus. Multiple loculations. Often requires decortication | Antibiotics + pleural drainage tube + fibrinolytics + VAT + other surgical procedures if VAT fails |

**Q. What are the indications of intercostal tube drainage in empyema?**

Indications for intercostal tube drainage are as following (Fig. 1.11):
- Loculated pleural fluid
- Pleural fluid pH <7.20
- Pleural fluid glucose <3.3 mmol/L (<60 mg/dL)
- Positive Gram's stain or culture of the pleural fluid
- Presence of gross pus in the pleural space.
- Recurrence despite two paracentesis mandates a tube thoracostomy
- Persistent fluid despite 24 hours requires
- Intrapleural thrombolytic therapy to break adhesions
- If persistent for >7 days, requires decortication

**Q. Describe tuberculous pleural effusion (TBPE).**
- Adenosine deaminase (ADA) remains the primary biomarker for TBPE with an overall sensitivity of 92% and a specificity of 90%. ADA has two isoforms: ADA1 and ADA2, and although ADA2 represents 88% of the total activity and is the predominant isoform in TBPE with a sensitivity and specificity of 97% and 94%, respectively, determination of ADA is recommended in clinical practice, as it is also a highly sensitive, low-cost and rapidly available option in biochemical analyses routinely performed on PF. In areas of high TB prevalence, PE containing predominantly lymphocytes associated with ADA >40 U/L has a positive predictive value of 98% and provides sufficient evidence to start anti-tuberculosis treatment.

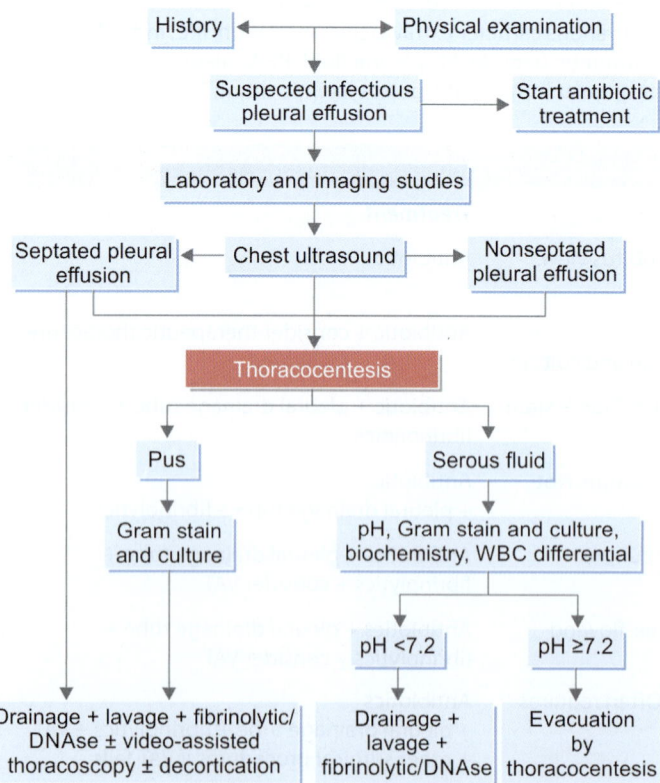

**Fig. 1.11:** Approach to empyema.

- A number of diseases can increase ADA levels in PF, including PPPEs, lymphomas, some solid tumors, and systemic rheumatic diseases (especially rheumatoid arthritis and systemic lupus erythematosus), as well as other rarer infectious diseases such as brucellosis, Q fever, histoplasmosis, or coccidioidomycosis. Despite a fixed cut-off, levels above 250 U/L suggest diagnoses other than TBPE.
- Interferon gamma (INF-γ) is a key cytokine in the immunopathogenesis of mycobacterial infection. It is released by activated CD4 lymphocytes and it primarily activates macrophages to increase their antimycobacterial activity. Concentrations may sometimes increase in blood cancers and empyema. The sensitivity and specificity of INF-γ are excellent for the diagnosis of TBPE, with some studies reporting values of above 85% and 95%, respectively.
- The tests known as INF-γ release assays (IGRAS) detect the release of INF-γ by sensitized T cells in peripheral blood or PF in response to specific antigens of encoded mycobacteria in the genome region known as the region of difference 1(RD1). Its sensitivity and specificity in PE appear to be similar to those of blood, and it has a sensitivity and specificity of 77% and 71% in tissue samples, and 78% and 72% in PE, respectively.
- In terms of microbiology, to be positive, a conventional sputum smear in PF requires a density of acid-alcohol-fast bacilli >10,000/mL, so this test has a low yield (<10%). Solid culture media have a low mycobacteria growth rate (<30%), while semiautomatic liquid culture media have higher yields in immunocompetent patients and in HIV patients: 56% and 75%, respectively. The use of polymerase chain reaction techniques has improved the cost-effectiveness of microbiological studies. Combining different samples also improves microbiological yield by up to 80% (**Fig. 1.12**).

**Q. What are the causes and mechanism of malignant pleural effusion?**
- Direct result
  - Pleural metastases with increased permeability
  - Pleural metastases with obstruction of pleural lymphatic vessels
  - Mediastinal lymph node involvement with decreased pleural lymphatic drainage
  - Thoracic duct interruption (chylothorax)
  - Bronchial obstruction (decreased pleural pressures)
  - Pericardial involvement
- Indirect result
  - Hypoproteinemia
  - Postobstructive pneumonitis
  - Pulmonary embolism
  - Postradiation therapy

**Q. What are the causes of malignant pleural effusion?**
- Lung carcinoma
- Breast carcinoma

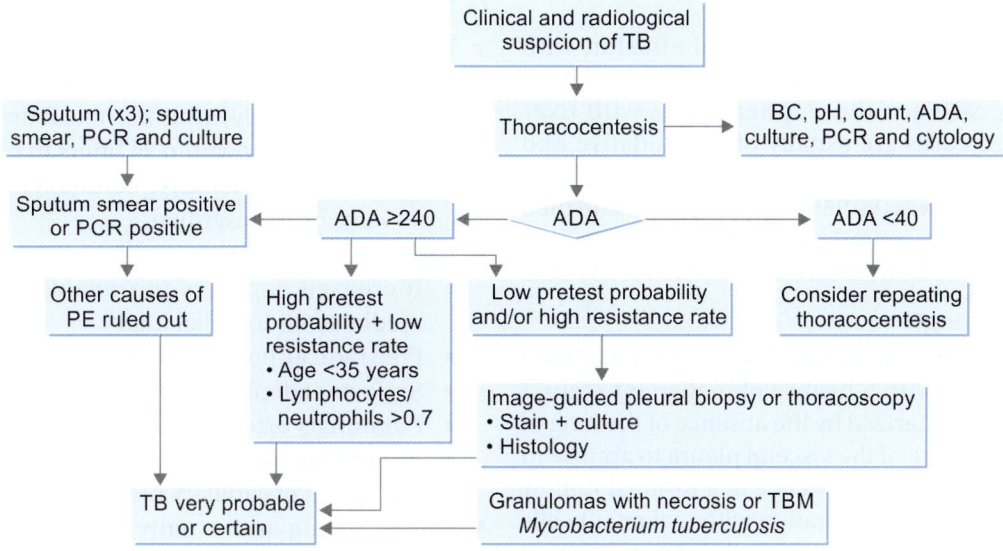

**Fig. 1.12:** Management of TB pleural effusion.

- Lymphoma and leukemia
- Ovarian carcinoma
- Sarcoma (including melanoma)
- Uterine and cervical carcinoma
- Stomach carcinoma
- Colon carcinoma
- Pancreatic carcinoma
- Bladder carcinoma
- Other carcinoma
- Primary unknown

**Q. Algorithm for the treatment of malignant pleural effusion (MPE).**

Refer **Figure 1.13**.

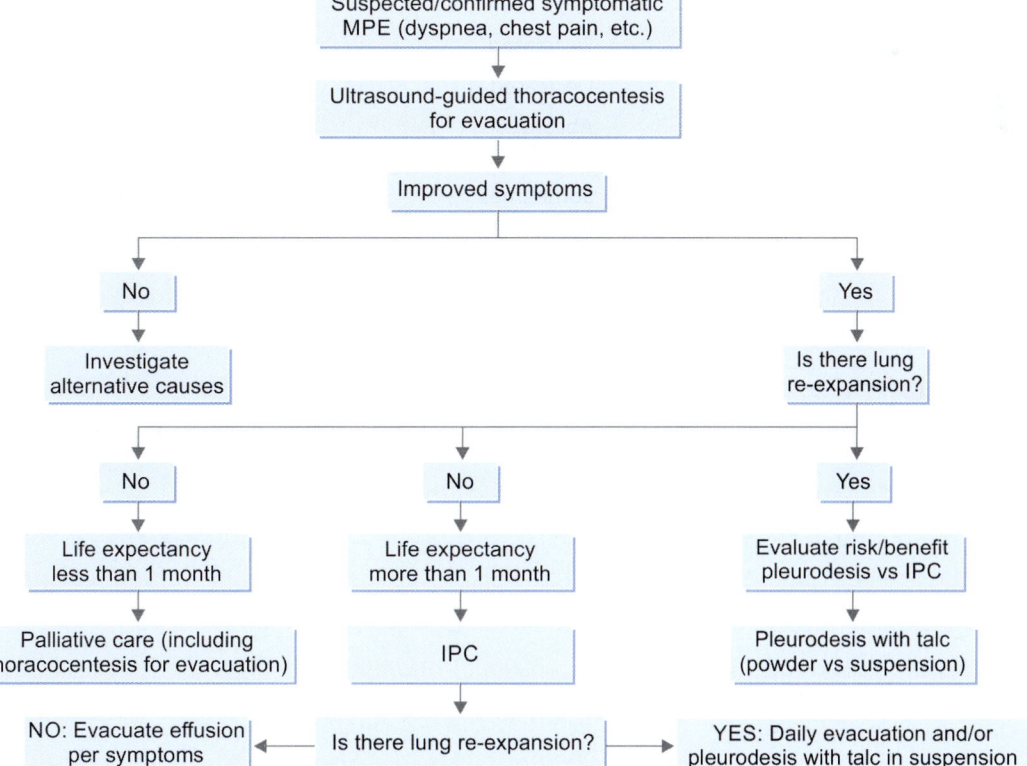

**Fig. 1.13:** Treatment of malignant pleural effusion.
(IPC: indwelling pleural catheter; MPE: malignant pleural effusion)

**Q. Define Contarini's syndrome.**

**Contarini's syndrome** is bilateral pleural effusion with different etiology. This is uncommonly reported. For example, malignancy with cardiac failure; pneumonia with liver cirrhosis. Reported cases are usually of an exudative and transudative effusion.

Francesco Contarini was the 95th Doge of Venice and died in 1625. His postmortem examination revealed that he had right hydrothorax due to heart failure as well as left empyema.

**Q. What is trapped lung?**

Trapped lung is used to describe an advanced state of lung pathology in a patient with a history of malignant pleural effusion, which is characterized by the absence of the lung to fully expanded, the failure of the visceral pleura to appose to the parietal pleura with the persistence of a residual hollow cavity, causes include direct infiltration with malignant cells or development of fibrotic tissue within the visceral pleura, presence of pleural carcinomatosis, radiation-induced fibrotic transformation, and proximal endobronchial obstruction causing distal lung collapse or chronic atelectasis with a concomitant malignant or paramalignant pleural effusion.

**Q. What is re-expansion pulmonary edema?**

- Drainage of more than 1.5 liters of fluid is associated with the development of re-expansion pulmonary edema.
- Develops frequently in the first hour following thoracentesis and tends to occur within 24 hours in most patients.
- Mostly unilateral edema is a common occurrence, bilateral cases have been described.
- Mechanisms:
  - Increased capillary permeability due to hypoxia-mediated endothelial injury
  - Free radical-mediated injury
  - Surfactant depletion
  - Pulmonary arterial pressure changes
  - A sudden increase in blood flow, and a sudden expansion of capillary blood.
- Self-resolving and usually resolves within 3–5 days of occurrence, but sometimes can cause ARDS and death.

**Q. How do you clinically co-relate the amount of pleural effusion?**

Refer **Table 1.12**.

**Table 1.12:** Summary of findings in pleural effusion based on the severity.

| Finding | Mild effusion (<300 mL) | Moderate effusion (300–1,500 mL) | Massive effusion (>1,500 mL) |
|---|---|---|---|
| Tachypnea | No | Present | Significant |
| Chest expansion | Normal | Decreased on the affected side | Significantly decreased on the affected side |
| Tactile fremitus | Normal | Decreased | Absent |
| Breath sounds | Vesicular | Decreased | Absent or bronchial |
| Contralateral tracheal or mediastinal shift | Absent | Absent | Present |
| Bulging intercostal spaces | No | Sometimes | Present |
| Egophony | No | Yes | Yes |

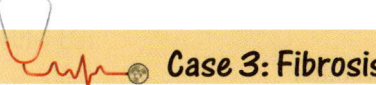

## Case 3: Fibrosis

### Brief History
A 45-year-old male with past history of pulmonary tuberculosis presents with dyspnea on exertion for 6 months.

### General Examination
- Moderately built and poorly nourished
- BMI: 13.67
- Pallor, and grade 2 clubbing present
- BP: 110/70 mm Hg
- PR: 110 b/min regular rhythm, character and volume.

### Systemic Examination
### Respiratory System Examination Inspection:
- Shape of chest bilateral symmetrical
- Trail's sign + with prominence of left SCM
- Bilateral supraclavicular hollowing and infraclavicular flattening
- Reduced chest expansion bilateral with more on left side.

### Palpation:
Trachea shifted to left.
Chest expansion 2 cm, 1.5 cm on right side and 0.5 cm on left side.

### Percussion
Impaired note heard over left infraclavicular and supraclavicular area.

### Auscultation
Cavernous bronchial breathing in left infraclavicular and axillary area with fine crepitations. Other areas normal vesicular breath sounds heard.

### Diagnosis
Left upper lobe fibrocavitary disease, possibly post-tuberculae sequelae, no evidence of cor pulmonale or respiratory failure.

## DISCUSSION

**Q. Why there is bronchial breath sounds in axilla?**
Bronchial BS heard in the axilla may be due to a cavitary lesion in left upper lobe associated with fibrosis.

**Q. What are the features of adrenal tuberculosis?**
Adrenal TB is a manifestation of disseminated disease presenting rarely as adrenal insufficiency.

The clinical features of Addison's disease include weakness, weight loss, low blood pressure, amenorrhea and gastrointestinal symptoms.

A characteristic hyperpigmentation of the skin, most notably over the elbows and the lower back, occurs in fair-skinned persons. Pigmented patches also occur in the mouth, a useful sign in dark-skinned patients.

Diagnosis of hypoadrenalism is confirmed by tests of adrenal function and tuberculosis is suggested by the presence of calcification in the adrenals visible on abdominal X-rays. Hormonal replacement, in addition to antituberculosis therapy, is required.

**Q. What are the manifestation in straight back syndrome?**
Tall, thin, ectomorphic, asthenic, apparently healthy patients who had a very straight thoracic vertebral column, an anterior-posterior/transverse thoracic diameter less than expected, and sometimes pectus excavatum, which causes the heart being squeezed between the sternum and the straight back and leads to apical systolic murmur.

**Q. List the external markers of tuberculosis.**
- **Eyes: Choroid tubercles**, painful hypersensitivity-related **phlyctenular conjunctivitis**.
- **Ear:** Hearing loss, otorrhea, and tympanic membrane perforation.
- **Throat:** In the nasopharynx, TB may simulate granulomatosis with polyangiitis (Wegener's).
- **Skin: Scrofuloderma, lupus vulgaris** (a smoldering disease with nodules, plaques, and fissures), miliary lesions, and **erythema nodosum, extensive tinea corporis**.
- **Lymph node:** Lymph node TB presents as painless swelling of the lymph nodes, most commonly at posterior cervical and supraclavicular sites (a condition historically referred to as **scrofuloderma**. **Tuberculous mastitis** results from retrograde lymphatic spread, often from the axillary lymph nodes.
- **Spinal TB (Pott's disease)** or tuberculous spondylitis, with advanced disease, collapse of vertebral bodies results in kyphosis **(gibbus)**.

**Q. What are the diseases affecting various radiological zones of the lung?**

### Upper zones
- Tuberculosis
- Chronic sarcoidosis
- Extrinsic allergic alveolitis
- Langerhans' cell histiocytosis
- Subacute silicosis
- Progressive massive fibrosis

### Middle zones
- Pulmonary edema
- Alveolar proteinosis
- *Pneumocystis carinii* infection

### Lower zones
- Cryptogenic fibrosing alveolitis
- Asbestosis
- Bronchopneumonia

- Collagen diseases
- Tropical eosinophilia

### Q. List the drugs causing lung fibrosis.
- Cytotoxics
- Nitrofurantoin
- Sulfasalazine, salicylates
- Gold
- Penicillamine
- Amiodarone

### Q. List the causes of interstitial lung diseases.

**Occupational and environmental**
- Asbestos
- silicates
- Beryllium
- Bauxite
- Coal, graphite
- Cobalt, antimony

**Organic dusts**
- Microorganisms
- Fungal spores
- Actinomycetes
- Animal protein
- Bird bloom
- Small mammal protein

**Collagen diseases**
- Rheumatoid
- Systemic sclerosis
- Lupus erythematosus
- Sjögren's syndrome

**Inherited disorders**
- Tuberous sclerosis
- Neurofibromatosis
- Ankylosing spondylitis
- Familial pulmonary fibrosis
- Weber-Christian disease
- Hermansky-Pudlak syndrome

**Vasculitis/granulomas**
- Churg-Strauss syndrome
- Polyarteritis nodosa
- Wegener's granulomatosis

**Toxic fumes and vapors**

*Oxygen*
- Chlorine, fluorine and other gases
- Nitrogen dioxide
- Lipids
- Drugs
- Poisons
- Paraquat
- Toxic oil syndrome

**Miscellaneous**
- Radiation
- Cryptogenic fibrosing alveolitis
- Sarcoidosis
- Langerhans' cell histiocytosis
- Hemosiderosis
- Amyloidosis
- Lymphangioleiomyomatosis

### Q. What are the causes of clubbing in long-standing fibrosis?
- Bronchiectasis
- Scar carcinoma.

### Q. What are the ocular manifestations of bronchogenic carcinoma?
- Horner's syndrome causing ptosis, miosis **(Figs. 1.14A and B)**
- Conjunctival chemosis, proptosis secondary to superior vena caval obstruction in lung cancer.

### Q. What are the paraneoplastic syndromes of lung cancer?

Paraneoplastic syndromes occur in approximately 10–20% of lung cancer patients.
- Endocrine syndromes include hypercalcemia, the syndrome of inappropriate antidiuretic hormone secretion, and ectopic adrenocorticotropic hormone secretion.
- Neurologic syndromes are relatively rare, are most commonly associated with SCLC, and may have autoimmune mechanisms. Such syndromes include Eaton-Lambert syndrome, limbic encephalopathy, cerebellar degeneration, subacute sensory neuropathy, autonomic neuropathy, and optic neuritis.
- Skeletal manifestations include digital clubbing and hypertrophic pulmonary osteoarthropathy.
- Hematologic and vascular syndromes include hypercoagulable states, migratory thrombophlebitis (Trousseau's syndrome), and nonbacterial thrombotic endocarditis.
- Cutaneous manifestations include dermatomyositis, acanthosis nigricans, erythema gyratum repens, and hyperkeratosis of the palms and soles of the feet [Ref: Harrison's internal medicine].

### Q. What is Kronig's isthmus?

A band of resonance about 5–6 cm width connecting the resonant areas of lung on the anterior and posterior chest in the apex of the lung bounded by:
- Medially—neck muscles
- Laterally—ipsilateral shoulder joint
- Anteriorly—clavicle and posteriorly—trapezius

Kronig's isthmus is elicited by percussion over the apex of the lung where the note is normally resonant. The area becomes dull on percussion in the presence of the apical tuberculosis, pancoast's tumor or apical pneumonia.

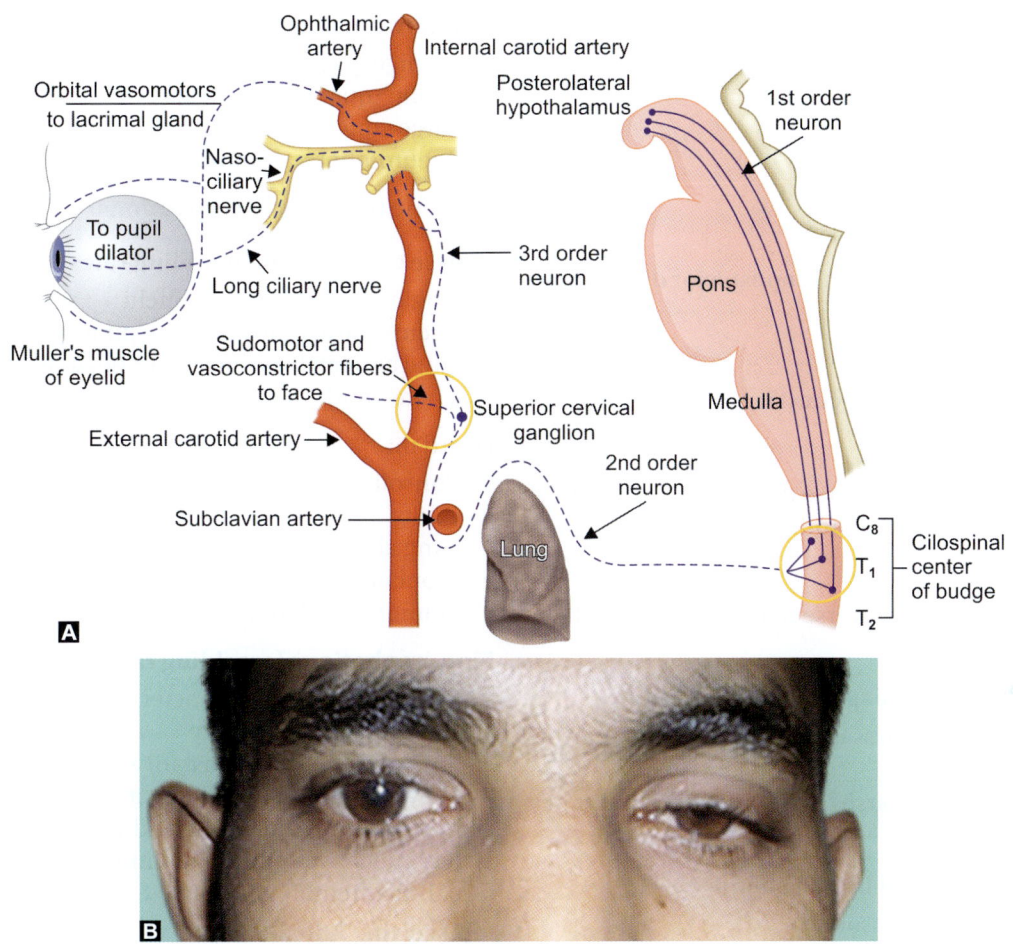

**Figs. 1.14A and B:** Left Horner's syndrome.

### Q. What is Pemberton's sign?

Pemberton's sign is the development of facial flushing, distended neck and head superficial veins, inspiratory stridor and elevation of the jugular venous pressure (JVP) upon raising both of the patient's arms above his/her head simultaneously, as high as possible (Pemberton's maneuver).

A positive Pemberton's sign is a sign of superior vena cava syndrome, possibly from a mass in the mediastinum, such as a tumor, or goiter (thoracic inlet obstruction due to retrosternal goiter or mass).

Apical lung cancers often cause a positive Pemberton's sign and a high index of suspicion should be maintained in patients with symptoms of dyspnea and facial plethora with an extensive smoking history.

### Q. Name the features of SVC syndrome.

Neck and facial swelling (especially around the eyes), dyspnea, and cough. Hoarseness, tongue swelling, headaches, nasal congestion, epistaxis, hemoptysis, dysphagia, pain, dizziness, syncope, and lethargy. Bending forward or lying down may aggravate the symptoms. The characteristic physical findings are dilated neck veins; an increased number of collateral veins covering the anterior chest wall; cyanosis; and edema of the face, arms, and chest. More severe cases include proptosis, glossal and laryngeal edema, and obtundation.

### Q. What are the respiratory causes of clubbing?
- Bronchogenic carcinoma
- Bronchiectasis
- Lung abscess
- Empyema
- Cystic fibrosis
- Interstitial lung disease
- Mesothelioma
- Sarcoidosis.

### Q. What is Trail's sign?

It is the undue prominence of the sternal head (lower end) of the sternocleidomastoid on the side to which the trachea is deviated. The pretracheal fascia encloses the clavicular head of the sternocleidomastoid on both sides. When the trachea is shifted to one side the pretracheal fascia covering the sternomastoid on that side relaxes, making the clavicular head more prominent.

### Q. What are the respiratory causes of cyanosis?
- Pulmonary edema
- Pulmonary thromboembolism
- High altitude sickness
- Severe pneumonia
- Acute severe attack of asthma
- Chronic obstructive lung disease

### Q. What is the normal ratio of anteroposterior diameter to the transverse diameter?
Normal—5:7.

### Q. What is flat chest and barrel chest?

#### Flat chest
- The anteroposterior to transverse diameter ratio is 1:2
- Seen in pulmonary TB and fibrothorax.

#### Barrel chest
- The anteroposterior to transverse diameter ratio is 1:1
- Seen in COPD.

### Q. What is bronchial breathing?
- It is produced due to the passage of air through the narrow air passages.
- It is less intense and less harsh than heard over the trachea and is of a higher pitch.

#### Characteristics of bronchial breath sound
- A high-pitched inspiratory sound
- A pause between inspiration and expiration
- A harsh and high-pitched expiratory sound
- Marked prolongation of expiration

#### Types
- Tubular
- Cavernous
- Amphoric

#### Tubular bronchial breathe sounds
It is a high-pitched bronchial breathing with characteristic "tubular" or "aspirate" quality. It is present in:
- Pneumonic consolidation
- Collapsed lung or lobe when a large draining bronchus is patent
- Above the level of pleural effusion.

#### Cavernous bronchial breathing
It is a low-pitched bronchial breathing with characteristic "hollow" character, normally heard with a stethoscope over the occipital region of the skull. When heard over the chest, it indicates:
- Underlying cavity in the lung
- An open pneumothorax
- Pulled trachea syndrome

#### Amphoric bronchial breathing
It is a high-pitched bronchial breathing with characteristic "metallic" quality. It is present in:
- Large smooth walled cavity
- Pneumothorax communicating with bronchus

### Q. Name the types of crepitations.

#### Coarse crepitations (bubbling rales)
- Originates from large bronchi
- Occurs during the end of inspiration
- Loud enough to be heard without a stethoscope or felt with a bare hand

Heard in:
- Consolidation
- Cavity
- Lung abscess
- Bronchiectasis
- Pulmonary edema

#### Fine crepitations (crackling rales)
- Lack the bubbling character
- Has a 'crackling' quality
- They are localized, constant and accentuated by coughing
- They are due to sudden separation of sticky alveolar walls by inrushing of air at the end of inspiration
  It is indicative of fluid exudation within the alveoli, usually of inflammatory origin.

It is seen in:
- First stage of pneumonia
- Early pulmonary tuberculosis
- Collapse of lung (Fig. 1.15)
- Bronchitis
- Pulmonary edema.

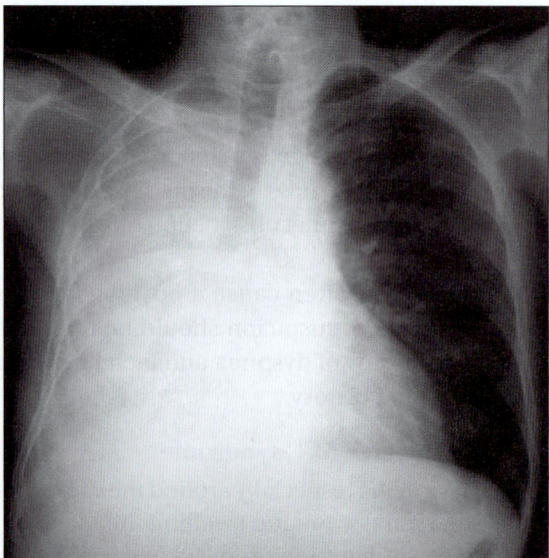

**Fig. 1.15:** Chest X-ray shows collapse of the right lung.

**Q. What are the differences between collapse and fibrosis?**
Refer **Table 1.13**.

**Table 1.13:** Differences between collapse and fibrosis.

| Features | Fibrosis | Collapse |
|---|---|---|
| Onset | Chronic | Sudden |
| Clubbing | Present | Absent |
| Percussion | Impaired | Dull |
| Breath sounds | Decreased | Absent |
| Added sounds | Crepitations | None<br>Monophonic rhonchus if bronchial obstruction |

**Q. What are the causes of fibrosis?**

**Upper lobe pulmonary fibrosis—causes**
- Tuberculosis
- Cystic fibrosis
- Ankylosing spondylitis
- Silicosis
- Sarcoidosis
- Langerhans cell histiocytosis
- Bronchopulmonary aspergillosis
- Radiotherapy

A useful **mnemonic** for pulmonary predominantly upper zone involvement (infiltration/shadowing/fibrosis) causes include:

**Mnemonic (BREASTS)**
- **B:** berylliosis
- **R:** radiation
- **E:** extrinsic allergic alveolitis
- **A:** ankylosing spondylitis/aspergillus
- **S:** sarcoidosis
- **T:** tuberculosis
- **S:** silicosis.

Mnemonics for conditions with a lower lobe predominance in chest radiology include:
- CIA
- BADAS
- RASCO

**Mnemonic (CIA)**
- **C:** collagen vascular disease
- **I:** idiopathic pulmonary fibrosis
- **A:** asbestosis

**Mnemonic (BADAS)**
- **B:** bronchiectasis
- **A:** aspiration pneumonia
- **D:** drugs; desquamative interstitial pneumonia
- **A:** asbestosis
- **S:** scleroderma and collagen vascular disease

**Mnemonic (RASCO)**
- **R:** rheumatoid arthritis
- **A:** asbestosis
- **S:** scleroderma
- **C:** collagen vascular disease
- **O:** other (drugs, e.g., busulfan, bleomycin, nitrofurantoin, hydralazine, methotrexate, amiodarone)

**Lower lobe pulmonary fibrosis—causes**
- Cryptogenic fibrosing alveolitis
- Rheumatoid arthritis
- Asbestosis
- Bleomycin toxicity
- SLE
- Scleroderma

**Q. What are the types of scoliosis?**

**Scoliosis may be:**
- Functional (nonstructural or postural)
- Structural

**Causes of scoliosis**
- Idiopathic—80%
- Secondary scoliosis—20%

**Nonstructural (postural)**
- Compensatory (short leg)
- Sciatica
- Hysterical
- Postural

**Structural**
- Idiopathic
- Bone disorders
- Congenital hemivertebra
- Osteogenesis imperfecta
- Osteoporosis
- Bone lysis
- Tuberculosis
- Malignancy
- Spondylolisthesis
- Neurological disorders
  - Syringomyelia
  - FrIedreich's ataxia
  - Poliomyelitis
- Muscular disorders
  - Duchenne's muscular dystrophy
  - Fasciohumeroscapular dystrophy
- Connective tissue disease
  - Marfan syndrome
  - Ehlers-Danlos syndrome
  - Homocystinuria
  - Morquio's syndrome
- Thoracic disorders
  - Thoracoplasty

- Fibrothorax (secondary to empyema)
- Lung fibrosis
- Pneumonectomy
- Thoracic burns
- Chest irradiation.

**Q. How will you differentiate whether scoliosis is functional or structural?**

**Forward Bend test:** Functional scoliosis is reversible, the curvature being abolished by forward flexion of spine whereas in structural scoliosis the deformity persists on forward flexion.

**Q. When will you say chest is barrel shaped?**
- Anteroposterior diameter is increased often to equal transverse diameter
- Subcostal angle is wide and horizontal position of ribs is accentuated
- Presence of upper thoracic kyphosis
- Sternum is arched

**Q. What is egophony? Where it is heard? What is mechanism behind?**
- When spoken voice sounds during auscultation display a peculiar quivering, nasal quality, like the bleating of a goat.
- It is heard
  - In pleural effusion just above level of percussion dullness
  - Over pleural effusion overlying area of consolidation
  - Over a cavity half filled with secretion

**Mechanism**
- Interposition of thin layer of fluid between lung and chest allowing transmission of overtones damping off lower fundamental tunes.
- Partial compression of lung tissue underneath the upper part of effusion altering the normal relationship between bronchi and lung parenchyma, so it causes reinforcement of high-pitched nasal sounds.

**Q. What is bronchophony? Where it is heard?**

When spoken voice sounds appear unduly loud or intense, clear and sound close to the ear ("chest voice"). The individual words or syllables, however, remaining indistinguishable, referred as bronchophony.

It is heard in:
- **Lung consolidation:** Lobar pneumonia, massive bronchopneumonia, caseous or tuberculous pneumonia
- Above level of pleural effusion
- Tuberculous or bronchiectatic cavity located superficially or surrounded by consolidation.

**Q. Can long-standing fibrosis cause malignancy?**

Yes, it can cause scar carcinoma—adenocarcinoma. Carcinoma arising from scar anywhere is squamous cell carcinoma but in lung scar carcinoma is adenocarcinoma.

**Q. What is significance of right supraclavicular lymph node enlargement in lung carcinoma?**
- Right supraclavicular lymph node signifies pathology in right upper, middle, lower lobe and left lower lobe.
- Left supraclavicular lymph node enlargement signifies intra-abdominal, testis, lung or breast carcinoma. In lungs it signifies left upper lobe involvement.

**Q. What are the accessory muscles of respiration?**
- External intercostals (inspiration) and internal intercostals (expiration)
- Sternocleidomastoid muscle (inspiration)
- Anterior serrati (inspiration)
- Scaleni (inspiration)
- Rectus abdominis—abdominal thoracis with the external and internal obliques (expiration)

**Q. What is postural drop and what are the causes of postural hypotension?**

It is defined as a sustained drop in systolic (>20 mm Hg) or diastolic (>10 mm Hg) BP after 2–3 minutes of standing from supine position.

**Neurogenic causes:** Autonomic neuropathy, i.e., diabetes, demyelinating disorders, parkinsonism, etc.

**Non-neurogenic causes**
- **Cardiac pump failure:**
  - MI, myocarditis
  - Constrictive pericarditis
  - Aortic stenosis
  - Tachyarrhythmias and bradyarrhythmias
  - Salt losing nephropathy
  - Adrenal insufficiency
  - Diabetes insipidus
  - Venous obstruction
- **Reduced intravascular volume:** Straining, dehydration, hemorrhage, burns, diarrhea, emesis

**Metabolic causes**

Adrenal insufficiency, hypoaldosteronism, pheochromocytoma, severe potassium depletion.

**Venous pooling**

Alcohol, postprandial dilation of splanchnic vessels, vigorous exercise with skeletal vessel vasodilation, fever, hot environment, hot bath, prolonged supine or standing position, sepsis.

**Medications**
- Antihypertensives
- Diuretics
- Vasodilators (nitrates, hydralazine)
- Alpha and beta blockers
- CNS sedatives: Barbiturates, opiates
- Tricyclic antidepressants
- Phenothiazines

**Q. What are the abnormal pulses in relation to respiratory system?**

**Pulsus paradoxus:**

It is the exaggeration of normal inspiratory decline in systolic arterial pressure >10 mm Hg indicating a decline of 7% in LV stroke volume.

If the decline in systolic arterial pressure is >20 mm Hg then the inspiratory decline in the amplitude of pulse is evident by normal palpation of radial or brachial pulse without sphygmomanometer.

If the decline is <20 mm Hg then it can be detected by sphygmomanometry by inflating the cuff 20 mm Hg above the systolic pressure and slowly deflating the cuff at a rate of 2 mm Hg/beat. First the Korotkoff sounds are heard only in expiration. The point at which it is equally heard in both inspiration and expiration is noted and difference in 2 pressures is the magnitude of pulsus paradoxus and patient must be breathing normally during the procedure.

**Causes**

Cardiac tamponade, constrictive pericarditis, restrictive cardiomyopathy, massive pulmonary embolism, severe hypovolemic shock, COPD, acute severe asthma, upper airway obstruction.

Bounding pulses in carbon dioxide retention.

**Q. What is pulsus alternans?**

It is regular rhythm in which a strong beat alternated with a weak beat and it is a sign of severe LV dysfunction **(Fig. 1.16)**.

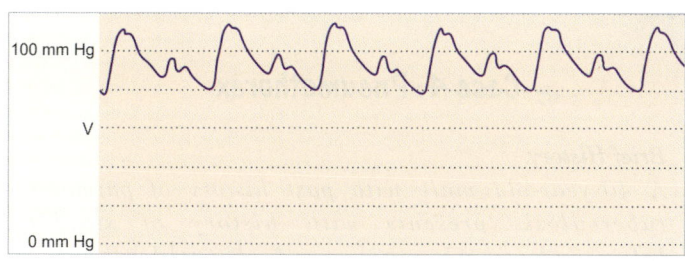

**Fig. 1.16:** Pulsus alternans.

Pulsus alternans is associated with myocardial damage. The damage is usually severe enough to cause gross heart failure. However, it may be present without heart failure when it is secondary to cardiac hypertrophy and increased afterload, as in hypertension or aortic stenosis, but with the addition of some minor myocardial damage, such as the scar of an old infarction.

**Q. What are the causes of decreased and increased vocal fremitus?**

- Fremitus is decreased or absent when the voice is soft or when the transmission of vibrations from the larynx to the surface of the chest is impeded. Causes include an obstructed bronchus; COPD; separation of the pleural surfaces by fluid (pleural effusion), fibrosis (pleural thickening), air (pneumothorax), or an infiltrating tumor; and also, a very thick chest wall.
- Vocal fremitus is increased in consolidation of lung.

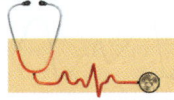

## Case 4: Pneumothorax

### Brief History
A 40-year-old male with past history of pulmonary tuberculosis presents with history of stabbing left-sided chest pain and breathlessness of 4 days duration.

### General Examination
- Middle aged male
- Conscious
- Cooperative
- Obeying commands
- Moderately built and nourished
- Height: 170 cm, weight: 57 kg
- BMI: 19.7 kg/m$^2$

### Vitals
- Pulse: 100/min
  - Regular rhythm, normal volume, character, all peripheral pulses well felt
- Blood pressure: 107/70 mm Hg
- Temp: 98.5°F
- Respiratory rate: 22/min
  - Regular, abdominothoracic
  - Usage of accessory muscles present
- Jugular venous pulse—not elevated
- SpO$_2$: 97% on room air

### Physical Examination
- Pallor: Absent
- Icterus: Absent
- Cyanosis: Absent
- Clubbing: Absent
- Lymphadenopathy: Absent
- Edema: Absent
- No external markers of tuberculosis/HIV/malignancy/CTD

### Systemic Examination
**Upper Respiratory Tract Examination**
- Flaring of ala n\asi
- Nasal septum central, normal
- No sinus tenderness
- Tonsils appear normal
- Postpharyngeal wall normal

**Lower Respiratory Tract Examination**

### Inspection
- Shape and symmetry: Left hemithorax appears bulged
- Spine: Central
- Trachea: Trail sign positive on the right side
- Apex beat not visualized
- Respiratory movements are reduced on the left side
- No visible pulsations/sinus/scars
- Gauze-pad dressing noted in the left infrascapular region

### Palpation
- Spine: Central
- Trachea: Deviated to the right side
- Apex beat could not be localized
- Respiratory movements: Reduced on the left side
- AP: 19 cm, transverse: 28 cm AP: transverse: 0.67
- Chest circumference 88 cm, chest expansion 3.5 cm
- Right hemithorax: 42.5 cm, left hemithorax: 45.5 cm hemithorax expansion: 3 cm right side, 0.5 cm left side
- Vocal fremitus reduced in the left supraclavicular, infraclavicular, mammary, axillary, infra-axillary, interscapular and infrascapular areas
- Tactile fremitus: absent

### Percussion
- Increased resonance in the left infraclavicular, mammary, axillary, interscapular areas. Stony dullness in the left infrascapular and infrascapular areas.
- Straight line dullness noted (7th, 8th and 9th intercostal spaces in the midclavicular, midaxillary and infrascapular regions respectively)
- Shifting dullness present
- Liver dullness: Left 5th intercoastal space midclavicular line
- Traube's space percussion: Dull

### Auscultation
- Breath sounds: Normal vesicular in all areas on the right, reduced intensity vesicular in the left supraclavicular and suprascapular regions, absent breath sounds in the infraclavicular, axillary, infra-axillary, interscapular, infrascapular regions.
- Vocal resonance: Reduced in the left supraclavicular, infraclavicular, mammary, axillary, infra-axillary, interscapular and infrascapular areas
- Succussions splash present Adventitious sounds: Absent

### Other Systems
- Cardiovascular system: Apex not localized, S1, S2 soft, no murmurs
- Gastrointestinal system: Soft, nontender, no hepatomegaly, no splenomegaly, no free fluid, normal bowel sounds
- Nervous system: Conscious, well oriented, no focal deficits, bilateral plantars flexors

### Diagnosis
Left sided pleural disease— hydropneumothorax, likely etiology traumatic—post-tubercular, no signs of respiratory failure.

## DISCUSSION

**Q. How do you classify pneumothorax? List the common etiologies of pneumothorax.**
Refer **Figure 1.17**.

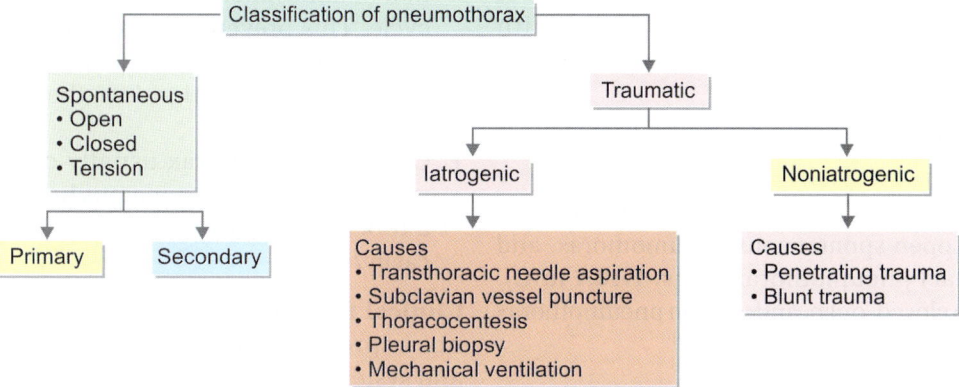

**Fig. 1.17:** Classification of pneumothorax.

## Etiology

### Spontaneous Pneumothorax

- **Primary (simple) spontaneous pneumothorax** occurs in the absence (no evidence) of overt lung disease.
  - It occurs in individual without any underlying lung disease or any trauma.
  - **Age:** Commonly occurs between the age group of 20–40 years.
  - **Risk factors:** Smoking, tall stature, and the presence of apical subpleural blebs, mostly familial.
  - About 50% of patients will have a recurrence. Both lungs are affected with equal frequency
- **Secondary spontaneous pneumothorax** occurs in the presence of an underlying lung disease.
  - **Causes:** Most common causes are **COPD** (chronic bronchitis and emphysema) and cavitary active pulmonary **TB**. It occurs due to rupture of emphysematous bullae and subpleural TB focus. Other causes include bronchial asthma, suppurative diseases of lung and pleura, cystic fibrosis, and *P. jirovecii* pneumonia (**Box 1.8**).

### Traumatic Pneumothorax

***Traumatic pneumothorax*** results from penetrating or nonpenetrating injuries to the chest.
- **Iatrogenic:** Following diagnostic or therapeutic interventions. These include transthoracic and transbronchial needle aspiration/biopsy (24%), subclavian vessel puncture (22%), thoracocentesis (22%), pleural biopsy (8%), and mechanical ventilation (7%).
- **Noniatrogenic:** Blunt and penetrating injuries to the chest wall, bronchi, lung or esophagus.

**Box 1.8:** Causes of secondary spontaneous pneumothorax.

**Airway disease**
- Chronic obstructive pulmonary disease
- Asthma
- Cystic fibrosis

**Infections**
- Necrotizing bacterial pneumonia, lung abscess
- *Pneumocystis jirovecii* pneumonia
- Tuberculosis

**Interstitial lung disease**
- Sarcoidosis
- Idiopathic pulmonary fibrosis
- Lymphangiomyomatosis
- Tuberous sclerosis
- Pneumoconioses

**Neoplasms**
- Primary lung cancers
- Pulmonary or pleural metastases

**Miscellaneous**
- Connective tissue diseases
- Pulmonary infarction
- Endometriosis, catamenial pneumothorax

**Q. What are the physical signs of pneumothorax?**

**General examination**

Patient will be cyanosed, tachypneic, peripheral pulses may be feeble, and hypotension may be present.

*Respiratory system*
- Inspection and palpation
  - **Accessory muscles of respiration in action**, **trachea and mediastinal** (apex beat) **shift to the opposite side.**
  - **On the affected side:** Fullness of the chest, diminished chest movements, increase in the size and diminished expansion of the hemithorax, increased spinoscapular distance, and markedly diminished vocal fremitus. Subcutaneous emphysema may be present.

- **Percussion:** Hyper-resonant note over the affected hemithorax.
- **Auscultation**
  - **On the affected side:** Markedly diminished/absent of breath sounds and vocal resonance, absence of adventitious sounds. Open pneumothorax with a bronchopleural fistula, there may be amphoric bronchial breathing.

### Q. List the differences between the types of spontaneous pneumothorax.

There are three types namely: (1) closed spontaneous pneumothorax, (2) open spontaneous pneumothorax, and (3) tension (valvular) pneumothorax **(Figs. 1.18A to C)**. Differences between closed, open, and tension pneumothorax are listed in **Table 1.14**.

#### Closed spontaneous pneumothorax

Pneumothorax where the communication between pleural space and the lung seals off and does not reopen. The mean pleural pressure remains negative and air can neither enter nor leave the pleural cavity/space. The trapped air is slowly and spontaneously reabsorbed and the lung re-expands completely in 2–4 weeks. Infection of the pleural cavity is uncommon.

**Clinical features:** Trivial breathlessness that gradually abates over a few days.

#### Open spontaneous pneumothorax

- Pneumothorax where the communication between bronchus and pleura does not seal off and remains patent and air continues to pass freely between the bronchial tree and pleural space. It results in a bronchopleural fistula.
- Free flow of air through the bronchopleural fistula results in intrapleural pressure (normally negative) same as that of atmospheric pressure throughout the respiratory cycle. This prevents the re-expansion of the collapsed lung. Development of bronchopleural fistula facilitates the spread of infection into the pleural space causing empyema.
- Open pneumothorax usually develops secondary to rupture of an emphysematous bulla, a small pleural bleb, a tuberculous cavity or a lung abscess into the pleural cavity/space.

**Clinical features:** Presents with breathlessness that does not improve. If there is infection of pleural space, fever and systemic features are observed. The physical signs are those of hydropneumothorax (air and fluid in the pleural space).

### Q. What is tension pneumothorax?

In tension pneumothorax, the pressure in the pleural space is positive throughout the respiratory cycle.

- Pneumothorax where communication between pleura and lung persists. This is due to formation of a valvular mechanism (one-way valve through) in which air is sucked into the pleural space during inspiration (coughing, sneezing and straining) but not expelled during expiration. Large quantity of air gets "trapped" in the pleural space/cavity and raises the intrapleural pressure much higher than the atmospheric pressure.

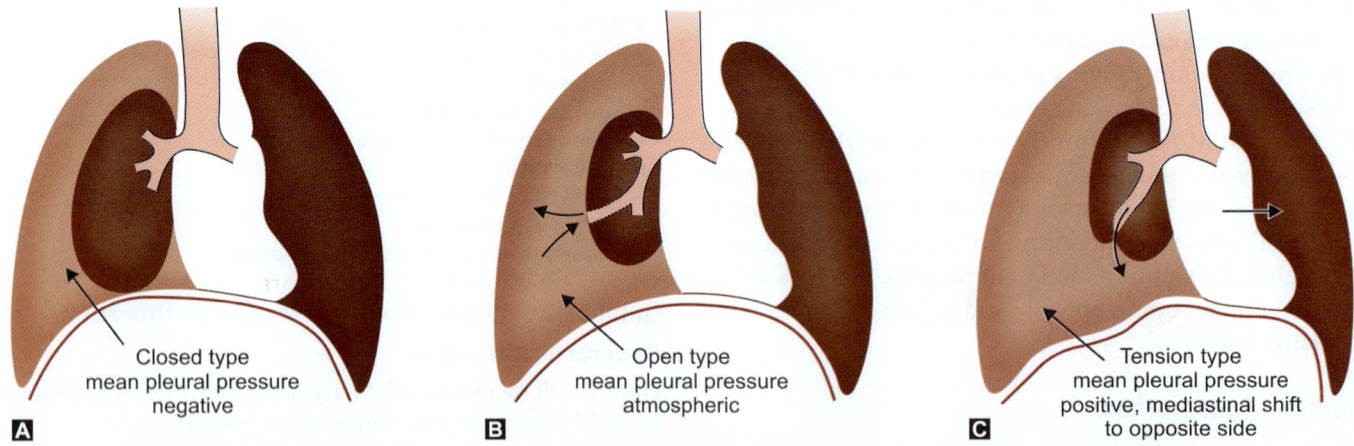

**Figs. 1.18A to C:** Types of spontaneous pneumothorax: (A) Closed type; (B) Open type; (C) Tension (valvular) type.

**Table 1.14:** Differences between closed, open, and tension pneumothorax.

| Closed pneumothorax | Open pneumothorax | Tension pneumothorax |
|---|---|---|
| The pleural tear is **sealed** | The pleural tear is **open** | The pleural tear acts as a **ball and valve** mechanism |
| The pleural cavity pressure is less than the atmospheric pressure | The pleural cavity pressure is equal to the atmospheric pressure | The pleural cavity pressure is more than the atmospheric pressure |

- The high intrapleural pressure causes compression of the underlying lung, shifts the mediastinum to the opposite side with consequent compression of the opposite lung also. It also decreases venous return to the heart by compressing the vena cava resulting in reduced cardiac output.

**Clinical features:** Rapidly progressive breathlessness, central cyanosis, rapid thread pulse, and signs of peripheral circulatory failure. Signs of pneumothorax are present **(Fig. 1.19)**.

> **Treatment**
> - Tension pneumothorax should be treated as an acute medical emergency.
> - Emergency treatment: Insertion of a large-bore needle into the pleural space through the second anterior intercostal space. The diagnosis is confirmed, if large amounts of air escape through the inserted needle. The needle should be left in place till a thoracostomy tube can be inserted. Cover the open end of the needle with a glove finger. Other methods:
>   - Insertion of wide-bore plastic cannula. The opposite end is attached to long rubber tubing, the end of which is placed underwater in a bottle.
>   - Introduction of an intercostals catheter connected to a water-seal drainage system.
>   - If above methods cannot be performed, simple stab on chest wall to release pressure.

**Q. What are the causes for recurrent pneumothorax?**
- After primary spontaneous pneumothorax, recurrence occurs within a year in about 25% of patients.
- Recurrent pneumothorax is common with emphysematous bullae. The recurrence usually occurs on the same side. It can also occur with lymphangioleiomyomatosis (LAM).

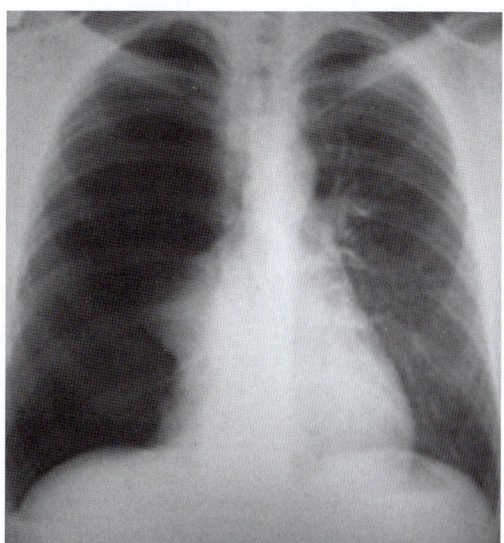

**Fig. 1.19:** Chest X-ray shows right-sided pneumothorax.

> **Treatment**
> - Obliteration of the pleural space by artificial pleurodesis. This can be accomplished by intrapleural instillation of an irritant like tetracycline hydrochloride of talc powder.
> - Pleurodesis is recommended for all patients following a second pneumothorax. Pleurodesis is achieved by pleural abrasion or parietal pleurectomy at thoracotomy or thoracoscopy.

**Q. What is catamenial pneumothorax?**
- Rare condition occurring in females above the age of 25–30 years.
- It presents with repeated attacks of spontaneous pneumothorax usually on the right side, in association with menstruation. Attacks usually occur within 2 days before or after the onset of menstruation. Hemoptysis may also develop. Most frequently associated with endometriosis of thorax.

> **Treatment**
> Ovulation-suppressing drugs, surgical exploration, and pleurodesis.

**Q. What is clicking pneumothorax?**

In clicking pneumothorax, a small left-sided pneumothorax gets localized in front of the pericardium. This produces alteration of the heart sounds so that the sound becomes loud and resonant ("clicking").

**Q. List the complications of pneumothorax.**
- **Pyopneumothorax:** It is caused by aspiration or intercostal chest tube insertion (iatrogenic). It may also result from necrotic pneumonia, lung abscess, or caseous pneumonia. Its causes are listed in **Box 1.9**.
- Hydropneumothorax
- **Hemopneumothorax:** Bleeding in pleural space and commonly caused due to rupture of vessels in adhesions. When lung re-expands, bleeding will stop. If bleeding persists, surgical ligation may be required.
- Mediastinal and subcutaneous emphysema.

**Q. What are the causes and clinical features of hydropneumothorax?**

Similar findings as pneumothorax except the following findings:
- **Percussion note** is **hyper-resonant over the upper air-containing part** and **stony dull over the lower fluid-containing part**.
- Treatment

**Box 1.9:** Causes of pyopneumothorax.

> - Complication of pneumothorax
> - Thoracocentesis
> - Trauma to thorax
> - Bronchopleural fistula
> - Esophagopleural fistula

- **Straight line dullness. Shifting dullness** can be elicited.
- **Amphoric bronchial breathing** in case of bronchopleural fistula.
- **Coin-test** is positive over the upper air-containing part.
- **Succussion splash** can be elicited on the affected side.

**Causes of hydropneumothorax**
- Trauma
- Thoracentesis
- Tuberculosis
- COPD
- Pneumonia
- Prior surgery
- Bronchopleural fistula
- Malignancy

**Figure 1.20** shows the X-ray of left hydropneumothorax.

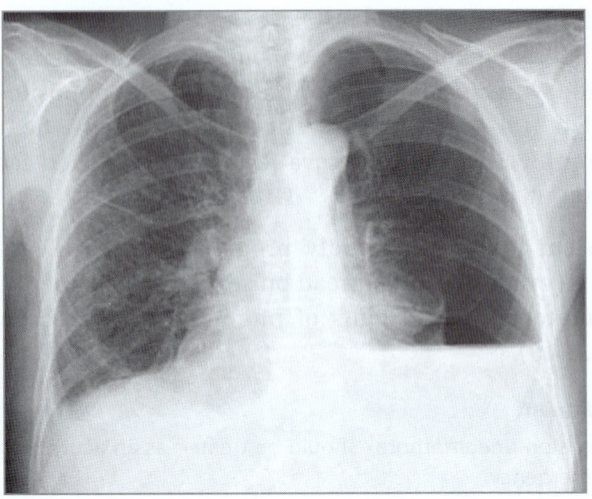

**Fig. 1.20:** X-ray of left hydropneumothorax.

## Case 5: Suppurative Lung Disease

### Brief History
A 24-year-old male with history of cough with copious amounts of purulent sputum for 1 month and episode of hemoptysis three days ago.

### General Examination
- Young male
- Conscious
- Cooperative
- Obeying commands
- Moderately built and poorly nourished
- Height: 150 cm, weight: 37 kg
- BMI: 16.44 kg/m$^2$

Vitals:
- Pulse: 110/min
  - Regular rhythm, normal volume, character, all peripheral pulses well felt
- Blood pressure: 106/74
- Temperature: 100.6°F
- Respiratory rate: 20/min
  - Regular, thoracoabdominal
  - No usage of accessory muscles
- Jugular venous pulse—not elevated

On Physical Examination:
- Pallor: Present
- Icterus: Absent
- Cyanosis: Absent
- Grade 2 pandigital clubbing
- Lymphadenopathy: Absent
- Edema: Absent
- No external markers of tuberculosis
- Ridging of nails
- Normal tongue, oral mucosa
- Skin, normal hair

Others
No features suggesting respiratory failure at the time of examination

### Systemic Examination
Upper Respiratory Tract Examination
- No flaring of ala nasi
- Nasal septum central, normal
- Nasal polyps present on the right side
- No sinus tenderness
- Tonsils appear normal
- Postpharyngeal wall is granular

Lower Respiratory Tract Examination Inspection:
- Shape and symmetry: Normal
- Spine: Central
- Trachea: Central
- Apex beat not visualized
- Bilateral respiratory movements are equal but reduced
- No visible pulsations/sinus/scars palpation:
- Spine: Central
- Trachea: Central
- Apex: Could not be localized
- Respiratory movements: Reduced in all areas
- AP: 16 cm, transverse: 24 cm AP: transverse: 0.66
- Chest circumference 74, chest expansion 2 cm
- Hemithorax: 37 cm, hemithorax expansion 1 cm both sides
- Vocal fremitus bilateral equal reduced in all areas
- Tactile fremitus: Present in bilateral infraclavicular areas

Percussion
- Resonant in all areas
- Liver dullness: Left 5th intercoastal space midclavicular line

Auscultation
- Breath sounds: Bilateral vesicular in all areas with prolonged expiration, normal intensity
- Vocal resonance: Bilateral equal, reduced in all areas

Adventitious Sounds
- Bilateral infraclavicular and mammary areas: Coarse crackles
- Bilateral diffuse rhonchi

Other Systems
- Cardiovascular system: Apex not localized, normal S1, loud P2, no S3/S4, no murmurs
- Gastrointestinal system: Soft, nontender, mild hepatomegaly, no splenomegaly, no free fluid, normal bowel sounds
- Nervous system: Conscious, well oriented, no focal deficits, bilateral planter's flexors, no flaps

### Diagnosis
Acute infective exacerbation of a diffuse lung disease with predominantly upper lobe bronchiectasis likely etiology being cystic fibrosis with pulmonary hypertension, no signs of corpulmonale, no signs of respiratory failure, with anemia.

## DISCUSSION

### Bronchiectasis

**Q. Define bronchiectasis.**

Bronchiectasis is defined as an **irreversible** (permanent), **abnormal dilation of the cartilage-containing airways bronchi or bronchioles.**

**Q. Classify bronchiectasis.**

- **According to the shape of the bronchial dilation**—based on the bronchographic appearance (Reid's classification) (Figs. 1.21A to C):
  - **Tubular (cylindrical):** Characterized by smooth dilation of the bronchi. It is the most common form.
  - **Varicose (bulbous):** In which the bronchi are dilated with multiple indentations.

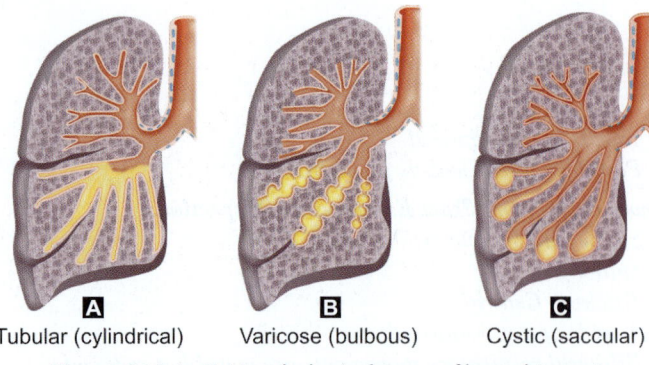

**Figs. 1.21A to C:** Morphological types of bronchiectasis: (A) Cylindrical type; (B) Varicose (bulbous) type; (C) Saccular.

- **Cystic (saccular/balloon appearance):** In which dilated bronchi terminate in blind ending sacs.
♦ **According to the extent of involvement**
  - **Diffuse (generalized) bronchiectasis:** Characterized by widespread bronchiectatic changes throughout the lung. It is **usually bilateral** and commonly affects the **lower lobes**. **Left lobe is more commonly involved than the right**. It is most severe in the distal bronchi and bronchioles.
  - **Focal (localized) bronchiectasis:** Bronchiectatic change is **restricted to a** localized area of the lung **(single segment of the lung)** and usually occurs in association with obstruction of the airway (parenchymal tumor or aspiration of foreign bodies).
♦ **According to the underlying disease/mechanism**
  - Congenital/acquired
  - Cystic fibrosis (CF) associated and noncystic fibrosis bronchiectasis
  - Associated with post fibrosis: Traction bronchiectasis
  - Without much expectorant: Dry bronchiectasis.

**Q. Which is the commonest site of involvement in bronchiectasis?**
♦ Lower lobes > middle and lingular lobe > upper lobes
♦ Left lower lobe is the most common site.

**Q. What are the causes of bronchiectasis?**
Refer **Box 1.10**.

**Q. What is proximal bronchiectasis?**
In which, dilatation involves larger airways:
♦ Allergic bronchopulmonary aspergillosis (ABPA)
♦ **Brock's syndrome/middle lobe syndrome:** Primary TB/foreign body/tumor compressing main bronchus.
♦ **Lady Windermere syndrome (LWS):** These women have the habit of voluntarily suppressing cough. It results in inability to clear the secretions from the right middle lobe and lingual leading to infection and later bronchiectasis.
♦ **Congenital syndromes: Kartagener's syndrome, yellow nails syndrome, Chandra–Khetarpal syndrome** (immunodeficiency associated with levocardia,

**Box 1.10:** Causes of bronchiectasis.

**Congenital**
✦ Cystic fibrosis (CF)
✦ Ciliary dysfunction syndromes
  - Primary ciliary dyskinesia (immotile cilia syndrome), Young's syndrome
  - Kartagener's syndrome (sinusitis and transposition of the viscera)
✦ Primary hypogammaglobulinemia, alpha-1 antitrypsin deficiency
✦ *Others:* Bronchial cysts, cul-de-sacs, bronchomalacia, atopic bronchial asthma, pulmonary sequestration, Mounier–Kuhn syndrome or tracheobronchomegaly, Williams–Campbell syndrome (bronchomalacia)

**Acquired: Children**
✦ Pneumonia (complicating whooping cough or measles)
✦ Primary tuberculosis
✦ Inhaled foreign body

**Acquired: Adults**
✦ Pulmonary tuberculosis, *Mycobacterium avium* complex (MAC)
✦ Suppurative pneumonia
✦ Allergic bronchopulmonary aspergillosis (ABPA) complicating asthma
✦ Postobstructive bronchiectasis: Partial or total obstruction of the bronchial lumen, e.g., endobronchial tumors or foreign bodies, enlarged hilar lymph nodes or tumor masses and bronchostenosis following endobronchial tuberculosis
✦ Autoimmune diseases, e.g., rheumatoid arthritis, Sjögren's syndrome, systemic lupus erythematosus, inflammatory bowel disease
✦ *Others:* Repeated aspiration of gastric juice, inhalation of toxic gas (ammonia), HIV infection, interstitial lung fibrosis (traction bronchiectasis), radiation fibrosis, sarcoidosis, chronic hypersensitivity pneumonitis, bronchiolitis obliterans after lung transplantation

bronchiectasis, and paranasal sinus anomalies), **Young's syndrome, cystic fibrosis, Chédiak–Higashi syndrome**.

**Q. What are the theories of bronchiectasis?**
♦ **Atelectasis theory:** Aspiration of viscid material into peripheral parts of the bronchial tree may result in atelectasis and dilatation of the bronchi in the collapsed area, which is compensatory, in turn reduces lung volume and increases intrapulmonary negative pressure, these in turn dilates any bronchi proximal to the block, as these remain in communication with the atmosphere.
♦ **Pressure of secretions theory:** Following mucous plug obstruction of a bronchi, secretions distal to the obstruction accumulate and mechanically distend the bronchi beyond the block.
♦ **Traction theory:** Bronchial dilatation occurs secondary to fibrosis of lung parenchyma, the resulting scar tissue requiring high inflation pressures on inspiration to overcome abnormally high retractive forces.

## Q. What are the symptoms of bronchiectasis?

- **Severe persistent (chronic) productive cough: It is the most common symptom.** Cough is chronic, daily, and persistent. **Paroxysm of cough develops when the patient rises in the morning** because the postural changes drain the collections of pus and secretions into the bronchi. Sputum production varies with posture.
- **Sputum:** It is **foul-smelling** (due to anaerobic infections), thick, copious, tenacious, and continuously purulent, sometimes bloody.
- **Hemoptysis:** Streaks of blood is common with exacerbations of infection and is commonly recurrent. Rarely massive hemoptysis occurs. Hemoptysis occurs due to rupture of the thin-walled blood vessels present on the walls of dilated bronchi.
- **Pleuritic (chest) pain:** It may be caused due to infection of pleura, or due to segmental collapse caused by retained secretions.
- **Infective exacerbation:** Increased sputum volume with fever, malaise, and anorexia are precipitated by upper respiratory tract infections.
- **General debility:** In severe/widespread bronchiectasis, the patient presents with difficulty maintaining weight, anorexia, exertional breathlessness/dyspnea, wheezing, and orthopnea.
- **Bronchiectasis sicca/dry bronchiectasis:** Occasionally, the patient is asymptomatic or has nonproductive cough. It is termed bronchiectasis sicca and commonly follows TB of upper lobe. Only manifestation will be hemoptysis.
- Situs inversus is found in 50% cases of ciliary dyskinesia.

## Q. Discuss radiological features of bronchiectasis.

Plain chest radiograph
- Sensitivity 87.8%, specificity 74.4%
- Ring shadows—produced by dilated bronchi seen end-on—honeycomb lung, cystic lung
- Parallel lines—produced by dilated bronchi viewed side-on—tram lines
- Solid tubular opacities—finger in glove appearance
- Features of PHTN—prominent proximal pulmonary artery trunks with cardiac enlargement—extensive disease
  - Dextrocardia, situs inversus **(Fig. 1.22)**.

## Computed Tomography

- HRCT is the investigation of choice
- Sensitivity: 82 to 97%
- False-positive and false-negative rates of 1 and 2%
- 1–2 mm cuts at 10 mm intervals, reducing to 5 mm intervals at areas of particular interest
- The two main features are bronchial dilatation and bronchial wall thickening
  1. A bronchus is said to be dilated if its internal diameter is greater than that of the accompanying pulmonary artery (broncho-arterial ratio >1)

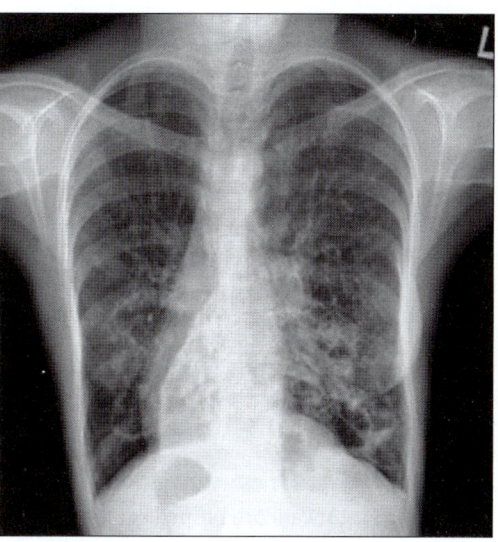

**Fig. 1.22:** Chest X-ray (CXR) showing bilateral bronchiectasis with dextrocardia with situs inversus.

  2. Bronchial wall thickening is said to be present if the thickness of the wall is at least equal to the diameter of the adjacent pulmonary artery branch.

**Table 1.15** shows the direct and indirect signs of bronchiectasis.

### Q. What are the specific examination findings you get in a case of bronchiectasis?

It may reveal anemia, **pandigital clubbing** (7% cases), fever, weight loss, night sweat, weakness, **halitosis** (may accompany purulent sputum) and sinusitis. Signs and symptoms of lung infection, such as fever may not be present.

## Respiratory System

- Nasal polyps and signs of chronic sinusitis may be present.
- Signs may be unilateral, but are usually bilateral and basal. In dry bronchiectasis, no abnormal physical signs may be found.
- **Auscultation:** Reveals **crackles** and wheezing. Presence of large amounts of secretion is responsible for the characteristic **"bilateral, coarse, leathery crepitations"** of bronchiectasis which may be palpable (tactile fremitus).

**Table 1.15:** Direct and indirect signs of bronchiectasis.

| Direct signs | Indirect signs |
|---|---|
| • Bronchial dilatation | • Bronchial wall thickening |
| • Signet ring sign | • Fluid or mucus filled bronchi |
| • Tram tracts sign | • Mosaic perfusion |
| • Varicose appearance **(Fig. 1.23)** | • Centrilobular nodules |
| • Air filled cysts **(Fig. 1.24)** | • Atelectasis/consolidation |
| • Lack of tapering >2 cm distal to bifurcation | • Air trapping on expiratory scan |
| • Visibility of the peripheral airways thickening | |

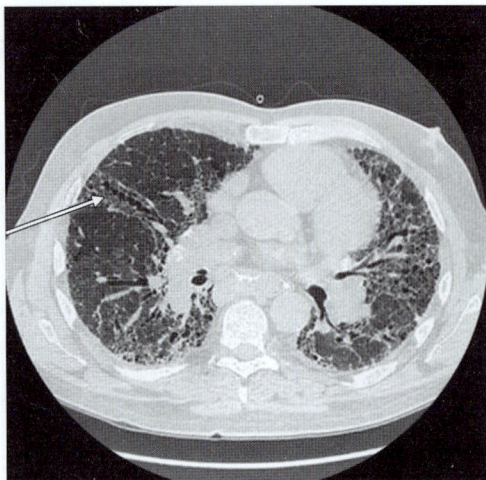

**Fig. 1.23:** Varicose bronchiectasis.

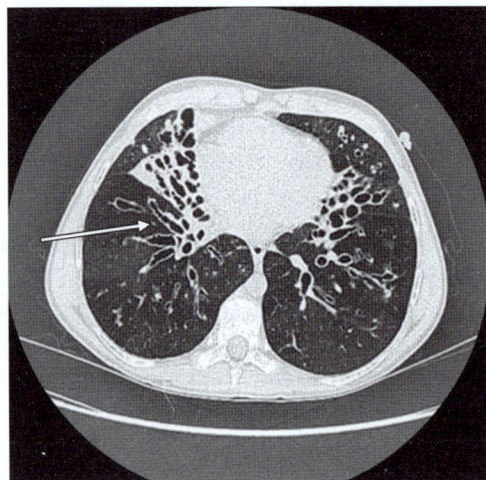

**Fig. 1.24:** HRCT showing cystic bronchiectasis.

**Q. What are the complications of bronchiectasis?**
Complications of bronchiectasis are shown in **Table 1.16**.

**Q. What is pseudobronchiectasis?**
Pseudobronchiectasis (functional bronchiectasis) is characterized by dilated bronchi and is reversible. It is common in patients with pneumonia of any cause. But re-expansion of the collapsed lung in atelectasis and regeneration of the mucosa in tracheobronchitis leads to reversal of the bronchographic findings. This reversible dilatation of bronchi is termed as pseudobronchiectasis.

**Q. What is postobstructive bronchiectasis?**
- It is bronchiectasis that develops distal to a bronchial obstruction.
- **Causes: Partial or total obstruction of the bronchial lumen due to endobronchial tumors, foreign body aspiration, mucus plugs, enlarged hilar lymph nodes or tumor masses, and bronchostenosis (due to endobronchial TB).**

**Q. What is bronchiectasis sicca?**
- Usually, bronchiectasis presents with copious sputum.
- **Bronchiectasis sicca** is a condition where bronchiectasis presents with repeated episodes of hemoptysis without sputum production.
- It usually occurs in bronchiectasis of upper lobe following TB.

**Q. Name the severity scoring of bronchiectasis.**
Severity scoring

**FACED score includes:**
- F: FEV1
- A: Age
- C: *Pseudomonas aeruginosa* colonization
- E: Extent of bronchiectasis
- D: Dyspnea
- Each variable is scored as 0, 1 or 2
- The 5 year mortality in mild (0–2), moderate (3–4) and severe (5–7) disease is 4%, 25% and 56%

**BSI score:**
- Includes age, BMI, FEV1, previous hospitalization, exacerbation frequency, colonization status, radiological appearances
- The score was designed to predict future exacerbations, hospitalizations, health status and death over 4 years

**Table 1.16:** Complications of bronchiectasis.

| | |
|---|---|
| • Hemoptysis | • Metastatic abscesses (e.g., brain abscess) |
| • Pneumonia | • Generalized edema (100 mL sputum/4–5 g protein)—protein loosing pneumopathy |
| • Lung abscess | |
| • Empyema | |
| • Cor-pulmonale | • Generalized amyloidosis |
| • Septicemia | • Aspergilloma |
| • Meningitis | • Respiratory failure |
| • Osteomyelitis | • Microbial resistance to antibiotics |

# LUNG ABSCESS

**Q. What is lung abscess?**
Lung (pulmonary) abscess is defined as a severe, **local suppurative process within the lung** associated with cavity formation. It is characterized by necrotic area of lung parenchyma containing **pus accompanied by the destruction of lung tissue. Necrotizing pneumonia:** Often used to describe similar pathologic process with multiple small (<2 cm) cavities in contiguous are as of the lung (**Fig. 1.25**).

**Q. What are causes of lung abscess?**
Refer **Box 1.11**.

**Q. Define post-tussive suction.**
Post-tussive suction is the sucking sound produced by the gushing of air into a thin-walled collapsible cavity communicating with a bronchus during inspiration after a bout of coughing.

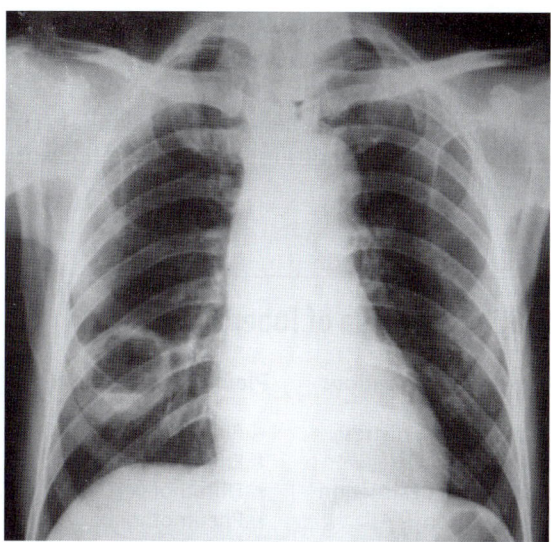

**Fig. 1.25:** Chest X-ray shows lung abscess in right lower zone.

**Q. What are the requisites of post-tussive suction.**
- Empty cavity with thin collapsible walls in communicating with a bronchus
- Absent in thick-walled cavities—abscess and cavitation tumors
- Present in thin-walled cavities—TB cavity.

**Q. What is the classical percussion note obtained over a cavity?**

Cracked pot resonance.

**Q. What are the clinical features of lung abscess?**

Lung abscess may present either as an acute (symptoms <1 month) or chronic (symptoms >1 month).
- **Acute:**
  - Majority present acutely with dry **cough**, high-grade **fever**, chills, rigors, and pleuritic chest pain.
  - After a few days, when the abscess ruptures into a patent bronchus, the patient suddenly starts expectorating **large amounts of foul-smelling purulent or sanguineous sputum.** The sputum may often be blood-tinged and expectoration **varies with posture.**
- **Chronic:** Lung abscess secondary to aspiration often presents as chronic, insidious in onset with low-grade fever, malaise, weight loss, anorexia, and a deep-seated chest **pain**/discomfort.

## Physical Findings

### General Examination

Anemia, fever, **clubbing of the fingers and toes** (may develop rapidly), **halitosis,** and oronasal sepsis.

### Respiratory System Examination

- **Early stages:** May be normal
- Later:
  - **Signs of consolidation:** Dullness of percussion, increased vocal fremitus and vocal resonance, bronchial breathing, crepitations, and pleural rub.
  - **Signs of cavitation:** Once the abscess opens into a bronchus, signs of cavitation like cavernous or amphoric bronchial breathing and coarse post-tussive crepitations are heard on auscultation.

**Q. What are the complications of lung abscess?**

Refer **Box 1.12**.

## CYSTIC FIBROSIS

**Q. What is cystic fibrosis?**

Cystic fibrosis is a fatal multisystem genetic disorder because of abnormal ion transport function causing inability to adequately hydrate mucus.

**Box 1.11:** Causes of lung abscess.

A. **Infectious causes**
   **Bacteria**
   - **Usual:** Mouth flora anaerobes, most frequently isolated anaerobes: *Peptostreptococcus, Fusobacterium nucleatum, Prevotella melaninogenica*
   - **Less common:** *Staphylococcus aureus, Streptococcus pyogenes, Pseudomonas aeruginosa, Klebsiella pneumoniae, Streptococcus pneumoniae,* gram-negative bacilli, such as *Escherichia coli, Haemophilus influenzae* type B, *Legionella, Nocardia asteroides*. Mixed infections occur when lung abscess develops due to inhalation of foreign material
   - **Mycobacteria:** *Mycobacterium tuberculosis, M. avium* complex, *M. kansasii*, other mycobacteria

   **Fungi:** *Aspergillus* spp., *Histoplasma capsulatum, Pneumocystis jirovecii, Coccidioides immitis, Blastocystis hominis, Cryptococcus*

   **Parasites:** *Entamoeba histolytica, Paragonimus westermani, Strongyloides stercoralis* (postobstructive)

B. **Noninfectious causes**
   - **Neoplasms:** Primary lung cancer, metastatic carcinoma, lymphoma
   - **Pulmonary infarction:** Due to bland embolus (may be secondarily infected in <5%)
   - **Septic embolism:** Tricuspid endocarditis due to S. aureus and others (typically with positive blood cultures), jugular venous septic phlebitis due to **Fusobacterium necrophorum (Lemierre's syndrome)**
   - **Vasculitis:** Wegener's granulomatosis, rheumatoid lung nodule
   - **Developmental:** Pulmonary sequestration
   - **Airway disease:** Bullae, blebs, or cystic bronchiectasis (usually thin-walled)
   - **Other:** Sarcoidosis, transdiaphragmatic bowel herniation giving appearance of cavity with air fluid level

**Box 1.12:** Complications of lung abscess.

- Extension of the infection into the pleural cavity: Leading to empyema/pneumothorax/pyopneumothorax/bronchopleural fistula/pleural effusion/pleurocutaneous fistula
- Hemorrhage into the abscess cavity
- Hemoptysis
- Septic emboli may cause metastatic brain abscesses or meningitis
- Secondary amyloidosis (type AA)
- Aspergilloma
- Residual fibrosis and bronchiectasis

**Q. What is the genetic defect in cystic fibrosis?**

It is transmitted as an autosomal recessive disorder and characterized by mutation in a gene on the long arm of chromosome 7. This gene codes for a chloride channel known as cystic fibrosis transmembrane conductance regulator (CFTR). This influences salt and water movement across epithelial cell membranes.

## CFTR Protein

- Normally present in epithelia and functions as cAMP-regulated chloride ion channel and as inhibitor of $Na^+$ channels.
- Mutation in CFTR gene causes intracellular degradation of CFTR. Thus, epithelial membranes are unable to secrete chloride ion in response to cAMP-mediated signals.

**Q. What are the organs involved in cystic fibrosis?**

- **Volume-absorbing epithelia:** Airways and distal intestinal epithelium.
  - In cystic fibrosis, **$Na^+$ absorption increased and chloride ion secretion is decreased.** This leads to reduced volume of periciliary fluid (with relative dehydration of the airway epithelium), thickening of mucus, adhesion and failure to clear mucus from the airway lumen. Mucus stasis and mucus hypoxia predispose to chronic bacterial infection (favors *Pseudomonas* growth) and ciliary dysfunction. It can lead to bronchiectasis.
- **Salt-absorbing epithelia:** In the sweat duct epithelium, cystic fibrosis is associated with increased sodium and chloride content in sweat. Aquagenic wrinkling of the palms (wrinkling and nodules) that develop after several minutes of immersion in water is quite characteristic.
- **Volume secretary epithelia:** Epithelium of proximal intestine and pancreas
  - **Pancreas:**
    - Failure of $Cl^-HCO_3$ and water exchanger to secrete $Na^+$, $HCO_3$ and water
    - Enzymes retained
    - Steatorrhea, azotorrhea, and pancreatic destruction.
  - **Intestine:**
    - Reduced bicarbonate secretion
    - Low pH in duodenum
    - Thick intestinal mucus
    - Predisposition to obstruction.
  - **Hepatobiliary system:**
    - Retention of biliary secretion, focal biliary cirrhosis, bile duct proliferation, chronic cholecystitis, and cholelithiasis.

# MISCELLANEOUS

## Complications/Sequela of Tuberculosis

| Parenchymal complications | Pleural complications |
|---|---|
| ♦ Acute respiratory distress syndrome<br>♦ Extensive lung destruction and cicatrization<br>♦ Cystic lesions<br>♦ Aspergilloma<br>♦ Tuberculoma<br>♦ Bronchogenic carcinoma | ♦ Pleurisy<br>♦ Empyema<br>♦ Fibrothorax<br>♦ Pneumothorax<br>♦ Bronchopleural fistula |
| **Airway complications** | **Chest wall complications** |
| ♦ Bronchiectasis<br>♦ Bronchiolitis obliterans<br>♦ Tracheobronchial stenosis<br>♦ Broncholithiasis | ♦ Osteomyelitis<br>♦ Spondylitis<br>♦ Empyema necessitatis |
| **Vascular complications** | **Other complications** |
| ♦ Arteritis and thrombosis<br>♦ Hypertrophied bronchial arteries<br>♦ Pulmonary artery pseudoaneurysm | ♦ Iatrogenic: Lung resection<br>♦ Cor pulmonale<br>♦ Secondary amyloidosis<br>♦ Type 2 respiratory failure |
| **Mediastinal complications** | |
| ♦ Esophagomediastinal and/or esophagobronchial fistula<br>♦ Lymph node calcification<br>♦ Fibrosing mediastinitis<br>♦ Constrictive pericarditis | |

**Q. What are the radiological features of active and healed (inactive) tuberculosis?**

Refer **Figure 1.26**.

# CONSOLIDATION

**Q. What are signs of consolidation?**

- No mediastinal/tracheal shift
- Woody dullness
- Tubular bronchial breathing bronchophony
- Whispering pectoriloquy

**Q. What are the stages of consolidation?**

- Stage of congestion
- Stage of red hepatization

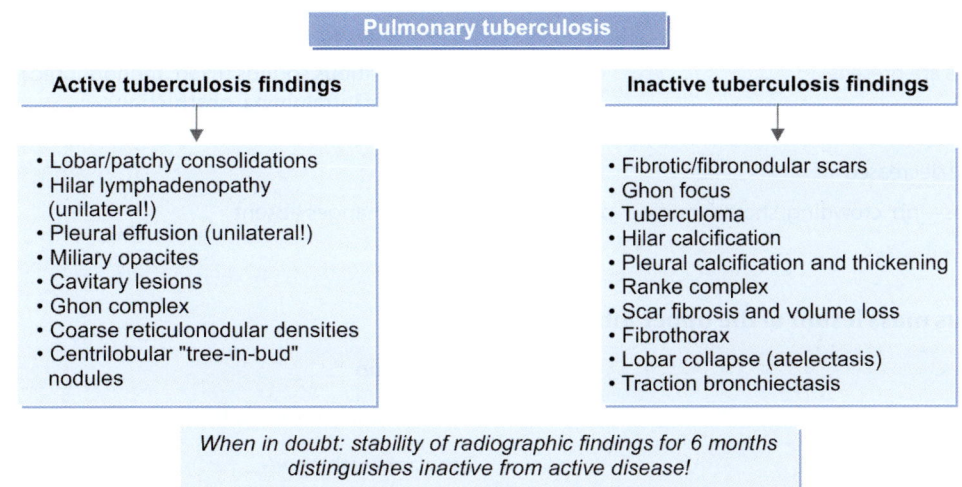

**Fig. 1.26:** Radiological features of active and healed (inactive) tuberculosis.

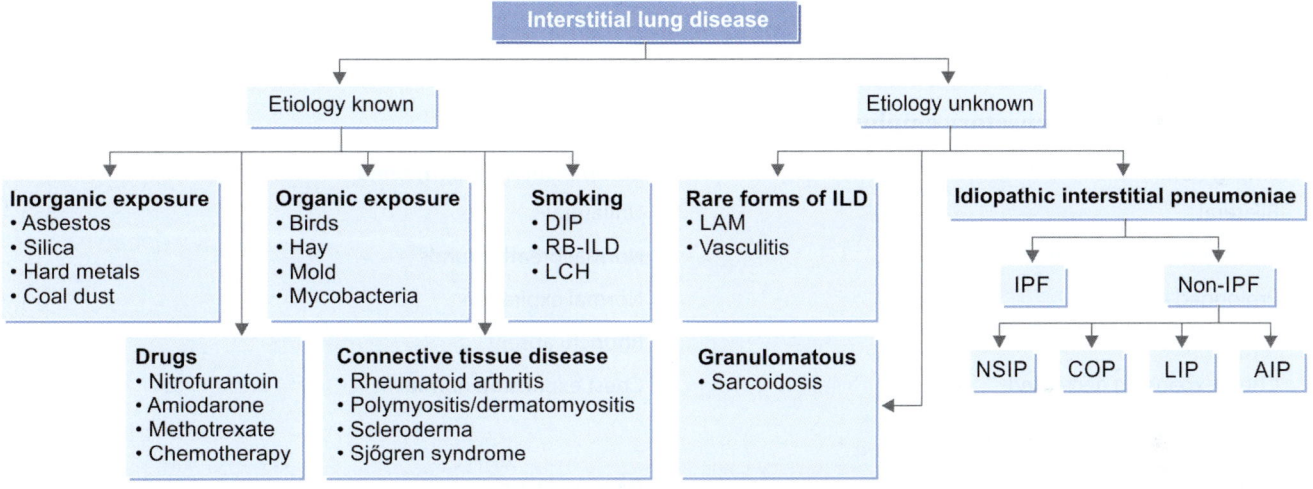

**Fig. 1.27:** Classification of interstitial lung disease.

- Stage of gray hepatization
- Stage of resolution.

### Q. Correlate the signs with the stages of consolidation.

- Fine late inspiratory crepitations (indux crepitations)— **stage of congestion**
- Tubular breathing with bronchophony and whispering pectoriloquy—**stages of red and gray hepatization**
- Coarse late inspiratory crepitations (redux crepitations) with bronchophony and no tubular breathing—**stage of resolution**

### Q. What are the classification of interstitial lung disease?

Refer **Figure 1.27**.

### Q. What are the differential diagnosis of respiratory diseases?

**Fibrosis versus collapse**

| Fibrosis | Active collapse |
| --- | --- |
| Past history of TB | Absent |
| Chronic >6 months | Acute |
| Breath sounds are decreased | Breath sounds absent |

| Fibrosis | Active collapse |
|---|---|
| Fine crepitations are present | No adventitious sounds (fixed monophonic rhonchus may be heard if intraluminal obstruction) |
| Vocal resonance decreased | Absent |
| Skeletal changes—rib crowding, shoulder droop present | Skeletal changes absent |

## Consolidation versus mass lesion of the upper lobe

| Consolidation | Mass lesion |
|---|---|
| Nontracheal shift | Tracheal shift present to the opposite side |
| Tubular breathing | Tubular breathing +/- |
| VR is increased | Variable |
| Crepitations present | Monophonic rhonchus +/- |
| Clubbing absent | Clubbing + |
| High-grade fever + | Cachexia, wasting, + |

## Emphysema versus compensatory emphysema

| Emphysema | Compensatory emphysema |
|---|---|
| Bilateral | Unilateral |
| Decreased breath sounds | Normal breath sounds |
| Prolonged expiration | Normal expiration |
| Rhonchi present | Rhonchi absent |
| Chest expansion decreased | Chest expansion normal |

## Emphysema versus pneumothorax

| Emphysema | Pneumothorax |
|---|---|
| No mediastinal/tracheal shift | Shift to opposite side |
| Breath sounds decreased bilateral | Decreased unilaterally |
| Rhonchi present | Absent |

## Mass lesion versus encysted pleural effusion

| Mass lesion | Loculated effusion |
|---|---|
| Dull percussion note | Stony dull percussion note |
| Mediastinal shift to opposite side | No mediastinal shift |

# Respiratory System: Summary of Findings in Common Respiratory Diseases

| | Findings | Fibrosis | Collapse | Pleural effusion | Pneumo-thorax | Hydropne-umothorax | Consoli-dation | Cavity | Emphysema | ILD |
|---|---|---|---|---|---|---|---|---|---|---|
| **Inspection** | Trachea/ mediastinum | Pulled to same side | Pulled to same side | Pushed to opposite side | Pushed to opposite side | Pushed to opposite side | Central | Central | Central | Central |
| | Retraction/ bulge | Retraction on the affected side | Retraction on the affected side | Bulging/ fullness on the affected side | Bulging/ fullness on the affected side | Bulging/ fullness on the affected side | — | — | Barrel-shaped chest | Bilaterally diminished movements |
| **Palpation** | Chest expansion | Reduced on the affected side | Reduced on the affected side | Reduced on the affected side | Reduced on the affected side | Reduced on the affected side | Reduced on the affected side | Reduced on the affected side | Reduced bilaterally | Reduced bilaterally |
| | Hemithorax dimension | Reduced on the affected side | Reduced on the affected side | Increased on the affected side | Increased on the affected side | Increased on the affected side | Normal dimensions | Normal dimensions | Bilaterally inflated lungs with AP:T diameter = 1:1 | Decreased or normal chest dimensions |
| | Vocal fremitus | Reduced | Reduced | Reduced | Reduced | Reduced | Increased | Increased in the presence of communication with bronchus | Bilaterally equal | Bilaterally equal |
| **Percussion** | Percussion note | Impaired note over fibrosed lung | Dull note over the collapsed lung | Stony dull note over the pleural effusion and skodaic resonance at the level of pleural effusion | Hyper-resonant note over the pneumothorax | Hyper-resonant note above the air fluid level and dull note below the air fluid level | Woody dull note over the consolidation | Large cavity gives resonant note | Hyper-resonant note over bilateral lung fields | Resonant note heard over bilateral lung fields |
| | Special findings | William's tracheal resonance | | Ellis curve pattern of upper level of effusion Grocco's triangle Obliteration of Traube's space Garland's triangle | Bell tympany can be appreciated (Coin test positive) | Shifting dullness, straight line dullness, succussion splash, Bell tympany can be appreciated (Coin test positive) | | Wintrich's sign (cavity communicating with bronchus) Friedreich's sign Gerhardt's sign | Liver dullness is pushed down Negative for tidal percussion | |
| **Auscultation** | Breath sounds | Diminished breath sounds | Absent breath sounds | Absent breath sounds | Absent breath sounds | Absent breath sounds | Tubular breath sounds | Cavernous breath sounds | Vesicular breath sounds with prolonged expiration | Vesicular breath sounds |
| | Adventitious sounds/ special findings | Fine crepitations | — | — | Bell tympany can be appreciated (Coin test positive) | Bell tympany can be appreciated (Coin test positive) | Crepitations heard | Post-tussive suction (in superficial cavity) | Rhonchi heard over the bilateral lung fields | Fine Velcro crepitations |
| | Vocal resonance | Reduced | Reduced | Reduced | Reduced | Reduced | Increased (bronchophony, egophony, whispering pectoriloquy) | Increased in the presence of communication with bronchus | Bilaterally equal | Bilaterally equal |

# SECTION 1: Respiratory System

## Schematic Approach to Clinical Diagnosis in Respiratory System

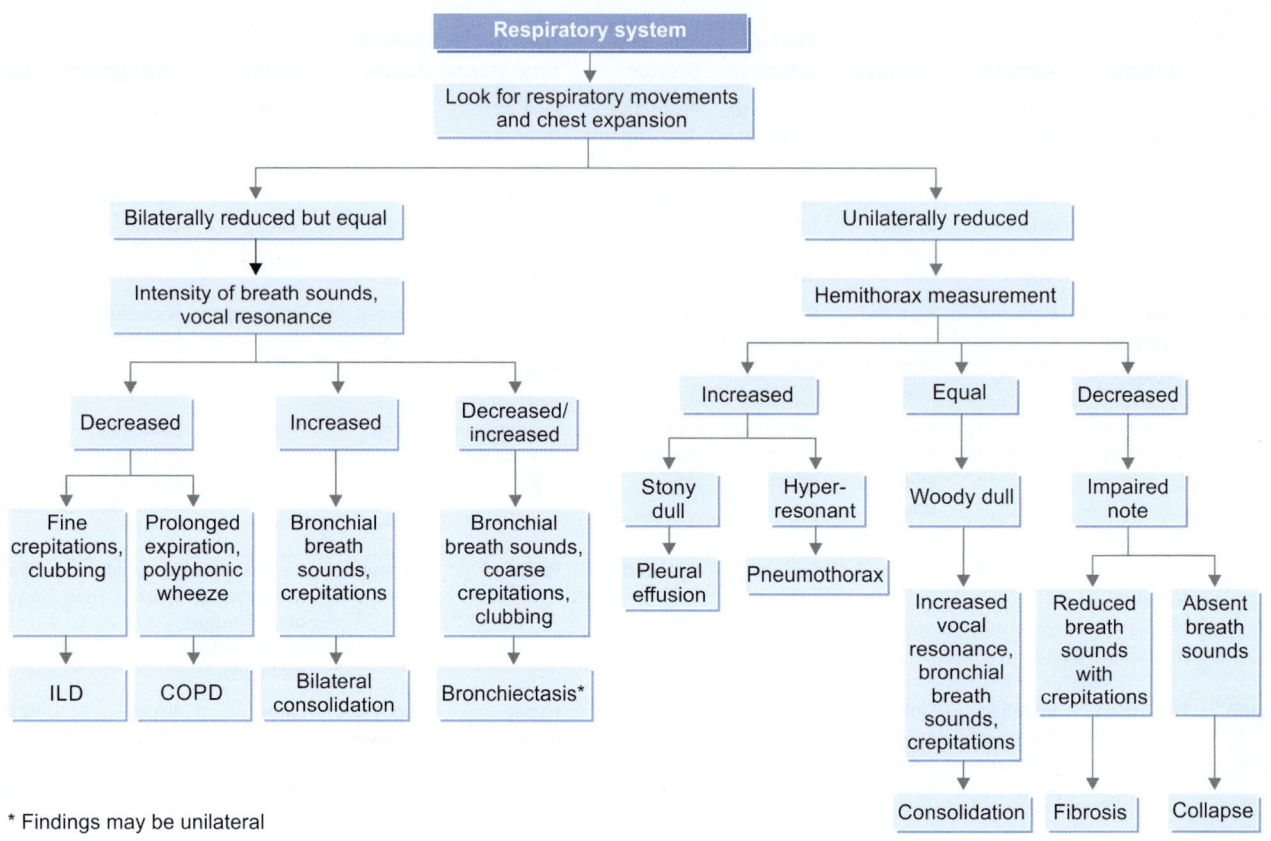

* Findings may be unilateral

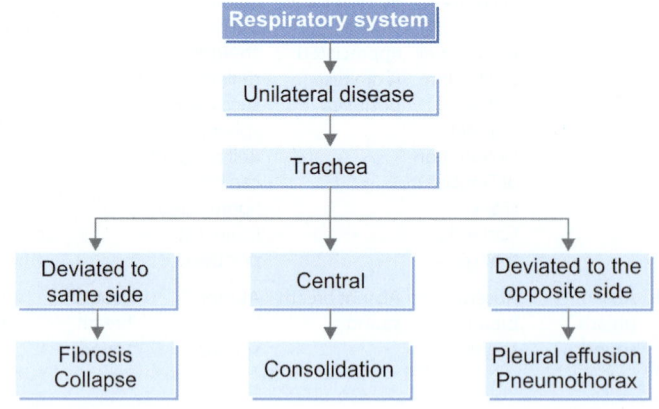

# Section 2: Cardiovascular System

## Section Outline

- **Case Sheet Format**
- **Diagnosis Format**
- **Sample Case Sheet and Discussion**
  - Valvular Heart Disease
    - Mitral Stenosis
    - Mitral Regurgitation
    - Aortic Stenosis
    - Aortic Regurgitation
  - Congenital Heart Disease
    - Atrial Septal Defect
    - Ventricular Septal Defect
    - Patent Ductus Arteriosus
    - Eisenmenger's/Cyanotic Heart Disease
- **Schematic Approach to Clinical Diagnosis in Cardiovascular System**

# Case Sheet Format

## HISTORY TAKING

Name:

Age:

Sex:

Residence:

Occupation:

**Chief complaints (describe in chronological order):**

1. _____ × days
2. _____ × days
3. _____ × days

**Dyspnea:**
- Duration
- Onset
- Grade
- Progression
- Aggravating factors
- Relieving factors
- Orthopnea
- Trepopnea
- Platypnea
- Bendopnea
- Paroxysmal nocturnal dyspnea
- Associated symptoms
  - Wheeze
  - Cough with expectoration

**Chest pain:**
- Duration
- Onset
- Site
- Type of pain
- Radiation
- Diurnal variation (nocturnal angina)
- Aggravating factors
- Relieving factors
- **Associated symptoms:** Nausea, vomiting, sweating
- Dyspepsia
- Local tenderness
- Angina equivalents.
  - Dyspnea
  - Diaphoresis
  - Discomfort in lower jaw
  - Dyspeptic symptoms
  - Fatigue

**Palpitations:**
- Duration
- Onset
- Fast or slow
- Regular or irregular
- Precipitating factors
- **Associated symptoms:** Stoke Adams
- Post-palpitation diuresis

**Syncope:**
- Duration
- Onset
- No of attacks
- Awareness
- Precipitating factors
- Associated symptoms

**Pedal edema:**
- Duration
- Onset
- Progression
- Aggravating factors
- Relieving factors
- Is it preceded by facial puffiness or followed by facial puffiness?
- Abdominal distension

**Other symptoms:**
- Hemoptysis
- Cyanosis
- Decreased urine output
- Gastrointestinal symptoms
- Right hypochondrial pain
- Fatigability
- Fever
- Rheumatic fever history
- Infective endocarditis
- Cyanotic spells
- Squatting after exertion

**Past history:**
- Asthma
- Chronic obstructive airway disease
- Tuberculosis
- History of contact with tuberculosis
- Diabetes mellitus
- Hypertension
- Ischemic heart disease (IHD)
- Seizure disorder
- History of sudden cardiac death.

**Family history:**

Three generation pedigree chart to be drawn

**Personal history:**
- Bowel habits
- Bladder habits
- Appetite
- Loss of weight
- Occupational exposure
- Sleep
- Dietary habits and taboo
- Food allergies
- Smoking index or pack years
- Alcohol history (if yes mention in grams of alcohol)

**Treatment history:**
- Drugs using
- Frequency of drug (e.g., drug taken 5 times a week most likely to be digoxin)
- Duration of usage
- Any blood test to be monitored (e.g., INR for warfarin)
- Any intramuscular injections (once in 3 weeks IM injection most likely to be benzathine penicillin for rheumatic heart disease prophylaxis)

**Menstrual and obstetric history:**
- Gravida, parity, live births, abortions (GPLA)
- Age of menarche
- Menopause at
- Duration
- Peripartum worsening of underlying heart diseases.

**Summarize:**

**Differential diagnosis:**

1.
2.
3.

# GENERAL EXAMINATION

**Patient**
- Conscious
- Coherent
- Cooperative
- Obeying commands

**Body Mass Index (BMI)**
- Weight (kg)/H² (meters)
- Arm span
- Upper segment/lower segment ratio

**Vitals Examination**
- **Pulse**
  - Rate
  - Rhythm
  - Volume
  - Character
  - Vessel wall thickening
  - Radioradial delay and radiofemoral delay
  - Peripheral pulses
- **Blood pressure**
  - Right arm
  - Left arm
  - Leg—right and left
  - Postural drop in BP
- **Respiratory rate**
  - Regular/irregular
  - Abdominothoracic (male) or thoracoabdominal (female)
  - Usage of accessory muscles
- **Jugular venous pressure:** Centimeter (cm) of water (blood) above sternal angle (+ 5 cm from the right atria)
- **Jugular venous pulse:** Waveform
- Pulse oximetry

**Physical Examination**
- Pallor:
- Icterus:
- Cyanosis:
- Clubbing:
- Lymphadenopathy:
- Edema:

**Others**
- Signs of infective endocarditis
- Signs of rheumatic fever
- Any dysmorphies/stigmata of congenital heart disease

# SYSTEMIC EXAMINATION

**Inspection**
- Chest shape and symmetry
- Breast abnormalities
- Spine deformity
- Scars
- Precordial prominence
- Cardiovascular pulsations
  - Apical pulse
  - Pulsation in aortic and pulmonary area
  - Sternoclavicular pulsations
  - Left parasternal pulsations
  - Epigastric pulsations
  - Ectopic pulsations
- Distended veins

**Palpation**
- Confirmation of shape and symmetry
- Palpation of precordium
- Palpation of cardiovascular pulsation for sounds, thrills and rubs
- Tracheal tug
- Parasternal heave

**Percussion**
- Right heart border

- Left heart border
- 2nd IC space
- Sternal percussion

**Auscultation**
- **Apex (mitral area)**
  - S1
  - S2
  - S3, S4
  - OS/clicks
  - Murmur
    1. Timing
    2. Grade
    3. Quality
    4. Pitch
    5. Configuration
    6. Radiation
    7. Best heard with diaphragm or bell
    8. Patient position
    9. With breath held in inspiration or expiration
    10. Dynamic auscultation
- **Tricuspid area**
  - S1
  - S2
  - S3, S4
  - OS/clicks
  - Murmur
    1. Timing
    2. Grade
    3. Quality
    4. Pitch
    5. Configuration
    6. Radiation
    7. Best heard with diaphragm or bell
    8. Patient position
    9. With breath held in inspiration or expiration
    10. Dynamic auscultation
- **Erb's neoaortic area**
  - S1
  - S2
  - S3, S4
  - OS/clicks
  - Murmur
    1. Timing
    2. Grade
    3. Quality
    4. Pitch
    5. Configuration
    6. Radiation
    7. Best heard with diaphragm or bell
    8. Patient position
    9. With breath held in inspiration or expiration
    10. Dynamic auscultation.
- **(R) 2nd intercostal space (aortic area)**
  - S1
  - S2
  - S3, S4
  - OS/clicks
  - Murmur
    1. Timing
    2. Grade
    3. Quality
    4. Pitch
    5. Configuration
    6. Radiation
    7. Best heard with diaphragm or bell
    8. Patient position
    9. With breath held in inspiration or expiration
    10. Dynamic auscultation.
- **(L) 2nd intercostal space (pulmonary area)**
  - S1
  - S2
  - S3, S4
  - OS/clicks
  - Murmur
    1. Timing
    2. Grade
    3. Quality
    4. Pitch
    5. Configuration
    6. Radiation
    7. Best heard with diaphragm or bell
    8. Patient position
    9. With breath held in inspiration or expiration
    10. Dynamic auscultation.
- **Other areas**
  - Axilla
  - Epigastrium
  - Clavicle
  - Carotid
  - Back (interscapular area)

## OTHER SYSTEM EXAMINATION

**Respiratory:**
- Inspection:
- Palpation:
- Percussion:
- Auscultation:

**Gastrointestinal system:**
- Inspection:
- Palpation:
- Percussion:
- Auscultation:

**Nervous system:**
- Higher mental functions:
- Cranial nerves:
- Sensory system:
- Motor system:
- Reflexes:
- Cerebellar system:
- Meningeal signs:

# Diagnosis Format

## ACQUIRED/CONGENITAL HEART DISEASE

### For Acquired Heart Disease

- Acquired heart disease possible etiology (rheumatic/ischemic/cardiomyopathy/degenerative)
- Valvular involvement (MS/MR/AS/AR/others) with severity grading
- With/without evidence of pulmonary artery hypertension (grading)
- Patient in or not in atrial fibrillation (if AF present look for signs of thromboembolism)
- With or without evidence of heart failure (right/left/congestive)
- With or without signs of infective endocarditis
- With or without signs of active rheumatic carditis
- Patient is in NYHA (New York Heart Association) class (I/II/III/IV)

**Example:** Acquired valvular heart disease, possibly rheumatic etiology, with severe mitral stenosis and moderate mitral regurgitation, with severe pulmonary artery hypertension, patient in atrial fibrillation and congestive cardiac failure, with no signs of infective endocarditis, thromboembolism or active rheumatic carditis. Patient is in NYHA class III.

### For Congenital Heart Disease

- Congenital cyanotic/acyanotic heart disease
- Type of defect (shunt/obstructive)
- With/without evidence of pulmonary artery hypertension (grading)
- Patient in or not in atrial fibrillation (if AF present look for signs of thromboembolism)
- With or without evidence of heart failure (right/left/congestive)
- With or without signs of infective endocarditis
- Patient is in NYHA class (I/II/III/IV).

**Note:** Mention if any features of dysmorphic facies or syndromes.

**Example:** Congenital acyanotic heart disease, atrial septal defect with pulmonary artery hypertension, with left to right shunt, patient not in atrial fibrillation, no evidence of heart failure or infective endocarditis. Patient in NYHA class II. Patient has features of Holt–Oram syndrome.

# Sample Case Sheet and Discussion

## Valvular Heart Disease

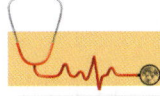

### Case 1: Mitral Stenosis

**Brief History:**
Middle-aged male with history of progressive exertional dyspnea and palpitations of 7 years duration, now presents with worsening dyspnea and leg swelling for 3 weeks.

**General Examination**
- Height: 150 cm
- Weight: 42 kg
- BMI: 18.6
- Moderately built and moderately nourished
- No pallor, icterus, cyanosis clubbing, lymphadenopathy. Bilateral pitting pedal edema present.
- BP: 104/70 mm Hg (in right arm supine position average of 3 reading)
- Pulse: Irregularly, irregular. 74/minutes
- No special character, apex pulse deficit of 12
- No radioradial and radiofemoral delay, all peripheral pulses well felt.
- RR: 24/min
- Temp: 98.4°F
- JVP: 6 cm from sternal angle, a wave absent.

**Systemic Examination**

**Cardiovascular Examination**

*Inspection:*
- No precordial bulge
- No suprasternal and epigastric pulsation
- Left parasternal pulsations visible
- No scars, no sinuses
- Apex beat 5th ICS ½ inch medial to left midclavicular line.

*Palpation:*
- Apex: 5th ICS ½ inch medial to midclavicular line tapping in nature
- Left parasternal heave grade 3
- Palpable P2

*Percussion:*
- Right heart border corresponds to right sternal edge.
- Left heart border corresponds to apex.
- Left second ICS dull to percuss.

*Auscultation:*
- Mitral area:
  - Loud S1 with varying intensity
  - Opening snap present
  - S2 heard, no S3/S4
  - Soft mid-diastolic murmur of grade 2/4, no presystolic accentuation best heard with bell of stethoscope in left lateral position with breath held at expiration.
- Tricuspid area—S1 variable, S2 heard, no S3/S4.
- Pulmonary area—S1 variable Loud P2.
- Aortic area—S1 variable S2 heard.

**Diagnosis:**
Acquired valvular heart disease, rheumatic mitral stenosis, moderate in severity, patient in atrial fibrillation with pulmonary arterial hypertension and right heart failure, no signs of infective endocarditis or active rheumatic carditis (NYHA Class 3).

## DISCUSSION

**Q. What are the characteristics of normal apical impulse?**

- Apical impulse is the lower most and outer most point of definite cardiac impulse with a maximum perpendicular thrust to the palpating finger.
- Normal apical impulse is produced by left ventricle and the left ventricular portion of the interventricular septum.
- Normal site of the apical impulse is about 1 inch medial to midclavicular line or 10 cm lateral to midsternal line at the left 5th intercostal space in adults.
- Normal displacement is 1 cm laterally in left lateral decubitus position.
- Normal apical impulse is confined to one intercostals space and has an area of 2.5 cm².
- Normal duration of thrust of apical impulse is less than 1/3 of systole.
- Mildly tapping in character

**Q. What are the differentiating features between A2-OS and A2-S3?**

Refer **Table 2.1**.

| Table 2.1: Features of A2-OS and A2-S3. | | |
|---|---|---|
| **Features** | **A2-OS** | **A2-S3** |
| Interval | 30–150 m sec | >150 m sec |
| Site | Mid or entire precordial | Apical |
| Pitch | High | Low |
| Character | Snapping | Thudding |

| Features | A2-OS | A2-S3 |
|---|---|---|
| Associations | Loud S1<br>Mid-diastolic murmur<br>MS or TS | Normal or soft S1<br>Pansystolic murmur<br>MR or TR |
| Variation on standing | A2-OS interval increases | No change |

### Q. What are the causes of mitral stenosis with shifted apex?
- MS with MR
- MS with AS/AR
- MS with HTN
- MS with IHD/cardiomyopathy
- MS with acute rheumatic myocarditis

### Q. What is pulse deficit (apex-pulse deficit)?
It is the difference between the heart rate and the pulse rate, when counted simultaneously for one full minute.

### Q. What are the causes for irregularly irregular pulse and how do you differentiate it from each other?

**Causes**
- Sinus arrhythmia
- Ectopics
- Atrial fibrillation
- Multifocal atrial tachycardia
- Atrial flutter with variable block.

**Differentiating features between VPC and AF (Table 2.2)**

**Table 2.2:** Features of VPC and AF.

| Features | Ventricular premature beats (VPCs) | Atrial fibrillation (AF) |
|---|---|---|
| Pulse deficit | Less than 10 per min/ | More than 10 per min |
| 'a' wave in JVP | Present | Absent |
| On exertion | Decreases or disappears | Persists or increases |
| Rhythm | Short pause (between normal beat and VPC) Followed by a long pause (following VPC) | Pauses are variable and chaotic |

### Q. Describe the mechanism of PND.
Paroxysmal nocturnal dyspnea is the occurrence of dyspnea during sleep, commonly 2–3 hours after going to bed. It is often associated with sweating, wheezing, and coughing and is usually relieved by assuming upright position for 5–15 minutes.

PND strongly suggest PVH. It is due to interstitial edema and sometimes due to intra-alveolar edema usually secondary to LVF. MS is the commonest cause for PND.

Other valvular heart diseases, DCM and CAD may also give rise to PND but are often late in occurrence. Patients with PND are functionally classified into NYHA class III. Once right ventricular failure develops (CHF), PND disappears.

**Pathogenesis**
Absorption of edema fluid from the interstitial compartments of lower limbs during supine position increases the venous return to the right heart and subsequently increases RV output which cause overfilling of the lungs leading to pulmonary interstitial edema.

**Other mechanisms**
- Decreased sympathetic drive during sleep which may decrease left ventricular contractility.
- Nocturnal arrhythmias, sleep apnea and dreams may also precipitate PND.

**Conditions simulating PND**
Nocturnal episodes of bronchial asthma (typically occurs in early mornings, 4–6 AM). Other COPDs may also wake up the patient in the night. However, cough and expectoration precede dyspnea and SOB is often relieved only once he takes the inhalers.
- Nocturnal episodes of recurrent pulmonary emboli.
- Postnasal discharge with associated severe cough.
- GERD
- OSA
- Anxiety with hyperventilation.
- Nocturnal hypoglycemia
- REM sleep phenomenon
- Nightmares

### Q. What are the causes of orthopnea?
It is dyspnea that occurs in supine position and is promptly relieved by assuming upright position. Orthopneic patients are functionally graded into NYHA class IV. Similarly, it is related to an increased venous return to the right heart in supine position and subsequently to increase RV output which further increases the pulmonary venous congestion.

**Etiology**
- Orthopnea is characteristic of LVF but can also occur in
- Chronic obstructive pulmonary disease (COPD)
- Bilateral weakness or paralysis of diaphragm.
- Large ascites often due to constrictive pericarditis, chronic renal failure and sometimes associated with congestive heart failure.

Difference between PND and orthopnea is given in **Table 2.3**.

### Q. Define palpitations. What are the causes?
It is an unpleasant awareness of the forceful or rapid beating of the heart. It is the increased motion of the heart within the chest that is perceived as palpitation rather than the increase in cardiac contractility which explains the absence of palpitation in conditions characterized by an increased force of cardiac contraction, such as, PS and severe systemic or pulmonary hypertension.

| Table 2.3: PND versus orthopnea. | | |
|---|---|---|
| | **Paroxysmal nocturnal dyspnea** | **Orthopnea** |
| **Definition and timing** | Episodes of sudden onset dyspnea<br>Occurs few hours after sleep<br>Patient wakes up from REM sleep<br>Sometimes may be unrecognized by patient | Dyspnea in recumbent posture<br>Occurs soon after lying posture |
| **How is it relieved?** | Air hunger, self-ventilates to comfort | Gets up, sleeps in erect posture, use more pillows |
| **Patient profile** | Often healthy, otherwise class I and are in early stages of cardiac compromise with underlying SHT, valvular (mitral, aortic) or myocardial disease | Common in established CHF<br>Often class 3–4, edema legs, renal dysfunction |
| **Differential diagnosis** | Panic attacks/nightmares<br>Obstructive sleep apnea | COPD/acute asthma/gross obesity |
| **Mechanism** | Depressed respiratory center, sudden awakening from REM sleep, catecholamine surge (?nightmare). Heart rate suddenly increases. Lung congestion—interstitial (non-alveolar) respiratory center lags behind and acute dyspnea is perceived. Fluid shift less contributory<br>*(PND is akin to doing a sudden exercise during sleep)* | Mechanical: Compression of diaphragm V/Q mismatch Hemodynamic: Shifting of venous blood into pulmonary circulation<br>(>400 mL on lying posture) |
| **Associated symptoms** | Angina (rarely),* sweating, palpitation | Baseline symptoms of CHF |
| **$O_2$ saturation cyanosis** | Transient hypoxia rare | Normal<br>Nil, may be peripheral |
| **Effect on PCWP** | Transient sudden raise | Slow sustained raise |
| **Risk to life** | Rarely kills, but SCD possible<br>Hypoxia and catecholamine surge can be trigger for ventricular arrhythmias | Less risk for SCD<br>Usually poor long-term outcome |
| **Echocardiographic correlates** | Early diastolic dysfunction, hypertensive heart disease | Often advanced systolic dysfunction as well as restrictive filling pattern |
| **Diagnostic evaluation** | Needs more extensive/occult CAD has to be ruled out | Rarely a difficult issue as diagnosis is already established |
| **Newer concepts** | PND may be anginal equivalent especially in diabetic with silent critical CAD | Postural diastolic dysfunction |

*Can be an anginal equivalent.

**Note:** Sometimes PND and orthopnea occur in a same patient, but usually they are temporally separated by at least few months.

## Cardiac causes

- **Valvular heart disease:** Due to increased stroke volume AR, MR, TR.
- Acyanotic congenital heart disease
  - With shunts; PDA, VSD, ASD.
  - Arrhythmogenic right ventricular dysplasia.
- Cyanotic congenital heart disease
  - With increased pulmonary blood flow: TAPVC, PAPVC, TGA with VSD without PS.
  - Arrhythmogenic: Ebstein's anomaly, after mustard operation.
- Arrhythmias
  - Tachyarrhythmias; VT, SVT, atrial fibrillation, atrial flutter, PAT, PAC, PVC.
  - Bradyarrhythmias: CHB, sick sinus syndrome.
  - Pacemaker malfunctioning.

MVP, HCM, CAD, Prolong QT syndrome, prosthetic heart valves.

## Non-cardiac causes

- Hyperkinetic circulatory states
  - Anemia
  - AV fistula
  - Fever
  - Thyrotoxicosis
  - Pheochromocytoma.
- Arrhythmogenic
  - Thyrotoxicosis
  - Hypoglycemia
  - Orthostatic hypotension
- Drugs
  - Caffeine, alcohol (holiday heart syndrome) nicotine, cocaine, amphetamines

- Sympathomimetic drugs
- Digitalis
- Vasodilators (calcium channel blockers)
- Tricyclic antidepressants.
♦ **Psychiatric:** Anxiety, depression, panic disorders, bereavement, and somatization.

### Q. What is the approach to palpitation?

History remains the most important and valuable mode of examination to distinguish cardiac from non-cardiac causes of palpitation.
♦ *Duration and frequency.*
♦ *Mode of onset.*
♦ *Nature or character.*
♦ *Relieving factors.*
♦ *Associated symptoms.*

### Duration and frequency
♦ Acute or chronic
♦ Persistent or non-persistent.
♦ If it is non-persistent, then how frequently it occurs.

### Persistent palpitations
Suggest volume overload conditions such as:
♦ **Valvular heart disease:** AR, MR, TR.
♦ **Acyanotic CHD:** PDA, VSD, ASD.
♦ **Cyanotic CHD:** TAPVC, PAPVC, TGA, with VSD without PS.
♦ Persistent arrhythmia like atrial fibrillation.
♦ Anemia, AV fistula, thyrotoxicosis, psychiatric illness.

In these conditions exertion results in exaggeration, and some patients may not experience palpitations at rest but may manifest it on exertion. Patients with chronic AF may not experience palpitations at all.

Non-persistent or paroxysmal palpitations are usually arrhythmogenic origin due to:
♦ Arrhythmias.
♦ **Noncardiac causes:** Thyrotoxicosis, hypoglycemia, addictions, and drugs. Psychiatric illness may also cause paroxysmal palpitations.

Similarly, recurrent palpitations with perspiration in a HTN patient suggest pheochromocytoma.

### Mode of onset
♦ Whether palpitation occurred spontaneously or was precipitated or exaggerated by exertion?
♦ If it begins suddenly and ends abruptly: Often due to paroxysmal atrial or junctional tachycardia, atrial flutter, or fibrillation.
♦ Gradual onset and cessation of the palpitation suggests; sinus tachycardia or anxiety.

### Nature/character of palpitation
The patient may describe symptoms of palpitation as pounding, stopping, jumping, racing, floating or flopping sensation in the chest.

♦ When palpitation lasts for an instant, it is often described as skipped beats or flopping in the chest which is commonly due to premature beats. The premature beats may be perceived as floating sensation in the chest.
♦ A pounding sensation in the chest occurs due to paroxysmal tachycardia.
♦ The sensation that the heart has stopped beating correlates with the compensatory pause following a premature beat.
♦ Regular rapid palpitation may be due to sinus tachycardia, SVT, or paroxysmal atrial tachycardia.
♦ Irregular rapid palpitation may be due to atrial fibrillation, atrial flutter, or atrial tachycardia with a varying block.
♦ Slow palpitations with slow heart rate may suggest AV block or sinus node disease.

### Relieving factors/how it stops
It stops spontaneously in most of the paroxysmal arrhythmias. However, if it relieved by vagal maneuvers such as stooping, breath holding or inducing gagging or vomiting it suggests a diagnosis of paroxysmal SVT.

### Associated symptoms
♦ **Syncope:** Stoke–Adams attack, severe bradycardia, pheochromocytoma, hypoglycemia.
♦ **Chest pain:** MI
♦ **Dyspnea:** HF, acute pulmonary embolism, bronchial asthma.
♦ **Polyuria:** Paroxysmal atrial tachycardia, paroxysmal atrial fibrillation.
♦ **Sweating:** MI, most arrhythmias, pheochromocytoma, hypoglycemia.
♦ **Deafness:** Prolong QT syndrome.
♦ **Diarrhea:** Thyrotoxicosis, hypokalemia-induced arrhythmias, irritable bowel syndrome.

### Q. Why the internal jugular vein is preferred to external jugular vein in measuring JVP?
♦ Anatomically the IJVs are closer to the right atrium as they take a direct course (straight line) through innominate veins to the superior vena cava and right atrium, while the external jugular veins follow a more circuitous route, and hence IJVs more accurately reflect the dynamics of the right heart.
♦ Transmission of RA pulsations prevented by prominent valves at the proximal IJV.
♦ Other structures of neck and upper thorax causes extrinsic compression of EJV.
♦ Increased sympathetic activity causes vasoconstriction of EJV and pulsations become barely visible.

### Q. Why the right IJV is preferred to left IJV?
♦ Right IJV and innominate vein extend in an almost straight line from the SVC and RA, while the left innominate into which left IJV drains, does not extend in a straight line from the SVC and RA.

- The left innominate vein may be kinked or compressed by a variety of normal structures by a dilated aorta or by an aneurysm.

  However, if there is any difficulty in visualization of JVP on the right side, both sides of the neck should be carefully examined.

### Q. What is the etiology of AF?
- 10% of elderly >75 years.
- Lone AF <65 years (normotensive with normal heart).
- Valvular heart disease.
- Hypertensive heart disease.
- Coronary heart disease.
- Myocarditis and cardiomyopathy.
- Cardiac surgery.
- Hypothyroidism.
- Hyperthyroidism.
- Pheochromocytoma.
- Pericarditis.
- Alcohol intake (holiday heart syndrome)
- Post-CABG
- Drugs, such as digoxin and sympathomimetics.

### Q. What are the signs of activity in acute rheumatic fever?
- Fever
- Tachycardia
- Leukocytosis with high ESR.

### Q. What is the clinical evidence of rheumatic carditis?
- **Pericarditis:** Pericardial rub, pericardial effusion.
- Myocarditis
  - Relative tachycardia (pulse rate raises by >10/min per degree rise of temperature
  - Tic-tac quality of heart sound
  - S1 muffled or soft (reflected as prolonged PR interval)
  - S3 gallop rhythm due to heart failure.
  - Congestive heart failure
  - Heart size—enlarged (apex goes down and outwards due to cardiac dilatation). It is very imp bedside clinical test.
  - Conduction defects—dropped beat in pulse due to heart block.
  - Arrhythmias—may occur.
- Endocarditis
  - Soft systolic murmur due to mitral incompetence.
  - Soft early diastolic murmur in the aortic area due to acute involvement of the aortic valve.
  - Carey-Coombs murmur—due to mitral valvulitis (temporarily producing MS as a result of edema of the mitral valve cusps).
  - Change in the character of existing organic murmurs.

### Q. What are the characteristics of rheumatic arthritis?
- Most common in children (5–15 years); commonest major manifestation (75%).
- Big joints are involved (knee (MC), ankle, hip, elbow); but no joint is immune to inflammatory process. Small joints of hand and feet may be affected as seen in rheumatoid arthritis. Joint involvement is usually asymmetrical. Involved joints are red, hot, swollen, painful and tender.
- Typically, it is fleeting or migratory in nature (as the inflammation of one joint is subsided, others tend to become affected. The affection of joints in rheumatoid arthritis is additive in nature).
- Spine, sternoclavicular and temporomandibular joints are rarely affected
- Recovery is complete.
- Usually there is no residual deformity
- Rarely recurrent attacks of arthritis may lead to minor deformities of joints at MCP joints—Jaccoud's arthritis.
- No radiological abnormalities.

### Q. Discuss management of acute rheumatic fever.
- Bed rest—specially for fever, arthritis, arthralgia, carditis and heart failure.
- High calorie salt restricted diet.
- Chorea—reassurance, sedatives, such as clonazepam or chlorpromazine, and in severe cases haloperidol, sodium valproate or carbamazepine is used.
- Symptomatic treatment:
  - Arthritis, arthralgia, fever—aspirin in a dose of 80–100 mg/kg/day in children and 4–8 g/day in adults in 4–5 divided doses is started and continued for 2 weeks. If symptoms subside, a lower dose of 60–70 mg/kg/ day (in children) is continued for a further 2–4 weeks. Naproxen at a dose of 10–20 mg/kg/day gives good symptomatic response.
  - Patient without carditis—aspirin is preferred.
  - Patient with carditis but without heart failure.
    - Aspirin +/– glucocorticoid (role of corticosteroids are doubtful in carditis but majority of cardiologists believe that they help in rapid resolution of heart failure). Prednisolone 1–2 mg/kg/day (maximum of 80 mg) is given orally for a period of 2 weeks and tapered over next 2 weeks.
  - Patient with carditis and heart failure:
    - Majority say that corticosteroid is mandatory over and above aspirin.
    - Antibiotics: Single injection of 1.2 million units of benzathine penicillin, IM (after proper skin test) is given to eradicate group A streptococcal infection, if present. Oral penicillin (penicillin V) 500 mg BD orally for 10 days, or erythromycin 40 mg/kg/day orally may be used for 10 days in patients allergic to penicillin.
    - Secondary prevention of acute rheumatic fever:
      - The mainstay of controlling rheumatic heart disease is secondary prevention. The dose of injection

benzathine penicillin is 1.2 million units, IM given at 4 weekly intervals (in endemic areas and high-risk cases, the interval is 2–3 weekly). Dose of penicillin in children (<27 kg) is 0.6 million units. Instead, oral penicillin V may be used 250 mg BD or oral erythromycin 250 mg bd.

- Rheumatic fever without proven carditis—5 years after the last attack or until the age of 21 years whichever is longer.
- Rheumatic fever with carditis but having no residual valve damage—10 years after the last attack or 21 years of age, whichever is longer.
- Rheumatic fever with carditis along with residual heart disease—10 years after last episode or until the age of 40, whichever is longer. Few clinicians prefer to give penicillin lifelong in this situation.
- If valvular surgery is done—penicillin prophylaxis is continued lifelong.

**Q. What are the heart failure symptoms and signs present in this case?**
- Progressive exertional dyspnea
- Bilateral pedal edema
- Raised JVP

**Q. Prophylaxis for rheumatic heart disease.**
Refer **Table 2.4**.

**Table 2.4:** Prophylaxis for rheumatic heart disease.

| Antibiotics | Continuous regimen | |
|---|---|---|
| Injection benzathine penicillin (IM) Penicillin V oral | Adults >27 kg 1.2 million units every 21–28 days 250 mg twice daily | Children <27 kg 6,00,000 units every 21–28 days 250 mg twice daily |
| Erythromycin (if allergic to penicillin) | 250 mg orally once daily | 5 mg/kg orally once daily |

**Q. In which condition do we give injection benzathine penicillin at a dose of 2.4 million units?**

**Primary, secondary, early latent syphilis—injection benzathine penicillin G** 2.4 MU I/M **once.**

**Late latent and tertiary syphilis—injection benzathine penicillin G** 2.4 I/M **once weekly for 3 weeks.**

Neurosyphilis:

Injection aqueous penicillin G 3–4 million units every 4 hours × 14 days

(OR)

Injection procaine penicillin G **2.4 MU** once daily + oral probenecid 500 mg QID × 14 days

**Q. Discuss the pathogenesis of mitral stenosis.**
- Mitral stenosis clinically manifests after a latent period about 20 years from the first episode of acute rheumatic fever **(Fig. 2.1)**. Its symptoms usually start when the mitral valve surface area reduces to 2.5 cm$^2$.

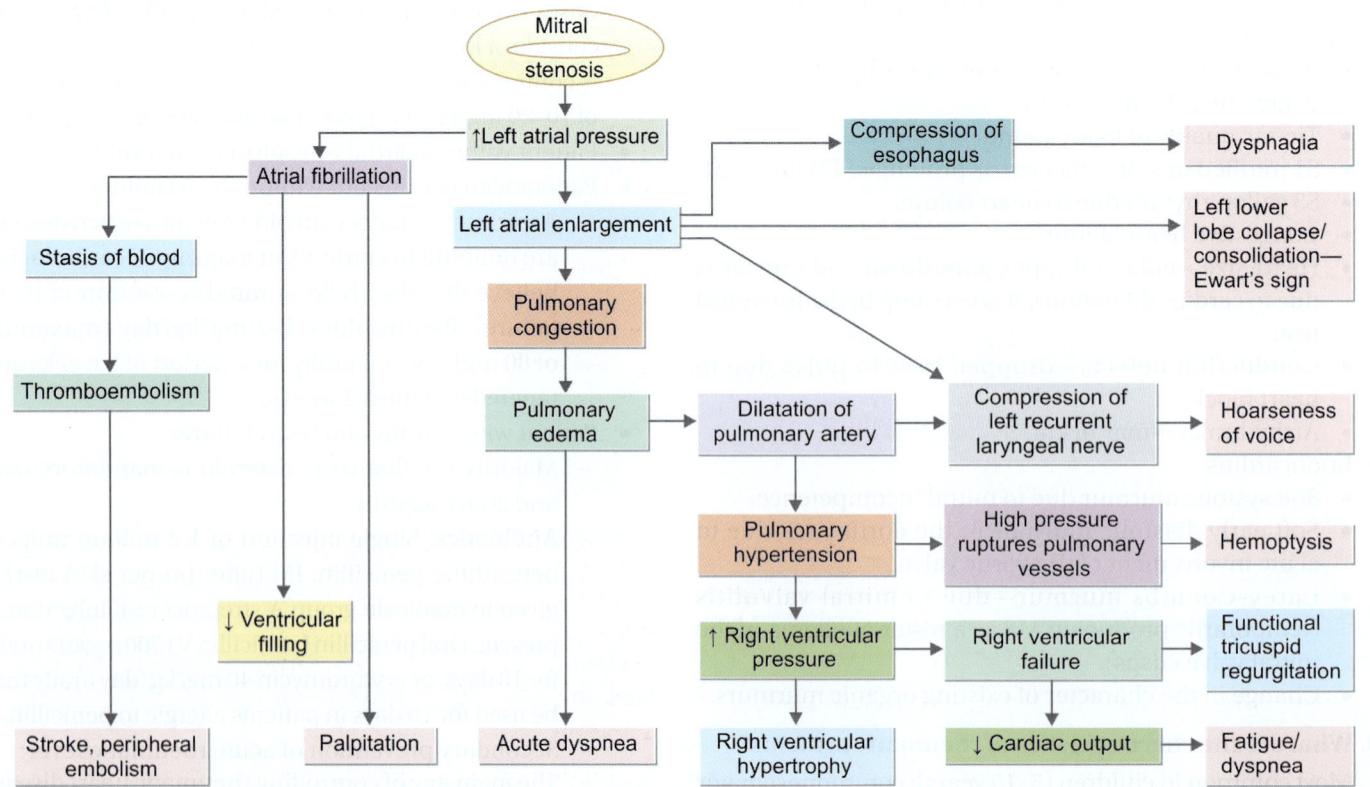

**Fig. 2.1:** Pathogenesis of mitral stenosis.

- Normally, the mitral valve opens during (left ventricular) diastole and allows the flow of blood from left atrium to the left ventricle. During ventricular diastole, the pressures in the left atrium and the left ventricle are equal.
- Mitral stenosis obstructs the blood flow from left atrium to left ventricle and raises the pressure in the left atrium (up to 25 mm Hg in severe stenosis). Initially, this rise in left atrial pressure may occur only during exercise, but later it is raised even during rest.
- Raised left atrial pressure is reflected back in the pulmonary veins that produce pulmonary venous hypertension and subsequently pulmonary arteries which produce pulmonary arterial hypertension.
- The symptoms consist of episodes of paroxysmal nocturnal dyspnea (PND) evident as pulmonary edema and hemoptysis, i.e., Winter bronchitis.
- Repeated episodes of PND produce arteriolarization of pulmonary capillaries and veins → pulmonary arterial hypertension.
- During this period, there may be resolution of symptoms and signs of pulmonary venous hypertension. Patient develops progressive exertional dyspnea. Patient feels better in terms of symptoms, although the disease has progressed.
- Pulmonary arterial hypertension (pulmonary hypertension) progressively increases in severity over the next 10–15 years till finally the right ventricle fails (early fourth decade).

**Q. What are types of pulmonary hypertension in mitral stenosis (MS)?**
- **Passive pulmonary hypertension:** Due to passive backward transmission of elevated left atrial pressure by venous and capillary.
- **Reactive pulmonary hypertension:** Due to reflex spasm of pulmonary arterioles in response to elevate pulmonary venous and left atrial pressure.
- **Obliterative pulmonary hypertension:** Due to chronic hypertension producing fibrosis of pulmonary bed.

**Q. What is the classical triad of pulmonary hypertension?**
Exertional dyspnea + Exertional fatigue + Exertional angina

**Q. What are the consequences of chronic pulmonary hypertension?**
- Hypertrophy of right ventricle: Which may later undergo dilatation → right ventricular failure
- Functional tricuspid regurgitation due to dilatation of tricuspid valve ring secondary to dilatation of right ventricle
- Pulmonary valve incompetence (regurgitation) may develop due to dilatation of pulmonary valve rim.

**Q. What are the causes of angina in mitral stenosis?**
- Decrease in cardiac output
- Pulmonary hypertension
- Embolism to coronary arteries

**Q. What are the consequences of raised left atrial pressure?**
Causes left atrial dilatation and this enlarged left atrium is prone to:
- Atrial fibrillation
- Stasis of blood with thrombus formation
- Detachment of the thrombus resulting in systemic embolism

Reduced ejection fraction of left ventricle is found in one-third of patients due to:
- Decreased preload due to impaired filing.
- Increased afterload secondary to reflex vasoconstriction (secondary to decreased cardiac output)

**Q. What is the cause of variable S1 in this patient?**
Atrial fibrillation

**Q. How to say whether heart sounds are loud?**
In general, S1 is always loud in mitral area, similarly A2 is always loud in pulmonary area.
- If S1 is louder than A2 in Aortic area: Definitely S1 is loud
- If A2 is louder than S1 in mitral area: Definitely loud A2
- If P2 is louder than A2 in pulmonary area: Definitely loud P2

**Q. How do you assess severity of mitral stenosis?**

**According to valve area and symptoms (Table 2.5):**

**Table 2.5:** Severity of mitral stenosis according to valve area and symptoms.

| Valve area | Symptoms | Severity |
| --- | --- | --- |
| >2.5 cm² | None | |
| 1.5–2.5 cm² | Dyspnea on severe exertion | Mild MS |
| 1–1.5 cm² | PND +/- pulmonary edema | Moderate MS |
| <1 cm² | Orthopnea | Severe MS |

**According to A2-OS gap (Table 2.6)**

**Table 2.6:** Severity of mitral stenosis according to A2-OS gap.

| Severity | A2-OS Gap |
| --- | --- |
| Mild MS | >120 ms |
| Moderate MS | 60–80 ms |
| Severe MS | 40–60 ms |

**According to stenotic gradient across mitral valve (Table 2.7)**

**Table 2.7:** Severity of mitral stenosis according to stenotic gradient across mitral valve.

| Severity | Gradient |
| --- | --- |
| Normal | 0 mm Hg |
| Mild MS | <5 mm Hg |
| Moderate MS | 5–15 mm Hg |
| Severe MS | >15 mm Hg |

Duration of the diastolic murmur is directly proportional to the severity.

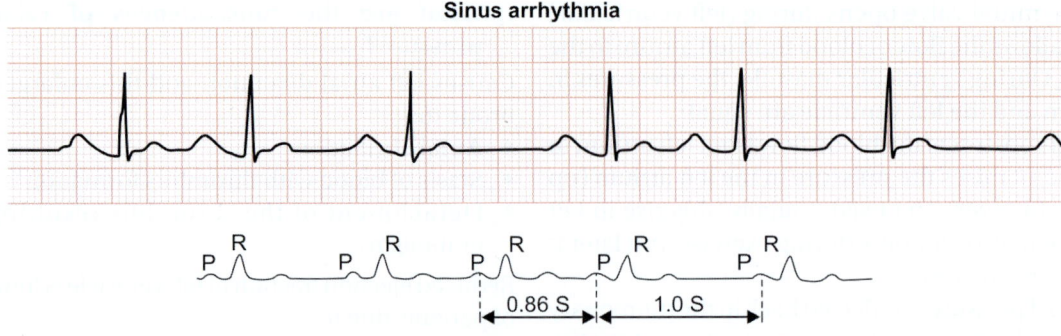

**Fig. 2.2:** ECG showing sinus arrhythmia.

**Q. What is the importance of sinus arrhythmia?**
- There is a slight beat-to-beat variation which is normally present in healthy individuals.
- When this variability is more accentuated, the term *sinus arrhythmia* is used **(Fig. 2.2)**.
- The heart rate normally increases slightly with inspiration and decreases slightly with expiration because of changes in vagal tone that occur during the different phases of respiration.
- During inspiration, parasympathetic tone falls and heart rate increases, while in expiration heart rate decreases.
- Absence of sinus arrhythmia will be seen in:
  - Autonomic neuropathy
  - Cardiac failure

**Q. Within how much time will the patient lose consciousness in ventricular fibrillation?**
6–8 seconds.

**Q. Name the conditions where opening snap is present.**
- MS, pure MR (10–20%)
- TS, TR
- Large VSD, large ASD
- HCM
- PDA
- Ebstein anomaly

**Q. What are causes of MS?**
- Rheumatic heart disease—most common
- Mitral annular calcification
- Congenital—four categories which included typical MS with short chordae tendineae, obliteration of interchordal spaces and reduction of interpapillary distance; hypoplastic congenital MS almost always associated with a hypoplastic left heart syndrome; supramitral ring; and parachute mitral valve.
- Mucopolysaccharidoses type 1 and 4.
- Radiation, infective endocarditis, endomyocardial fibroelastosis, malignant carcinoid syndrome, systemic lupus erythematosus, Whipple disease, Fabry disease, and rheumatoid arthritis.
- Methysergide treatment

**Q. What are the features of mitral stenosis?**
Salient features of mitral stenosis (MS) is shown in Box 2.1.

**Box 2.1:** Salient features of mitral stenosis (MS).

- First chamber to fail in MS: Left atrium
- Ventricle to fail in MS: Right ventricle
- Atria that fibrillates in MS: Affects both right and left atria
- Left ventricle in MS: Left ventricular end-diastolic volume (LVEDV) is reduced in 15%, while it is normal in the rest
- The most common complication of MS: Atrial fibrillation (AF)

**Q. What are the normal mitral valve areas and classify mitral stenosis?**
Refer Table 2.8.

**Table 2.8:** Classification of mitral stenosis.

| Stage | Definition | Valve anatomy | Valve hemodynamic | Hemodynamic consequence | Symptoms |
|---|---|---|---|---|---|
| A | At risk of MS | Mild valve doming during diastole | Normal transmitral flow velocity | None | None |
| B | Progressive MS | Rheumatic valve changes with commissural fusion and diastolic doming of the mitral valve leaflets Planimetered mitral valve area >1.5 cm² | Increased transmitral flow velocities Mitral valve area >1.5 cm² Diastolic pressure half-time <150 ms | Mild to moderate LA enlargement Normal pulmonary pressure at rest | None |

| Stage | Definition | Valve anatomy | Valve hemodynamic | Hemodynamic consequence | Symptoms |
|---|---|---|---|---|---|
| C | Asymptomatic severe MS | Rheumatic valve changes with commissural fusion and diastolic doming of the mitral valve leaflets Planimetered mitral valve area ≤1.5 cm² | Mitral valve area ≤1.5 cm² Diastolic pressure half-time ≥150 ms | Severe LA enlargement Elevated PASP >50 mm Hg | None |
| D | Symptomatic severe MS | Rheumatic valve changes with commissural fusion and diastolic doming of the mitral valve leaflets Planimetered mitral valve area ≤1.5 cm² | Mitral valve area ≤1.5 cm² Diastolic pressure half-time ≥150 ms | Severe LA enlargement Elevated PASP >50 mm Hg | Decreased exercise tolerance |

- Normal valve area: 4–6 cm²
- Mild MS: 1.5–2.5 cm²
- Moderate MS: 1.0–1.5 cm²
- Severe MS: <1.0 cm²
- Tight (critical) MS: <1.0 cm²
- Symptomatic MS: <2.5 cm²
- Hemodynamically significant MS: <1.5 cm²

### Q. What are symptoms of MS?
- Dyspnea, orthopnea, PND and acute pulmonary edema
- Edema and abdominal distension
- Chest pain, palpitation, hemoptysis and hoarseness
- Recurrent chest infections—pneumonia, bronchitis

### Q. How do you correlate LA pressures with severity of MS?
- Normal—12 mm Hg
- Symptomatic MS—18 mm Hg
- Critical MS—20 mm Hg
- Acute pulmonary edema—25 mm Hg

### Q. What is the mechanisms of dyspnea in MS?
Elevated pulmonary venous pressure.

### Q. What is the mechanisms of orthopnea in MS?
- Increased venous return
- Increases area of lung in dependent position
- Increased pressure in diaphragm

### Q. What is the mechanisms of chest pain in MS?
- RV ischemia secondary to PAH
- Concurrent coronary atherosclerosis identical
- Pulmonary embolism due to AF (from right side source)

### Q. What is the mechanisms of palpitations in MS?
- Atrial fibrillation
- Pulmonary hypertension
- Right ventricular hypertrophy

### Q. What is the causes of hemoptysis in MS?
- Rupture of bronchial veins or of pulmonary vein or bronchial vein collaterals—pulmonary apoplexy
- Rupture of pulmonary capillaries during pulmonary edema
- Pulmonary congestion, embolism, and infarction
- Winter bronchitis
- Pulmonary hemosiderosis due to chronic recurrent pulmonary edema
- Anticoagulant use

### Q. What is the mechanisms of hoarseness of voice in MS?
It is a very rare complication of severe pulmonary hypertension secondary to mitral stenosis.

It is characterized by paralysis of left recurrent laryngeal nerve due to compression between the enlarged tense pulmonary artery and the aorta at ligamentum arteriosum.

Earlier it was thought to be due to compression of recurrent laryngeal nerve by the enlarged left atrium.

## EXAMINATION FINDINGS IN MS

### Q. What is mitral facies?
Pinkish purple appearance of the face due to decreased blood flow + cyanosis secondary to AV anastomoses and vascular statistics.

### Q. What are findings in pulse in MS?
- Usually normal
- Irregularly irregular in atrial fibrillation
- Low volume in severe MS
- Peripheral pulses may be absent in embolism due to atrial fibrillation

### Q. What are findings in BP in MS?
- Usually normal
- Low pulse pressure in severe MS

**Q. What are findings in JVP in MS?**
- Usually normal.
- Prominent a waves (due to vigorous right atrial systole) observed when there is pulmonary hypertension without atrial fibrillation,
- Absence of waves in atrial fibrillation,
- Prominent V waves (C-V waves) and rapid descent when there is development of functional tricuspid regurgitation.

**Q. What are findings in apex beat in MS?**
- It is not shifted and is tapping character of S1 at apex (closing snap).
- Apex beat is shifted when there is coexistent of MS with mitral regurgitation (MR)/aortic stenosis (AS)/systemic hypertension/ischemic heart disease (IHD)/myocarditis **(Table 2.9)**.

**Table 2.9:** Characteristics of apex beat.

| Loud SI | Soft SI | Variable SI |
|---|---|---|
| • Valvular lesions—MS, TS | • Valvular lesions—MR, AR, AS, TR | • Atrial fibrillation |
| • Hyperkinetic states | • Depressed contractility—LV dysfunction, acute myocardial infarction | • Second- and third-degree AV block |
| • Tachycardia | | • Multiple ventricular premature beats and ventricular tachycardia |
| • Short PR interval | | |
| • Left atrial myxoma | • Bradycardia | |
| • Mitral valve prolapse | • Prolonged PR interval | • Pulsus alternans |
| • ASD | • Obesity, pericardial disease | |
| • Ebstein's anomaly | | |

**Q. What is the mechanism of taping apex beat in MS?**
- Due to loud palpable SI
- Loud SI implies a pliable anterior valve leaflet.

**Q. What are the causes of loud SI in MS?**
- Sudden closure of the leaflets which are partially open at the start of the ventricular systole over a long distance.
- The stiff non-complaint leaflets resonate with high amplitude.
- In mitral stenosis, the forces that open and close the mitral valve increase as left atrial pressure increases.

**Q. What are the causes of abnormal wide split SI?**
- RBBB
- LV premature beat
- LV pacing

**Q. What is the basis of intensity of SI in MS?**
Related to mobility of the anterior mitral leaflet

**Q. What is the soft SI in MS?**
- Associated dominant MR /AR/AS
- MS with cardiac failure/PAH
- MS with extensive valve calcification
- Prolonged PR

**Q. What is the mechanism of opening snap?**
High-pitch snapping sound produced by the sudden tensing of the mitral/tricuspid valve leaflets as they try to open in early diastole.

**Mechanism:**
- In mitral/tricuspid stenosis is due to the elevated right/left atrial pressures and change in gradient across AV valves.
- It is the most important auscultatory sign of valvular involvement in MS.
- Absent OS indicates the calcification of body of the leaflets.

**Characteristics of OS**
- Medium—high-pitch sound
- 0.05–0.12 sec after S2
- Best heard medial to apex

**Q. What are the causes of the OS?**

**Mitral OS**
- MS
- MR
- VSD
- PDA

**Tricuspid OS**
- TS
- TR
- ASD

**Q. What are the factors decreasing intensity of OS?**
- Associated valvular disease
  - Dominant MR
  - AS
  - AR
- Poor flow states
  - Cardiac failure
  - PAH
- MS with extensive valve clarification

**Q. What is the correlation between soft OS and S1?**
- Reciprocal sounds produced by termination of the movement of the mitral valve complex.
- Calcification of the valves commissures—soft S1
- Calcification of the valve body—soft OS

**Q. What are the factors affecting A2-OS?**
- **Severity of MS:** Severe MS = short A2-OS interval
- Associated valvular heart disease
  - AS, AR—prolonged A2-OS
  - MR—narrow
- **Increased LVEDP:** LV dysfunction and increased LVEDP—long A2-OS interval
- **Heart rate:** Bradycardia = long A2-OS interval

**Q. What are the causes of absent OS in mitral stenosis?**
- Severe MS with calcification of valve

- Congenital MS
- Associated valvular heart disease—MR, AS and AR

### Q. What is Wells index in MS?
- Prolongation of Q-S1 interval. As the LA pressure rises, the LA-LV pressure crossover occurs late.
- Q-S1 interval minus A2-OS interval and is expressed in units of 0.01 seconds. More than 2 units indicate MVA <1.2 cm$^2$.

### Q. Describe the murmur in MS.
Low-pitched rough and rumbling mid-diastolic murmur with presystolic accentuation best heard with bell at the mitral area with the patient in the left lateral position the murmur is not conducted (Fig. 2.3).
- In MS coexisting with MR—a loud pansystolic murmur which radiates to the axilla and is heard at the left lower sternal border.
- Duration of murmur depends on the severity of stenosis.
- Increases after isotonic exercises (squatting, hand grip)

### Q. What are the components of murmur in MS?
**Mid to moderate MS**
- Mid-diastolic murmur
- Presystolic murmur

**Severe MS**
Holodiastolic murmur

### Q. Mechanism of presystolic accentuation in mitral stenosis.
- Atrial contraction
- The valve leaflets tending to close towards the end of diastole

### Q. What are the conditions where the presystolic accentuation is absent?
Atrial fibrillation.

**Mechanism of preserved presystolic accentuation in some cases of mitral stenosis with fibrillation**
- The valve leaflets pending to close towards the end of the diastole
- Persistent diastolic gradient.

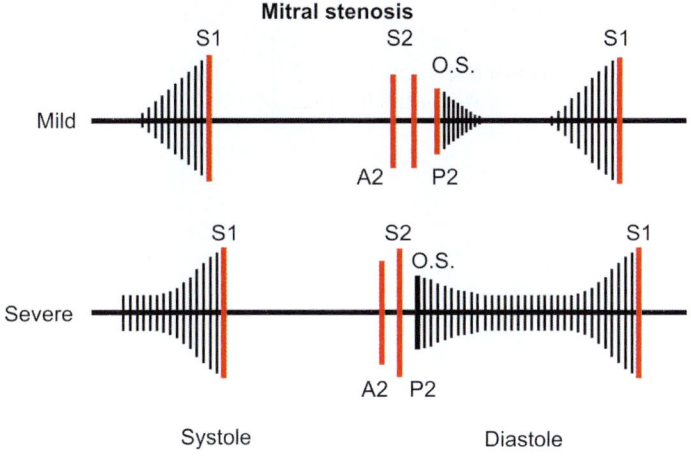

**Fig. 2.3:** Murmur in mitral stenosis.

**Basis of left lateral position to be used in auscultation**
- Left right position accentuates the low frequency vibration.
- Left lateral position increases the heart rate and transvalvular flow.

**Other murmurs in mitral stenosis**
- **Systolic murmur:** In pulmonary hypertension leading to RVH and dilatation, there will a secondary tricuspid regurgitation producing a pansystolic murmur accentuated during inspiration (de Carvallo's sign) audible best in the 4th left ICS along the parasternal region; along with giant "v" waves in the JVP. **S3** will also be present.
- **Pulmonary murmurs:** Ejection systolic murmur in early cases. Later early diastolic murmur (Graham-Steel murmur) of severe pulmonary regurgitation.

**Table 2.10** shows the variations in mid-diastolic murmur (MDM). **Table 2.11** shows the effect of other coexisting cardiac conditions on MS.

### Q. What are the causes of absent MDM in MS?
- Thick chest wall
- Emphysema
- COPD
- Dampened MS (due to severe PH)
- Low CO
- RV apex

### Q. What are the complications of MS?
- Atrial fibrillation
- Thrombus formation
- Systemic embolization (10–25%)
- Pulmonary hypertension
- Heart failure—right heart failure
- Ortner's syndrome
- Hemoptysis

**Table 2.10:** Variations in mid-diastolic murmur (MDM).

| Conditions where MDM is decreased in intensity | Conditions where MDM is increased in intensity |
| --- | --- |
| ✦ **Low flow states**<br>– Severe MS<br>– Cardiac failure<br>– PAH | ✦ Combined MS and MR<br>✦ Tachycardia |
| ✦ **Silent MS:** MS with counterclockwise rotation of the heart (Dampened MS)<br>✦ **Associated valve lesions**<br>– AS<br>– AR<br>– ASD<br>✦ **Miscellaneous**<br>– Obesity<br>– COPD | |

**Table 2.11:** Effect of other coexisting cardiac conditions on MS.

| Effect of coexistent MR on MS | Effect of coexistent AS on MS | Effect of coexistent AR on MS |
|---|---|---|
| • Soft S1<br>• Soft OS<br>• Narrow A2-OS<br>• MDM intensity increased | • Soft S1<br>• Soft OS<br>• Long A2-OS<br>• MDM intensity decreased | • Soft S1<br>• Soft OS<br>• Long A2-OS<br>• MDM intensity decreased |

- Dysphagia
- Pulmonary edema
- Cardiac cirrhosis
- Pulmonary hemosiderosis
- Lower lobe pneumonia
- Infective endocarditis (rare)

**Q. What is the effect of atrial fibrillation (AF) in MS?**

- The most common complication of MS prevalence and incidence varies according to age and roughly parallels the age of the patient (e.g., second decade—10% and sixth decade and beyond—80%).
- AF worsens symptoms of MS by: (1) Decreasing diastolic filling time—leads to increased LA pressure, (2) loss of atrial contribution to LV filling—leads to increased LA pressure, and (3) LA thrombus leading to systemic embolization.
- Prognosis: A 5-year survival of AF without MS is 85% and with MS is 64%
- AF causes decrease in cardiac output by 20% in MS.

**Q. What is the basis of deterioration by atrial fibrillation in MS?**

- Rapid ventricular rate lead to shortening of diastole. This leads to decrease ventricular filling.
- Rapid ventricular rate leads to increase flow rate and elevated transvalvular pressure gradient and their by left atrial pressure. The elevated LA pressure may precipitate pulmonary edema.
- Atrial booster effect on ventricular filling is lost.

**Q. What are the causes/differential diagnosis of MDM?**

- Mitral stenosis
- Tricuspid stenosis
- Flow murmurs—VSD, PDA, and MR
- Austin Flint murmur
- Atrial myxoma
- Cor-triatriatum
- Ball valve thrombus
- Carey Coombs murmur
- Rytand murmur

| Mitral stenosis | Flow murmur of VSD and PDA |
|---|---|
| Loud S1 | Absent |
| Opening snap present | Absent |
| Presystolic accentuation present | Absent |

| Mitral stenosis | Austin Flint murmur |
|---|---|
| Atrial fibrillation +/– | Usually absent |
| PAH common | Uncommon |
| Loud S1 absent | Soft S1 |
| S3 absent | Present |
| Opening snap present | Absent |

**Q. What are ECG finding in MS?**

- LAE-P mitrale in II and positive Morris index in V1
- RVH
- RAD
- AF

**Q. What will you examine in other systems in patient with MS?**

- **CNS:** To look for stroke (hemiplegia/focal neurological deficits), hoarseness of voice (Ortner's)
- **Eye:** To look for Roth spots, pallor
- **Palms and soles:** To look for Janeway lesions, splinter hemorrhages and clubbing.
- **GIT:** Splenomegaly, hepatomegaly, ascites
- **RS**—basal crepitations, left lower lobe pneumonia.

**Q. Discuss the X-ray finding in MS.**

Refer **Figures 2.4 and 2.5**.

**Chest X-ray (PA view):**

- Slight increase in transverse diameter of heart (due to RVH)
- 'Mitralization' of heart means straightening of the left border of heart (from above downwards) is due to:
  - Aortic knuckle—small.
  - Convexity due to dilated pulmonary artery.
  - Left atrial appendage—becomes prominent and produces a convexity.
  - Left border of left ventricle—**no change**.
- Double contour of the right border of heart (shadow within shadow): The outer and upper border is due to LA, and the inner and lower border is due to RA enlargement.

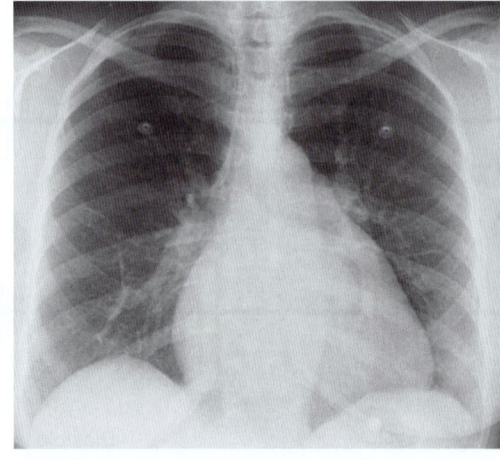

**Fig. 2.4:** Pulmonary venous hypertension on X-ray.

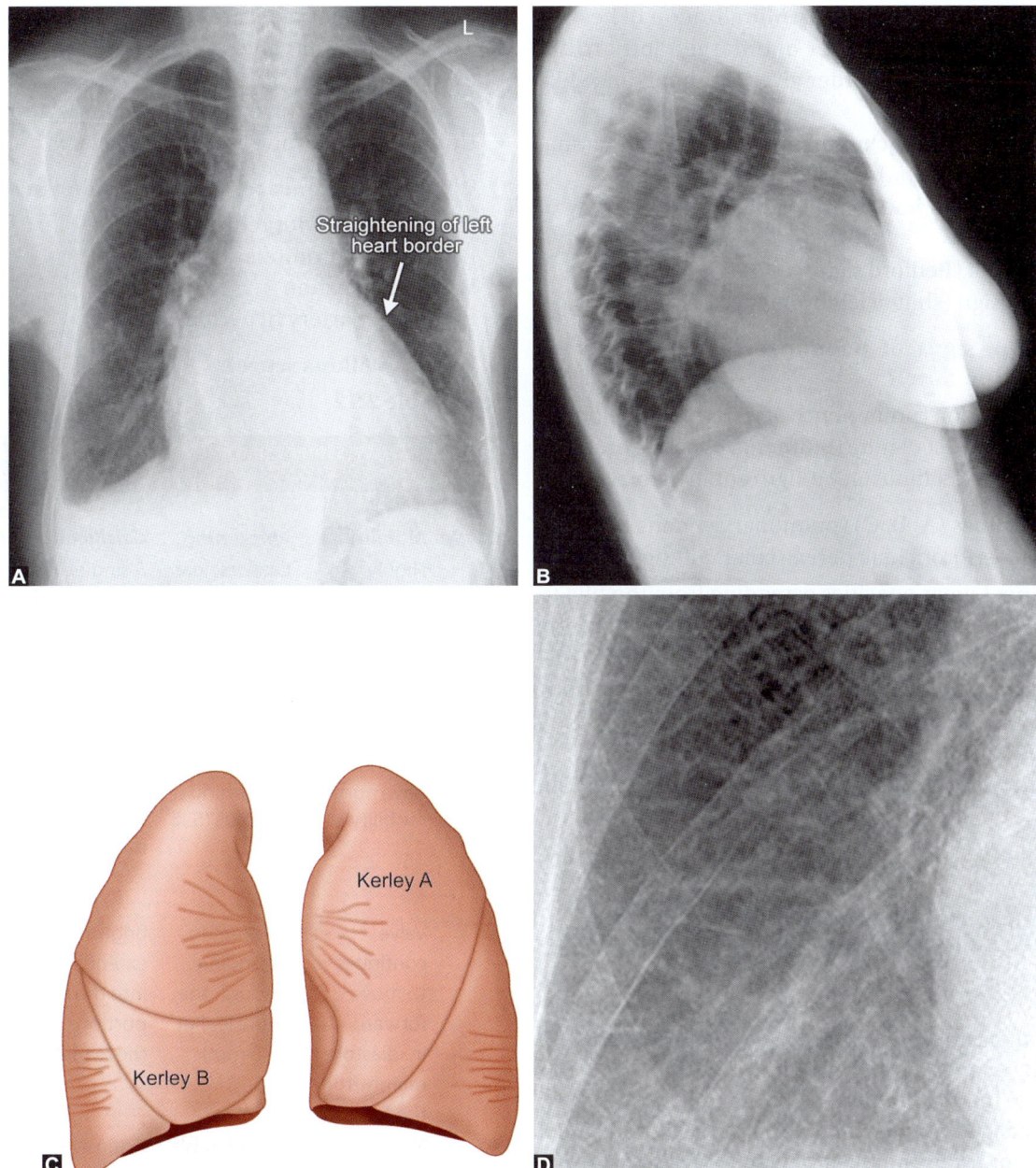

**Figs. 2.5A to D:** (A) X-rays of mitral stenosis showing double atrial shadow and straightening of left heart border; (B) Lateral X-ray showing walking man sign; (C) Schematic representation of Kerley lines; (D) X-ray showing Kerley B lines.

- Evidence of 'pulmonary hypertension': Dilated pulmonary arteries at hilum with peripheral pruning (i.e., peripherally pulmonary arteries taper sharply).
- Dilatation of upper lobe pulmonary veins (earliest X-ray feature of pulmonary venous hypertension).
- Fan-shaped opacity from parahilar region to periphery indicates pulmonary edema.
- Kerley's B lines—fine, dense horizontal lines at the base of the lung due to distension of interlobular septa and lymphatics, with edema.
- Mitral valve calcification—best seen in fluoroscopy.
- Elevation of left upper lobe bronchus (due to LA enlargement).
- Multiple small opacities due to pulmonary hemosiderosis (subjects who had multiple hemoptysis may show hemosiderin deposits in the lungs) and parenchymal ossification—rare.

**Q. What are the chest X-ray signs due to enlargement of left atrium?**

- Enlarged left atrial appendage causes filling up of normal concavity between pulmonary artery shadow and the left ventricle.

- Straightening of left heart border: Mitralization of heart
- Double atrial shadow: Border of enlarged left atrium together with right atrial border gives an appearance like atrium within an atrium.
- Pushing of left main bronchus upward causing wide carinal angle (splaying of carina)
- Pushing esophagus backward visible in lateral view of chest X-ray
- Left shift of aorta (Bedford sign)
- Walking man sign (shift of left bronchus forward)

### Q. What are the signs of pulmonary venous/capillary hypertension on X-ray?

**Grade 1:** Cephalization (prominence of veins of upper lobe of lung) of pulmonary vasculature (pulmonary venous pressure ≤20 mm Hg) (inverted moustache sign/antler's horn sign).

**Grade 2:** Kerley lines (A, B, C) (pulmonary venous pressure 20–25 mm Hg), peribronchial, perivascular cuffing.
- **Kerley A line:** Linear opacities extending from the hila to periphery; they are caused by distension of anastomotic channels between periphery and central lymphatics.
- **Kerley B line:** Short horizontal lines situated perpendicularly to the pleural surface at the lung base; they represent edema of interlobar septa.
- **Kerley C line:** Reticular opacities at lung base, representing Kerley B line en face.

**Grade 3:** Batwing opacities (pulmonary venous pressure >25 mm Hg).

### Q. What are the indicators of severity in mitral stenosis?
- Symptoms
- Signs
  - Length of diastolic murmur
  - Proximity of opening snap to S2
  - Signs of pulmonary hypertension/congestion
  - Functional pulmonary incompetence (Graham-Steel murmur) or tricuspid incompetence
- CXR
  - Left atrial/right ventricular enlargement.
  - Pulmonary hypertension and congestion
- ECG
  - Atrial enlargement
  - Right ventricular strain pattern
- Echo: M-mode
  - Flattering of EF slope: More than 30 min/s is mild, less than 10 mm/s is severe.
- Catheter
  - Mitral valve gradient
  - Elevated right heart pressures.
  - Decreased cardiac output during exercise.

### Q. How is severity of mitral stenosis assessed by 2-D echocardiography?

- Cross-sectional valve area >2.5 cm$^2$—asymptomatic
- Cross-sectional valve area 1.5–2.5 cm$^2$—symptoms on exercise only
- Cross-sectional valve area 1–1.5 cm$^2$—symptoms at rest
- Cross-sectional valve is <1 cm$^2$—severe.

### Q. What is the echocardiography finding in MS?
- Stenotic valve with reduced area
- Left atrium thrombus
- Valve calcification
- Pulmonary artery hypertension

### Q. What is Wilkins score?
Refer **Table 2.12**.

**Table 2.12:** Assessment of mitral valve anatomy according to the Wilkins score.

| Grade | Mobility | Thickening | Calcification | Subvalvular thickening |
|---|---|---|---|---|
| 1 | Highly mobile valve with only leaflet tips restricted | Leaflets near normal in thickness (4–5 mm) | A single area of increased echo brightness | Minimal thickening just below the mitral leaflets |
| 2 | Leaflet mid and base portions have normal mobility | Mid leaflets normal, considerable thickening of margins (5–8 mm) | Scattered areas of brightness confined to leaflet margins | Thickening of chordial structures extending to one-third of the chordial length |
| 3 | Valve continues to move forward in diastole, mainly from the base | Thickening extending through the entire leaflet (5–8 mm) | Brightness extending into the mid-portions of the leaflets | Thickening extended to distal third of the chordae |
| 4 | No or minimal forward movement of the leaflets in diastole | Considerable thickening of all leaflet tissue (>8–10 mm) | Extensive brightness throughout much of the leaflet tissue | Extensive thickening and shortening of all chordal structures extending down to the papillary muscles |

The total score is the sum of the four items and ranges between 4 and 16.

### Q. What are the indications for cardiac catheterization prior to surgery in MS?
- Age >40 in males and >50 in females
- Suspected associated CAD
- Suspected associated valvular heart disease
- Borderline echo results

### Q. Discuss the treatment of mitral stenosis.

Rheumatic fever prophylaxis to be given. However, infective endocarditis prophylaxis is not necessary **(Fig. 2.6)**.

**Indications for anticoagulation:** (1) Atrial fibrillation (persistent or paroxysmal), (2) embolic events, (3) left trial thrombus, (4) left atrial diameter >55 mm, and (5) spontaneous echo contrast.

- Restrict/decrease sodium intake.
- Diuretics: Early symptom such as mild dyspnea (due to pulmonary congestion) is usually treated with low doses of diuretics.
- Beta-blockers or non-dihydropyridines (DHP) calcium channel blockers (e.g., verapamil or diltiazem) to reduce heart rate (even in sinus rhythm, more useful in atrial fibrillation).
- Digoxin if atrial fibrillation with right heart failure. Atrial fibrillation also needs anticoagulation to prevent atrial thrombus and systemic embolization.

**Surgical management:**

Four operative measures are available.

1. **Trans-septal balloon mitral valvotomy (BMV):**
   - Also known as percutaneous balloon valvuloplasty (PBV) is the treatment of choice.
   - **Procedure:** Under local anesthesia, a catheter is passed through the femoral vein into the right atrium. The interatrial septum is punctured and the catheter is passed into the left atrium and across the mitral valve. A balloon is passed over the catheter across the valve, and briefly inflated to split the valve commissures.
   - **Indications:** Pliable mitral valves with little involvement of the subvalvular apparatus and minimal mitral regurgitation.
   - **Contraindications:** Moderate or severe mitral regurgitation, severe calcification, severe subvalvular fibrosis, thrombus in left atrium or ventricle, recent embolism, bleeding disorders, and interatrial septal thickness >3 mm (relative contraindication).
   - **Complications:** Mitral regurgitation may be severe enough to need surgery (2%), mortality (1–2%), cardiac perforation (1%), and cerebral embolism (1%).

2. **Closed mitral valvotomy (CMV):**
   - **Indication:** Mobile, noncalcified mitral valves without regurgitation
   - **Contraindication:** Left atrial thrombus, mitral valvular calcification, severe subvalvular disease, or moderate or severe mitral regurgitation
   - **Advantages:** Cardiopulmonary bypass is not required and good result is obtained for 10 years or more.
   - **Disadvantage:** The valve cusps may refuse necessitating another operation.

3. **Open mitral valvotomy (OMV):**
   - It is usually performed and is preferred over closed valvotomy or mitral valve replacement.
   - **Procedure:** Under direct view, the valvular cusps are carefully separated from each other and commissures are incised.
   - **Advantage:** Less chances of traumatic mitral regurgitation, concurrent annuloplasty can be done for mitral regurgitation. Removal of LA thrombus (if present), calcium in leaflets, amputation of LA

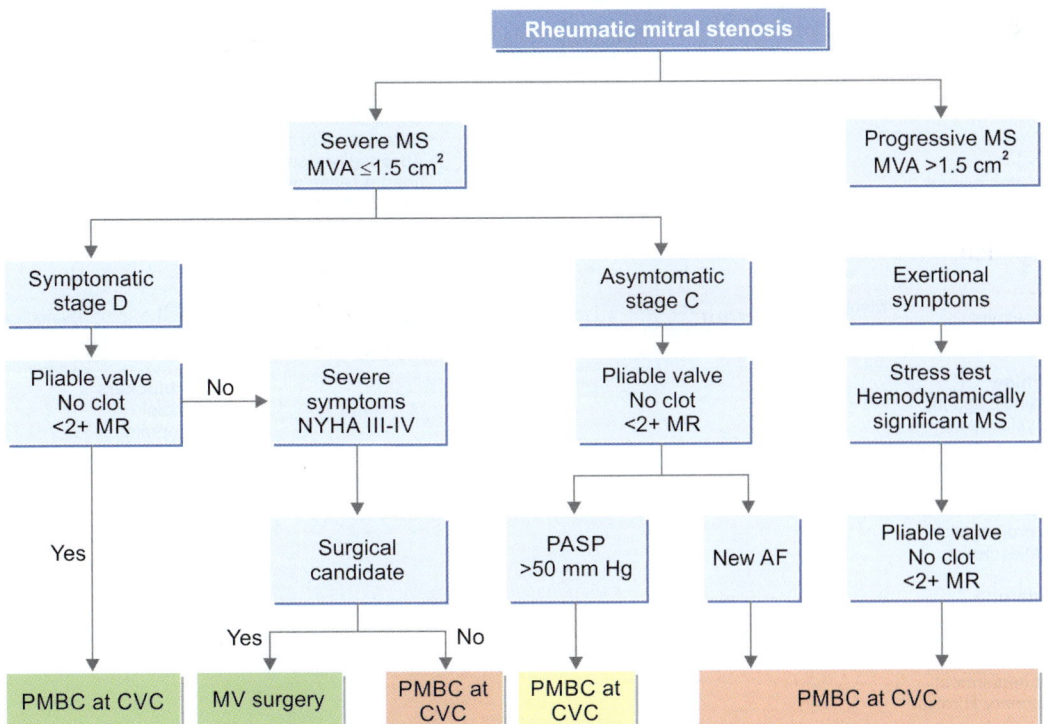

**Fig. 2.6:** Management of MS.

appendage, and separation of fused chordae can also done along with this surgical procedure.
- **Disadvantage:** Needs cardiopulmonary bypass.
4. **Mitral valve replacement (MVR)**
   - Indications:
     – Mitral stenosis associated with mitral regurgitation
     – Severely damaged or severely calcified stenotic valve which cannot be reopened without producing significant mitral regurgitation
     – Moderate or severe mitral stenosis and presence of thrombus in the left atrium even after anticoagulation therapy

- Type of prosthesis: Mechanical prosthesis if age is <65 years and bioprosthesis if age is >65 years.
- Artificial valves usually work successfully for >20 years and anticoagulants are usually given postoperatively to prevent thrombus formation and its embolization.

**Q. Discuss management of atrial fibrillation in structural heart diseases.**

Refer **Figures 2.7 to 2.9**.

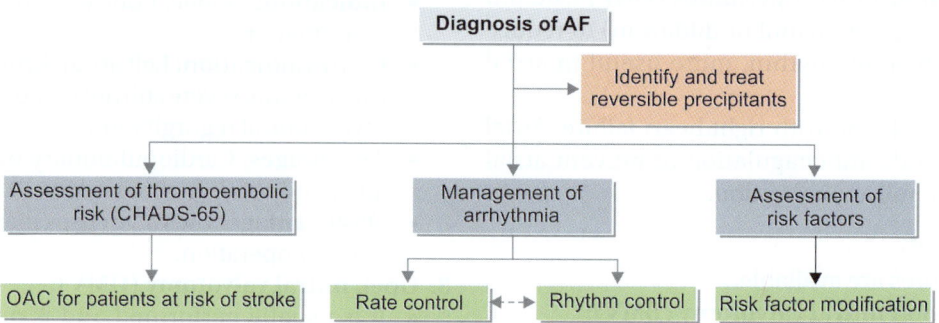

**Fig. 2.7:** Diagnosis of atrial fibrillation.

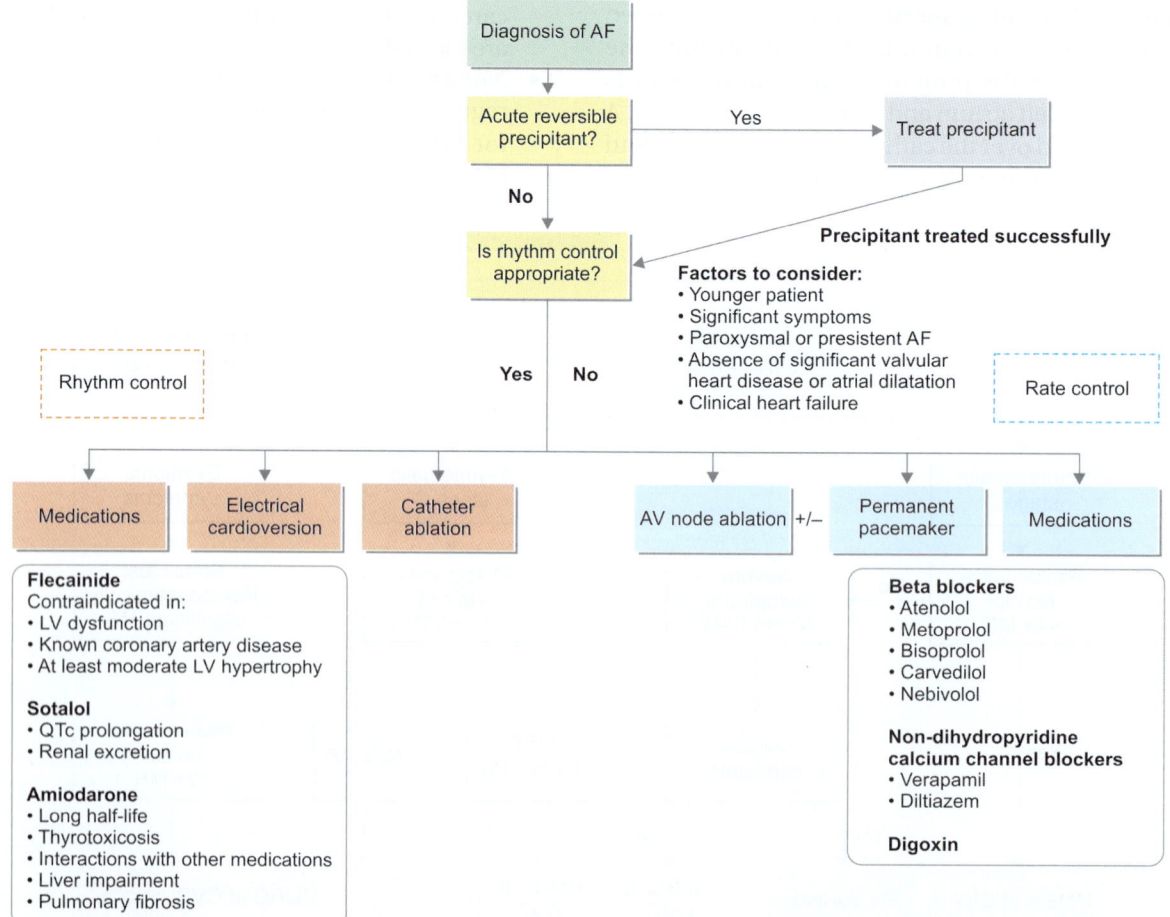

**Fig. 2.8:** Approach to management of AF.

| Anticoagulation | | |
|---|---|---|
| $CHA_2DS_2$-VA (Congestive heart failure, **H**ypertentsion, **A**ge >75 years (2 points), **D**iabetes, Stroke/transient ischemic attack (2 points/1 point respectively), **V**ascular disease, **A**ge >65 years)<br>• $CHA_2DS_2$-VA = 0: Oral anticoagulants (OACs) are not recommended<br>• $CHA_2DS_2$-VA = 1: OACs should be considered<br>• $CHA_2DS_2$-VA = 2: OACs are recommended. | **High $CHA_2DS_2$-VASC**<br><br>Stroke risk: 2.2–11.4%/year<br><br>NOAC and VKA | **Hypertrophic cardiomyopathy**<br><br>Stroke risk: ~3.75%/year<br><br>NOAC and VKA |
| | **Mitral stenosis**<br><br>Stroke risk: 4–17%/year<br><br>NOAC: mild MS<br>VKA: Moderate or severe MS | **Mechanical heart valve**<br><br>Stroke risk: Extremely high<br><br>VKA only |

**Fig. 2.9:** Use of anticoagulants in AF.

## Case 2: Mitral Regurgitation

*Brief History:*
A 34-year-old male presented with dyspnea on exertion, palpitations and leg swelling.

*Examination*
- Patient is conscious and oriented, moderately built and moderately nourished with height—156 cm, weight—40 kg BMI—16.4.
- Upper segment—76 cm, lower segment— 80 cm
- Upper segment-lower segment ratio—0.95, arm span—158 cm

*Vitals:* Pulse rate—76 /min irregularly irregular with variable volume and no special character, normal condition of vessel wall, no radioradial or radiofemoral delay and all peripheral pulses are felt with an apex pulse deficit of 12.

- Blood pressure (average of 3 readings).
- Right upper limb—126/70 mm Hg, supine position
- Right lower limb—136 mm Hg of systolic
- Left upper limb—120/70 mm Hg, supine position
- Left lower limb—138 mm Hg systolic

Respiratory rate—24 breaths/min thoracoabdominal
Temperature—98.6°F
JVP—8 cm above the sternal angle with earlobe pulsations in 45 degrees recumbent position with absent 'a' waves.

*General Examination*
- Arcus senilis—present
- Pallor, icterus, cyanosis, clubbing, lymphadenopathy —absent
- Bilateral pitting type of pedal edema present in both lower limbs
- No evidence of infective endocarditis

*Cardiovascular System Examination*
Inspection:
- Precordium—no precordial bulge
- Apex beat—visible in left 6th intercostal space, 2.5 cm lateral to midclavicular line. Parasternal pulsations are seen.
- Anterolateral scar of 10 cm extending from left lower sternal border towards the midaxillary line just below the left 6th intercostal space.
- No visible suprasternal pulsations, sinuses.

Palpation:
- Apex beat—felt in the left 6th ICS, 2.5 cm lateral to MCL, hyperdynamic in character
- Parasternal heave present—grade 2
- Palpable P2 in the left 2nd ICS
- No thrills

Percussion:
Dull note present in the left 2nd ICS.

Auscultation:
Mitral area:
- S1—variable and diminished
- S2—loud (loud P2)
- Mid-diastolic murmur of Grade 3 best heard in left lateral position in expiration with bell of stethoscope
- Pansystolic murmur of Grade 3, radiating to left axilla
- Opening snap—not heard

Tricuspid area:
- S1 S2 heard
- Pansystolic murmur grade 3 present

Pulmonary area:
- S1 heard loud P2 heard
- Early diastolic murmur best heard in inspiration Aortic area:
  – S1 S2 heard and normal
  – No additional sounds and murmurs
  – No venous hum

Respiratory System
- Bilateral normal vesicular breath sounds
- No added sounds

Per Abdomen
- Soft, hepatomegaly present
- Tenderness present in the right hypochondrium
- Epigastric pulsations felt over the tip of the finger
- No splenomegaly, no free fluid

Central Nervous System
- Higher mental functions—normal
- No neurological deficits
- Fundus in both eyes normal

*Diagnosis*
Mitral re-stenosis with mitral regurgitation and tricuspid regurgitation with pulmonary hypertension and atrial fibrillation in right heart failure without any signs of infective endocarditis (NYHA Class 3)

## DISCUSSION

**Q. What are the types of scars over the chest and surgeries performed?**

- **Medial sternotomy scar indications:** In open heart surgeries, such as valve replacement, CABG, cardiac transplant and arterial and venous cannulation for bypass.
- **Left infraclavicular region:** Pace maker incision scar of about 4–5 cm.
- **Thoracotomy scars**
- **Posterolateral scars indications:**
  - Persistent ductus arteriosus
  - Coarctation of aorta
  - Creation of systemic—pulmonary anastomoses

- Aneurysms and traumatic ruptures of the descending thoracic aorta
- **Anterolateral scar indications:**
  - On left:
    - Closed mitral valvotomy
    - Banding of pulmonary artery
  - On right:
    - Intra-atrial correction of transposition of great arteries
    - Closure of atrial septal defects mitral valve repair
- **Axillary scar indications:** Pneumonectomy and pneumothorax operations.
- **Importance of scars in apex beat:** Apex beat moves downward and outward in anterolateral scars. So position of apex beat cannot be told only the character of apex is to be considered.

**Q. What are the causes of pansystolic murmur?**
Refer **Table 2.13**.

**Table 2.13:** Features MR, TR, VSD.

| Features | MR | TR | VSD |
|---|---|---|---|
| Site | Apex | Left lower sternum | Left parasternal 3rd |
| Conduction | To axilla, base, back | Right lower sternum | Throughout the precordium |
| Accentuation with respiration | In expiration | In inspiration | ? In expiration |

**Q. Name the cause of diastolic murmur in pulmonary area.**
- Graham steel murmur
- A high-pitched decrescendo diastolic murmur along left sternal border in 2nd ICS.

**Q. Describe the grading of murmurs.**

**Levine and Freeman's grading of murmurs systolic murmurs:**
- **Grade 1:** Very soft (heard in quiet room)
- **Grade 2:** Soft
- **Grade 3:** Moderate
- **Grade 4:** Loud with thrill
- **Grade 5:** Very loud with thrill (heard with stethoscope partly off chest wall)
- **Grade 6:** Very loud with thrill (heard even when stethoscope is slightly away from the chest wall)

**Diastolic murmurs**

Diastolic murmurs are usually not graded but can be described as:
- Very soft
- Soft
- Moderate
- Loud or associated with palpable thrill.

**Q. What are the features of JVP in irregularly irregular pulse?**
- In irregularly irregular pulse (AF), there is no atrial contraction and 'a' wave will be absent and JVP will loose its double wave form pattern.
- In case of tricuspid regurgitation—prominent and distended jugular veins that is very pulsatile and may be confused with carotid pulse.
- There is a distinct "C-V"(regurgitant) wave due to systolic regurgitation into right atrium.
- Jugular venous distension may be more prominent with inspiration—Kussmaul's sign.

**Q. What are the precipitating factors for heart failure?**
Refer **Tables 2.14 and 2.15, and Figure 2.10**.

**Table 2.14:** Clinical features of right heart failure versus left heart failure.

| Cardiac | Metabolic | Patient-related |
|---|---|---|
| Acute ischemia | Anemia | Dietary/fluid non-adherence |
| Arrhythmia | Hyperthyroidism | HF therapy non-adherence |
| Endocarditis | Thyrotoxicosis | Cardiotoxins<br>✦ Cocaine<br>✦ Chronic alcoholism<br>✦ Amphetamines<br>✦ Sympathomimetic |
| Myocarditis | Infection | Medications<br>✦ NSAID<br>✦ COX-2 inhibitors<br>✦ Steroids<br>✦ Lithium<br>✦ β-blockers<br>✦ Calcium channel blockers<br>✦ Antiarrhythmics<br>✦ Thiazolidinediones |
| Pulmonary embolus | Pregnancy | |
| Uncontrolled hypertension | Worsening renal function | |
| Valvular disorders | | |

**Table 2.15:** Clinical features of heart failure.

| Signs/symptoms | Left-sided heart failure | Right-sided heart failure |
|---|---|---|
| Pitting edema | Mild to moderate | Moderate to severe |
| | Pulmonary edema | Ascites |
| Fluid retention | Pleural effusion, pericardial effusion | Congestive Hepatomegaly |
| Jvp | Mild to moderate raised | Grossly raised JVP |

| Signs/symptoms | Left-sided heart failure | Right-sided heart failure |
|---|---|---|
| Neck veins | — | Neck veins distended |
| Dyspnea | Prominent (PND) | Present but not as prominent |
| Gastrointestinal | Present | Prominent GI symptoms (loss of appetite, bloating, constipation) |

**Q. What are the causes of raised JVP?**

- **P**ericardial effusion/**P**ulmonary embolism/**P**ericardial constriction
- **Q**uantity of fluid raised (fluid overload)
- **R**ight heart failure
- **S**uperior vena caval obstruction
- **T**ricuspid stenosis/**T**ricuspid regurgitation/**T**amponade

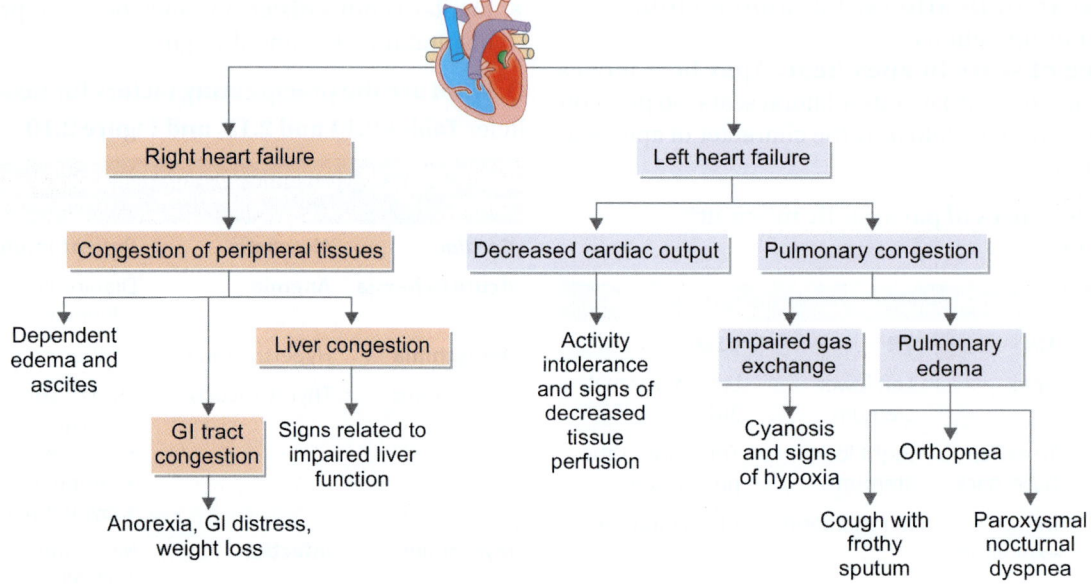

**Fig. 2.10:** Clinical features and mechanism of left and right-sided heart failure.

**Q. What are the causes of cardiac failure?**

Refer **Table 2.16**.

| Table 2.16: Etiologies of heart failure. | |
|---|---|
| Depressed ejection fraction | ◆ Coronary artery disease (myocardial infarction or ischemia)<br>◆ Chronic pressure and volume overload (hypertension, obstructive valvular disease, regurgitant valvular disease, shunting)<br>◆ Nonischemic dilated, or idiopathic cardiomyopathy*<br>◆ Disorders of rate and rhythm (chronic<br>◆ brady- and tachyarrhythmias) |
| Preserved ejection fraction | ◆ Primary hypertrophic cardiomyopathy<br>◆ Secondary hypertrophy (hypertension)<br>◆ Restrictive cardiomyopathy (infiltrative or storage disease)<br>◆ Fibrosis |
| Pulmonary heart disease | ◆ Cor pulmonale<br>◆ Pulmonary vascular disease |
| High-output states | Metabolic disorders (hyperthyroidism, nutritional disorders (beri-beri))<br>Excessive blood-flow requirements (systemic arteriovenous shunting, chronic anemia) |

*Infections, toxins, genetic defects of cytoskeletal proteins

### Q. What is Ewart's sign?

Ewart's sign is a finding on physical examination seen in patients with pericardial effusions **(Fig. 2.11)**. Sometimes, a large pericardial effusion may produce an area of dullness near the lower angle of the scapula. This sign is known as Ewart's sign. It is a combination of dullness to percussion over the left scapula, aegophony, bronchial breath sounds over the left lung.

### Q. What is the etiology of mitral regurgitation?

**Acute**
- Infective endocarditis
- Rupture of papillary muscle
  - Acute MI
  - MVP
  - Trauma
  - Cardiac surgery
  - Acute rheumatic carditis
  - Prosthetic valve dysfunction

**Chronic**
- Damage to valve leaflets
  - RHD
  - Myxomatous degeneration
  - MVP
  - IE
  - SLE
- Damage to annulus
  - Abscess (IE)
  - Annular calcification
  - Dilated cardiomyopathy
- Damage to chordae tendineae
  - Myxomatous degeneration
  - Marfan's, Ehrler-Danlos
  - IE
  - Acute rheumatic fever
- Damage to papillary muscles
  - Coronary artery disease
  - Dilated cardiomyopathy
- Damage to left ventricle
  - Ischemia
  - Dilated cardiomyopathy

### Q. What is primary MR and secondary MR?

**Primary mitral regurgitation**

Caused by a primary abnormality of one or more components of the valve apparatus.
- Leaflets
- Chordae tendineae
- Papillary muscles
- Annulus

**Secondary mitral regurgitation**
- Caused by another cardiac disease such as coronary heart disease or a cardiomyopathy.
- Identification of the cause and type (primary or secondary) of MR is required for appropriate management of MR as well as any associated conditions.

*Loud P2*
- Hyperkinetic states
- Thin chest wall
- Straight back syndrome
- Ostium secundum ASD—due to dilated pulmonary artery.

### Q. What are the causes of parasternal pulsations?
- Right ventricular hypertrophy:
  - Pulmonary hypertension
  - Pulmonary stenosis
  - Tricuspid regurgitation
  - ASD, VSD, mitral stenosis
- Normal right ventricle:
  - Moderate to severe mitral regurgitation
  - Regional wall motion abnormality of left ventricle.
  - Children and thin adults
  - Anemia
- Hyperdynamic circulations like pregnancy, thyrotoxicosis, fever
- Thin chest wall.

### Q. What is diastolic shock?

Palpable P2 is called as diastolic shock.

### Q. Name the cause of diastolic knock.

Constrictive pericarditis.

### Q. When is P2 said to be loud?

When P2 is as loud as A2 in pulmonary area then we can say P2 is loud.

### Q. Describe the abnormal "a" waves in JVP.
- Large "a" wave:
  - Tricuspid atresia
  - Tricuspid stenosis
  - Pulmonary hypertension

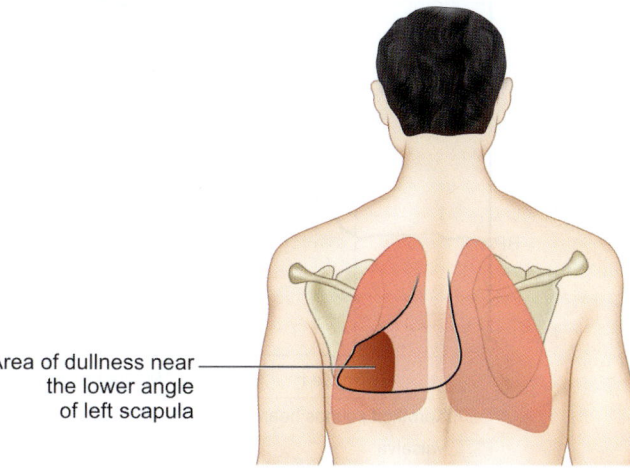

**Fig. 2.11:** Ewart's sign.

- Pulmonary stenosis
- Acute pulmonary embolism
- Right ventricular cardiomyopathy or infraction.
- Right atrial myxomas.
♦ **Cannon a wave:**
  - Complete heart block
  - Isorhythmic AV dissociation
  - Ventricular tachycardia
  - Junctional rhythm VT 1:1 retrograde conduction
♦ **Absent a wave:** Atrial fibrillation.

### Q. What are the cardiovascular changes in anemia?

♦ **Blood pressure:** Systolic blood pressure will be high but diastolic blood pressure will be normal. Hence there will be wide pulse pressure.
♦ **Pulse:** Usually tachycardia. However, it can be normal in chronic anemia.
♦ **Inspection:** Parasternal pulsations can be seen. Apex beat is in deviated outward and downward direction.
♦ **Palpation:** Palpable P2 (pulmonary artery dilatation) and apex beat shifted down and outward.
♦ **Percussion:** Second left intercostal space is dull (due to pulmonary artery dilation).
♦ **Auscultation:**
  - Ejection systolic murmur in aortic and pulmonary areas.
  - Pansystolic murmurs in mitral and tricuspid areas (due to annular dilatation of mitral and tricuspid valves of dilated heart).
  - Early diastolic murmurs are seen in pulmonary and aortic areas due to both pulmonary and aortic artery dilatation.
  - Muffled heart sounds due to dilatation all valve annulus.
  - Ejection clicks due to opening of valve in case of dilated valve. S3 and S4 can be heard.

### Q. In anemia, murmurs are best heard in which areas of heart?

Murmurs are best heard in aortic and pulmonary areas because of small size valves when compared to mitral and tricuspid areas which are huge valves that can tolerate increased flow. Hence, murmurs are not well appreciated in mitral and tricuspid areas.

### Q. Which murmur is highly unlikely in anemia?

Mid-diastolic murmur.

### Q. How to differentiate between congestive state and congestive heart failure?

Valsalva maneuver is the procedure to differentiate congestive state from congestive heart failure.

This maneuver is performed by blowing into a blood pressure manometer to maintain a level of 40 mm Hg for 30 seconds or taking a relatively deep inspiration followed by forced expiration against a closed glottis for 10–20 seconds. It consists of four phases which records the changes in blood pressure and heart rate in each phases of maneuver (**Figs. 2.12 and 2.13**).

**Phase I**: As deep inspiration commences intrathoracic pressure increases which is associated with a transient rise of left ventricular output and systemic arterial pressure followed by a reflex bradycardia.

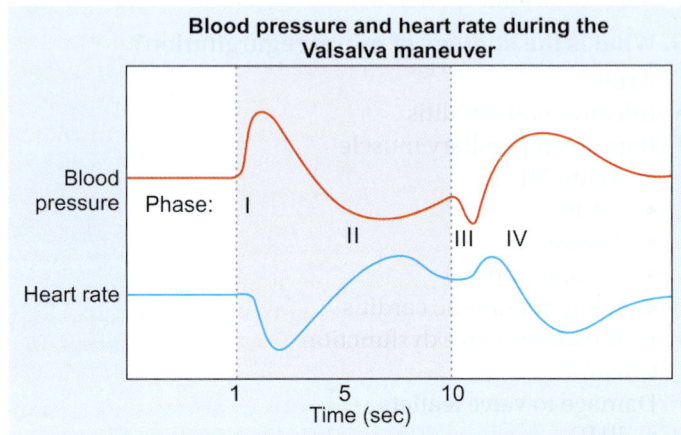

**Fig. 2.12:** In Valsalva maneuver sympathetic activity gets activated in phase II and shows its action in phase III.

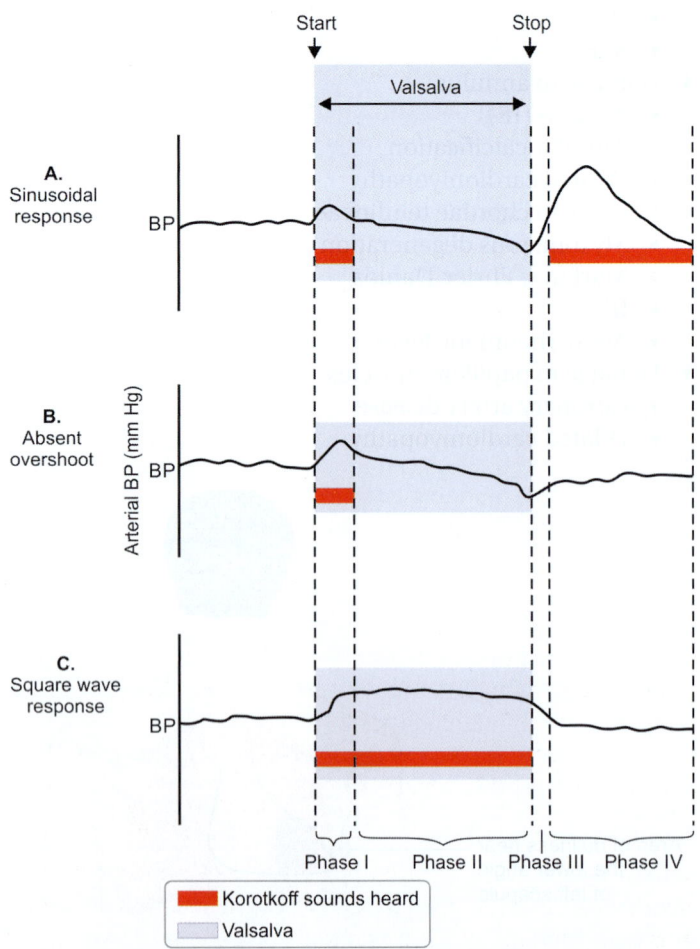

**Fig. 2.13:** Responses during Valsalva maneuver.

**Phase II:** It is associated with perceptible decreases in systemic venous return and stroke volume which results in decrease in systolic and diastolic and pulse pressure and reflex tachycardia.

**Phase III:** (release of Valsalva maneuver) cessation of inspiration results in sudden increase in systemic venous return but there is an abrupt transient decrease in arterial pressure equivalent to the fall in intrathoracic pressure.

**Phase IV:** (over shoot phase) return of events to pre-Valsalva levels after 6–8 beats with transient overshoot of systemic arterial pressure, wide pulse pressure and reflex bradycardia.

**Graph A:** Indicates normal response to Valsalva maneuver in normal person.

**Graph B:** Indicates Valsalva maneuver changes in congestive heart failure where there is absence of overshooting of blood pressure in phase 4.

**Graph C:** Indicates Valsalva maneuver changes in congestive heart failure where there is blunting of phase 2 resulting in square root pattern to the graph because of overactivity of sympathetic system in failing heart.

## Q. What are the types of angina?

### Angina pectoris/Heberden's angina

Angina pectoris is a clinical syndrome that presents as paroxysmal and recurrent attacks of substernal or precordial chest discomfort due to transient myocardial ischemia which falls short of inducing necrosis of myocardial cell.

### Stable angina

It is characterized as chest pain classically described as constricting discomfort/squeezing/tightening/heaviness/aching in the front of chest. Pain may radiate to left arm, neck, jaw, less commonly to right arm, back, epigastrium lasting for 2–5 minutes brought on by physical exertion such as heavy meals, walking in cold weather which gets relieved by rest or sublingual glyceryl trinitrate.

### Prinzmetal angina

It is a vasospastic angina which occurs without exertion and usually at rest. It is due to spasm of coronary artery and more frequent in women. Characteristically, it is associated with transient ST segment elevation on the ECG during the pain.

Provocation tests (e.g., hyperventilation, cold pressure testing or ergotamine challenge) may be needed for establishing the diagnosis. Prognosis is usually better than those with fixed significant obstructive lesions. Usually the response to beta blockers may be poor. Calcium channel blockers are used for the treatment.

### Unstable angina

Unstable angina includes patients with acute coronary syndrome but with normal ECG, without elevation of cardiac markers. Management of unstable angina is same as non-ST elevation myocardial ischemia.

- Rest angina: Angina occurring at rest and prolonged usually more than 20 min.
- New onset angina: New onset angina of at least Canadian classification class 3 severity.
- Increasing angina: Previously diagnosed that has become distinctly more frequent, longer in duration or lower in threshold class to at least CCS class 3 severity.
- ECG changes without elevation of cardiac injury markers.
- Patients with unstable angina have a high risk of developing MI or sudden death when compared to patients of stable angina.

### Abdominal angina

Abdominal angina is postprandial abdominal pain after eating that occurs in individuals with chronic mesenteric ischemia due to occlusion of mesenteric vessels that has advanced to the point where blood flow cannot increase enough to meet visceral demands.

### Vincent's angina

Vincent's angina is a fusospirochetal infection of the pharynx and palatine tonsils causing ulceromembranous pharyngitis and tonsillitis characterized by superficial ulceration and necrosis of the tonsils and pharynx that often results in formation of a pseudomembrane, foul smelling, odynophagia, submandibular lymphadenopathy.

## Q. What are the differences between the holosystolic murmur and pansystolic murmur?

Both are high-pitched murmurs that begin with S1 and occupy all of systole and ends with S2.

These are regurgitant murmurs produced by retrograde flow from chamber of high pressure to a chamber of low pressure. Hence timing of murmur with systole has to be made. Holosystolic murmur is of same intensity throughout the systole but pansystolic murmur can have midsystolic accentuation of intensity.

## Q. What are the components of mitral valve apparatus?

The main feature of the mitral valve is the mitral apparatus, which is composed of the left atrial wall, left ventricle wall, the mitral annulus, the anterior and posterior leaflets, chordae tendinae and papillary muscles **(Figs. 2.14A to F)**.

## Q. What are the causes of MR?

### Cuspal lesions

- Rheumatic heart disease
- Mitral valve prolapse
- Infective endocarditis
- Trauma

### Annual lesions

- Dilation dilated cardiomyopathy
- Ischemic heart disease
- Calcification—mitral valve annular calcification

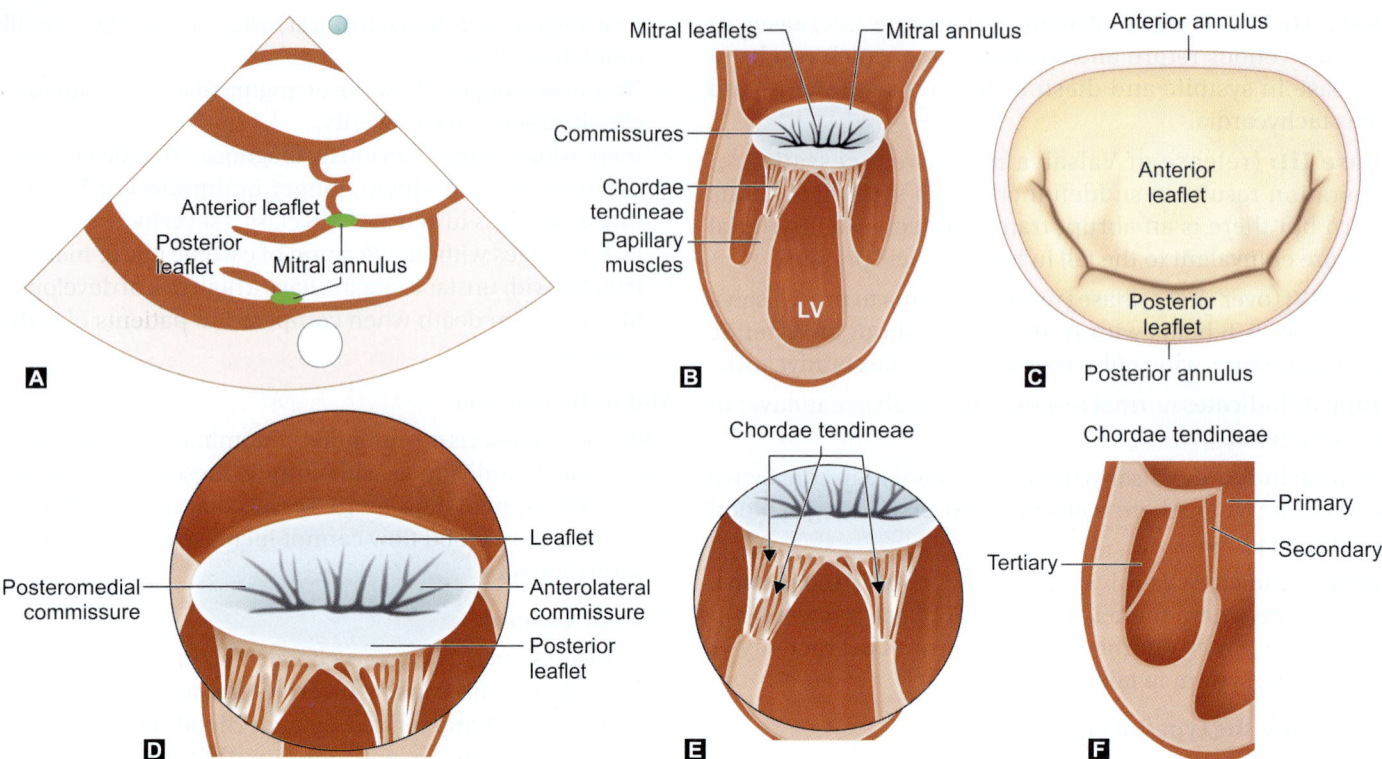

**Figs. 2.14A to F:** Mitral valve apparatus—annulus: (A and B) Mitral leaflets: There are two thin leaflets. One is located anteriorly and is thicker and larger. The other is posteriorly located and is thinner and more flexible; (C) A fibroelastic structure separating LA from LV; (D) Commissures is the sites where the leaflets insert and joint to annulus; (E and F) Tendinous chords: Fibrous strings that attach specific portions of mitral leaflets to papillary muscle tips.

**Chordal lesions**
- Mitral valve prolapse
- Trauma
- Infective endocarditis

**There are three types of chordae based on the location of insertion:**

a. **Primary (marginal):** Attaches at the leaflet tip. It is primary function is to maintain coaptation of leaflets. Failure of the primary chords, either elongated which leads to leaflet prolapse, or primary chord rupture leading to flail leaflet are concerning.
b. **Secondary:** Attaches at mid-body of leaflets.
c. **Tertiary:** Attaches at base of leaflets and provides structural support.

**Papillary muscles (PM):** Large trabeculated muscles to which tendinous chords are attached.

**Papillary lesions**
- Myocardial infarction
- Angina

**LV lesions**
- Aneurysm
- Hypertrophic cardiomyopathy

**Connective tissue diseases**
- Marfan syndrome
- Ehlers-Danlos syndrome
- Rheumatoid arthritis
  **Box 2.2** shows the etiology of acute and chronic MR.

**Q. What is the hemodynamic impact of MR?**

The burden of MR on the heart is volume overload.

**Acute severe MR**

This produces surplus of volume within LA, builds up a high pressure and therefore LAP is acutely increased, leading to development of acute pulmonary edema and cardiogenic shock.

**Chronic MR**

Here, cardiac remodeling takes place over time as a compensatory mechanism in response to chronic volume overload, leading to development of left atrial and left ventricular enlargement.

The more severe the MR, the more severe LV geometry alteration would be.

While during earlier stages of chronic MR, the remodeling process is accommodative and patients remain asymptomatic (at the expense of left-chambers dilation), later on during advanced stages of chronic MR, the high build-up of

**Box 2.2:** Etiology of acute and chronic MR.

- **Acute MR**
  - Endocarditis
  - Papillary muscle rupture: AMI, chest trauma
  - Chordal rupture (flail leaflet): Myxomatous disease, rheumatic heart disease, spontaneous rupture
  - Dynamic LVOT (especially in stress CM)
  - Iatrogenic, e.g., after removal of transaortic left ventricular assist device
- **Chronic MR**
  - Chronic primary MR
    » MVP
    » Rheumatic valve disease, connective tissue disease, e.g., Marfan syndrome, systemic inflammatory disorders, e.g., SLE
    » HOCM (systolic anterior movement of mitral valve)
    » MV annulus calcification: Idiopathic, CKD, hyperparathyroidism
    » Congenital: MV clefts, Parachute MV, endocardial cushion defects
  - Chronic secondary MR
    » Chronic ischemic heart disease
    » Dilated CM
    » Long-standing AF
    » Left ventricular aneurysm

**Box 2.3:** Pulse, BP, JVP and precordium signs in MR.

**Pulse in MR**
- Normal in mild MR
- Hyperkinetic in moderate to severe MR
- Quick rising with normal volume
- Hyperkinetic pulse is indicative of significant MR
- Irregularly irregular in atrial fibrillation
- Peripheral pulses may be absent in embolism due to atrial fibrillation

**Blood pressure in MR**
- Usually, normal
- In severe mitral regurgitation: Wide pulse pressure
- Three recordings are necessary if patient has atrial fibrillation (AF)
- Pulsus alternans in acute MR

**JVP in MR**
- Usually, normal
- Prominent a waves in PAH
- Prominent v waves in TR

**Apex beat in MR**
- Hyperdynamic—forceful apex beat
- Cardiomegaly—shifted down and out in moderate to severe MR

**Left parasternal heave**
- Late systolic lift by enlarged left atrium
- Pansystolic lift due to PAH

pressure within the enlarged chambers puts patient at risk of developing acute pulmonary edema and cardiogenic shock following a clinical trigger.

In chronic primary MR, presence of the following factors imply severity of the MR:
- LAE, LVE
- PH (type 2).
- AF

**Q. What does MR beget MR mean?**
- MR leads to LV dilatation which leads to future MR
- MR leads to LV dilatation and papillary muscle dysfunction.

**Q. Discuss the pulse, BP, JVP and precordium signs in MR.**
Refer **Box 2.3**.

**Q. Discuss the heart sounds abnormalities in MR.**
Refer **Table 2.17**.

**Table 2.17:** Heart sounds abnormalities in MR.

| S1 | S2 |
|---|---|
| **S1 is soft**<br>+ Incomplete apposition of the valve cusps<br>+ Partial closure of the mitral valve orifice by the time ventricular systole begins<br>**Loud S1 in MR**<br>+ Associated MS<br>+ MVP—MR<br>+ MR—papillary muscle dysfunction | **Pulmonary component (P2)** of S2 is loud and palpable in pulmonary hypertension and also due to anterior displacement of pulmonary artery caused by dilated LA.<br>Widely split second heart sound (S2) is due to aortic valve closure (A1) occurring early but the split is mobile. |
| **S3** | **S4** |
| **LV S3 in MR**<br>+ Increased LVEDV<br>+ LV dysfunction | **Acute MR**<br>S4 is a sign of acute MR as left atrium is not dilated in acute MR. |

**Q. Discus the murmurs in MR.**
Refer **Table 2.18**.

**Table 2.18:** Murmurs in MR.

| Type | Causes |
|---|---|
| Holosystolic murmur | Rheumatic MR<br>Regurgitation starts during isovolumetric contraction and continues till isovolumetric relaxation |
| Late systolic murmur | MVP and papillary muscle dysfunction |
| Holosystolic with late systolic accentuation | MVP and papillary muscle dysfunction |
| Holosystolic with midsystolic accentuation | Severe MR |
| Tapering holosystolic murmur | Acute MR; trivial MR<br>Severe MR with small left atrium |

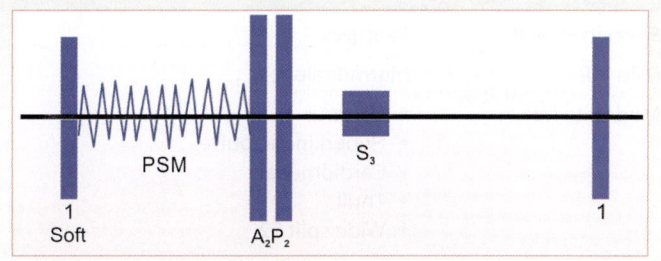

### Q. What are the causes of soft murmur in MR?

**Low flow states**
- LV dysfunction
- PAH

**Etiology of the MR**
- MR in acute myocardial infarction
- MR in LV dilatation
- MR due to papillary muscle dysfunction

**Associated valve lesions**
Mitral stenosis.

**Miscellaneous**
- Obesity
- COPD.

### Q. Describe the characteristic murmur of MR.

- High-pitched, blowing, and usually holosystolic/pansystolic loudest at the apex
- Plateau-shaped, best heard with diaphragm of stethoscope
- Commonly radiates widely over the precordium and into the axilla and left interscapular area (if anterior leaflets involved as in rheumatic) or radiating to base (if posterior leaflets involved). Conducted to entire vertebral column in large left atrium
- It may be accompanied by a thrill.
- No beat to beat variation of the murmur in MR with ventricular premature beats (beat to beat variation present in aortic stenosis)
- Best heard in left lateral position with breath held in expiration

### Q. What is the significance of S3 and S4 in MR?

Presence of S3 and S4 rules out significant associated MS. S4 is never found in chronic rheumatic MR. S4 is common in acute MR.

### Q. List the complications of MR.

- Cardiac failure
- Infective endocarditis
- AF
- PAH
- Embolism
- Recurrent infections

### Q. How do you assess the severity of MR?
Refer **Table 2.19**.

**Table 2.19:** Severity of MR.

| Severity of MR | Features |
|---|---|
| Mild MR | Murmur alone |
| Moderate MR | ◆ Murmur<br>◆ Hyperkinetic pulse<br>◆ Cardiomegaly<br>◆ Thrill<br>◆ Wide split S2 |
| Severe MR | ◆ Murmur<br>◆ Hyperkinetic pulse<br>◆ Cardiomegaly<br>◆ Thrill<br>◆ Wide split S2<br>◆ LVS3<br>◆ Flow MDM at mitral area |

### Q. What is the importance of dynamic auscultation in MR?
Refer **Table 2.20**.

**Table 2.20:** Importance of dynamic auscultation in MR.

| Procedure | RHD-MR | MVP-MR |
|---|---|---|
| Standing | Decrease | Increase |
| Sitting | Increase | Decrease |
| Isometric exercise | Increase | Decrease |

### Q. What are the differences between MR and AS?
Refer **Table 2.21**.

**Table 2.21:** Differences between MR and AS.

| Feature | Mitral regurgitation | Aortic stenosis |
|---|---|---|
| Pulse | Hyperkinetic pulse, AF common | Anacrotic pulse |
| BP | Normal to wide pulse pressure | Reduced pulse pressure |
| JVP | Normal JVP | Prominent a waves |
| APEX | Forceful hyperdynamic apex | Heaving apex |
| Thrill | Systolic thrill apex | Systolic thrill 2nd Right ICS |
| LPH | LPH present | Absent |
| S1 | Soft S1 | Normal S1 |
| S2 | Normal S2 | Soft A2 |
| Split of S2 | Wide split | Paradoxical split |
| Ejection Click | absent | Present |
| S4 | Only in acute MR | Present |
| Murmur | PSM mitral area<br>No change with PVC | ESM aortic area<br>Changes after PVC |

### Q. What are the differences between MR and TR?
Refer **Table 2.22**.

**Table 2.22:** Mitral regurgitation (MR) versus tricuspid regurgitation (TR).

| MR | TR |
|---|---|
| Hyperkinetic pulse | Normal pulse |
| Normal JVP | Prominent V wave |

| MR | TR |
|---|---|
| Forceful apex | RV apex |
| P2 not palpable | P2 palpable |
| Systolic thrill at apex present | Absent |
| LPH present | LPH present |
| PSM mitral area—conducted to axilla | PSM tricuspid area—increasing with inspiration |
| Hepatic pulsations absent | Present |

### Q. What are the differences between MR and VSD?
Refer **Table 2.23**.

**Table 2.23:** MR versus VSD without PAH.

| MR | VSD without PAH |
|---|---|
| Systolic thrill apex | Thrill LLSB |
| LPH present | LPH absent |
| PSM mitral area | PSM LLSB |

### Q. What are the differences between MR and HOCM?
Refer **Table 2.24**.

**Table 2.24:** MR versus HOCM.

| MR | HOCM |
|---|---|
| Forceful apex | Double apex |
| Wide split S2 | Paradoxical S2 |
| S4 rare | Common |
| PSM mitral area conducted to axilla | ESM LLSB |
| PSM decreased with standing and increased with isometric exercise | PSM increased with standing and decreased with isometric exercise |
| Associated valvular heart disease present | Absent |

### Q. What are the ECG findings in MR?
- Left atrial enlargement—p mitrale in II and positive Morris index in VI
- LVH (33%)
- RVH (15%)
- Atrial fibrillation

### Q. What are the X-ray findings in MR?
- **Left atrial enlargement**
  - Enlargement of left atrial appendage
  - Shadow in shadow appearance
  - Elevation of left bronchus
  - Esophageal compression in barium swallow
- **Cardiomegaly**
- **Pulmonary field changes** (less prominent)
  - Inverted mustache appearance of prominent upper lobe veins
  - Kerley B lines
  - Bats wing (pulmonary edema)
  - Peripheral hypertranslucency of pulmonary hypertension
- Calcification of mitral valve
- Differentiate between MS and MR by CXR finding **(Table 2.25)**

**Table 2.25:** Differentiate between MS and MR by CXR finding.

|  | MS | MR |
|---|---|---|
| LAE | Present | Marked |
| Cardiomegaly | Minimal | Marked |
| Lung field changes | More Prominent | Less Prominent |

### Q. What are the ECHO findings in MR?
- Regurgitant mitral value
- Left atrium, LV dilated
- Etiology of MR (2D echo)

### Q. Discuss the management in MR.
- **Prophylaxis** of rheumatic fever avoidance/correction of **precipitating factors**
  - Exertion
  - Anemia
  - Thyroid disease
  - Infective endocarditis
  - Rheumatic fever
  - Arrhythmias
- **Afterload reduction** with ACE inhibitors or nifedipine
- **Symptomatic** patients with diuretics and digoxin
- **Atrial fibrillation**
  - Rate reduction
  - Anticoagulants
  - Cardioversion
- **Anticoagulants**
  - Patients with atrial fibrillation
  - Embolic episodes

### Q. What are the indicators of mitral valve replacement?
- Class III/IV symptoms
- Severe MR with LV dysfunction of LV ejection fraction <60% or LV end-systolic diameter >40 mm by echo.

### Q. What are the indicators of MV repair (valvuloplasty/annuloplasty)?
- MVP
- Mitral valve annular calcification
- Chordal rupture
- Papillary muscle rupture

### Q. What are the causes and clinical presentation of acute MR?
- Myocardial infarction
- MVP
- Infective endocarditis
- Trauma
- Prosthetic valve dysfunction

**Presentation of acute MR**
- Acute pulmonary edema
- Hypotension

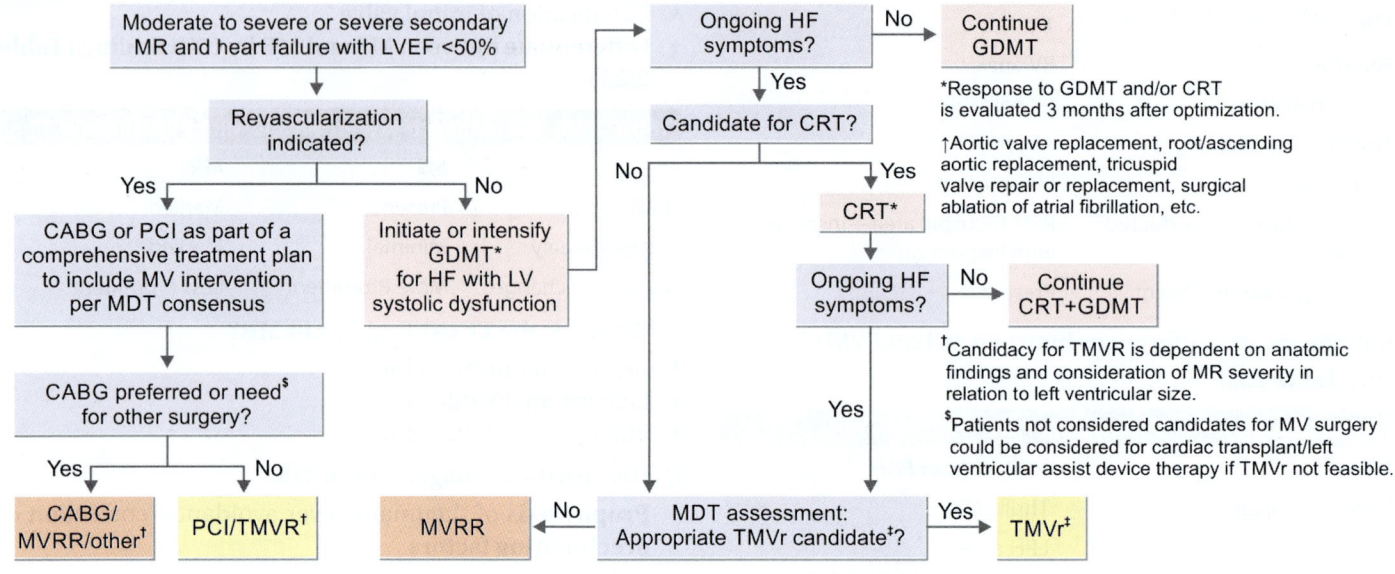

**Fig. 2.15:** Intervention for symptomatic secondary MR.
(AAD: anti-arrhythmic drug; AF: atrial fibrillation; CABG: coronary artery bypass graft; CRT: cardiac resynchronization therapy; GDMT: guideline-directed management and therapy; HF: heart failure; LVEF: left ventricular ejection fraction; MDT: multidisciplinary team; MR: mitral regurgitation; MV: mitral valve; MVRR: mitral valve repair or replacement; PCI: percutaneous coronary intervention; TMVr: transcatheter mitral valve repair)

**Signs of acute MR**
- Hypotension
- Absence of cardiomegaly
- PAH
- LVS4
- Decrescendo murmur

**Q. What is the intervention for symptomatic secondary MR?**
Refer **Figure 2.15**.

**Q. List the difference between acute MR and chronic MR.**
Refer **Table 2.26**.

**Table 2.26:** Differences between acute and chronic mitral regurgitation (MR).

| Characters | Acute MR | Chronic MR |
|---|---|---|
| Pulse | Alternans | High volume |
| Atrial fibrillation | Absent | + |
| Jugular venous pressure (JVP) | Grossly elevated | Mild elevation |
| Cardiomegaly | Absent | Present |
| Pulmonary hypertension | Very severe | Variable |
| S1 | Normal | Soft |
| S2 | Present | +/− |
| S4 | Present | Can never be present |
| Murmur | Late systolic | Pan systolic |

**Q. What are the signs of papillary muscle dysfunction producing MR?**
- LV S4 is classical
- Late systolic murmur or pan systolic murmur with late systolic accentuation.

**Q. What is the influence of associated AR on MR?**
- Increased symptoms due to MR
- Loud S3
- Loud PSM
- Loud flow MDM

**Q. What are the signs which reveal the dominant lesion in combined MS and MR?**
Refer **Table 2.27**.

**Table 2.27:** Clinical assessment of the dominance of lesions in the presence of combined mitral stenosis and mitral regurgitation.

| Parameter | Predominant mitral regurgitation | Predominant mitral stenosis |
|---|---|---|
| Pulse volume | High | Low |
| Blood pressure | Wide pulse pressure | Narrow pulse pressure |
| Cardiomegaly | ++ | − |
| $S_1$ | Soft | Loud |
| LVS3 | ++ | − |
| Mid-diastolic murmur | Short | Long, loud with presystolic accentuation |

### Q. List MVP syndromes.

- Mitral valve prolapse (MVP) is an abnormal movement of one or both of the mitral valve leaflets >2 mm beyond annular plane into the left atrium during systole with or without mitral regurgitation.
- MVP syndrome is also called as systolic click-murmur syndrome/Barlow's syndrome.
- MVP is one of the more common causes of mild mitral regurgitation
  **Figure 2.16** shows the dynamic auscultation in MVP MR.

### Q. What are differences between mitral regurgitation (MR) due to mitral valve prolapse and that due to rheumatic heart disease?

Refer **Table 2.28**.

**Table 2.28:** Differences between mitral regurgitation (MR) due to mitral valve prolapse and that due to rheumatic heart disease.

| Characters | Mitral valve prolapse MR | Rheumatic heart disease MR |
|---|---|---|
| Leaflets affected | Any | Posterior |
| $S_1$ | Loud | Soft |
| Click | Midsystolic click | No |
| Murmur | Midsystolic | Holosystolic |
| Squatting and isometric handgrip | Decrease murmur | Increase murmur |
| Association | Atrial septal defect (ASD) and polycystic kidney disease | Mitral stenosis |

### Q. What are the chances of mitral re-stenosis?

- Mitral re-stenosis occurs at a rate of 2% per year post-valvotomy—10% at the end of 5 years.
- The cause of re-stenosis is persistent rheumatic activity.

### Q. What is Carpentier classification of MR?

**Carpentier classification** divides **mitral valve regurgitation** into three types based on leaflet motion (**Fig. 2.17**):

- **Type I:** Normal leaflet motion
  - Annular dilation, leaflet perforation
  - Regurgitation jet directed centrally

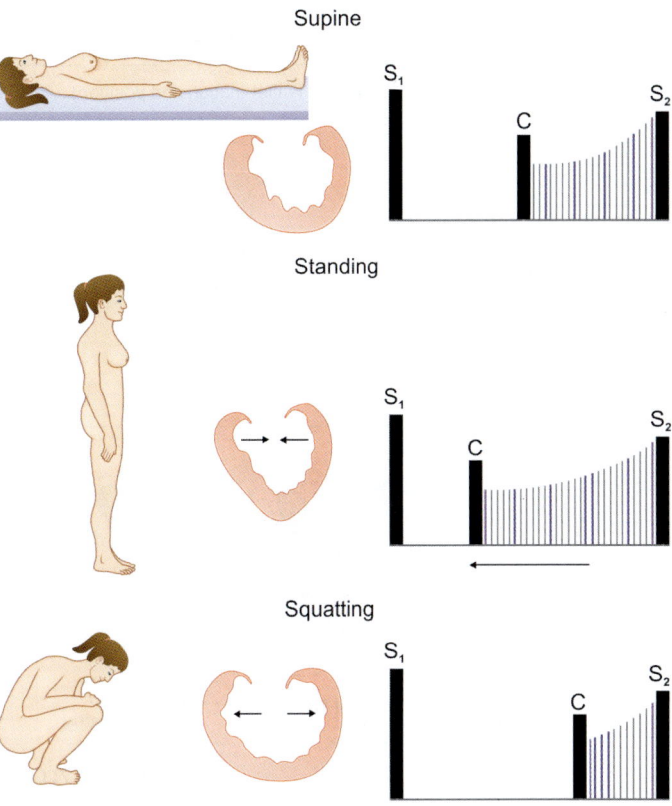

**Fig. 2.16:** Dynamic auscultation in MVP MR.

- **Type II:** Excessive leaflet motion
  - Papillary muscle rupture, chordal rupture, redundant chordae
  - Eccentric jet, directed away from involved leaflet
- **Type III:** Restricted leaflet motion
  - **IIIa:** Leaflet motion restricted in both systole and diastole
    - Rheumatic heart disease
    - Jet may be centrally or eccentrically directed
  - **IIIb:** Leaflet motion restricted in diastole
    - Papillary muscle dysfunction, left ventricular dilation
    - Jet may be centrally or eccentrically directed

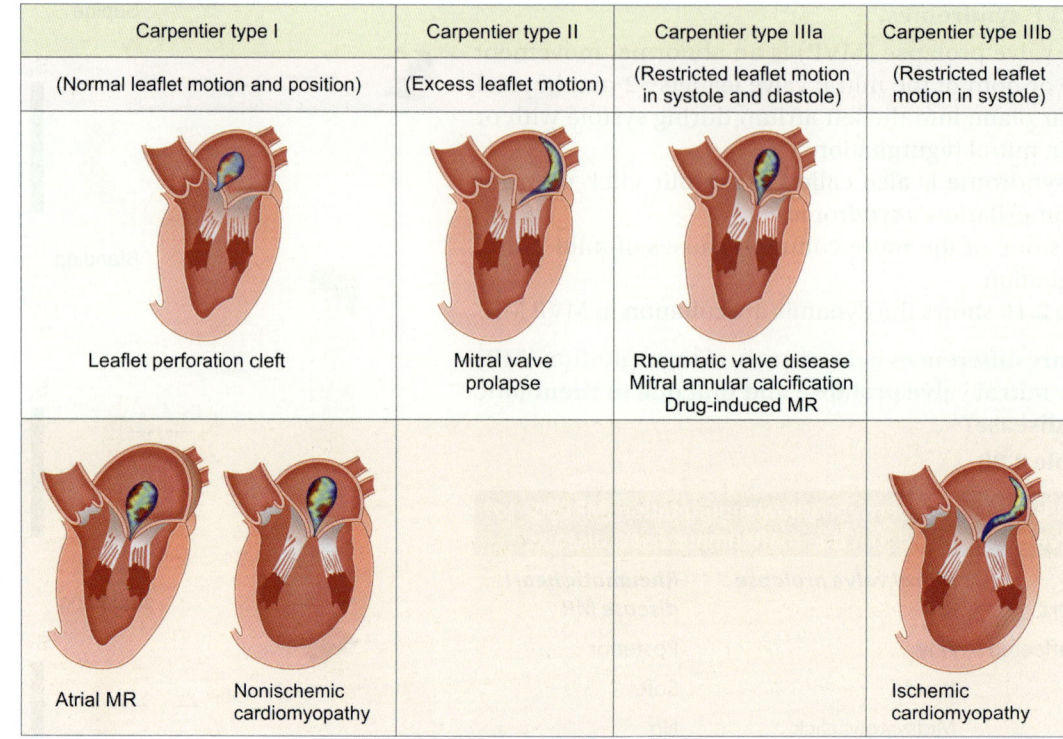

**Fig. 2.17:** Carpentier classification.

## Case 3: Aortic Stenosis

*Brief History*
Elderly male, with history of dyspnea on exertion and episodes of syncope.

*Examination*
- Patient is conscious, cooperative
- Height—178 cm
- Weight—81 kg
- BMI—25.56 kg/m²
- Pulse—68/min, regular in rhythm, pulsus parvus et tardus (character), all peripheral pulses felt, no radioradial or radiofemoral delay
- BP—110/90 mm Hg in right arm, supine position, no postural drop
- Respiratory rate—20/min, abdominothoracic type
- Temperature—afebrile (98.6°)
- JVP—not elevated
- No pallor, icterus, cyanosis, clubbing, lymphadenopathy, pedal edema
- No peripheral signs of infective endocarditis

*Systemic Examination*
CVS examination
Inspection
No precordial bulge, apical impulse not seen, no other pulsations seen.

*Palpation*
Apical impulse palpable in left 5 ICS in the left lateral position in the midclavicular line, heaving type, no parasternal heave.

*Percussion*
Left 2nd intercostal space—resonant.

*Auscultation*
- Mitral area—S1, S2 heard—normal intensity, long systolic murmur heard, Grade 3, no radiation.
- Tricuspid and pulmonary area—S1, S2 heard, no murmur.
- Aortic area—S1, S2 present, normal intensity. Harsh ejection systolic murmur present, Grade 3/6 intensity, best heard in the sitting and bending forward position with the diaphragm of the stethoscope, with breath held in expiration. The murmur is conducted to the carotids.

*Respiratory System*
Features of COPD present (barrel-shaped chest, AP/transverse ratio—1:1, chest expansion—3 cm, cardiac dullness—obliterated).

*Provisional Diagnosis*
Acquired valvular heart disease, aortic stenosis, moderate severity. Etiology—degenerative or bicuspid aortic valve; no signs of CHF or infective endocarditis; patient in sinus rhythm (NYHA Class 3).

## DISCUSSION

**Q. What is pulsus parvus et tardus?**

Slow rising, late peaking and low volume pulse. 'Parvus' means low volume and 'tardus' means slow or late.

**Q. What is pulsus bisferiens?**

High volume, double beating pulse. It is more easily detected in the brachial or radial artery than in the carotid artery.

**Causes:** Aortic regurgitation, combined AS and AR, HOCM. A bisferiens contour occasionally may be detected in high output states in subjects with a normal heart.

**Q. What is difference in the arm and leg pressure?**

The arterial pulse wave contour changes as the distance from the aortic valve increases. The systolic upstroke becomes steeper, and peak systolic pressure is greater in the distal arteries, although mean arterial pressure remains constant.

A progressive increase in systolic pressure normally occurs as the point of measurement is moved peripherally from the central aorta. Direct recordings of femoral and brachial artery pressures (systolic, diastolic and mean) in adults and children and indirect measurement of popliteal and brachial artery pressures have demonstrated that mean pressures are equal at these sites.

Systolic leg pressures may exceed arm pressures by as much as 20 mm Hg. However, it is believed to be due to a sphygmomanometric artifact.

**Q. What is the normal arm span in adults?**

Arm span or reach (**Fig. 2.18**) is the physical measurement of the length from one end of an individual's arms (measured at the fingertips) to the other when raised parallel to the ground at shoulder height with a 90° angle. The average reach correlates to the person's height.

**Q. When is arm span significant?**

When the arm span is **more than 5 cm** than the height/length then it is significant.

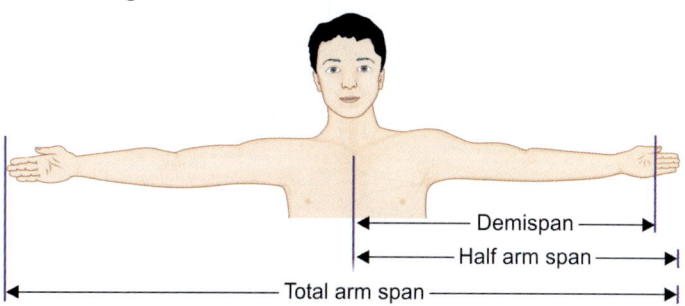

**Fig. 2.18:** Arm span in adults.

**Q. Why do you measure upper segment/lower segment ratio? What is the normal valve?**

**Upper segment:** Measured from the top of the head to the upper border of the symphysis pubis.

**Lower segment:** Measured from the top of symphysis pubis to the soles of stature = US + LS = distance between the TIPS of the fingers of the two outstretched hands.

Normally the span and stature are about equal and so are the upper and lower measurements **(Fig. 2.19)**.

**In premature epiphyseal union** (e.g., adrenal cortex tumor)— stature > span.

**In delayed epiphyseal union** (e.g., Marfan's, homocystinuria, Klinefelter's, hypogonadism—span > stature.

**Q. What are the cardiac lesions expected in Marfan's syndrome?**
- Dilatation of ascending aorta + AR
- Dissection of ascending aorta
- MVP + MR
- Calcification of mitral annulus
- Dilatation of main pulmonary artery in the absence of valvular or peripheral PS
- Thoracic or abdominal aortic dissection/dilatation.

**Q. What is the importance of pulse pressure?**
- Pulse pressure is an objective measurement of pulse volume.
- Pulse pressure = SBP-DBP
- Normal pulse pressure is 30–60 mm Hg
- Small volume pulse <30, e.g., AS
- Large volume pulse >60, e.g., AR

**Q. What does parasternal heave suggest? Demonstrate parasternal heaving? Which part of the hand is used?**
- Left parasternal heave suggests right ventricular hypertrophy and left atrial hypertrophy

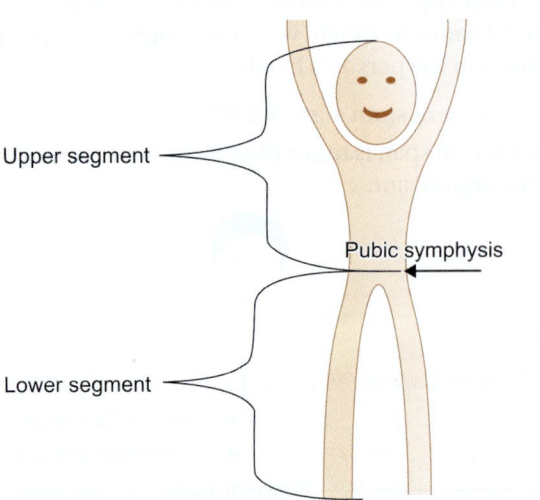

**Fig. 2.19:** Upper segment/lower segment ratio.

- It is done using the HEEL of the hand with fingers cocked upwards.
- Ulnar border of the hand also can be used.
- It is better **seen** than felt.

**Q. What other ways you can demonstrate parasternal heave?**
- A pen can be kept on the left parasternal border and it movements observed.
- Parasternal heave is better **seen** than felt.

**Q. What is the importance of left 2nd ICS dullness?**
Dull note in left 2nd ICS is heard in:
- Dilated pulmonary artery
- PDA
- Enlarged left atrial appendage.

**Q. What is S3? Significance of hearing S3.**
S3 is produced by the initial rapid filling of the ventricle in diastole. It is a protodiastolic sound or ventricular gallop.

**Causes of pathological S3**
- High output states
- ASD, VSD, PDA
- Regurgitation lesions AR, MR, TR
- Hypertrophic cardiomyopathy
- Ischemic heart disease
- Constrictive pericarditis
- Systemic hypertension
- Pulmonary hypertension

**Q. What is the difference between LV-S3 and RV-S3?**
Refer **Table 2.29**.

| Table 2.29: Difference between RV-S3 and LV-S3. | | |
|---|---|---|
| Features | RV-S3 | LV-S3 |
| Site | Tricuspid area | Mitral area |
| Accentuates with | **Inspiration** | Expiration |

**Q. What is S4? What is the significance of hearing S4?**
- S4 is caused by atrial contraction against a STIFF ventricle (diastolic dysfunction of the ventricle).
- S4 is also known as presystolic gallop or atrial gallop
- Causes of pathological S4
  - Hypertrophic cardiomyopathy
  - Systemic hypertension leading to LVH
  - Coronary artery disease

**Q. Which do you hear in young adults—S3 or S4?**
- S3 is heard in young adults <40 years
- S4 is recordable, but inaudible in young adults.

**Q. Name the causes of left ventricular hypertrophy.**
- **Concentric LVH**
  - Aortic stenosis
  - Systemic hypertension
  - Idiopathic hypertrophic subaortic stenosis (IHSS)
  - Coarctation of aorta

- **Eccentric LVH**
  - MI or AR
  - IHD
  - Severe anemia
  - Thyrotoxicosis
  - Cardiomyopathy—dilated
  - VSD, PDA

### Q. What are the causes of AS?

**Young adults**
- Congenital valvular
- Congenital supravalvular
- Congenital subvalvular

**Middle aged**
- Bicuspid aortic valve
- Rheumatic AS

**Elderly**
- Bicuspid aortic valve
- Rheumatic AS
- Senile degenerative AS

### Q. What is the normal aortic valve area?
- Normal valve area 3–4 cm$^2$
- **Severe AS:** <1 cm$^2$

### Q. What are the symptoms of AS?
*The SAD triad—Syncope, Angina, Dyspnea*
- Exertional angina
- Exertional syncope
- Exertional dyspnea

### Q. How do you classify AS?
Refer **Box 2.4**.

### Q. What is the mechanism of angina in AS?
**Imbalance in the supply demand ratio**
- Increased demand due to LV hypertrophy
- Decreased supply due to decreased coronary perfusion gradient caused by increased LV EDP

### Q. What is mechanism of syncope in AS?
Decreased cerebral blood flow
- Systemic vasodilation against a fixed cardiac output
- Transient atrial/ventricular arrhythmias
- Transient AV blocks
- Vasodepressor response due to baroreceptor malfunction

### Q. What is the mechanism of dyspnea in AS?
LV dysfunction.

### Correlate symptoms with survival in AS (Fig. 2.20)
- Angina—5 years
- Syncope—3 years
- Dyspnea—2 years
- CCF—1.5 years

---

**Box 2.4:** Classification and etiology of aortic stenosis.

**Valvular aortic stenosis:**
- **Acquired:** Rheumatic aortic stenosis (young adults, middle-aged, elderly), **calcific aortic valvular disease** (CAVD—in middle-aged to elderly), systemic lupus erythematosus (SLE), Fabry disease, chronic kidney disease, Paget's disease of bone, rheumatoid arthritis, infective endocarditis, senile degenerative aortic stenosis (middle-aged to elderly), previous radiation exposure, homozygous familial hypercholesterolemia, and ochronosis
- **Congenital:** Congenital aortic stenosis (infants, children, adolescents), bicuspid aortic valve (BAV), calcification and fibrosis of congenitally **bicuspid aortic valve** (young adults to middle-aged)

**Subvalvular aortic stenosis:**
- Membranous diaphragm
- Hypertrophic cardiomyopathy
- Congenital subvalvular aortic stenosis (infants, children and adolescents)

**Supravalvular aortic stenosis:**
- Hourglass constriction of aorta
- Congenital supravalvular aortic stenosis (infants, children and adolescents)
- Williams syndrome

**Williams syndrome:** Characterized by Elfin facies, supravalvular aortic stenosis, idiopathic hypercalcemia, mental retardation, and behavioral profile. On examination, the right upper limb blood pressure may be a higher than the left upper limb and the pulse volume on the right arm better than left. This is called *Coanda effect* **Shone's complex:** It is a rare combination of four left-sided congenital cardiac anomalies including parachute mitral valve, supravalvular ring, coarctation of the aorta, and subaortic obstruction.

### Q. Mention the other presentation in AS.
- Cardiac failure
- Infective endocarditis—especially in young patients with mild valve deformity
- Sudden death
- CVA/TIA
- GI bleeding = Angiodysplasia especially in patients with calcific AS—**Heyde's syndrome** associated with acquired von Willebrand syndrome (AVWS).

### Q. When do you suspect associated mitral valve disease in AS?
- Duration of dyspnea >5 years
- Atrial fibrillation
- PAH
- RVF

### Q. List the characteristic signs you would get in AS.
- Anacrotic pulse
- Low pulse pressure
- Heaving apex beat
- Basal systolic thrill

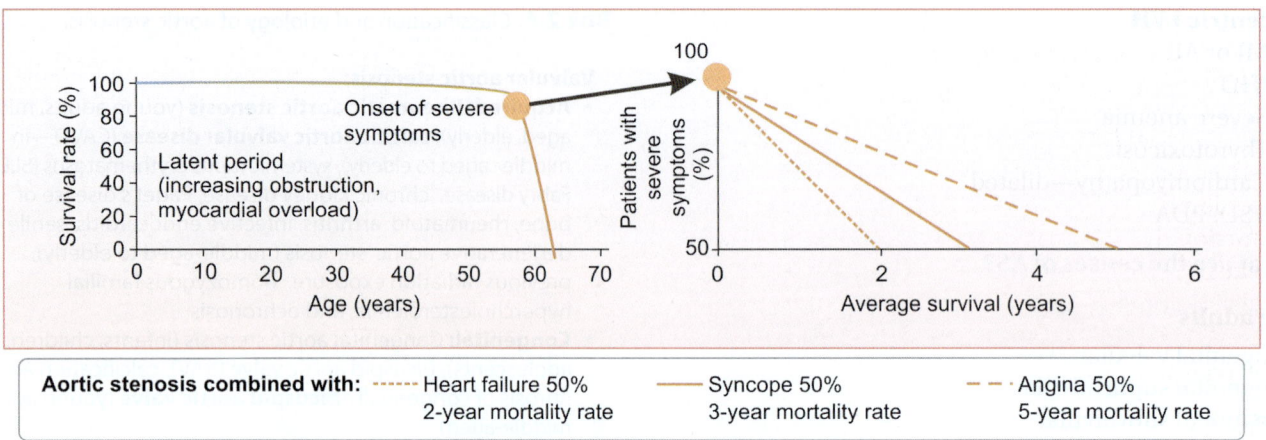

**Fig. 2.20:** Symptoms with survival in AS.

- Paradoxical split
- LV S4
- EC at apex and right 2nd ICS.
- High-pitched rough crescendo-decrescendo ejection systolic murmur at the aortic area/apex conducted to the carotids
- Severe AS produces "Dresden China" look—asthenic appearance with pale skin and light flush.

### Q. What are the pulse abnormalities you may get in AS?

- Anacrotic pulse (severe AS)
- Pulsus parvus et tardus—slow rising pulse with a delayed sustained peak
- Carotid shudder (anacrotic notch with coarse systolic vibrations).
- Pulsus bisferiens if associated with AR
- Coanda effect in supravalvular AS
- Normal pulse if there is coexistent AR, hypertension (HTN)

### Q. What are the BP abnormalities you may get in AS?

- Low pulse pressure
- Systolic pressure >200 mm Hg excludes severe AS
- Systolic BP >140 mm Hg—associated AR/hypertension

### Q. What are the JVP abnormalities you may get in AS?

- Usually normal
- Prominent a waves—Bernheim effect

### Q. What is Bernheim effect?

Septal bulge into the right ventricle producing prominent a waves in JVP. Due to the hypertrophied bulging septum producing decreased RV compliance. Also seen in HOCM **(Figs. 2.21A to C)**.

### Q. What is reverse Bernheim effect?

- Septal bulge into the left ventricle
- Seen in:
  - ASD

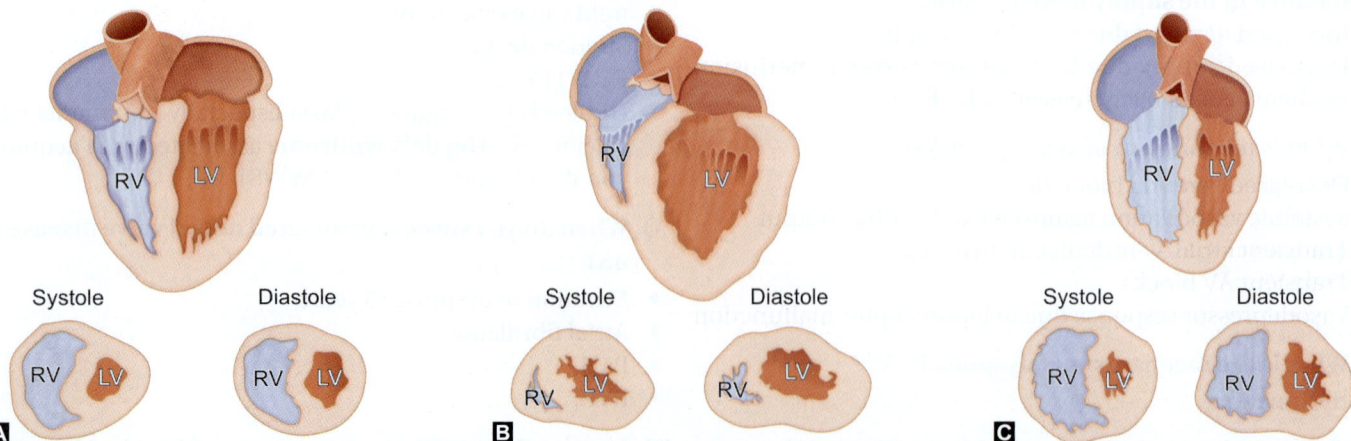

**Figs. 2.21A to C:** An illustration of the spectrum of ventricular interdependence. (A) Depicting the normal concavity of the IVS toward the LV throughout the cardiac cycle; (B) Outline of the original description of Bernheim effect wherein concentric LVH detrimentally affects the RV function owing to exaggerated rightward movement of the IVS; (C) Reverse-Bernheim effect wherein RV pressure or volume overload tends to result in septal flattening and a consequential "D"-shaped LV in setting of RV dysfunction.
(IVS: interventricular septum; LV: left ventricle; LVH: left ventricular hypertrophy; RV: right ventricle).

- RV myocardial infarction
- Pulmonary thromboembolism
- Cardiac tamponade

### Q. Mention the factors which affect the pulse in AS.
- Hypertension
- Hypovolemia
- LV function
- Presence of PAH
- Mitral valve disease
- Age
- Aortic regurgitation

### Q. Mention the factors which will apparently normalize the pulse in AS.
- Hypertension
- Elderly
- Presence of AR

### Q. Mention the factors which will apparently exaggerate the low pulse volume in AS.
- Hypovolemia
- Cardiac failure
- Presence of PAH
- Associated valve lesions—severe MS

### Q. What is the comment about the apex beat in AS?
Undisplaced heaving apex. Displaced in associated aortic regurgitation or mitral regurgitation and in LV dysfunction.

### Q. What are the palpatory findings in AS?
- Heaving apex
- Palpable S4
- Systolic thrill 2nd Right ICS

### Q. Comment on S1 in AS.
- Usually normal/decreased
- Due to the partial closure of the mitral valve in presystole. Loud S1—associated MS
- Comment on A2 in AS
- Loud A2—pliable valve especially congenital AS
- Soft A2—rigid calcified valve

### Q. Comment on split in AS.
- Normal split
- Paradoxical split
- Single S2

### Q. Name the conditions of normal split in AS.
- Mild-moderate AS
- Split is normal in congenital AS even when severe

### Q. What is the significance of paradoxical split in AS?
Refer **Figure 2.22**.
- Signifies severe AS in the absence of LBBB/LV dysfunction.
- Other causes producing paradoxical split
  - LBBB

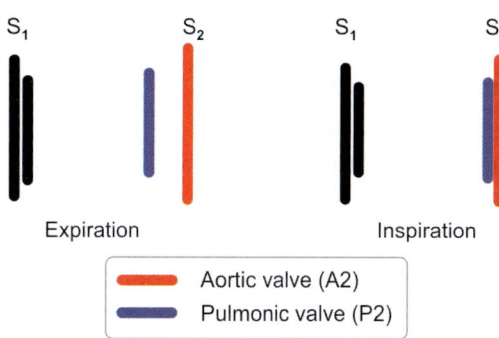

**Fig. 2.22:** Paradoxical split S2.

  - HOCM
  - Severe AR
  - Large PDA
- Seen only in 25% of *elderly* with severe AS
- Significance of single S2 in AS
- Seen in 66% of elderly with severe AS
- Signifies either absent A2 or masked P2 by the murmur

**Basis of paradoxical split**

Prolonged LV electromechanical systole producing delayed A2.

### Q. Where do you get a paradoxical split?
- LBBB
- AS
- HOCM
- Hypertension
- Large PDA
- Severe AR
- LV dysfunction

### Q. What is the significance of S4 in AS?
Presence of S4 is indicative of severe AS except in CAD/hypertension. However, palpable S4 always indicates severe AS.

### Q. What are the characteristics and importance of aortic ejection click (AEC)?
- High-pitched sound produced by the snapping open of the stenotic thickened aortic valve
- Indicates valvular AS with mobile valves
- Especially common in congenital AS and bicuspid aortic valve
- No correlation with severity
- Disappears with valve calcification
- Rare in the elderly

**Features of Aortic EC**
- 0.06 sec after S1
- Best heard at the apex/aortic area
- No variation with respiration
- High pitched

**Q. What are the features identifying the severity of AS?**

**Criteria to say severe AS**
- Pulsus parvus et tardus
- Systolic BP and pulse pressure may be reduced
- Palpable thrill or carotid shudder in the carotids
- Prominent 'a' wave
- Single S2 or paradoxical splitting of S2
- Louder and later peaking ejection systolic murmur

**Q. How do you assess severity of AS?**
- According to S2 **(Table 2.30)**

**Table 2.30:** Severity of aortic stenosis.

| | |
|---|---|
| Mild stenosis | A2 followed by P2 |
| Moderate stenosis | A2 is delayed giving rise to single S2 |
| Severe stenosis | Reverse/paradoxical splitting of S2 (P2-A2). |

According to valve area **(Table 2.31)**

**Table 2.31:** Severity of AS based on valve area.

| | |
|---|---|
| Normal aortic valve area | 3 cm$^2$–4 cm$^2$ |
| Severe aortic stenosis | <1 cm$^2$/m$^2$ body surface area |
| Critical aortic stenosis | <0.5 cm$^2$/m$^2$ body surface area |

Long murmur and late peaking of murmur indicate severe AS.
- According to the gradient across aortic valve **(Table 2.32)**

**Table 2.32:** Severity of AS based on gradient.

| Severity | Gradient |
|---|---|
| Normal | 0 mm Hg |
| Mild AS | <25 mm Hg |
| Moderate AS | 25–40 mm Hg |
| Severe AS | >40 mm Hg |

Presence of S4 and **absent A2** indicate severe AS.
- Presence of S3 in AS means severe systolic dysfunction and elevated filling pressure **(Table 2.33)**.

**Table 2.33:** Severity of AS based on clinical signs.

| Severity | Features |
|---|---|
| Mild AS | Murmur |
| Moderate | ◆ Anacrotic pulse<br>◆ Long murmur<br>◆ Late peaking<br>◆ Loud murmur<br>◆ Thrill |
| Severe AS | ◆ Anacrotic pulse<br>◆ Long murmur<br>◆ Late peaking<br>◆ Loud murmur<br>◆ Thrill<br>◆ Paradoxical split S2<br>◆ LVS4 |

**Q. What is classical murmur in AS?**

High-pitched rough crescendo-decrescendo ejection systolic murmur in the aortic area conducted to the carotids. Heard best with the patient leaning forward and the breath held in expiration. May be heard at the apex also.

**Q. What is Gallavardin phenomenon?**
- Selective line of progression of high-pitched components of the ESM towards the apex with increased/same intensity. Especially in elderly patients.
- Due to periodic wake phenomenon
- Seen both in aortic stenosis and aortosclerosis.

**Q. What is the effect of other valvular diseases on AS?**

Refer **Table 2.34**.

**Table 2.34:** Effect of other valvular diseases on AS.

| Effect of MS on AS | Effect of MR on AS |
|---|---|
| ◆ Decreased severity of angina and syncope<br>◆ Atrial fibrillation<br>◆ Early onset PAH<br>◆ Decreased length and intensity of ejection systolic murmur | ◆ Decreased severity of angina and syncope<br>◆ Atrial fibrillation<br>◆ Early onset PAH<br>◆ Decreased length and intensity of ejection systolic murmur |
| **Effect of AR on AS**<br>◆ Pulse may be normal<br>◆ Pulse pressure may be normal<br>◆ Apex may be normal in character<br>◆ Increased length and intensity of ejection systolic murmur | |

**Q. Mention the clinical picture in AS with failure.**
- Low pulse volume is exaggerated
- Pulse pressure is lower
- Heaving character of apex in exaggerated
- Murmur becomes softer and shorter

**Q. What are the causes for absent murmur in AS?**
- **Low flow states**
  - Cardiac failure
  - PAH
- **Additional valve involvement**
  - MS
  - MR
- **Miscellaneous**
  - COPD
  - Obesity

**Q. What are the ECG findings in AS?**
- LVH ± strain
- Pseudoinfarction pattern—loss of "r" waves in precordial leads
- Left atrial overload
- Atrial fibrillation in 10–15%
- AV conduction defects and IVCD in 5% of calcific AS due to extension of calcium to conduction system
- Ventricular arrhythmias

**Q. What are the X-ray findings in AS?**
- Normal sized heart with post-stenotic dilatation. Cardiomegaly—associated AR/cardiac failure. Left atrial enlargement—associated MS
- Calcification of aortic valve

**Q. What are the ECHO findings in AS?**
- Stenotic valve
- LVH
- Pressure gradient

**Dobutamine stress echo:**
- **Severe AS:** Increase in gradient. No change in valve area
- **Mild AS:** Increase in valve area
- Also assesses contractile reserve and predicts improvement in LV function after surgery

**Q. What is the indication of coronary angiography in AS?**

**Cardiac catheterization in AS:** Coronary angiography is needed before aortic valve surgery and for detecting any associated coronary artery disease.

**Q. Discuss the management of AS.**

**Asymptomatic patients:** Irrespective of the severity of AS, asymptomatic patients have a good immediate prognosis. Hence, should be managed conservatively with regular review for assessment of symptoms and echocardiography.

**Medical treatment**
- Avoid vigorous physical activity in patients with severe AS.
- Diuretics decrease dyspnea but may also reduce cardiac output.
- **ACE inhibitors:** To be used with caution and given only if there is LV failure
- **Avoid beta-blockers:** Because they produce LV failure.
- **Vasodilators for other purposes, such as angina:** Be careful in titration as there will be no compensatory increase in cardiac output.
- **Atrial fibrillation:** Cardioversion can be tried.
- Infective endocarditis prophylaxis for those who have undergone valvular replacement
- Rheumatic fever prophylaxis

**Surgical indications**
- **Symptomatic patients:** Symptoms are a good index of severity in aortic stenosis, and all symptomatic patients should undergo aortic valve replacement.
- **Asymptomatic patients:** Surgical intervention for severe aortic stenosis is recommended in patients with:
  - Symptoms during an exercise test or with a fall of blood pressure
  - Left ventricular ejection fraction of <50%
  - Moderate-to-severe aortic stenosis undergoing CABG, surgery of the ascending aorta, or other cardiac valve

**Surgical aortic valve replacement (SAVR)**
- Historically the treatment of choice
- **Risks:** Periprocedural stroke, major bleeding.
- Mechanical valves require long-term anticoagulation, while bioprostheses only need 3 months aspirin.
- Mechanical valves are more suitable for younger patients, as they are more durable.

**Transcatheter aortic valve implantation (TAVI)**
- Initially only for higher risk patients unfit for SAVR, but increasingly used even in low-risk individuals.
- **Procedure:** Under anesthesia Entry can be transluminal, through the femoral (common) or subclavian artery, or transapical, which involves a mini-thoracotomy through the left ventricle. Balloon dilates the prosthetic valve, pushing the existing valve out of the way. Though sometimes called 'replacement' (TAVR), the old valve is not removed.
- **Risks versus SAVR:** Similar mortality, more aortic regurgitation, less periprocedural stroke, less major bleeding.
- **Postoperative antiplatelets:** Lifelong aspirin plus 3-6 months clopidogrel

**Balloon valvuloplasty**
- Can provide temporary relief (6-12 months).
- Only used as a bridge to TAVI in unstable patients

**ROSS procedure:** Replacement of deceased aortic valve by pulmonic valve and implantation of homograft instead of native pulmonic valve.

**Q. What is the rate of progression of aortic valve decreases?**
- Congestive heart failure: 50–60%.
- Infective endocarditis: 15–20%.
- Sudden death: 15–20%.
- Overall, on average, the aortic valve area decreases by approximately 0.1 cm$^2$/year and the peak instantaneous gradient increases by 10 mm Hg/year.
- However, in any individual patient, this is highly variable.

**Rapid versus slow progress**

There can be two distinct types of patients:
1. Those whose conditions progress slowly.
2. Others whose conditions progress rapidly.

There are no reliable clinical predictors to help us identify into which subgroup an individual patient will fall.

**Q. What are differences between aortic stenosis versus HOCM?**

Refer **Table 2.35** and **Figure 2.23**.

**Table 2.35:** Aortic stenosis versus HOCM.

|  | Aortic stenosis | HOCM |
|---|---|---|
| Pulse | Anacrotic pulse | Jerky |
| BP | Narrow pulse pressure | Normal |
| Apex | Heaving apex | Double apex |

|  | **Aortic stenosis** | **HOCM** |
|---|---|---|
| Thrill | Systolic thrill 2nd RICS | Absent |
| A2 | A2 soft | Normal |
| Click | AEC+ | Absent |
| Murmur | ESM aortic area Conducted to carotids | ESM LLB not conducted, PSM at apex |
| Association | Associated AR | Absent |

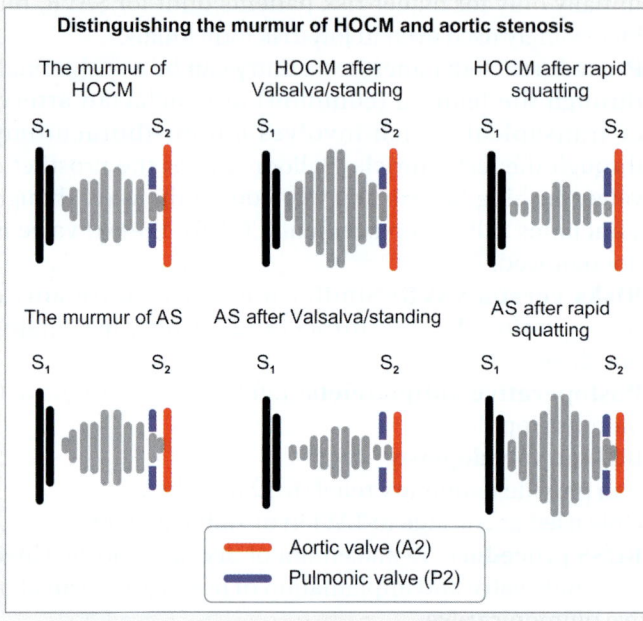

Fig. 2.23 Murmurs of HOCM versus aortic stenosis.

**Q. What are differences between aortic stenosis versus mitral regurgitation?**

Refer **Table 2.36**.

**Table 2.36:** MR versus AS.

|  | MR | AS |
|---|---|---|
| Pulse | Hyperkinetic pulse | Anacrotic pulse |
| BP | Normal/wide pulse pressure | Reduced pulse pressure |
| JVP | Normal JVP | A waves |
| Apex | Forceful hyperdynamic apex | Heaving apex |
| Thrill | Systolic thrill apex | Systolic thrill 2nd RICS |
| LPH | LPH present | Absent |
| S1 | Soft S1 | Normal S1 |
| S2 | Normal S2 | Soft A2 |
| S2 split | Wide split | Paradoxical split |
| Click | EC absent | Present |
| Murmur | PSM mitral area | ESM aortic area |
|  | Murmur radiates to axilla/base | Murmur conducts to carotid |
| Post-PVC | No change in murmur | Beat to beat change in murmur |

**Q. What are differences between aortic stenosis versus pulmonary stenosis?**

Refer **Table 2.37**.

**Table 2.37:** Aortic stenosis versus pulmonary stenosis.

|  | **Aortic stenosis** | **Pulmonary stenosis** |
|---|---|---|
| Pulse | Anacrotic pulse | Normal |
| BP | Narrow pulse pressure | Normal |
| JVP | Normal JVP | Prominent "a" wave |
| Apex | Heaving apex | Normal |
| thrill | Systolic thrill 2nd RICS | Systolic thrill 2nd LICS |
| LPH | LPH is absent | Present |
| S2 | A2 soft | P2 soft |
| S2 split | Paradoxical split | Wide mobile split |
| Click | AEC+ | PEC+ |
| Murmur | ESM aortic area conducted to carotids | ESM pulmonary area conducted to clavicle |
| AR | Associated AR | Absent |

**Q. What is the difference between aortic sclerosis and calcific aortic stenosis? How to differentiate between them clinically?**

Aortic sclerosis is typically seen in aged persons in which there is fibrosis, thickening, and calcification of bases of the aortic valve cusps. These give rise to harsh, ejection systolic murmur up to grade 4 in some cases. They can be differentiated from aortic stenosis by:

- No history of syncope, angina or heart failure
- Normal pulse volume, absent thrill
- No shift of apex, normal A2
- Murmur localized to aortic area
- Other features of atherosclerosis, such as thickened peripheral arteries, locomotor brachialis, suprasternal pulsations, xanthelasma, etc.
- **Valvular AS vs degenerative aortic sclerosis (Table 2.38)**
- About 25% patients are above the age 65 years and 40% over 85 years.
- Risk factors: Dyslipidemia, diabetes, hypertension, and smoking. Higher prevalence in Paget disease and end-stage renal disease (ESRD)
- There may be coexisting mitral annular calcification. Even if there is no AS, calcific aortic sclerosis increases cardiovascular death and MI by 50%.

**Q. What is the rate of aortic calcification after 60 years?**

Calcific aortic stenosis is invariable a progressive disease. Rate of progression from patient to patient is extraordinarily variable. Progression in the decrease in valve area is **0.1 cm$^2$ to as much as 0.3 cm$^2$ per year** while gradient may increase from less that 5 mm Hg to as much as 20 mm Hg per year. Survival is nearly normal as long as the patient is truly asymptomatic.

However, once the patient develops symptoms mortality rate soars to as much as 2% per month so that 3 years after the onset of symptoms, 75% of the patients with AS will have died unless the aortic valve is replaced.

**Q. What are the features of bicuspid aortic valve?**
- It is the most common congenital heart disease found in 1–2% of live births.
- Male-to-female ratio is 3:1.
- Some cases are inherited as autosomal dominant and *NOTCH1* gene mutation are found in some cases.
- **Associated conditions:** Other congenital cardiac diseases (e.g., dilatation of proximal ascending aorta secondary to abnormalities of the aortic media), coarctation of aorta, ventricular septal defect (VSD), and atrial septal defect (ASD).
- Calcification is common in adults with bicuspid aortic valve.
- **Auscultatory findings:** Ejection click best heard at the apex and may be associated murmurs of aortic stenosis or aortic regurgitation.
- **Diagnosis:** By echocardiography

**Complications**
- **Aortic regurgitation:** About 20% develop severe AR
- **Aortic stenosis:** Due to calcification and severe AS occurs after 50 years of age
- Infective endocarditis
- **Ascending aortic dilation:** Due to medial degeneration and is not related to severity of aortic stenosis
- **Aortic dissection:** Risk is increased by 5–9 times.

**Q. List the differences between valvular AS and degenerative aortosclerosis.**
Refer **Table 2.38**.

**Table 2.38:** Valvular AS versus degenerative AS.

| Feature | Valvular AS | Degenerative aortic sclerosis |
|---|---|---|
| Age | Young age | Old age |
| Pulse | Anacrotic, slow rising | Normal |
| Apex beat | Shifted down and outwards | Normally localized |
| Murmur | Radiates to carotids and lower down to apex | Localized |
| Other changes | Not present | Changes of old age, i.e., palpable vessels, arcus senilis, thin lax skin |
| Calcification | Uncommon | Common |
| Hypertension | Uncommon | Systolic hypertension common |

**Q. What are the features of supravalvular aortic stenosis, Williams syndrome?**
- Supravalvular aortic stenosis (SVAS) is an uncommon but well characterized congenital narrowing of the ascending aorta above the level of the coronary arteries. It can be a familial disorder, can occur sporadically, or associated with Williams syndrome (WS) which is a neurodevelopmental disorder affecting connective tissue and the central nervous system.
- Williams syndrome (also known as Williams-Beuren syndrome) is a autosomal dominant disorder associated with deletion of multiple genes on the long arm of chromosome 7.
- This patient presented to us with the characteristic 'elfin facies' having a large mouth, widely spaced eyes, mal-occluded teeth, patulous lips broad forehead with a short and upturned nose.
- Supravalvular aortic stenosis, pulmonary stenosis, ventricular septal defect and mitral valve prolapse are seen.
- **Infantile hypercalcemia**—the underlying abnormality causing hypercalcemia, which affects 5–50% of patients, remains unknown, but abnormal 1,25-dihydroxy vitamin D metabolism or decreased calcitonin production have been implicated.

**Q. What is Coanda effect?**
- In supravalvular aortic stenosis, the right upper limb blood pressure can be more than that in left upper limb **(anisosphygmia)** because the jet is directed towards the brachiocephalic artery. This is known as Coanda effect **(Figs. 2.24A and B)**.
- Coanda effect is the tendency of a jet stream to adhere to a wall, usually causing higher blood pressure in the right upper limb in supravalvular aortic stenosis.

**Q. How do you differentiate between valvular, subvalvular, and supravalvular AS?**
Refer **Table 2.39**.

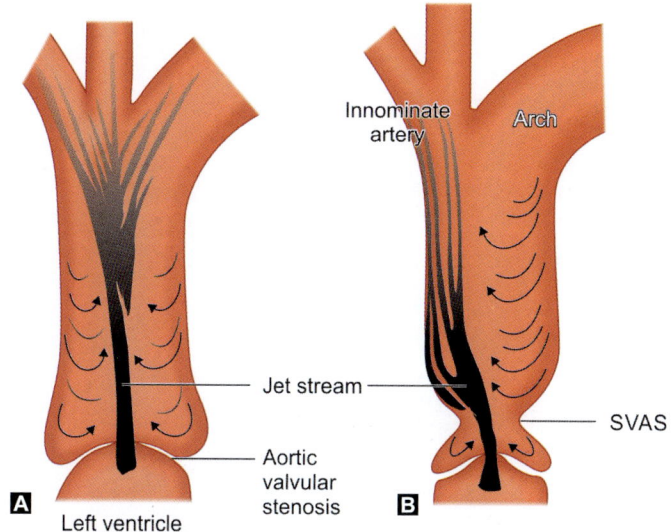

**Figs. 2.24A and B:** Coanda effect.

**Table 2.39:** Differences between valvular, subvalvular, and supravalvular AS.

| | Valvular AS | Subvalvular AS | Supravalvular AS | HOCM |
|---|---|---|---|---|
| Pulse | Low volume | Normal | Right UL > left UL (Coanda) | Spike and dome |
| Pulse volume after ectopic | Increases | | | Decreases (Brokenberg phenomenon) |
| A2 | Soft (degenerative/rheumatic) Loud (BAV) | Normal | Normal | Normal |
| S4 | Present | Absent | Absent | Rarely present |
| EC | Present (BAV) | Absent | Absent | Absent |
| Paradoxical split of S2 | Present | Absent | Absent | Rarely present |
| Murmur after Valsalva/standing | Decreases | Decreases | Decreases | Increases |
| Associated AR | + | | | |

### Q. What is Brokenberg phenomenon?

HOCM a paradoxical decrease in the arterial pulse pressure and an associated increase in the LV systolic pressure in the beat following a PVC, giving rise to the sign now called **Brockenbrough-Braunwald-Morrow**. After a PVC, there is a compensatory pause that causes an increase in diastolic filling time and therefore an increase in diastolic volume. The normal physiologic response to increased stretch according to Frank Starling's law is to increase stroke volume by an increase in contractility, causing the arterial pulse pressure to rise. In patients with HOCM, the increase in contractility after a PVC worsens the LVOT obstruction, causing a decrease in the arterial pulse pressure and the Brockenbrough-Braunwald-Morrow sign.

# Case 4: Aortic Regurgitation

*Brief History*
A 50-year-old male patient hailing from Puttur, manual laborer by occupation presented with.

*General Physical Examination*
Patient is conscious, cooperative and well oriented to time, place and person moderately built and nourished.
- Pulse: Rate—59/min, rhythm—regular, character—good volume pulse, condition of vessel wall—normal, no radioradial or radiofemoral delay and all peripheral pulses felt, collapsing pulse +, bisferiens pulse +.
- Blood pressure: Supine—100/50 mm Hg in both arm supine position, no postural drop, lower limb—systolic 150 mm Hg
- Respiratory rate: 18 cycles/min. Type of breathing—abdominothoracic
- Temperature: 98.6°F at the time of examination
- Height: 162 cm, Weight: 45 kg, BMI: 17.1 kg/m$^2$
- Jugular venous pulse—not elevated.
- Pallor present, bald tongue (+), angular stomatitis (+)
- No icterus, cyanosis, clubbing, lymphadenopathy
- Pedal edema present, pitting type up to middle of leg, facial puffiness and periorbital edema present.
- No evidence of infective endocarditis.
- No cranioskeletal dysplasia
- Arcus senilis present both eyes
- Right eye: Senile mature cataract
- Wasting of temporalis muscle (+)
- Peripheral signs of AR:
  - Hill's sign (+) difference between UL and LL BP is 50 mm Hg)
  - Collapsing/Water hammer pulse present.
  - Locomotor brachialis (+)
  - Corrigan's sign/dancing carotid (+)
  - Traube's sign (+)
  - Duroziez's sign (+)
  - Landolfi sign (+)
  - Quincke's sign (-)
  - De Musset sign (-)
  - Light house sign (-)
  - Muller's sign (-)
  - Becker's sign (-)
  - Rosenbach's sign (-)
  - Gerhardt's sign (-)

*Cardiovascular System Examination*
Inspection:
- Shape of chest is B/L symmetrical.
- Precordium normal
- Spine normal
- No scars, sinuses, dilated veins
- Carotid pulsation seen
- Apex beat: Visible in left 6th intercostal space about 1 cm lateral to midclavicular line
- No parasternal or epigastric pulsations

Palpation:
- Inspectory findings are confirmed
- Apex beat: Left 6th intercostal space about 1cm lateral to midclavicular line, localized, ill-sustained in nature. No thrill present
- No parasternal heave, pulsations and thrill. No epigastric pulsation
- Aortic area: No palpable heart sounds, thrill (+)
- Pulmonary area: No palpable heart sounds, no palpable P2, no thrill
- Tricuspid area: No palpable heart sounds, No palpable P2, No thrill
- Left 3rd ICS: Systolic thrill (+)

Percussion:
- Left heart border corresponds to apex
- Right heart border corresponds to right sternal margin
- No dullness in left second intercostal space
- Liver dullness on right side 5 intercostal space (ICS)

Auscultation: Aortic area:
- S1—heard
- A2—muffled

A harsh ejection systolic murmur of grade 4/6 crescendo-decrescendo type is present, murmur is radiating to apex and carotid area. Murmur increases on breath held in expiration and best heard in patient sitting and leaning forward, heard with diaphragm of the stethoscope.

A soft blowing early diastolic murmur of grade 2/4 which is best heard in sitting and leaning forward and breath held in expiration, best heard with the diaphragm of the stethoscope, murmur radiates to left 3rd intercostal space where it is best heard and also radiates to the apex.
- No ejection click
- Dynamic auscultation:
  - ESM murmur is augmented on squatting, reduces on standing and isometric hand grip.
  - ESM showing delayed return after Valsalva maneuver.

Pulmonary area:
- S1 S2+
- No loud P2

Tricuspid area—S1—normal, S2—normal. No murmur
Mitral area:
- S1 and S2 are heard normally.
- ESM and EDM are heard with less intensity.

*Respiratory System Examination*
- Bilateral normal vesicular breath sound
- No added sounds

*Gastrointestinal System*
- Soft
- Nontender
- No organomegaly
- No bruit

*Nervous System*
No focal neurological deficit

*Diagnosis*
- Acquired valvular heart disease? Degenerative aortic valve involvement with moderate AS and moderate AR, no signs of infective endocarditis.
- Not in failure
- No atrial fibrillation
- NYHA—Class 3

## DISCUSSION

### Q. What are the peripheral signs of AR?

- **Corrigan's pulse:** A rapid and forceful distension of the arterial pulse with a quick collapse.
- **De Musset's sign:** Bobbing of the head with each heartbeat (like a bird walking).
- **Light house sign/Morton and Mahon sign:** Alternating flushing and blanching of face.
- **Muller's sign:** Visible pulsations of the uvula
- **Quincke's sign:** Capillary pulsations seen on light compression of the nail bed
- **Traube's sign:** Systolic and diastolic sounds heard over the femoral artery ("pistol shots")
- **Duroziez's sign:** Is more specific of all the peripheral signs of AR. Paul Louis Duroziez described it in 1861. It is a *Bruit de tambour* and consists of:
  - Systolic murmur: A forward murmur perceived by pressing the femoral artery 2 cm above the stethoscope, which is due to powerful contraction of LV and increased stroke volume.
  - Diastolic murmur: A backward murmur perceived by pressing the femoral artery 2 cm below the stethoscope, which is due to the arterial recoil and back flow.
- **Hill's sign:** Hill and Rowlands in 1912 described the peak systolic pressure gradient between posterior tibial and radial arteries. It is due to greater velocity of blood in lower limb artery, which arises from the aorta in a straight course. Severity of AR from Hill's sign may be deduced: Systolic pressure difference of 20–40 mm Hg = angiographic 2+AR, 41–60 mm Hg systolic pressure difference = angiographic 3+AR, >60 mm Hg systolic pressure difference = angiographic 4+AR.
- **Shelly's sign/Dennison sign:** Pulsation of the cervix
- **Rosenbach's sign:** Hepatic pulsations
- **Becker's sign:** Visible pulsation of the retinal arterioles
- **Gerhardt's sign (Sailer's sign):** Pulsation of the spleen in the presence of splenomegaly
- **Mayne's sign:** A decrease in diastolic blood pressure of 15 mm Hg when the arm is held above the head (very non-specific)
- **Landolfi's sign:** Systolic contraction and diastolic dilation of the pupil
- **Lincoln sign:** Pulsatile popliteal artery
- **Ashrafian sign:** Pulsatile pseudoproptosis
- **Sherman sign:** Dorsalis pedis pulse is quickly located and unexpectedly prominent in age >75 years
- **Bozzolo's sign:** Pulsatile nasal mucosa
- **Drummond sign:** Systolic expulsion of air from nose when mouth is closed
- **Penny sign:** Flushing of wheals
- **Palmar click:** Pulsating palm
- **Julian sign:** Pulsation of retinal vessels
- **Minervini's sign:** Strong lingual pulsations. Tongue depressor moves up and down when tongue is depressed
- **Logue's sign:** Pulsation of sternoclavicular junction
- **Palfrey's sign** (Palfrey, 1952) is the pistol shot sounds heard over the radial artery.

### Q. How do you demonstrate Quincke's sign?

**Quincke's sign**—method of elicitation
Compress the skin of face or hands with a glass slide, or exert slight pressure on the nail beds and watch for intermittent flushing. We can also transilluminate the nail bed with a flashlight against the pad of the patient's finger while shading the finger with the other hand.

**Mechanism of capillary pulsations:**

The transmission of the arterial pulse through dilated capillaries to the subpapillary venous plexus. It is found in any condition that causes capillary dilatation, such as hot weather, a hot bath, fever, anemia, pregnancy or hyperthyroidism.

**Cardiac conditions that cause capillary pulsation:**

Any cardiac condition that causes large pulse pressure, such as AR, systolic hypertension, marked bradycardia as in complete AV block.

### Q. What is Harvey sign?

When aortic regurgitation is caused by primary valvular disease, the diastolic murmur is heard best along the left sternal border in the 3rd and 4th intercostal space. When murmur is caused mainly by dilation of the ascending aorta, the murmur is more readily audible along the right sternal border.

### Q. What is Hill's sign?

With the patient is horizontal (prone) position, compare the brachial artery systolic pressure with the popliteal (or dorsalis pedis) artery systolic pressure, indirectly determined by palpation or auscultation. Normally, the two indirectly determined pressures will be same, or the apparent systolic pressure in the lower extremity will be up to 20 mm Hg higher.

In aortic regurgitation, the indirect systolic pressure will be 20 mm Hg or higher in the lower limbs than the upper limbs. The degree of systolic pressure gradient is directly proportional to the degree of aortic insufficiency determined at cardiac catheterization.

### Q. List the causes of aortic regurgitation.

- Aortic valve involvement
  - Rheumatic heart disease
  - Infective endocarditis
  - Congenital bicuspid aortic valve
  - Congenital fenestration of AV
  - AV prolapse associated with VSD
  - Secondary AR in membranous subaortic stenosis.
- Aortic wall involvement
  - Syphilis
  - Rheumatoid arthritis
  - Ankylosing spondylitis
  - Marfan's syndrome
  - Ehlers-Danlos syndrome
  - Takayasu's arteritis
  - Aortic dissection
  - Systemic hypertension
  - Osteogenesis imperfecta
  - Idiopathic dilatation of aorta
  - Annuloaortic ectasia.

### Q. What is regurgitant fraction?

Regurgitant fraction (RF) = regurgitant volume/stroke volume
- Severe AR: RF >0.7
- Moderate AR: RF 0.3–0.6
- Mild AR: RF <0.3.

### Q. What is pathophysiology of AR?

**Figure 2.25** shows pathophysiology of aortic regurgitation.

### Q. What do you mean by AR Begets AR?

- Aortic regurgitation → increased LV systolic volume and annular dilatation → increases the regurgitation.
- Dilation of the ascending aorta leads to intensification of AR.

### Q. What is the mechanism of angina in AR?

- Increased demand due to LVH and increased cardiac output
- Decreased supply due to decreased coronary perfusion gradient caused by decreased aortic diastolic blood pressure +/− increased left ventricular end diastolic pressure (LVEDP).

### Q. List the complications of AR.

- Cardiac failure
- Infective endocarditis
- Arrhythmia

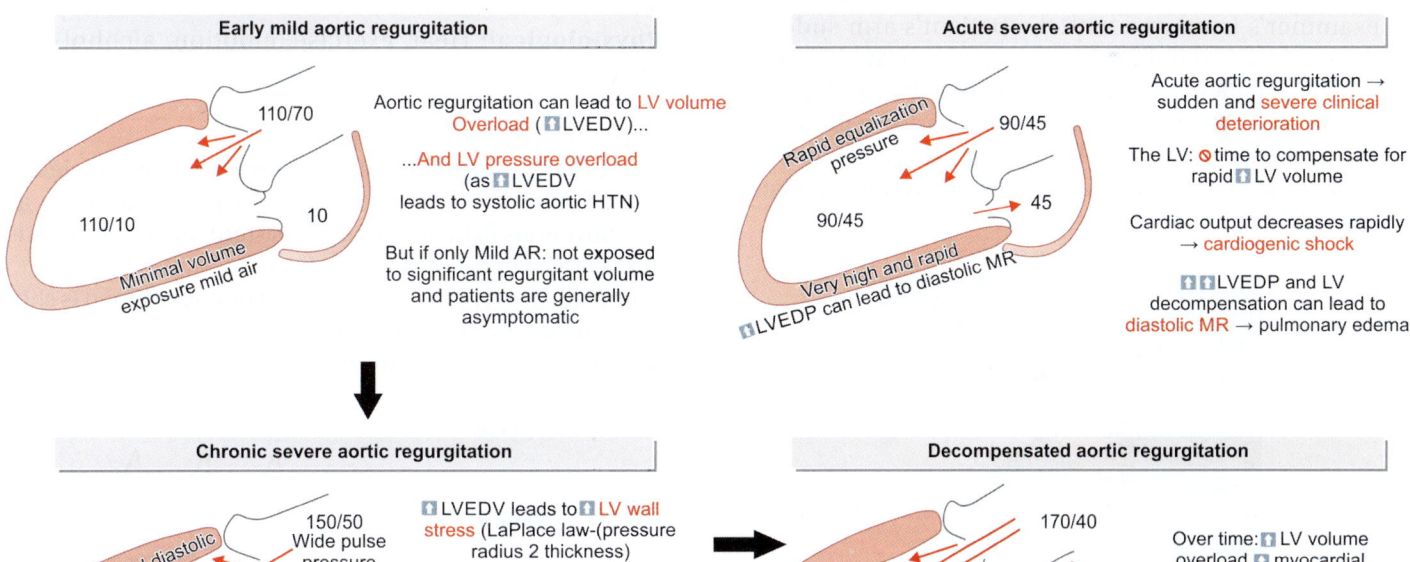

Fig. 2.25: Pathophysiology of AR.

### Q. What are the pulse abnormalities you will find in AR?

- **Collapsing pulse (Corrigan's pulse):** High volume pulse with rapid upstroke, rapid downstroke and ill-sustained peak
- Due to:
  - Early diastolic reflux of blood into the LV
  - Low systemic vascular resistance
- Bisferiens pulse may be felt in:
  - Moderate to severe AR
  - Moderate AR + mild AS
- Carotid shudder—coarse systolic vibrations may be felt. Carotid thrill or bruit may be felt.
- Factors decreasing pulse volume:
  - Hypovolemia
  - Acute AR
  - LV dysfunction/PAH
  - Associated valve lesions—AS

### Q. What is collapsing pulse?

**Collapsing pulse (Water-Hammer pulse and Corrigans pulse) (Figs. 2.26 and 2.27)**

The term was coined by Thomas Watson. Water hammer was a Victorian toy consisting of a glass vacuum tube containing a small amount of water. When the tube was turned on to one end the shock of the water falling could be felt and heard and was thought to represent the abrupt sensation under one's finger at the wrist.

It is best appreciated at radial pulse. Patients wrist is held in examiner's hand and with the patient's arm suddenly evaluated above shoulder. The percussion wave is abrupt, has an ill-sustained crest, and the collapse of the pulse is also rapid. The collapse occurs during systole, prior to the second sound and not, as commonly thought during diastole. No dicrotic notch is palpable but may be recordable displaced towards the base line.

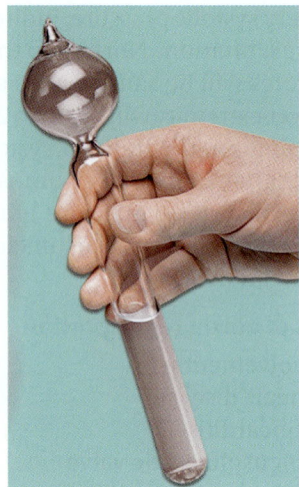

**Fig. 2.27:** Water hammer.

It is a large volume pulse with a rapid upstroke (systolic pressure is high) and a rapid downstroke (diastolic pressure is low) without dicrotic notch (low systemic vascular resistance). The rapid upstroke is because of an increased stroke volume. The rapid downstroke is because of diastolic run-off into the left ventricle, and decreased peripheral resistance and rapid run-off to the periphery **(Fig. 2.28)**.

Decreased peripheral resistance is due to large stroke volume stretching carotid and aortic sinus leading to reflex decrease in peripheral resistance.

**Causes**

- **Physiological:** Heat, exercise, emotion, alcohol and pregnancy.
- Hyperkinetic circulatory states
- Aortic and mitral incompetence
- Any leak in the arterial side of the circulation, if sufficiently great, will give rise to the same clinical findings, such as arteriovenous fistulae, a large persistent ductus arteriosus and a large ventricular septal defect
- Complete heart block: Here a large volume of blood is shot into a relatively empty reservoir.
- Rupture of sinus of Valsalva

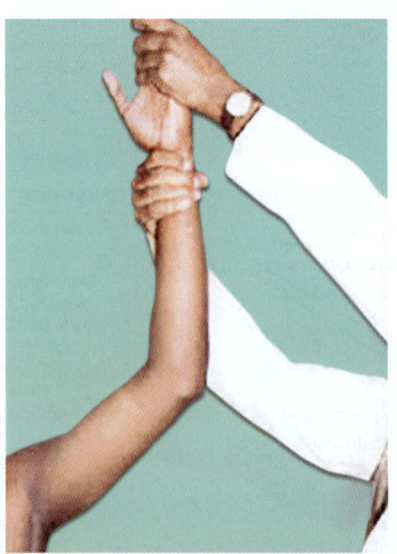

**Fig. 2.26:** Examination of collapsing pulse.

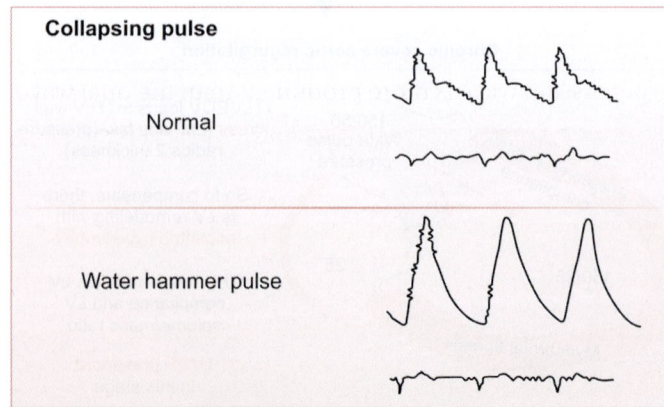

**Fig. 2.28:** Collapsing pulse.

- Truncus arteriosus with truncal sufficiency, pulmonary atresia with bronchopulmonary collaterals, tetralogy of Fallot (TOF) with bronchopulmonary collaterals, TOF after BT shunt.

### Q. What is bisferiens pulse? How to elicit bisferiens pulse? What are the conditions in which bisferiens pulse is seen?

Pulsus bisferiens is a single pulse wave with two peaks in systole separated by distinct midsystolic dip. This is best felt in brachial artery, apply graduated pressure or completely obliterate the pulse and gradually release it to appreciate two waves. It is due to ejection of rapid jet of blood through the aortic valve. During the peak of flow, Bernoulli's effect on the walls of ascending aorta causes a sudden decrease in lateral pressure on the inner aspect of the wall.

**Causes**
- Aortic stenosis and aortic regurgitation
- Hyperkinetic circulatory states
- Severe aortic regurgitation
- Hypertrophic obstructive cardiomyopathy (HOCM)
- Patent ductus arteriosus
- Dissection of aorta (unilateral bisferiens).

### Q. How do you differentiate between bisferiens pulse of AR and HOCM?

The two waves of bisferiens pulse are equal or tidal wave is prominent in AR, AR and AS. Whereas in HOCM, percussion is more prominent than tidal wave and it shows a "spike and dome" pattern.

However, it is usually recordable but not palpable. Pulse in HOCM (**Fig. 2.29**):
- The initial percussion wave is due to rapid ejection of blood into the ascending aorta during early systole.
- The midsystolic dip (negative wave) coincides with marked decrease in the rate of LV ejection, as the left ventricular outflow tract obstruction becomes manifest due to the thickening of interventricular septum and the systolic anterior motion (SAM) of anterior mitral leaflet.
- The second systolic (tidal) wave is most likely produced by reflected waves from the periphery.
- Hence, pulse of HOCM behaves partly like AR (initial component) and partly as AS (second component), but percussion wave is more prominent than the tidal wave.

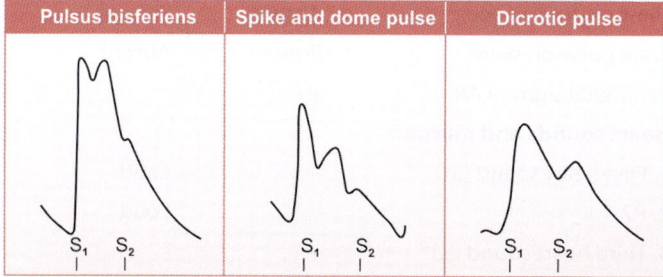

**Fig. 2.29:** Hypertrophic obstructive cardiomyopathy (HOCM).

### Q. What is the importance of checking BP in AR?
- Presence of a normal blood pressure in a patient with AR and good LV function rules out moderate to severe AR.
- Increased systolic pressure >140 mm Hg is suggestive of significant AR where pulse pressure is high.
- Diastolic blood pressure <50 mm Hg indicates severe AR irrespective of systolic pressure.
- Severe AR is unlikely when the diastolic blood pressure >60 mm Hg except in associated LV failure/systematic hypertension.

### Q. Describe the apical impulse in AR.
- Displaced forceful apex, hyperdynamic
- Gross cardiomegaly, apex beyond anterior axillary line, cor bovinum: Syphilitic AR
- Undisplaced forceful in mild-moderate AR

### Q. Describe the heart sounds in AR.

**S1 in AR**
- Usually decreased. Due to the partial closure of the mitral valve in presystole
- Loud S1-associated MS

**A2 in AR**
- Loud A2: AR due to aortic root dilatation. Tambour A2: Syphilitic AR
- Soft A2: Valvular causes decreased ability of the valve

**S3 in AR**
- LV S3: Seen in severe AR
- Commonly associated with Austin Flint murmur

**S4 in AR**

Common in severe AR.

**Aortic ejection click in AR**

Seen in patients with mild AR with normal LV function
- Valvular EC: AR due to bicuspid aortic valve
- Vascular EC: Aortic root dilatation

### Q. How do you assess severity of aortic regurgitation?

The presence of the following indicate significant AR (**Table 2.40**):
- Duration of murmur (>2/3 of diastole) is directly proportional to the severity. In moderate to severe AR, murmur becomes holodiastolic and may have a rough quality.
- Bisferiens pulse
- Hill's sign >60 mm Hg
- Apical impulse (down and out)
- Austin Flint murmur
- Marked peripheral signs (they are absent in depressed myocardial function).

### Q. What are the murmurs heard in AR?
- Early diastolic murmur

## SECTION 2: Cardiovascular System

| Table 2.40: Severity of aortic regurgitation. | |
|---|---|
| **Severity** | **Features** |
| Mild AR | Short EDM |
| Moderate AR | • Collapsing pulse<br>• Pulsus bisferiens<br>• Peripheral signs<br>• Soft S1<br>• Long EDM |
| Severe AR | • Collapsing pulse<br>• Bisferiens pulse<br>• Peripheral signs<br>• Hills sign<br>• Soft S1<br>• LVS3<br>• Long EDM<br>• MDM at apex |

- Ejection systolic flow murmur
- Mild diastolic flow murmur/Austin Flint murmur

### Early diastolic murmur

- High frequency EDM caused by the high velocity of flow and a small regurgitant volume
- Duration:
  - Mild AR—murmur confined to early diastole
  - Severe AR—holodiastolic and decrescendo
  - Free AR—murmur confined to early diastole
- Normally heard at the aortic area or neoaortic area
- Conducted down the left sternal border
- In elderly and CCF—may be best heard at the apex
- Increases by handgrip, squatting and simultaneous application of pressure cuffs to both arms for 20 seconds to a level 20 mm above the systolic blood pressure.

### Ejection systolic murmur

- In the aortic/neoaortic area
- Due to the rapid ejection of an increased stroke volume through an abnormal valve
- High-pitched, grade 1—4/6.
  Associated aortic stenosis is indicated only if:
- Long ESM
- Loud murmur >4/6
- Thrill
- Late peaking

### Q. What is the mechanism of Austin Flint murmur?

Austin Flint murmur is a functional murmur produced in AR due to the regurgitant jet of blood impinging on the anterior mitral valve leaflet in early-mid diastole. It is a functional MS murmur.

### Pathogenesis

From the phono-echocardiographic, echo-Doppler and MRI studies, the AFM in AR is due to the combination of the following:

- Regurgitant jet creating vibrations and turbulence in the following way:
  - Collision of the regurgitant jet with mitral inflow producing the turbulence
  - Regurgitant jet impinging on anterior mitral leaflet (AML) producing the vibrations of AML
  - Regurgitant jet impinging on the myocardial wall producing the vibrations
- Increased mitral inflow velocity creating a flow rumble
- Due to rapid closing motion of the mitral valve leaflets during mid diastole and presystole similar to MR and high output states
- Due to narrowing of the valve orifice by the regurgitant jet
- Incomplete valve opening during mid diastole and presystole
- Diastolic MR

### Q. How do you differentiate MDM at apex from MS and Austin Flint murmur?

Refer **Figure 2.30 and Table 2.41**.

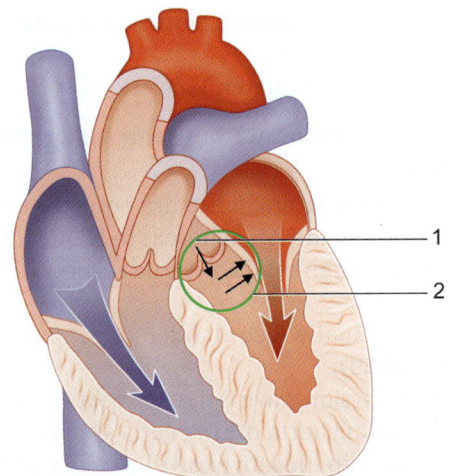

1. Regurgitant aortic valve
2. Anterior mitral leaflet

**Fig. 2.30:** Pathogenesis of Austin Flint murmur.

**Table 2.41:** Difference between Austin Flint murmur and mitral stenosis murmur.

| Features | Austin Flint murmur | Mitral stenosis murmur |
|---|---|---|
| Diastolic thrill at apex | Absent | Present |
| Wide pulse pressure | Present | Absent |
| Peripheral signs of AR | ++ | – |
| **Heart sounds and murmur** | | |
| 1. First heart sound (S1) | – | Loud |
| 2. P2 | – | Loud |
| 3. Third heart sound (S3) | + | – |
| 4. Opening snap (OS) | – | + |

| Features | Austin Flint murmur | Mitral stenosis murmur |
|---|---|---|
| 5. Presystolic accentuation | +/- | + |
| 6. Associated EDM in aortic area | ++ | - |
| 7. With amyl nitrate | Murmur decreases | No change |
| Evidence of PAH, RV enlargement and/or hypertrophy | Absent | Present |
| Evidence of LV enlargement and/or hypertrophy | Present | Absent |
| Atrial fibrillation | - | More common |

**Q. What is Cole-Cecil murmur?**

Occasionally, the murmur of aortic regurgitation is radiated to the left axilla, and is known as Cole-Cecil murmur. This is a useful way to differentiate AR from PR.

**Q. What is the effect of other valvular diseases on AR?**

Refer **Table 2.42**.

**Q. What are the ECG findings in AR?**

It shows the adaptive changes in the left ventricle due to the volume overload. These include:
- LV hypertrophy: Tall R waves and deeply inverted T waves in the left-sided chest leads
- Left axis deviation

**Table 2.42:** Effects of other cardiac conditions on AR.

| Effect of MS on AR | Effect of MR on AR | Effect of AS on AR |
|---|---|---|
| • Decreased symptoms due to AR<br>• Atrial fibrillation<br>• Early PAH<br>• Loud S1<br>• OS<br>• Masking of peripheral signs<br>• Apex may be normal in position<br>• Decreased length and intensity of EDM | • Decreased symptoms due to AR<br>• Dyspnea for long duration<br>• Atrial fibrillation<br>• Early PAH<br>• Masking of peripheral signs<br>• Apex shifted down and out<br>• Decreased length and intensity of EDM | • Pulse may be normal<br>• Pulse pressure may be normal<br>• Apex may be normal<br>• Increased length and intensity of ESM with thrill |

- Left atrial enlargement
- LV volume overload pattern (prominent Q waves in leads I, aVL, and V3 to V6 and relatively small r waves in V1)
- LV conduction defects (typically late in the disease process).

**Q. What are the chest X-ray findings in AR?**

- It shows cardiomegaly due to the enlargement/dilatation of the left ventricle in an inferior and leftward direction.
- The ascending aorta (and the aortic arch or knob) is also severely dilated. Left atrial enlargement is not found unless there is significant left ventricular dysfunction.
- Calcification of the ascending aortic wall and the aortic valve may be observed in syphilitic aortic regurgitation.
- Later, it may show features of left heart failure.

**Q. What are the echo findings in AR?**

- Aortic valve structure and morphology (e.g., bileaflet versus trileaflet, flail, thickening).
- Presence of vegetations or nodules (may require transesophageal echocardiography in selected cases)
- Quantitative measurements of regurgitant volume, fraction and orifice area assessment
- Fluttering anterior mitral leaflet
- Associated lesions of the aorta, e.g., dilation, aneurysm, dissection, or ectasia
- LV structure and function

**Q. What are the other investigations to be done in AR?**

- Coronary angiography: Indicated for the assessment of coronary anatomy prior to aortic valve surgery in patients with risk factors for coronary artery disease
- Other tests:
  - VDRL and TPHA: If syphilitic cause is suspected
  - RA factor, ANA, ESR and CRP: To exclude connective tissue disorders.

**Q. What is the medical management of AR?**

- Underlying cause of AR-like dissection, endocarditis, syphilis has to be treated.
- **Prophylaxis:** Rheumatic fever prophylaxis is needed if due to rheumatic. Infective endocarditis prophylaxis is not required.
- **Acute severe AR:** Surgical intervention is usually needed, but the patient may be medically supported with dobutamine to augment cardiac output and shorten diastole and sodium nitroprusside to reduce afterload in hypertensive patients.
- Chronic severe AR

**Medical treatment**

- Vasodilator therapy may be used in selected conditions to reduce afterload in patients with systolic hypertension to reduce wall stress and optimize LV function. In normotensive patients, vasodilator therapy may not be useful because it does not reduce regurgitant volume (preload) significantly.
- The acute administration of sodium nitroprusside, hydralazine, nifedipine, or felodipine reduced PVR and results in an immediate augmentation in forward cardiac output and a reduction in regurgitant volume. Nitroprusside and hydralazine induced acute hemodynamic changes lead to a consistent decrease in end-diastolic volume (EDV) and an increase in ejection fraction (EF).

**Q. What are the indications of aortic valve replacement in AR?**

- Patient is symptomatic (dyspnea, NYHA class IIIB, angina) with chronic severe aortic regurgitation.

- Patient is asymptomatic, with a resting left ventricular ejection fraction (LVEF) of <55%.
- Patient is asymptomatic, with left ventricular (LV) ejection fraction >55% but with left ventricle dilation (LV end-diastolic dimension >70 mm or end-systolic dimension >55 mm).
- Fractional shortening (FS) <0.27
- Acute severe aortic regurgitation, e.g., endocarditis
- If undergoing CABG, surgery of the ascending aorta or other cardiac valve.

AR usually requires replacement of the diseased valve with a prosthetic valve, although valve-sparing repair is available, such as transcatheter aortic valve replacement/implantation (TAVR/TAVI).

**Q. What are the differences between AR and PR?**
Refer **Table 2.43**.

**Table 2.43:** Differences between AR and PR.

|  | Aortic regurgitation | Pulmonary regurgitation |
|---|---|---|
| Pulse | Collapsing pulse | Normal |
| BP | Wide pulse pressure | Normal |
| JVP | Normal | Prominent A waves |
| Apex | Forceful apex | Normal |
| PAH | PAH absent | Present |
| Murmur | EDM 2nd aortic area conducted down Increases on expiration | EDM in pulmonary and localized Increases on inspiration |

**Q. What are the causes and signs of acute AR?**

**Etiology of acute AR**
- Infective endocarditis
- Aortic dissection
- Aortic valve damage caused by trauma

**Features of acute AR**
- Tachycardia
- Hypotension
- A wave in JVP
- No cardiomegaly
- Palpable P2
- LPH present
- Soft S1
- S2 single
- Soft A2
- LV S3—always
- LV S4—common
- Soft decrescendo murmur at apex

**Q. How to differentiate between acute AR and chronic AR?**
Refer **Table 2.44**.

**Table 2.44:** Acute versus chronic AR.

| Features | Acute AR | Chronic AR |
|---|---|---|
| Pulse pressure | Normal | Wide |
| Systolic pressure | Decreased (systolic decapitation) | Increased |
| Diastolic pressure | Decreased | Markedly decreased |
| Apex | Normal but not hyperdynamic | Hyperdynamic |
| S1 | Soft or absent | Normal |
| P2 | Normal or increased | Normal |
| S3 | Common | Uncommon |
| AR murmur | Short medium-pitched | Long high-pitched |
| Aortic systolic murmur | Grade 3 or less | Grade 3 or less |
| Austin Flint murmur | No presystolic murmur | Presystolic murmur may be heard |
| Peripheral signs | Absent | Present |
| ECG | Normal LV | LV enlargement |
| X-ray | Normal to moderately increased LV | Markedly increased LV |

**Q. What are the differences between rheumatic AR and syphilitic AR?**
Refer **Table 2.45**.

**Table 2.45:** Differences between rheumatic AR and syphilitic AR.

| Features | Rheumatic AR | Syphilitic AR |
|---|---|---|
| Age group | 10–40 years | Older than 40 years |
| Angina | Less common | More common |
| Early-diastolic murmur (EDM) best audible at | Erb's area | Aortic area |
| Character of EDM | Soft, blowing | Cooing dove or seagull |
| Character of $A_2$ | Soft | Loud and tambour |
| Association with aortic stenosis or mitral valve disease | May be associated | Not associated |
| Decompensation | Relatively late | Relatively early |
| Calcification aorta | Not seen | May be present |
| Features of underlying cause or etiology | Other features of rheumatic heart disease (RHD) may be present | Stigmata of syphilis present |

## MULTIVALVULAR HEART DISEASES (MVD)

- This is important as it impacts the disease progression and treatment approach

- The valve might not always be diseased but must exhibit significant functional impairment

### Q. What are the causes of MVD?
- Rheumatic heart disease (55%)
- Infective endocarditis
- Myocardial dysfunction (remodeled heart—MR, PR, TR)
- Aging and degenerative (calcific)—(43%)
- Other organ disorders—ESRD, carcinoid
- Myxomatous diseases—marfan, EDS
- Connective tissue diseases—SLE, APLA, RA
- Congenital diseases—subaortic stenosis, HOCM, Shone's complex, trisomy (13,15,18), alkaptonuria
- Endocardial disorders
- Thoracic/mediastinal radiation therapy
- Drugs—ergotamine, Fen-Phen, methysergide

*Note:*
- When multiple valves exhibit severe stenosis, it is typically due to rheumatic disease.
- Significant regurgitation across several valves generally points to a non-rheumatic cause.
- The presence of both significant stenosis and regurgitation simultaneously is most often associated with rheumatic heart disease.
- Quadrivalvular disease usually results from multiple causes: rheumatic, infective, congenital, inflammatory, or degenerative.
- A single cause of quadrivalvular disease is typically either rheumatic or myxomatous degeneration.

### Q. What is the pattern of valvular involvement in rheumatic fever with carditis?

**Clinical findings:**
- **Mitral valve (MV) involvement:** 70-75%
- **Combined mitral and aortic valve (MV + AV) involvement:** 20-25%
- **Aortic valve (AV) involvement alone:** 5-8%
- **Tricuspid valve (TV) involvement:** 1-2%
- **Pulmonary valve (PV) involvement:** Rare
- **Histopathological findings:** Overall valve involvement distribution: 30–35% (TV), 15–20% (PV)

| | |
|---|---|
| MS: 34.9% | MS+MR: 11.9% |
| MR: 14.8% | MS+AR: 21.1% |
| AR: 6.1% | MS+MR+TS: 4.8% |
| | MS+MR+TS+TR: 6.4% |
| | MS+AS+TS in 2.5% |

### Q. What are the non-valvular factors that trigger or worsen symptoms?
- Arrhythmias
- Infective endocarditis
- Recurrence of rheumatic fever leading to valvulitis and myocarditis
- Conditions causing excess blood volume, including anemia, deteriorating kidney function, and poor adherence to dietary guidelines
- Uncontrolled hypertension
- Reduced blood flow due to ischemic events such as coronary artery disease, acute coronary syndrome, respiratory illnesses, or high-altitude exposure
- Systemic inflammatory response syndrome (SIRS) often triggered by infections, with pneumonia being the most common cause.

### Q. In a patient with severe mitral regurgitation what findings suggest mitral stenosis be present?
- Palpable diastolic thrill at mitral area
- Long mid-diastolic murmur
- Characteristic opening snap
- Accentuated first heart sound (S1)
- Marked pulmonary arterial hypertension (PAH)

### Q. In a patient with severe aortic regurgitation what findings suggest aortic stenosis be present?
- Noticeable pulse abnormalities of AS
- Systolic decapitation of BP
- Murmur that peaks late, with a rougher and louder quality
- Prominent, forceful apical heartbeat
- Palpable systolic thrill in the aortic area

### Q. How do you identify tricuspid stenosis in a multivalvular disease?
- **Symptoms:** Increased fatigue, congestive heart failure (CHF), right ventricular failure (RVF), less paroxysmal nocturnal dyspnea (PND) and orthopnea.
- More common in females.
- Distal lesions may mask symptoms but signs remain prominent
- Jugular venous pressure (JVP) is crucial for diagnosis:
  - Giant a waves
  - Slow Y descent
- Presence of pulsatile liver
- Murmur characteristics in TS:
  - Location-specific
  - Pre-systolic or mid-diastolic timing
- TS often escapes easy detection
- Presence of loud T1, and tricuspid opening snap

### Q. How do you identify tricuspid regurgitation in a multivalvular disease?
- Always associated with MV disease in RHD
- Other causes—carcinoid, endomyocardial fibrosis, infective endocarditis, RV, myocardial infarction, dilated cardiomyopathy, traumatic
- Congenital conditions—ebstein anomaly, Marfan or Ehlers-Danlos syndrome
- TR can be primary/organic (intrinsic abnormality of valve apparatus) or secondary/functional (due to annular dilatation, RV dilatation, papillary muscle dysfunction)

- Symptoms
  - Weakness, fatigue—low cardiac output
  - Edema, ascites, painful hepatomegaly—RHF
  - Throbbing neck pulsations
  - Symptoms of pulmonary congestion.
- JVP in TR
  - Attenuation and obliteration of X descent
  - Dominant 'CV' systolic wave with ear lobe pulsations—Lancisi sign
  - Steep 'Y' descent – Friedrich's sign
  - Inspiratory rise of the venous pulse—Kussumal's sign
  - Absent 'A' wave in AF.
- Systolic hepatic pulsations
- Pansystolic murmur in LLSB which increases on inspiration/passive leg rising (Caravallos sign)
- RV S3, short MDM
- High pressure TR—features of pH—loud p2, prominent CV wave on JVP, high pitched PSM
- Low pressure TR—early systolic decrescendo low-pitched murmur, soft/inaudible in EMF, RV MI

**Q. How do you asses pulmonary venous hypertension based on dyspnea?**
- Dyspnea class:
  - Class II—mild PVH
  - Class III—moderate PVH
  - Class IV—severe PVH
- History of PND—moderate PVH
- History of orthopnea—severe PVH
- Pulmonary edema—severe PVH

**Q. What are the signs of pulmonary arterial hypertension?**
- Prominent "a" wave in JVP
- Parasternal heave, epigastric pulsations
- Pulmonary area pulsations, dullness in left 2nd ICS
- Loud, palpable P2,
- TR murmur,
- Ejection systolic murmur in pulmonary area in mild to moderate PAH
- PR—early diastolic murmur (Grahm Steel murmur) in severe PAH.

# SURGICAL MANAGEMENT FOR VALVULAR DISEASES

## American College of Cardiology (ACC)/American Heart Association (AHA) Guidelines

**Mitral Stenosis**
- **Symptomatic patients with severe MS (class I):** Patients with severe symptomatic MS (valve area ≤1.5 cm²) who are not candidates for PMBC due to unfavorable valve anatomy or those with contraindications such as left atrial thrombus should be considered for mitral valve repair or surgical commissurotomy.
- **Severe MS with new-onset atrial fibrillation (class IIa):** For patients with severe MS who develop new-onset atrial fibrillation or have recurrent systemic embolization, mitral valve repair or replacement should be considered if PMBC is not an option.
- **Pulmonary hypertension in severe MS (class IIa):** In patients with asymptomatic severe MS but who develop pulmonary hypertension, defined as a pulmonary artery systolic pressure >50 mm Hg, surgical intervention, including mitral valve repair, is recommended when PMBC is not appropriate.
- **Symptomatic moderate MS (class IIb):** Surgical mitral valve repair may be considered in patients with moderate MS (MV area >1.5 cm² but <2 cm²) who are symptomatic and have other cardiac indications for surgery, such as concomitant coronary artery bypass grafting (CABG).

**Mitral Regurgitation**
- **Symptomatic severe primary MR (class I):** Surgical mitral valve repair is recommended for symptomatic individuals with severe primary MR and preserved LV function [ejection fraction (EF) >30%].
- **Asymptomatic severe primary MR with LV dysfunction (class I):** In patients with severe primary MR who are asymptomatic but have evidence of LV dysfunction, defined as LVEF ≤60% or LV end-systolic diameter ≥40 mm, early surgical intervention with mitral valve repair is strongly recommended to prevent further LV remodeling and heart failure.
- **Severe primary MR with atrial fibrillation or pulmonary hypertension (class IIa):** Asymptomatic individuals with severe primary MR and preserved LV function who develop new-onset atrial fibrillation or resting pulmonary hypertension defined as above should be considered for mitral valve repair.
- **Asymptomatic severe primary MR with normal LV function and high likelihood of durable repair (class IIa):** Early mitral valve repair may be considered in patients with asymptomatic severe primary MR who have normal LV function and a high likelihood of successful and durable repair. This is especially relevant if the surgical team has a high success rate with repair procedures.
- **Severe secondary MR (class IIb):** For patients with severe secondary MR and heart failure, mitral valve repair may be considered if the patient is undergoing another cardiac surgery, such as CABG or aortic valve surgery. However, depending on the underlying cause and LV function, mitral valve replacement may sometimes be more appropriate, especially in patients with ischemic MR.
- **Moderate secondary MR in patients undergoing other cardiac surgery (class IIa):** In patients with moderate secondary MR undergoing surgery for another cardiac condition, such as CABG or aortic valve replacement, mitral valve replacement should be considered to address MR and improve long-term outcomes.

**Aortic Stenosis**
- Severe high-gradient AS with symptoms (class I recommendation, level B evidence)
- Asymptomatic patients with severe AS and LVEF <50 (class I recommendation, level B evidence)

- Severe AS when undergoing other cardiac surgery (class I recommendation, level B evidence)
- Asymptomatic severe AS and low surgical risk (class IIa recommendation, level B evidence)
- Symptomatic with low-flow/low-gradient severe AS (class IIa recommendation, level B evidence)
- Moderate AS and undergoing other cardiac surgery (class IIa recommendation, level C evidence)

**Aortic Regurgitation**

*Class I Indications (Strong Recommendations):*
- Symptomatic patients with severe AR:
  - Any patient experiencing symptoms (like shortness of breath, chest pain, or fatigue) due to severe aortic regurgitation should undergo AVR, according to the American Heart Association (AHA) and the American College of Cardiology (ACC).
- Asymptomatic patients with severe AR and LVEF ≤50% or LVESD >50 mm:
  - AVR is recommended for asymptomatic patients with severe AR and a reduced LVEF (below 50%), or with severe LV enlargement (end-systolic diameter greater than 50 mm), according to the Society of Thoracic Surgeons (STS) guidelines.

*Class IIa Indications (Reasonable Recommendations):*
- Asymptomatic patients with severe AR, normal LVEF, and severe LV dilation: AVR may be considered for asymptomatic patients with severe AR, a normal LVEF (above 50%), but significant LV enlargement (end-systolic diameter greater than 50 mm).

*Other Considerations:*
- Undergoing other cardiac surgery:
  - If a patient with severe AR requires another cardiac surgery, AVR should be considered at the same time.
- Progression of LV dysfunction:
  - Even in asymptomatic patients, close monitoring of LV function is crucial. If LV dysfunction (reduced LVEF or increased LV size) progresses, AVR may become indicated.

# CONGENITAL HEART DISEASE

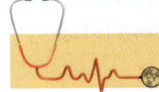

## Case 5: Atrial Septal Defect

*Brief History*
A 35-year-old with exertional fatigue and episodic palpitations.

*Examination*
- Conscious, cooperative
- Short built and poorly nourished
- Height = 158 cm, weight = 40 kg, BMI = 15.44 kg/m², arm span = 160, Height = 158, Ratio = 1.02
- Temperature = 36.8°C
- Pulse = 68/mt, normal rhythm and volume, character, no vessel wall thickening, no R-R delay, no R-F delay
- All peripheral pulses are well felt
- Blood pressure = 108/60 mm Hg in all four limbs, no postural drop
- Respiratory rate-16/mt, abdominothoracic
- Facial dysmorphism present, low set ears, low posterior hairline
- Chest hairs minimal but axillary and pubic hairs normal
- Skin and nail normal
- No pallor, icterus, cyanosis, clubbing, lymphadenopathy, pedal edema

*Systemic Examination*
Cardiovascular System Examination
Inspection:
- JVP not raised
- Precordial bulge present
- Apical impulse seen lateral to MCL in 5th intercostal space (ICS)
- Pulsations seen in left parasternal area, pulmonary area and suprasternal area
- No scars, engorged veins, sinus over chest
- No kyphoscoliosis, gibbus

Palpation:
- Apical impulse confirmed in 5th intercostal space 1 cm lateral to MCL. Hyperkinetic
- Left parasternal lift present grade 1
- Tricuspid area: No pulsations, no palpable S1, no Thrill
- Pulmonary area: Pulsations felt, palpable P2, Thrill present (systolic)
- Aortic area: No pulsations, no palpable a2, no Thrill

Percussion:
- Right heart border corresponds to right sternal margin and left border to apex
- Dullness in 2nd intercostals space

Auscultation:
- Mitral area—s1 s2 heard, mid systolic murmur heard, grade 1, not changing with posture or respiration
- Tricuspid area—s1 s2 heard, systolic murmur heard, grade 2, not changing with respiration and posture
- Pulmonary area—s1 loud, s2 wide and fixed split, ejection systolic murmur—crescendo decrescendo murmur, grade 4, increasing on sitting and height of inspiration, no associated click.
- Aortic area—s1 and s2 heard, systolic murmur radiating from pulmonary area

*Gastrointestinal System*
Hepatomegaly, 1 cm below costal margin, smooth surface, soft to firm consistency, nontender.

*Respiratory System*
NVBS, no added sounds.

*Nervous System*
No focal neurological deficit, WNL.

*Summary*
A 35-year-old male patient, low set ears, low posterior hairline and facial dysmorphism. CVS examination showed precordial bulge, LPH, hyperkinetic and ill-sustained apex, palpable P2 and thrill in pulmonary area.

On auscultation wide fixed S2 and ejection systolic murmur radiating to infraclavicular area and all over precordium.

*Diagnosis*
Congenital heart disease, ASD with pulmonary hypertension, no features of heart failure, or infective endocarditis, not in atrial fibrillation, NYHA class II.

*Points Favoring ASD:*
- Facial dysmorphism, low set ears, low posterior hairline (congenital HD)
- Precordial bulge (long-standing RVH)
- Left parasternal lift
- S2: Wide fixed split
- Ejection systolic murmur in pulmonary area
- Palpable P2 and loud P2 on auscultation

## DISCUSSION

**Q. What are the normal waves of JVP?**
- A wave—right atrial contraction, c wave—downward bulging of closed TV
- x descent—atrial relaxation, v wave—right atrial filling during RV systole when TV closed
- y descent—RA emptying during early RV diastole when TV opens

- Prominent a waves—tricuspid stenosis, tricuspid atresia, RA myxoma
- Bernheim effect due to severe AS and HOCM
- Cannon a waves—regular-junctional rhythm, irregular-CHB with AV dissociation, VPC
- JVP changes in tricuspid regurgitation—absent x descent, prominent v wave, rapid y descent

## Q. What are the normal cardiac chamber pressures?

- Right atrium-mean pressure = 1–5 mm Hg, left atrium = 2–12 mm Hg
- Right ventricle-peak systolic = 15–30 mm Hg, end diastolic = 1–7 mm Hg
- Pulmonary artery-peak systolic = 15–30 mm Hg, end diastolic = 4–12 mm Hg, mean = 9–19 mm Hg
- PCWP = 4–12 mm Hg
- Left ventricle-peak systolic = 90–140 mm Hg, end diastolic = 5–12 mm Hg
- Aorta-peak systolic = 90–140 mm Hg, end diastolic = 60–90 mm Hg, mean = 70–105 mm Hg

## Q. What is the difference between cardiac chamber enlargement and hypertrophy?

- In dilation of a chamber, heart muscle is stretched and the chamber becomes enlarged, e.g., congestive heart failure due to aortic valve regurgitation, atrial enlargements.
- In hypertrophy, the heart muscle fibers actually increases in size, with results in enlargement of chamber, e.g., aortic stenosis causes outflow obstruction which leads to hypertrophy of left ventricle.

## Q. What are the causes of left parasternal heave?

RVH and LAE, to differentiate:
- RVH—systolic, epigastric pulsations present
- LAE—diastolic

## Q. What is Lutembacher syndrome?

- Lutembacher syndrome is congenital ASD with acquired mitral stenosis. In 1916. Lutembacher described MS to be congenital.
- Ostium secundum ASD with rheumatic MS is classic case of Lutembacher syndrome.
- Lutembacher syndrome is also applied for ASD following Percutaneous mitral commissurotomies (PTMC) for rheumatic MS.
- Lutembacher syndrome is more common in females because ostium secundum ASD, and rheumatic MS are common in females.
- In underdeveloped countries 40% patient give antecedent history of rheumatic fever.
- MS is rheumatic even patient with familial ASD.

## Q. What is hemodynamic Lutembacher syndrome?

Coexistence of MS with ASD results in modification of symptoms and signs of both. Increased pressure of left atrium in MS has one more outlet, i.e., ASD, so gradient across mitral valve is reduced in presence of ASD with MS. Leading to masking signs and MS depending on whether ASD is restrictive or non-restrictive. Susceptibility of infective endocarditis is increased with this combination.

## Q. What happens to arterial pulse in ASD?

Pulse is small volume because of decreased stoke volume, due to left to right shunting.

## Q. What happens to jugular venous pulse in ASD?

JVP can be elevated and "a" wave may be prominent without right heart failure and pulmonary hypertension due left to right shunting

## Q. What is precordial examination?

This gives very valuable information, in case of Lutembacher syndrome. RV and pulmonary artery are dilated much more than isolated ASD, so left parasternal impulse is very prominent than isolated ASD and apex is formed by RV. Thrill across RVOT is present unlike isolated ASD. Diastolic thrill of MDM secondary to MS is rare in Lutembacher syndrome.

## Q. What are the effects on MS by ASD?

Depending on whether ASD is restrictive or nonrestrictive symptoms and signs of MS are further modified.

In patients with nonrestrictive ASD, symptoms and signs of MS are masked, i.e., hardly MDM of mitral valve is heard, instead MDM of tricuspid valve is heard due to increase flow, and first heart sound is not loud. Signs and symptoms of pulmonary venous hypertension are not present, i.e., orthopnea and PND, instead patient present with symptoms of easy fatigability, secondary to decreased cardiac output due to left to right shunting.

In patient with restrictive ASD with MS, signs and symptoms of MS still persist, with continuous murmur across ASD which increases with inspiration.

## Q. What are effects on ASD by MS?

Wide fixed second heart sound with more than grade four by six ejection systolic murmur (thrill) across RVOT is present (ASD alone usually is not associated with thrill).

## Q. Describe the ECG findings in ASD with MS.

- ECG in restrictive ASD with MS is predominate of MS, i.e., left atrial enlargement.
- ECG with nonrestrictive ASD is predominate of ASD.
- Atrial fibrillation is more frequent.

## Q. What are the chest X-ray findings of ASD with MS?

- Pulmonary venous hypertension is present in patient with restrictive ASD with MS but not in nonrestrictive ASD with MS.
- Left atrial enlargement is less than expected for MS but more than expected for ASD.
- RA and RV and PA dilatation is more than isolated ASD.
- **Echocardiogram:** It is very useful to identify ASD and MS.

**Q. What is the treatment of ASD with MS?**
- Right-sided heart failure: Diuretics
- **Atrial fibrillation:** Digoxin, beta-blockers, and calcium channel blockers used mainly for rate control, while amiodarone and sotalol used not only for rate control but also for conversion into and maintenance of normal sinus rhythm.
- Subacute bacterial endocarditis (SBE) prophylaxis

**Indications for surgery or percutaneous intervention**
- ASD with a Qp/Qs ratio of more than 1.5
- Moderate-to-severe mitral stenosis
- Any degree of pulmonary hypertension, except individuals with irreversible pulmonary hypertension (Eisenmenger syndrome)

Percutaneous closure of ASD and mitral balloon valvuloplasty, intervention is now performed early rather than late because the rates of heart failure and cardiac arrhythmia increase with age. Patients with pulmonary hypertension should demonstrate reversibility of pulmonary vascular resistance prior to surgical (or percutaneous) correction of ASD.

**Q. What is Shone complex?**

Shone's syndrome (also known as Shone's complex) is a rare combination of four left-sided congenital cardiac anomalies including parachute mitral valve, supravalvar ring, coarctation (narrowing) of the aorta, and subaortic obstruction. The mitral valve leaflets are abnormal, often thickened or immobile with fused commissures and thick, shortened cords, giving the valve a "parachute" shape **(Fig. 2.31)**.

Mitral regurgitation (leaking of blood back through the mitral valve) and stenosis (narrowing of the mitral valve) are characteristic of Shone's syndrome.

Supravalvar rings are made up of an abnormal ridge of connective tissue that obstructs blood flow through the mitral valve. Coarctation of the aorta prevents adequate blood flow from getting out of the left ventricle to the body. Subaortic obstruction due to narrowing of the left ventricular outflow tract may be worse if thickened papillary muscles are present. These left-sided heart problems and associated symptoms get worse over time without treatment. Shone's syndrome occurs in less than 1% of all congenital cardiac anomalies.

**Q. What is the physical examination/symptoms of Shone complex?**
- **Symptoms of congestive heart failure:** fatigue, tachypnea (fast breathing), tachycardia (fast heart rate), poor weight gain and edema (fluid retention).
- Loud first and second heart sounds, ejection click, and opening snap may be auscultated.
- Pulmonary regurgitation murmur may be present with long-standing pulmonary hypertension.

**Q. How do you diagnose Shone complex?**

**Chest X-ray**

Cardiomegaly due to enlargement of the right ventricle and left atrium. Pulmonary vasculature is prominent and pulmonary edema is present.

**EKG:** Left atrial hypertrophy, right ventricular hypertrophy, and right axis deviation are common.

**Echocardiogram diagnostic:** Cardiac catheterization or computed tomography angiogram (CTA).

**Q. What is the treatment of Shone complex?**
- For infants that are diagnosed prenatally with Shone's syndrome, it is recommended that delivery take place in a

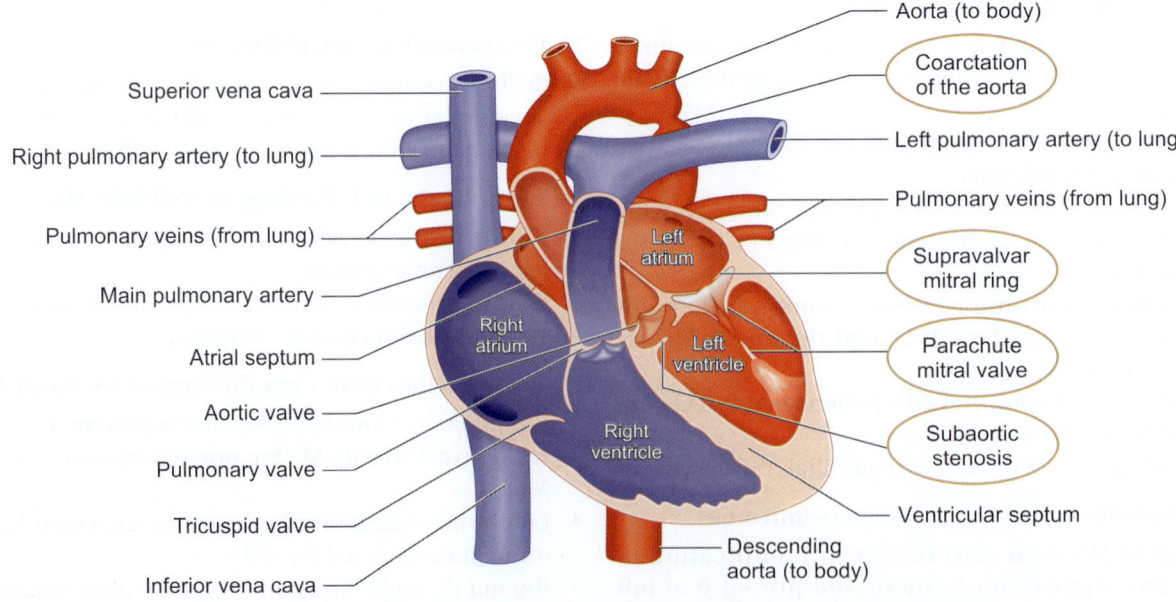

**Fig. 2.31:** Shone's syndrome.

tertiary care hospital with transfer to the neonatal intensive care unit (NICU) as soon as possible to initiate cardiology evaluation and medical interventions.
- When coarctation is present, prostaglandin E infusion is started as soon as possible to keep the ductus arteriosus open prior to surgery.
- Surgical intervention shortly after birth to repair coarctation of the aorta is usually necessary. Multiple surgical interventions may be needed to relieve left-sided obstructions.
- Medications may be needed to treat symptoms of congestive heart failure and/or pulmonary hypertension.
- Bacterial endocarditis antibiotic prophylaxis is required prior to any dental procedures.
- Life-long cardiology follow up is needed.

**Long-term outcomes**
- Infants with significant coarctation who do not undergo surgical intervention usually do not survive.
- Pulmonary hypertension may be a chronic problem requiring medications to manage.
- Growth and developmental outcomes vary depending on severity of disease and the presence or absence of other co-morbidities.

**Q. What are the types of atrial septal defects?**
- **Ostium secundum ASD (center):** Most common type of atrial septal defect. Ostium secundum defects result from shortening of the valve of the foramen ovale, excessive resorption of the septum primum, or deficient growth of the septum secundum.
- **Ostium primum ASD (big on medial side):** Also called atrioventricular septal defects because the atrioventricular septum is defective.
- **Sinus venosus ASD (all insertion of SVC, IVC):** Uncommon, constitute 2–3% of interatrial communications.
  Sinus venosus ASDs are of two types:
  1. Superior sinus venosus defects: Located in the atrial septum immediately below the orifice of the superior vena cava.
  2. Inferior sinus venosus defects: Located in the atrial septum immediately above the orifice of the inferior vena cava. These defects are also often associated with partial anomalous connection of the right pulmonary veins.

> The triad of partial anomalous pulmonary venous return, hypoplasia or aplasia of a lobe of the right lung (most often), and the presence of thoracic aorta to pulmonary artery collaterals to the small lung is referred to as the "**Scimitar syndrome.**" This syndrome may be associated with the development of pulmonary hypertension.

- **Coronary sinus ASD:** Defect is located at the site normally occupied by the right atrial ostium of the coronary sinus and is characterized by an opening in the wall of the distal end of the sinus or by unroofing caused by absence of the partition between the coronary sinus and left atrium.

**Q. What are the syndromes associated with atrial septal defects?**
- **Patau's syndrome (trisomy 13):** Polydactyly, flexion deformities of the fingers, palmar crease, microcephaly, holoprosencephaly, cleft lip, cleft palate, and low-set malformed ears.
- **Edward's syndrome (trisomy 18):** Clenched fists, rocker bottom feet, prominent occiput, low-set malformed ears, and micrognathia.
- **Axenfeld-Rieger anomaly:** Autosomal dominant disorder characterized by ocular abnormalities with glaucoma and monocular abnormalities that include maxillary hypoplasia, dental anomalies, umbilical hernia, and hypospadias.
- **Holt-Oram syndrome (also known as Hand Heart Syndrome):** Hypoplastic thumb with an accessory phalanx that results in triphalangism, a crooked appearance, and difficulty in apposition of thumb to fingertips. The thumb may be rudimentary or absent, and the metacarpal bone may be small or absent with hypoplasia extending to the radius.
- **Down's syndrome:** Congenital anomalies of the heart and gastrointestinal tract, epicanthal folds, flattened facial profile, small and rounded ears, up-slanted palpebral fissures, excess nuchal skin, and brachycephaly.
- **Familial atrial septal defect:** The first gene identified for familial ASD is NKX2-5 (CSX1), located on 5q35.
  The second causal gene for familial ASD with an autosomal-dominant mode of inheritance is GATA4 on chromosome 8p22-23.
  The third causal gene for familial ASD is MYH6, which is located in chromosome 14q12 and encodes myosin heavy chain 6.
- **Ellis–Van Creveld syndrome:** Autosomal-recessive skeletal dysplasia. Skeletal anomalies include short limbs, short ribs, postaxial polydactyly, and dysplastic nails and teeth. ASD and common atrium are the typical cardiac anomalies present in two-thirds of the cases.
- **TAR syndrome:** Thrombocytopenia with absent radius.

**Q. Why is the shunt left to right in ASD?**
- Compliance of right ventricle is more than left ventricle
- Larger size of tricuspid valve
- Compliance of the pulmonary veins

**Q. Mechanism of wide and fixed split in ASD.**
- Fixed—no change with respiration
- Wide—P2 delayed because of RV volume overload
- Wide fixed splitting is an auscultatory hallmark of atrial septal defect.
- Wide splitting is caused by a delay in the pulmonary component associated with an increase in pulmonary

vascular capacitance and an increase in "hangout interval" between the descending limbs of the pulmonary arterial and right ventricular pressure pulses.
- In inspiration increased venous return to right atrium is associated with decreased left-to-right shunt.
- In expiration decreased venous return is associated with increased shunting of blood from left to right atrium, resulting in wide fixed split.

### Q. What are the most common ECG change in ASD?
- Right bundle branch block (RBBB).
- Other ECG changes: Usually right axis deviation (ostium secundum, 85%); left axis deviation in ostium primum, and 10% having normal axis. RBBB is seen, which is partial or complete. Complete heart block may be revealed in ostium primum type; large ASD may have prolongation of P-R interval.

### Q. What is hangout interval?
The semilunar valves are expected to close at the point where the ventricular pressures fall below arterial pressures however they close slightly later, this interval from crossover of pressures and actual closure of valves is called hangout interval.

Due to higher pressures and lower compliance hangout interval on the aortic side is less than pulmonary side.

Hangout interval is measured between incisura of aorta and LV pressure at the same level on left side and between incisura of pulmonary artery and RV pressure at the same level on right side.
A. Hangout interval between LV and aorta **(Fig. 2.32A)**
B. Hangout interval between RV and pulmonary artery **(Fig. 2.32B)**

### Q. What is the importance of precordial bulge?
Precordial bulge indicates cardiac enlargement of long duration usually developing before puberty (16 years of age). Usually seen with RV dilatation.

**Causes:**
- Cardiac: Pericardial effusion, cardiomegaly.
- Noncardiac: Scoliosis, kyphoscoliosis, mediastinal growths, bronchogenic carcinoma.

### Q. Discuss the development of atrial septum.
Refer **Figure 2.33**.
- Septum secundum—upper part of septum
- Septum primum—lower part of septum

### Q. Mention the correlation of ASD with development.
- Ostium secundum—from septum secundum (fossa ovalis)
- Ostium primum—from septum primum

### Q. Mention the anatomy of ASD.
Refer **Figures 2.34A to G**.
- Ostium secundum
- Ostium primum—septum primum (partial AV canal defect)
- Sinus venosus—superior to fossa ovalis in relation to opening of superior vena cava into right atrium
- Coronary sinus—near opening of coronary sinus

### Q. What are the cardiac anomalies associated with ASD?
- Ostium secundum—MVP and partial anomalous pulmonary venous connection (right)
- Ostium primum—cleft mitral/tricuspid valve and 1st degree heart block
- Sinus venosus—partial anomalous pulmonary venous connection

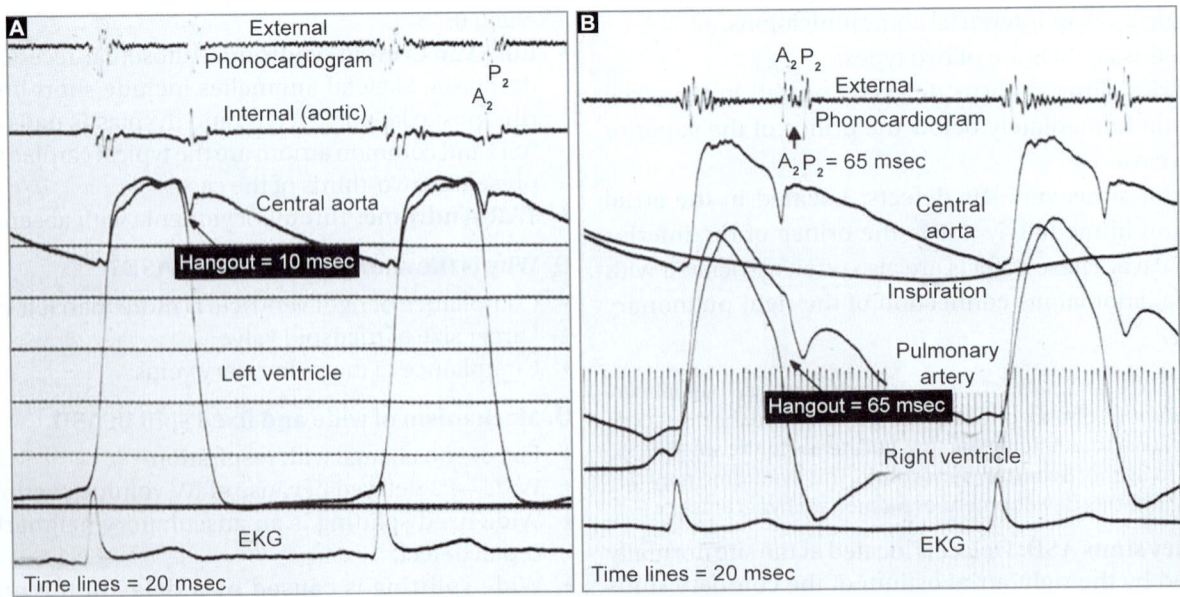

**Figs. 2.32A and B:** Hangout interval.

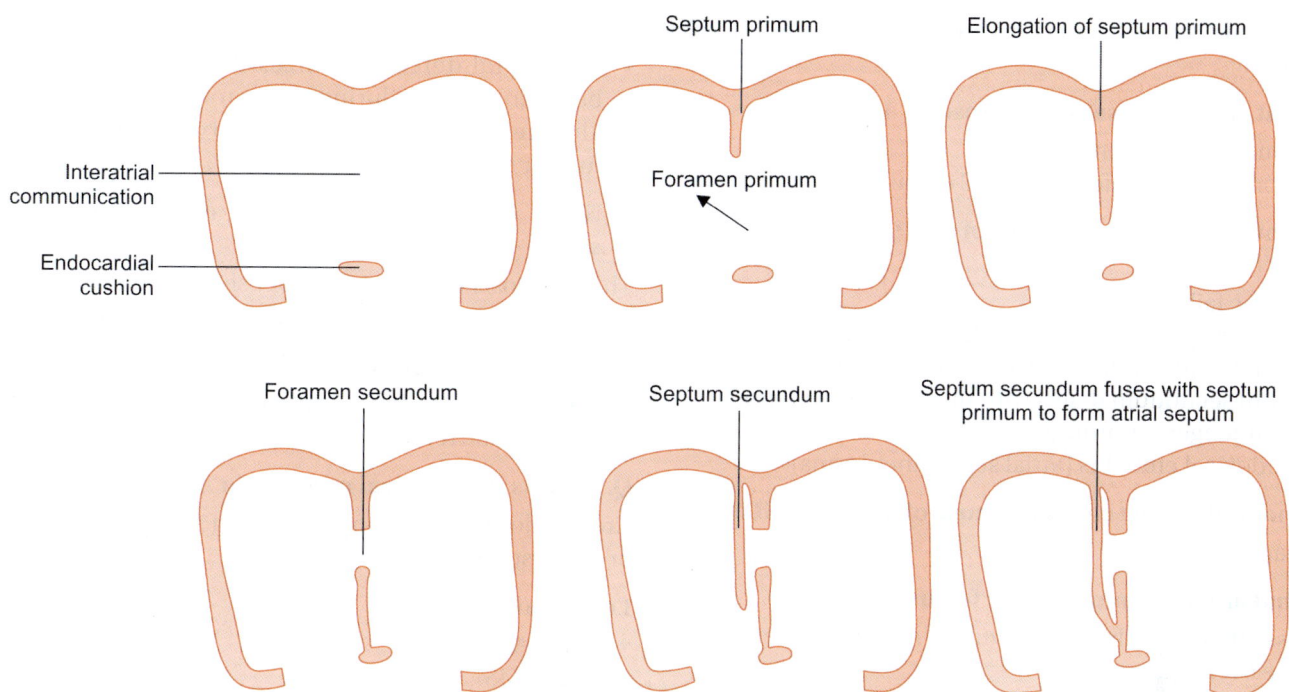

**Fig. 2.33:** Development of atrial septum.

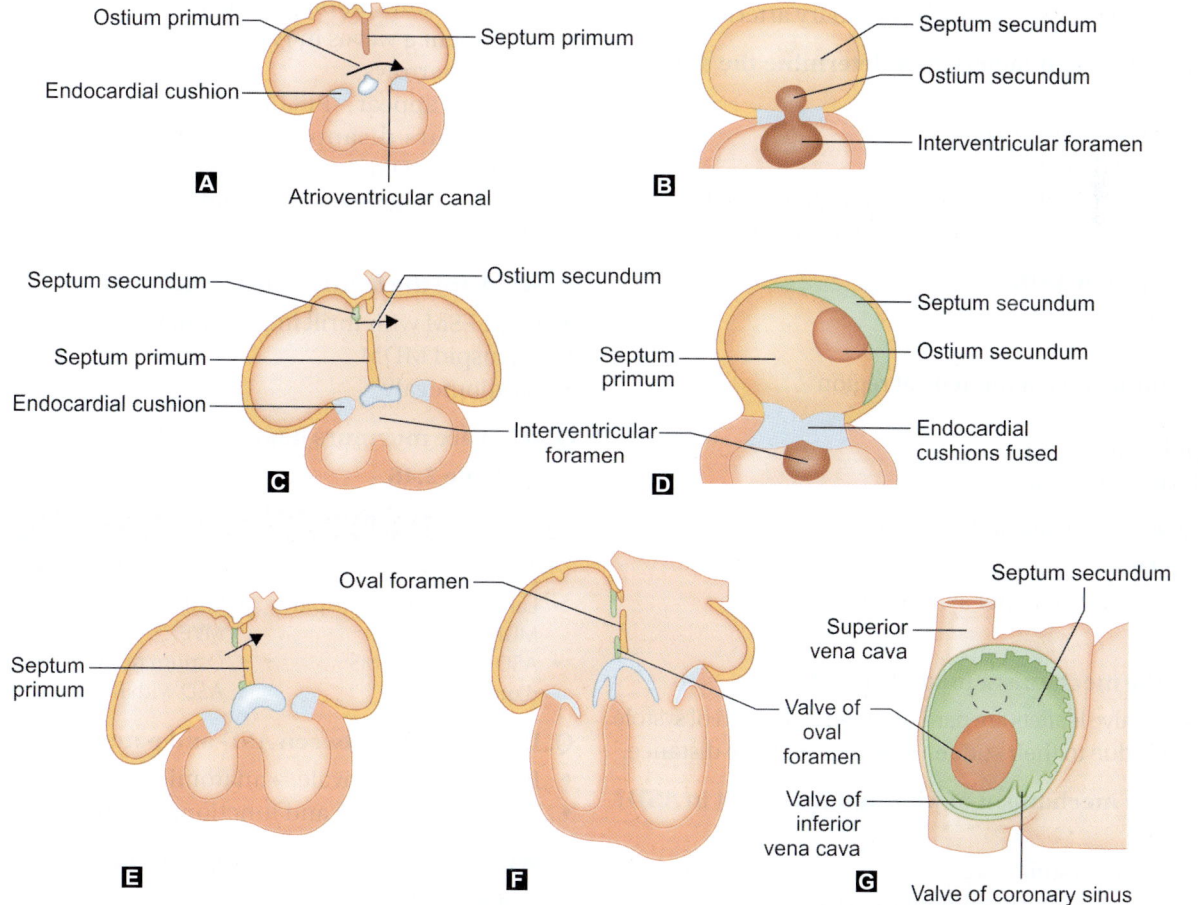

**Figs. 2.34A to G:** Anatomy of ASD.

- Coronary sinus—superior vena cava opening into left atrium

### Q. What are the causes for cyanosis in ASD?
- Eisenmenger syndrome
- Coronary sinus defect with SVC opening into left atrium

### Q. What are the complications of ASD?
- PAH (<10%)
- Cardiac failure
- Acute arrhythmias (atrial fibrillation and atrial flutter)
- Infective endocarditis (especially in ostium primum defect/ostium secundum defect with mitral valve prolapse)
- Eisenmenger syndrome
- Paradoxical embolus (atrial septal aneurysms)

### Q. What is the most common cause of death in ASD?
Cardiac failure

### Q. What are the hemodynamic features of ASD?
The essential hemodynamic feature of ASD is right ventricular volume overload.

When there is RV volume overload it produces the following effect:
- Right ventricle compress on the left ventricle producing reverse Bernheim effect on the interventricular septum.
- Right ventricle compress on the coronary arteries.

### Q. What are the main factors that determine the shunt in ASD?
Shunt in ASD is determined by:
- Size of septal defect
- Relative distensibility of the left and right ventricle.
- Pulmonary as well as systemic vascular resistance.

### Q. List the signs in ASD.
- Palpable P2
- LPH+
- Systolic thrill 2nd left intercostal region
- Wide fixed split S2
- ESM pulmonary area
- MDM tricuspid area

### Q. What are the causes of thrill in ASD?
- Large ASD
- ASD + MS (Lutembacher syndrome)
- ASD + PS

### Q. What is the mechanism loud S1 in ASD?
The tricuspid valve leaflets are partially open at the start of systole. The loud S1 is due to their sudden closure over large distance.

### Q. What is the mechanism of wide and fixed split in ASD?
**Wide split**
- Prolonged RV systole
- Prolonged pulmonary hangout interval
- RBBB

**Fixed split:**
- The septal defect equalizes the pressure differences between the atria during respiratory cycle.
- The already widened hangout interval cannot be increased further during inspiration.

### Q. Name the prerequisite before diagnosing wide fixed split.
The diagnosis of fixed/wide split should be made only after examining the patient in the sitting/standing position.

### Q. Why is P2 loud in ASD?
- Proximity of the dilated pulmonary trunk to the chest wall
- Brisk elastic recoil of the dilated pulmonary trunk

### Q. What is the classical murmur in ASD?
Crescendo-decrescendo ESM in the PA with peak in the early or midsystole.

**Loud murmur in ASD:**
- Large ASD
- ASD + MS
- ASD + PS

### Q. What are the changes in physical signs produced by PAH (Eisenmenger) in ASD?
- Cyanosis and clubbing appears
- Prominent a waves in JVP
- S2 split narrows
- 2 sounds appear—PEC and RVS4
- 2 murmurs disappear/soften—pulmonary ESM and tricuspid MDM
- 2 murmurs appear—tricuspid PSM of TR and pulmonary EDM of PR

### Q. What are the features of a large ASD?
- Loud ESM with thrill in pulmonary area
- Tricuspid MDM
- Cardiomegaly

### Q. What are murmurs heard in ASD in mitral area?
Refer **Table 2.46**.

**Table 2.46:** ASD murmurs.

| ASD with MDM at apex | ASD with PSM at apex |
|---|---|
| • Large ASD with tricuspid MDM<br>• ASD + acquired MS (Lutembacher) | • Ostium secundum ASD with MVP<br>• Ostium primum ASD with MR<br>• ASD with rheumatic MR |

### Q. Differentiate between ASD and patent foramen ovale.
- Patent foramen ovale—anatomical continuity
- ASD—anatomical and functional continuity

### Q. What are the chest X-ray findings in ASD?
Refer **Figure 2.35**.
- RA, RV enlargement

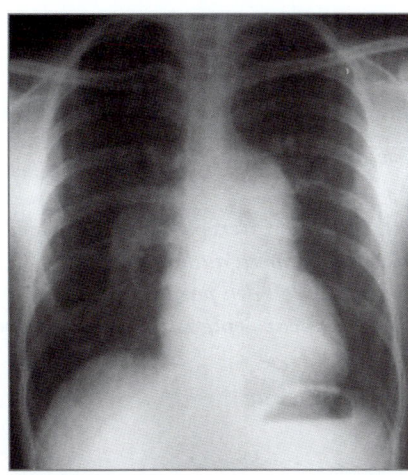

**Fig. 2.35:** Chest X-ray of atrial septal defect showing jug handle appearance.

- Prominent main pulmonary artery
- Prominent pulmonary plethora
- Hilar dance (on fluroscopy)

### Q. What are the echo findings in ASD?
- RV dilatation
- Paradoxical septal motion
- The defect best visualized with subcostal echo
- Confirmatory technique—2D echo with Doppler/contrast
- Transesophageal echo—diagnostic in ambiguous transthoracic echo

### Q. What are the indications for cardiac catheterization in ASD?
- Ambiguous echo
- Associated CAD
- Associated valve disease
- Associated PAH

### Q. Discuss the treatment of ASD.
- Median sternotomy with direct closure of small to moderate defect.
- Larger defects closed with autologous pericardium or synthetic patches, such as polyester polymer (Dacron) or polytetrafluoroethylene (PTFE).
- Surgical closure of the defect is done in patients above 3 years of age, provided there are no signs of pulmonary hypertension and the pulmonary flow is 50% more than the systemic blood flow (Qp:Qs>1.5/1).
- A transcatheter septal clamshell device closure may be used for most secundum ASDs (if suitable size).

**Indications for intervention**
- ASD with significant left to right shunting resulting in right atrial/ventricular enlargement irrespective of symptoms.
- Atrial septal defects in which pulmonary flow is increased 50% above systemic flow (i.e., flow ratio of 1.5:1).
- Thromboembolic events.

**Contraindications to treatment**
- Small defects with trivial shunts
- Severe PAH with right—left shunt (pulmonary vascular resistance: Systemic vascular resistance >0.7:1)

### Q. What is ASD with bidirectional shunt?
- ASD with shunt occurring in either direction depending on pulmonary vascular resistance and systemic vascular resistance.
- Patient has clubbing cyanosis only on exertion. There are clinical signs of ASD with left—right shunt pulmonary ESM and tricuspid MDM).

# 116 SECTION 2: Cardiovascular System

## Case 6: Ventricular Septal Defect

*Brief History*
A 46-year-old male with history of fever with chills and rigors, dyspnea, cough with expectoration of 2 weeks duration.

*General Examination*
- Middle-aged man
- Conscious and cooperative
- Febrile
- Weight—62 kg
- Height—164 cm
- BMI—23.1 kg/m²
- IV cannula in the left forearm; no signs of superficial thrombophlebitis
- No pallor/jaundice/cyanosis/clubbing/ lymphadenopathy/ pedal edema
- No thyroid swelling
- Gynecomastia present
- Vitals:
  - Temperature—101°F
  - Pulse—102/min, regular rhythm, normal volume and character, all peripheral pulses palpable, no radioradial and radiofemoral delay.
  - BP—130/90 mm Hg right upper arm supine position, no postural drop.
  - Respiratory rate—37/min

*Systemic Examination*
Cardiovascular System
Inspection:
- JVP—not raised
- Shape of precordium—normal
- Apical impulse—not visible
- No dilated veins/scars/pulsations.

Palpation:
- Apex felt at 6th left intercostal space 3 cm lateral to midclavicular line, hyperdynamic
- Thrill present in the left 4th parasternal area
- No left parasternal heave/epigastric pulsations/palpable P2

Percussion:
Pulmonary area—resonant.

Auscultation:
Mitral area:
- S1, S2—not heard
- A high pitched soft blowing pansystolic murmur grade 3 is heard; best heard with diaphragm of the stethoscope.
- Left 4 iCS parasternal area—pansystolic murmur, grade 4/6 intensity, heard with diaphragm of stethoscope, no change with respiration.

Tricuspid area:
- Pansystolic murmur with grade 4 intensity
- S1, S2—not heard.

Pulmonary area:
- Pansystolic murmur present of grade 3 intensity
- S2—heard; normal intensity.

Aortic:
- Pansystolic murmur, grade 2 intensity
- S1 and S2—soft; no carotid bruit.

*Diagnosis*
Ventricular septal defect with no evidence of pulmonary hypertension or heart failure, with possible infective endocarditis.

## DISCUSSION

**Q. What are the types of VSD?**

The types of VSD are (Figs. 2.36A to E):
1. **Infracristal/membranous**—below crista supraventricular located 1–2 cm below aortic valve cusps and occur just above the insertion of the septal leaflet of tricuspid valve. Rarely, high membranous infracristal VSD can result in communication between left ventricular outflow tract and right atrium. 80% in frequency.
2. **Muscular (5–20%)**—anterior aspect of trabeculated portion of muscular interventricular septum (multiple) anterior to papillary muscle of conus.
3. **Supracristal (5–7%)**—right ventricular outflow tract below pulmonic valve and above crista supraventricular. This type is common in Japan.

**Q. What are the associations of VSD?**
- **Aortic regurgitation**—acquired abnormality related to inadequate support of the semilunar valve ring of sinus of Valsalva because of contiguous VSD.
  Associated with supracristal defects mostly but also with high infracristal defects.
- Aneurysm of membranous septum associated with high VSD.
- Very large VSD with torrential left to right shunt, severe pulmonary vascular changes can result in markedly elevated pulmonary vascular resistance and subsequent reversal of L-R shunt (Eisenmenger syndrome).
- Tetralogy of Fallot.

**Q. What are the differences between mitral regurgitation and VSD?**
- In mitral regurgitation, pansystolic murmur is best heard in the mitral area that radiates to left axilla and left infrascapular areas.

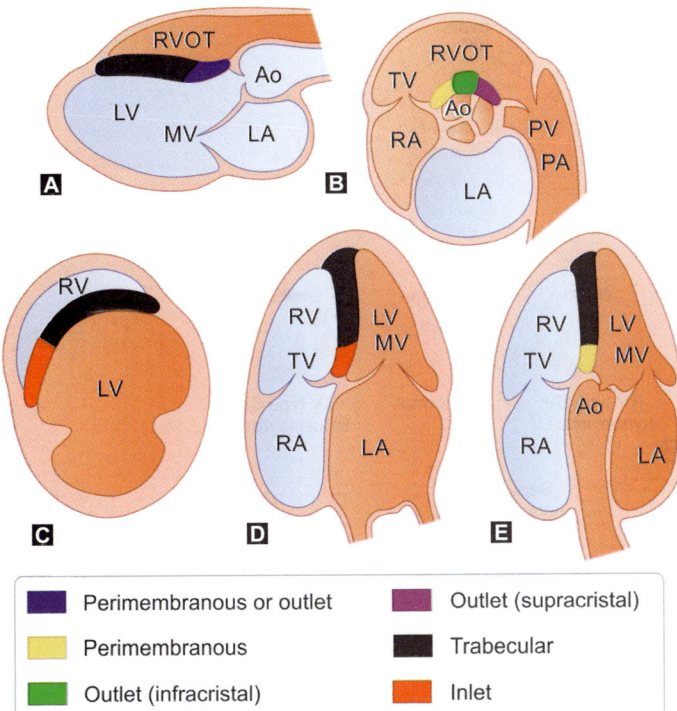

**Figs. 2.36A to E:** Types of VSD.

- In VSD, pansystolic murmur is best heard in the tricuspid area that radiates to right parasternal area, left axilla and left infrascapular areas.
- In MR, apex is LV type.
- In VSD, apex usually not displaced laterally. If there is pulmonary hypertension, apex will be shifted.

**Q. Discuss the development of ventricular septum.**

Refer **Figures 2.37A to H**.
- **Trabecular septum:** From primitive interventricular septum
- **Membranous septum:**
  - Proximal bulbar septum
  - Proliferation from AV cushions

**Q. What is the correlation of types of VSD with development of septum?**
- **Inlet type**—defect in the septum derived from AV cushions
- **Outlet type**—defect in the septum derived from proximal bulbar septum
- **Trabecular type**—defect of the septum derived from primitive ventricular septum

**Q. List the factors determining the shunt in VSD.**
- Size VSD
- Relative distensibility of the LV-RV
- Systemic and pulmonary vascular resistance

**Q. What are the factors facilitating the spontaneous closure of VSD?**
- Trabecular and perimembranous close preferentially.
- 5–10% nonrestrictive and 50–75% of restrictive close.
- 25% close in 1 year and 90% close by 8 years.

**Spontaneous closure of VSD:**
- Adherence of tricuspid valve leaflets to the defect
- Hypertrophy of septal muscle
- Ingrowth of fibrous tissue
- Prolapse of aortic cusp into the defect
- Ventricular septal symptoms

**Q. What do you mean by restrictive and nonrestrictive VSD?**

**Restrictive VSD**

Resistance to left–right shunt at the site of the defect. RV systolic pressure, LV systolic pressure. Moderate left–right shunt during systole and diastole. Low pulmonary vascular resistance. LV volume overload occurs. LV failure is the main complication.

**Nonrestrictive VSD**

The two ventricles act as a common chamber with equal systolic pressures. Shunt depends on the pulmonary and systemic resistance.

Pulmonary vascular resistance is elevated. Large left–shunt. LV volume overload occurs. Eisenmenger syndrome is common.

**Q. What are the symptoms of VSD?**
- Small VSD—asymptomatic.
- Moderate to large VSD
  - Dyspnea on exertion
  - Palpitation
  - Recurrent chest infections

**Q. List the signs of VSD.**
- Hyperkinetic pulse
- Forceful apex with cardiomegaly
- Systolic thrill LLSB
- Wide split S2
- LV S3
- PSM LLSB
- MDM mitral area

**Q. What are the murmurs you hear in VSD?**
- **Trivial defects**—high-pitched early systolic decrescendo murmur LLSB
- **Small defect**—high-pitched pansystolic murmur LLSB (Roger's murmur)
- **Moderate defect**—high-pitched PSM LLSB
- **Large defect**—high-pitched PSM LLSB
- **VSD with PAH**—high-pitched early systolic decrescendo murmur
- **Eisenmenger VSD**—high-pitched early systolic decrescendo murmur

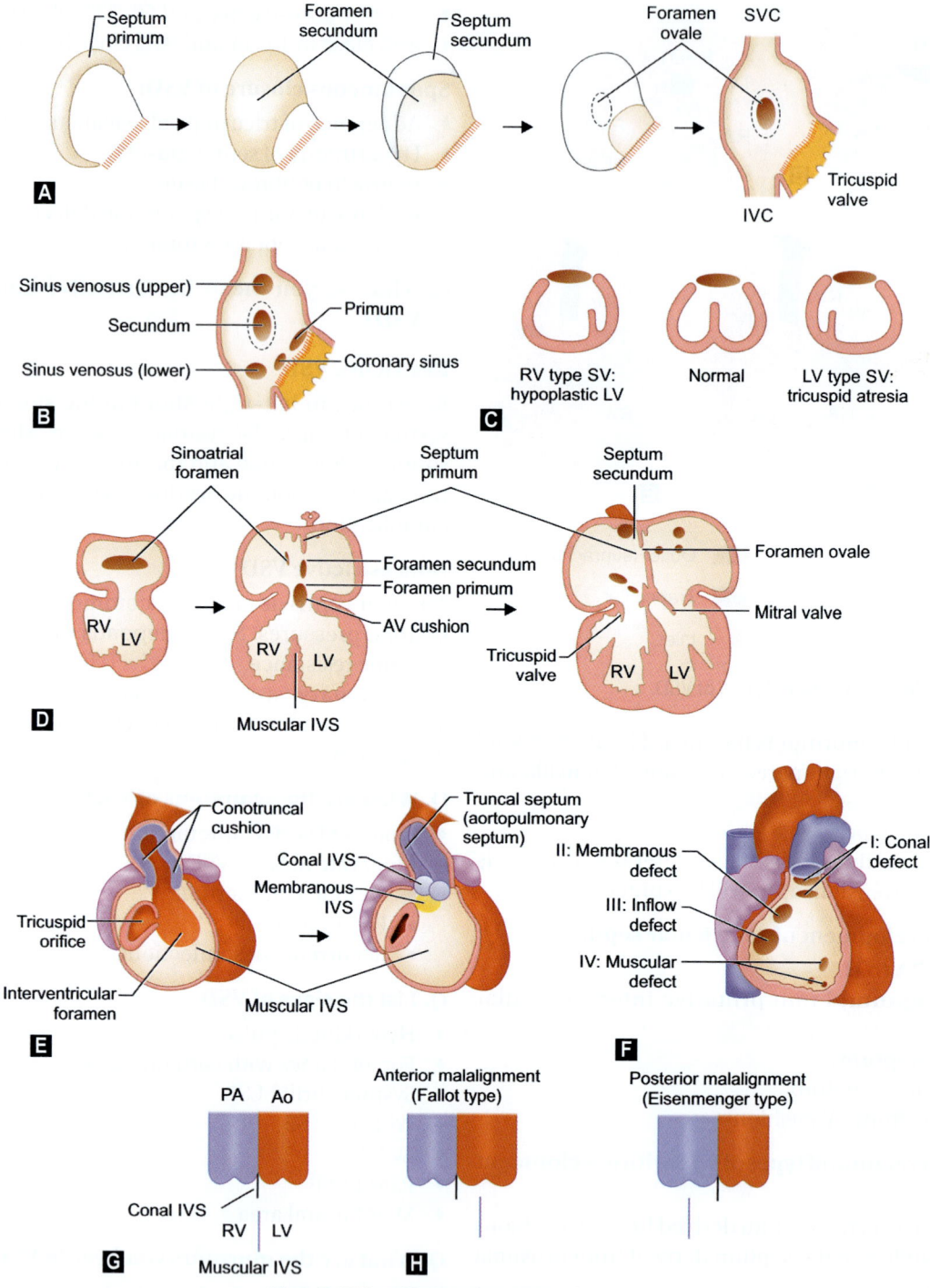

Figs. 2.37A to H: Development of septum.

**Q. What are the causes of VSD with early systolic murmur?**
- Trivial VSD
- VSD with PAH
- Eisenmenger VSD

**Q. What are the causes for absent murmur in VSD?**
- Newborn
- Spontaneous closure
- Eisenmenger syndrome
- RVOT obstruction

**Q. What are the signs of PAH development in VSD?**
- Prominent a waves in JVP
- LPH
- Loud P2
- S2 spit narrows or becomes single

- 2 sound appear—PEC and RV4
- 2 murmurs disappear/soften—PSM and mitral MDM
- 2 murmurs appear—PSM of TR and EDM of PR

### Q. How do you clinical correlate signs with the size of VSD?
Refer **Table 2.47**.

**Table 2.47:** Correlation of signs with the size of VSD.

| Size | Features |
|---|---|
| Small | Murmur alone |
| Moderate | • Hyperkinetic pulse<br>• Cardiomegaly<br>• Wide split S2 |
| Large | • Hyperkinetic pulse<br>• Cardiomegaly<br>• Wide split S2<br>• LVS3<br>• MDM mitral area |

### Q. How do you differentiate MR versus VSD?
Refer **Table 2.48**.

**Table 2.48:** MR versus VSD.

| MR | VSD |
|---|---|
| Systolic thrill apex | Thrill LLSB |
| LPH present | LPH absent |
| PSM mitral area | PSM at LLSB |

### Q. How do you differentiate TR versus VSD?
Refer **Table 2.49**.

**Table 2.49:** TR versus VSD.

| TR | VSD |
|---|---|
| Pulse normal | Hyperkinetic |
| JVP elevated with prominent "v" wave | Normal |
| Normal apex | Forceful apex |
| P2 palpable | Not palpable |
| No thrill | Systolic thrill LLSB |
| LPH present | Absent |
| Murmur increases with inspiration | No change |
| Hepatic pulsations present | Absent |

### Q. What are the ECG findings in VSD?
Refer **Table 2.50**.

**Table 2.50:** ECG findings in VSD.

| Small | Moderate VSD | Large | Essenmenger VSD |
|---|---|---|---|
| Normal | LAO | LAO and RAO | RAO |
| | LVH | LVH and RVH | RVH |
| | Left axis deviation (LAD) | Right axis deviation (RAD) | RAD |

**Katz-Wachtel phenomenon:** Tall diphasic QRS complexes (>50 mm in height) in the mid-precordial leads (leads V2, V3 or V4) typically associated with biventricular hypertrophy (BVH).

### Q. What are the X-ray signs in VSD?
Refer **Table 2.51**.

**Table 2.51:** CXR findings in VSD.

| Small | Moderate VSD | Large |
|---|---|---|
| Normal | • Cardiomegaly<br>• Left atrial and LV<br>• Enlargement | • Cardiomegaly<br>• Left atrial and LV<br>• Enlargement |
| | • Prominent main<br>• Pulmonary artery<br>• Pulmonary plethora | • Prominent main<br>• Pulmonary artery<br>• Pulmonary plethora |

### Q. Why there is no cardiomegaly in VSD—Eisenmenger?
- RV seldom dilates to cope with systemic vascular resistance.
- Little or no left atrial enlargement.

### Q. What are the complications of VSD?
- PAH and Eisenmenger syndrome
- Infective endocarditis
- Cardiac failure
- Aortic regurgitation
- RVOT obstruction

### Q. What are the features of RVOT obstruction in VSD?
- Seen in 5–10% of patients with VSD
- Resembles TOF.
- Physical signs in VSD with RVOT obstruction
  - Prominent a waves in JVP
  - LPH
  - Soft P2
  - 1 sound appears—RVS4
  - 2 murmurs disappear/become soft: PSM of VSD and MDM
  - 1 murmur appear crescendo-decrescendo: ESM of infundibular PS

### Q. What is the association of AR with VSD?
- Seen in 5% patients
- Usually noted after 5 years
- Detected by EDM and collapsing pulse
- Prolapse of aortic valve leaflet through the subpulmonic supracristal VSD
- Primary abnormality of the aortic valve leaflet—usually one defective commissure in cases of infracristal VSD

### Q. What is the approach to treatment of VSD?
Refer **Figure 2.38**.

# SECTION 2: Cardiovascular System

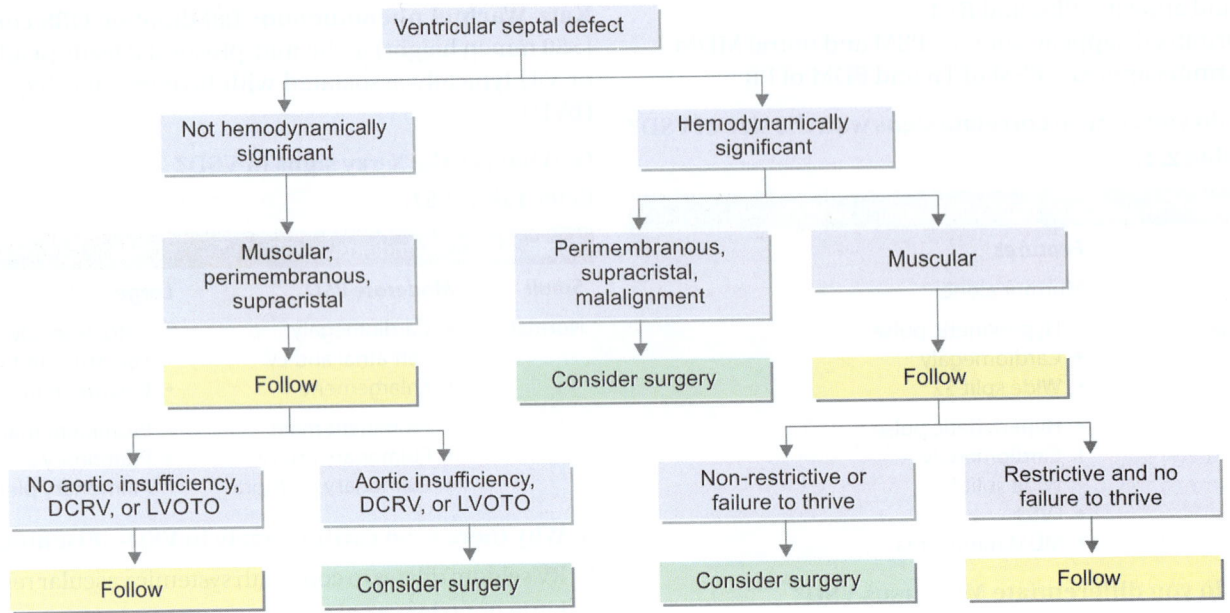

**Fig. 2.38:** Treatment of VSD.

### Q. Discuss the indications and contraindications for surgical correction of VSD.

**Indication of treatment**
- Significant left to right shunt with
- Pulmonary Systemic blood flow >1.5—2:1 **(Table 2.52)**

**Contraindications to treatment**
- Small defects with shunts <1.5—2:1
- Severe PAH with right–left shunt (pulmonary systemic vascular resistance >0.7:1).

| Table 2.52: Recommendations for VSD correction. | | |
|---|---|---|
| **Indications** | **Class** | **Level** |
| Patients with symptoms that can be attributed to L–R shunting through the (residual) VSD and who have no severe pulmonary vascular disease should undergo surgical VSD closure | I | C |
| Asymptomatic patients with evidence of LV volume overload attributable to the VSD should undergo surgical VSD closure | I | C |
| Patients with a history of IE should be considered for surgical VSD closure | IIa | C |
| Patients with VSD-associated prolapse of an aortic valve cusp causing progressive AR should be considered for surgery | IIa | C |

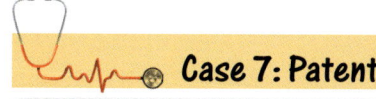

## Case 7: Patent Ductus Arteriosus

### Brief History
A one-month-old girl was referred to our hospital because of tachypnea and difficulty in breathing. The child was born via elective cesarean section at 37 weeks and 0 days of gestation, weighing 2,955 g, with Apgar scores of 6/9.

### Examination
Her weight was 3,015 g, body temperature was 37.3°C, blood pressure was 87/43 mm Hg, heart rate was 155 beats/min and regular, respiratory rate was 67 breaths/min, and blood oxygen saturation (lower extremity) was 96% (room air). A continuous murmur was heard at the left upper sternal border. Respiratory sounds were clear.

### Diagnosis
Congenital acyanotic heart disease—patent ductus arteriosus with no pulmonary hypertension.

## DISCUSSION

- Patent ductus arteriosus (PDA) represents 5–10% of all congenital heart defects.
- It can be associated with other cardiovascular anomalies, most importantly coarctation of the aorta, ventricular septal defect and aortic or pulmonary stenosis.
- PDA is most often diagnosed and surgically or percutaneously corrected in infancy, so a primary diagnosis is rare in adulthood.
- Left untreated, PDA can lead to pulmonary hypertension, Eisenmenger syndrome, heart failure and endarteritis. We report two adult patients diagnosed with PDA.
- When does the ductus close psychologically:
  - Within two hours of birth
  - 2 weeks usually can extend up to
    - 8 weeks in terms
    - 6 months is preterm

**Q. What is the development of ductus arteriosus?**
- Left 6th aortic arch factors which produce the closure of PDA
- Sudden increase in the partial pressure of oxygen
- Decrease in vasoactive prostaglandins

**Q. What are the symptoms of PDA?**
- Small PDA—asymptomatic
- Moderate to large PDA
  - Dyspnea on excretion
  - Palpitation
  - Recurrent chest infections

**Q. What are the signs of PDA?**
- Collapsing pulse
- Forceful apex with cardiomegaly
- Thrill in the infraclavicular area
- Paradoxical split
- LVS3
- Continuous murmuring in/above the 2nd LICS
- MDM in the mitral area.

**Q. What are the signs of PAH in PDA?**
- Prominent a waves in JVP
- LPH
- Loud P2
- S2 split normal
- 2 sounds appear—PEC and RVS4
- 2 murmurs disappear/soften—continuous murmur and mitral MDM
- 2 murmur appear—PSM of TR and EDM of PR

**Q. What are the clinical correlation with the size of the PDA?**

Refer **Table 2.53**.

**Table 2.53:** The clinical severity grading of the PDA in adults.

| Type of the PDA | Murmur | Wide pulse pressure | Dilated left ventricle | Pulmonary hypertension |
|---|---|---|---|---|
| Silent | – | – | – | – |
| Small | Continuous | – | – | – |
| Moderate | Continuous | + | + | + |
| Large | Systolic + | | | |
| | Diastolic ± | ± | ++ | ++ |
| Eisenmenger | Ejection murmur | – | ++ | +++ |

**Differential diagnosis of continuous murmur**
- PDA
- Venous hum
- Pulmonary AV fistula
- Bronchopulmonary collaterals in tetralogy of Fallot, tricuspid atresia
- Surgical Blalock–Taussig shunt
- Peripheral pulmonary artery stenosis
- RSOV
- ALCAPA
- AP window
- Coronary AV fistula
- Intercostal AV fistula

- Collaterals in coarctation of aorta
- Mammary souffle

### Q. What is the differences between venous hum versus PDA?

Refer **Table 2.54**.

| Table 2.54: Venous hum versus PDA. | |
|---|---|
| **Venous hum** | **PDA** |
| Disappears on lying down | No change |
| Disappears on applying pressure | No change |
| Increases with inspiration | No change |

### Q. What are the complications of PDA?
- PAH and Eisenmenger syndrome
- Infective endocarditis
- Cardiac failure
- Rupture of ductus

### Q. How do you treat PDA?

The definitive treatment of PDA is by closing it either by a transcatheter approach or by surgery. Transcatheter closure has been established to be the method of choice for treating a PDA in adults with very good outcome. However, surgical closure is still the method of choice for treating very large PDAs not amendable for catheter intervention
- Litigation/division of PDA
- Rashkind umbrella
- Operation deferred for several months after infective endocarditis because ductus is friable.

## Case 8: Eisenmenger's/Cyanotic Heart Disease

### Brief History
A 7-month-old boy presents with his mother, who reports episodes of tachypnea, cyanosis, and irritability during feeding. The mother explains that these episodes have become more frequent, with the patient becoming more cyanotic around the mouth and hands, but seem to resolve spontaneously. The patient currently appears comfortable, with no signs of respiratory distress, fever, or neurological impairment. The pregnancy and delivery of the patient were uncomplicated; the mother has had 2 prior pregnancies with no complications.

### Examination
The patient's vital signs include a pulse of 140 beats per minute, a respiration rate of 40 breaths per minute, and an oxygen saturation level of 80% (normal oxygen saturation levels: 95–100%). Lung sounds are normal to auscultation. Heart auscultation—single second heart sound with a systolic crescendo–decrescendo ejection murmur is heard most strongly in the pulmonary area.

### Diagnosis
Congenital cyanotic heart disease with decreased pulmonary blood flow possibly TOF.

---

Congenital heart disease (CHD) affects 8–12/1,000 live births in India, and approximately 25% are considered CCHD. The incidence of CHD increase to 2–6% for a second pregnancy after the birth of a child with CHD or if a parent is affected. Tetralogy of Fallot (TOF) is the most common CCHD (5% of all CCHD). Transposition of the great arteries (TGA) is the second most common CCHD (approximately 2% of all CCHD), and it is the most common CCHD manifesting in the first week after birth. It is estimated that 35% of infant deaths due to congenital malformations are related to cardiovascular anomalies **(Fig. 2.39)**.

### Q. Classify congenital heart diseases.

**CHD with increased pulmonary blood flow**
- Ventricular septal defect
- Atrial septal defect
- Patent ductus arteriosus

**CHD with decreased pulmonary blood flow**
- Pulmonary stenosis

**CHD with normal pulmonary blood flow**
- Aortic stenosis
- Coarctation of aorta

**CHD with increased pulmonary blood flow**
- Truncus arteriosus
- Total anomalous pulmonary venous connection
- Tricuspid atresia without pulmonary stenosis
- Transposition of great arteries without pulmonary stenosis
- Double outlet right ventricle without pulmonary stenosis

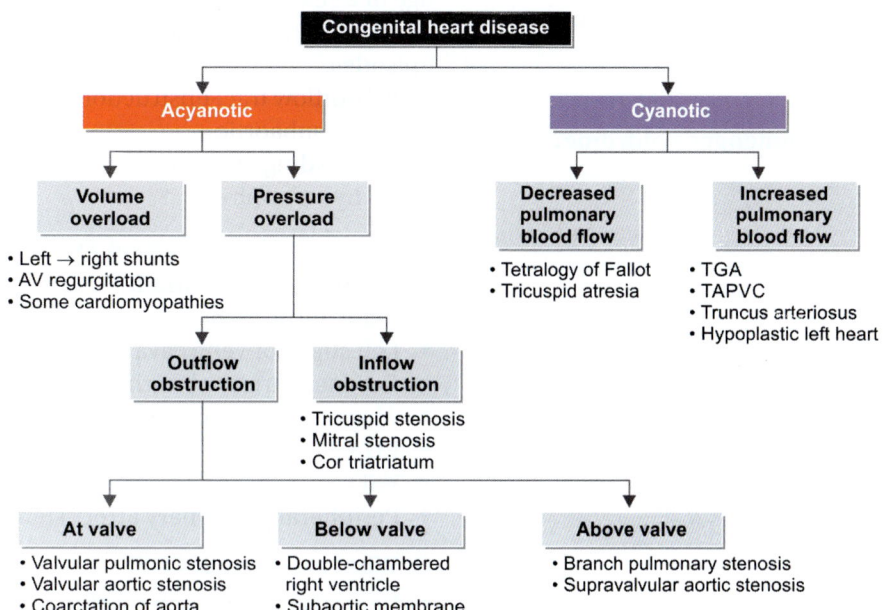

**Fig. 2.39:** Classification of CHD.

- Single ventricle without pulmonary stenosis
- Common atrium
- Hypoplastic left heart

**CHD with decreased pulmonary blood flow**
- Tetralogy of Fallot
- Tricuspid atresia + pulmonary stenosis
- Transposition of great arteries + pulmonary stenosis
- Double outlet right ventricle + VSD + pulmonary stenosis
- Single ventricle + pulmonary stenosis

### Q. What is Eisenmenger syndrome?

Syndrome resulting from bidirectional or right to left shunting of blood at the atrial, ventricular or arterial levels because of high resistance and obstructive pulmonary hypertension.

**Reversible**
- Delayed involution of the medial hypertrophy of the pulmonary vessels
- Pulmonary vasoconstriction

**Irreversible**
- Plexiform arteriopathy
- Necrotizing arteritis

### Q. What is the classification for vascular changes in pulmonary vascular disease?

**Heath and Edwards classification of vascular changes for assessing the potential reversibility of pulmonary vascular disease:**

**Grade 1:** Medial hypertrophy
**Grade 2:** Medial hypertrophy + intimal cellular proliferation
**Grade 3:** Medial hypertrophy + internal proliferation + concentric fibrosis
**Grade 4:** Plexiform arteriopathy
**Grade 5:** Complex plexiform, angiomatous and cavernous lesions
**Grade 6:** Necrotizing arteritis

### Q. What is the etiology of Eisenmenger syndrome?

**Pre-tricuspid shunts**
- ASD
- PAPVC

**Post-triscupid shunts**
- VSD
- PDA

### Q. List the signs of Eisenmenger syndrome.
- Central cyanosis and clubbing
- A wave in JVP
- P2 palpable
- LPH
- RVS4 and PEC
- Soft murmurs
- EDM of PR and PSM of TR

### Q. What are the examination findings?
- Central cyanosis and clubbing
- Differential cyanosis in PDA—Eisenmenger syndrome
- Pulse normal
- BP normal
- JVP prominent "a" waves
- No cardiomegaly
- Palpable P2
- Pulmonary artery pulsations
- No thrill
- LPH
- Loud P2
- Split variable
- RVS4
- Murmur of ASD/VSD/PDA—soft/absent
- Murmur of TR/PR

### Q. List the differences between ASD-ES, VSD-ES and PDA-ES.

Refer **Table 2.55**.

**Table 2.55:** ES in different cardiac conditions.

| ASD–ES | VSD–ES | PDA–ES |
|---|---|---|
| Onset of late age | Early | Early |
| Generalized cyanosis | Generalized | Only in the lower limbs |
| Prominent "a" waves in JVP | Absent | Absent |
| Cardiomegaly | Absent | Absent |
| LPH + | Absent | Absent |
| Narrow fixed split S2 | Single S2 | Single S2 |

### Q. What are components of TOF?

Most common congenital cyanotic heart disease above the age of 2 years.

Most common cyanotic heart disease with squatting episodes.
- RV outflow tract obstruction
- VSD—subaortic
- Over-riding of aorta
- RV hypertrophy

### Q. What are associations of TOF?

Refer **Figures 2.40A and B**.
- Right aortic arch
- Left superior vena cava
- Coronary artery abnormalities
- Absent left pulmonary artery
- PDA
- VSD
- Peripheral pulmonary artery stenosis

### Q. What are signs of TOF?
- Central cyanosis with clubbing
- No cardiomegaly

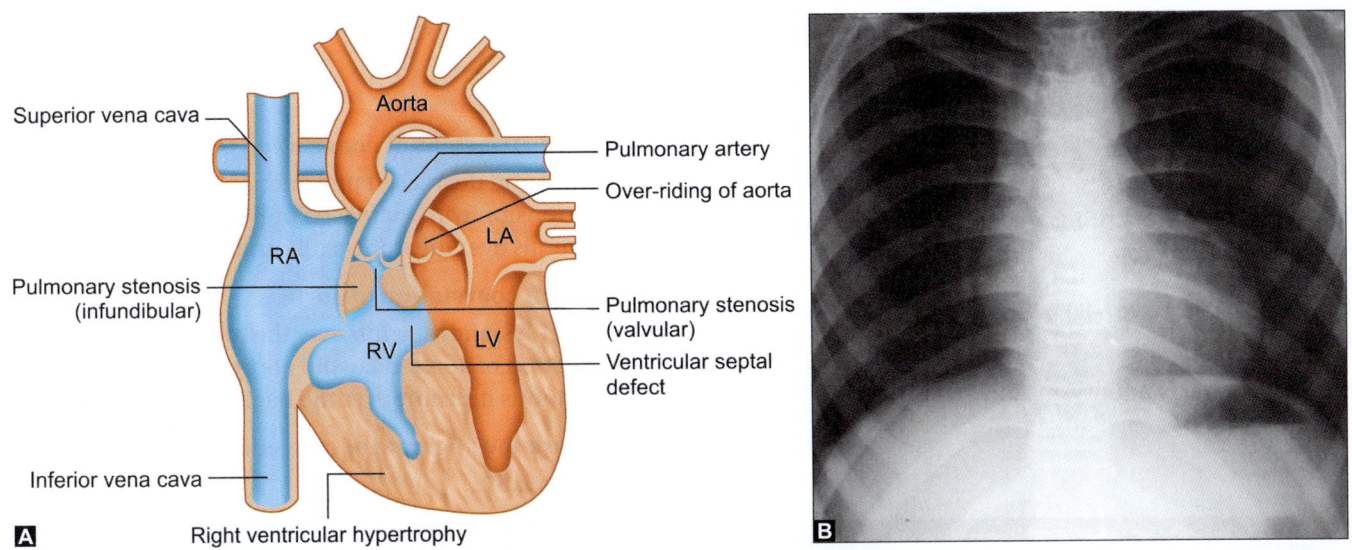

**Figs. 2.40A and B:** (A) Diagrammatic representation of tetralogy of Fallot; (B) Chest X-ray may classically showing "boot-shaped" heart with an upturned cardiac apex due to right ventricular hypertrophy and concave pulmonary arterial segment.

- No LPH/palpable P2
- S2 single and A2 loud
- ESM in the pulmonary area conducted to the left shoulder

### Q. What is pink Fallot?
Acyanotic Fallot with mild RV outflow tract obstruction.

### Q. What is Fallot spell?
- Cyanosis with crying/adrenergic stimulation
- Seen in 2 months—2 years of age

**Physiology of spells**

Increased right to left shunt due to:
- Increased infundibular stenosis due to adrenergic stimulation
- Decreased systemic vascular resistance due to lactic acidosis

### Q. What are the complications of TOF?
- Polycythemia and hyperviscosity states
- Paradoxical embolism
- Cerebral abscess
- Infective endocarditis

### Q. How do you manage TOF?
- Treatment of polycythemia
- Treatment of cerebral thrombosis/embolism and abscesses
- Prophylaxis of infective endocarditis

**Surgical management of TOF**
- Definitive
- Palliative

**Surgical shunts in TOF**
- Blalock-Taussig shunt (subclavian with pulmonary artery)
- Waterston shunt (ascending aorta with pulmonary artery)
- Potts shunt (descending aorta with pulmonary artery)

### Q. What is Fallot trilogy?
- Pulmonary stenosis
- RVH
- ASD

### Q. What is Fallot pentalogy?
- Pulmonary stenosis
- RVH
- ASD
- VSD
- Aortic overriding

### Q. What is Fallot physiology and what are the conditions causing it?
Nonrestrictive VSD + pulmonary stenosis.

**Conditions with a Fallot like physiology**
- TOF
- Tricuspid atresia + pulmonary stenosis
- Single ventricle + pulmonary stenosis
- Double outlet right ventricle + pulmonary stenosis
- Corrected transposition + VSD + pulmonary stenosis
- VSD + pulmonary stenosis

### Q. What are the differences between TOF versus Eisenmenger syndrome?
Refer **Table 2.56**.

| Table 2.56: TOF versus Eisenmenger syndrome. | |
|---|---|
| **TOF** | **Eisenmenger syndrome** |
| Early onset cyanosis | Late onset |
| Generalized cyanosis | Generalized ± |
| JVP is not elevated | "a" waves in ASD Eisenmenger |
| Cardiomegaly absent | Present in ASD—ES |

## SECTION 2: Cardiovascular System

| TOF | Eisenmenger syndrome |
|---|---|
| LPH and P2 not palpable | Palpable |
| | ◆ S2 single and loud—VSD<br>◆ Wide split loud P2—ASD<br>◆ Normal split loud P2—PDA |

**Q. What are the associations of coarctation of aorta?**

**Cardiac**
◆ Bicuspid aortic valve—80%
◆ VSD

**Extracardiac:** Berry aneurysms in the circle of Willis

**Q. What are the types of coarctation of aorta?**
1. Post-ductal
2. Pre-ductal

**Q. What are the signs of coarctation of aorta?**
◆ Delayed and decreased pulsations
◆ Hypertension with increased pulse pressure
◆ Collaterals over the front, axilla and back—Suzzman's sign

**Murmurs in coarctation of aorta**
◆ Ejection systolic murmur over the precordium and back—coarctation of aorta/bicuspid aortic valve
◆ Continuous murmur over the back due to collaterals

**Q. What are the stigmata of congenital heart disease?**
Refer **Table 2.57**.

**Table 2.57:** Stigmata of congenital heart disease.

| Syndrome | Cardiac defects | Other features |
|---|---|---|
| **Down syndrome (trisomy 21)**<br>(CHILD HAS MANY PROBLEM) | ECD, VSD | ◆ **C**ataract<br>◆ **H**ypotonia, **H**ypothyroidism<br>◆ **I**ncreased gap between 1st and 2nd toe (sandal gap)<br>◆ **L**eukemia<br>◆ **D**uodenal atresia<br>◆ **H**irschsprung's disease<br>◆ **A**lzheimer's disease<br>◆ **S**imian crease<br>◆ **M**ental retardation, **M**icrognathia<br>◆ **A**tlantoaxial instability<br>◆ **NY**stagmus<br>◆ **P**rotruding tongue, **P**oor hearing<br>◆ **R**ound face, **R**espiratory infections<br>◆ **O**cciput is flat, **O**blique palpebral fissure<br>◆ **B**rushfield spots, **B**rachycephaly<br>◆ **L**ow nasal bridge, **L**anguage problem<br>◆ **E**picanthic fold, **E**ar folded<br>◆ **M**ongolian slant, **M**yoclonus |
| **Marfan syndrome** | Aortic aneurysm, aortic and AML prolapse with MVP and MR | Arachnodactyly with hyperextensibility, subluxation of lens and other joint deformities |
| **William's syndrome** | Supravalvular AS<br>PA stenosis (peripheral PS most common) | Varying degrees of mental retardation, so-called elfin facies (consisting of some of the following: Upturned nose, flat nasal bridge, long philtrum, flat malar area, wide mouth, full lips, widely spaced teeth, periorbital fullness), hypercalcemia of infancy |
| **Rubella syndrome** | PDA and pulmonary stenosis (peripheral PS most common) | **Triad of the syndrome:** Deafness, cataract, and CHDs<br>Others include—intrauterine growth retardation, microcephaly, microphthalmia, hepatitis, neonatal thrombocytopenic purpura |
| **Noonan's syndrome (Turner-like syndrome)** | PS (dystrophic pulmonary valve), LVH (or anterior septal hypertrophy) | Similar to Turner's syndrome but may occur in phenotypic male and without chromosomal abnormality |
| **LEOPARD syndrome (multiple lentigines syndrome)** | PS, HOCM, long PR interval | Lentiginous skin lesion, ocular hypertelorism, pulmonary stenosis, abnormal genitalia, retarded growth, deafness |
| **Holt-Oram syndrome (cardiac-limb syndrome)** | ASD, VSD | Defects or absence of thumb or radius |

| Syndrome | Cardiac defects | Other features |
|---|---|---|
| Ellis–van Creveld syndrome (chondroectodermal dysplasia) | ASD, single atrium | Short stature of prenatal onset, short distal extremities, narrow thorax with short ribs, polydactyly, nail hypoplasia, neonatal teeth |
| DiGeorge syndrome | Interrupted aortic arch, truncus arteriosus, VSD, PDA, TOF | Hypertelorism, short philtrum, down slanting eyes, hypoplasia or absence of thymus and parathyroid, hypocalcemia, deficient cell-mediated immunity |
| Cornelia de Lange's (de Lange's) syndrome | VSD | Hirsutism, prenatal growth retardation, microcephaly, anteverted nares, downturned mouth, mental retardation |
| CHARGE syndrome | TOF, truncus arteriosus, aortic arch anomalies (e.g., vascular ring, interrupted aortic arch) | Coloboma, choanal atresia, growth or mental retardation, genitourinary anomalies, ear anomalies, genital hypoplasia |
| Ehlers-Danlos syndrome | TOF, ASD, great vessel aneurysms | Joint hypermobility, easy bruisability, hernia, kyphoscoliosis |

(AS: aortic stenosis; ASD: atrial septal defect; ECD: endocardial cushion defect; HOCM: hypertrophic obstructive cardiomyopathy; LVH: left ventricular hypertrophy; PA: pulmonary artery; PS: pulmonary stenosis; TOF: tetralogy of Fallot; VSD: ventricular septal defect; CHDs: congenital heart diseases; PDA: patent ductus arteriosus)

# HEART SOUNDS

## S1

- Produced by the closure of mitral and tricuspid valves
- Corresponds to the end of diastole, beginning of ventricular systole and precedes the upstroke of carotid.
- M1 is best heard over the apex of the heart
- T1 is best heard over the 4th ICS at the left sternal border
- High pitch sound best heard with diaphragm of the stethoscope
- S1 is louder than A2 at the apex and equal or exceed the intensity of S2 at the base
- Intensity of S1 depends on:
  - Length of the PR interval—indirectly proportional
  - Strength of the ventricular contraction—directly proportional
  - Stenosis—loud S1
  - Regurgitation—muffled
  - Distance between the 2 leaflets—directly proportional
  - Distance of the heart from the chest wall—indirectly proportional
  - Pliability of the cusps—diminished if its lost

Table 2.58 shows differences between loud and soft S1.

**Table 2.58:** Differences between loud and soft S1.

| Loud S1 | Soft S1 |
|---|---|
| Short PR interval | Long PR interval >200 msec |
| Tachycardia or hyperkinetic states | Depressed left ventricular contractility |
| Stiff left ventricle | Premature closure of mitral valve (acute AR) |
| Mitral stenosis | Left bundle branch block |
| Left atrial myxoma | Extracardiac factors—obesity, muscular chest, COPD, large breasts |
| Holosystolic mitral valve prolapsed | Flail mitral leaflet |

### Split S1

- PVC
- RBBB
- ASD
- LV pacing
- Ebstein anomaly

### Reverse split S1

- LBBB
- RV pacing
- Severe MS
- Left atrial myxoma

### Variable S1

- Whenever the relationship between the position of the mitral valve leaflets and LV pressure is inconsistent this will occur.
- Causes: Second or third degree heart block, AV dissociation, ventricular arrhythmias with dissociated atrial rates.

## S2

- Produced by the closure of aortic and pulmonary valves
- High pitch, best heard with diaphragm of the stethoscope
- Normally heard as single sound, with inspiration two components can be heard
- A2 best heard in aortic area (2nd right ICS)

- P2 best heard in pulmonary area (2nd left ICS) and left 4th intercostal space.
- P2 is softer than A2 even in pulmonary area
- Average split is 30–40 msec can be as great as 70–80 msec S2 heard as a single sound when the A2 and P2 distance is <20 msec
- Splitting is best heard in left 2nd ICS
- Intensity of S2 is more than S1
- Intensity depends on:
  - Valvular factors
  - Transvalvular gradient
  - Mechanical factors
  - Size of the great vessels
- Elevation of pressure in great vessels produces loud s2.
- Valvular diseases produces soft S2

**Wide split S2**

A2 and P2 distance is more than 30 msec:
1. Inspiration
2. RBBB
3. LV pacing
4. PVC from left ventricle
5. Delayed closure of PV-RV outflow obstruction, pulmonary hypertension,
6. Early closure of AV -MR, VSD with L–R shunting

**Wide and fixed split S2**

Defined as ≤20 msec of variation in the A2-P2 interval between inspiration and expiration:

- ASD WITH L-R shunt
- RV failure

**Reverse S2 split**
- LBBB
- RV pacing
- PVC from RV
- Delayed emptying of LV–AS
Various characteristics of S2 is shown in **Figure 2.41**.

## S3

- Produced by the rapid entry of blood from atrium to ventricle
- Low pitch, early diastolic sound
- Best heard with bell of the stethoscope
- When arised from LV best heard at the apex with patient in left lateral decubitus position at the end of expiration
- When arised from RV best heard at the left lower sternal border or xiphoid with patient in supine position
- Physiological in <40 years

### Pathological S3
- Systolic or diastolic ventricle dysfunction
- IHD
- MR/TR
- Hyperdynamic states
- Systemic/pulmonary hypertension
- Acute AR
- Volume overload

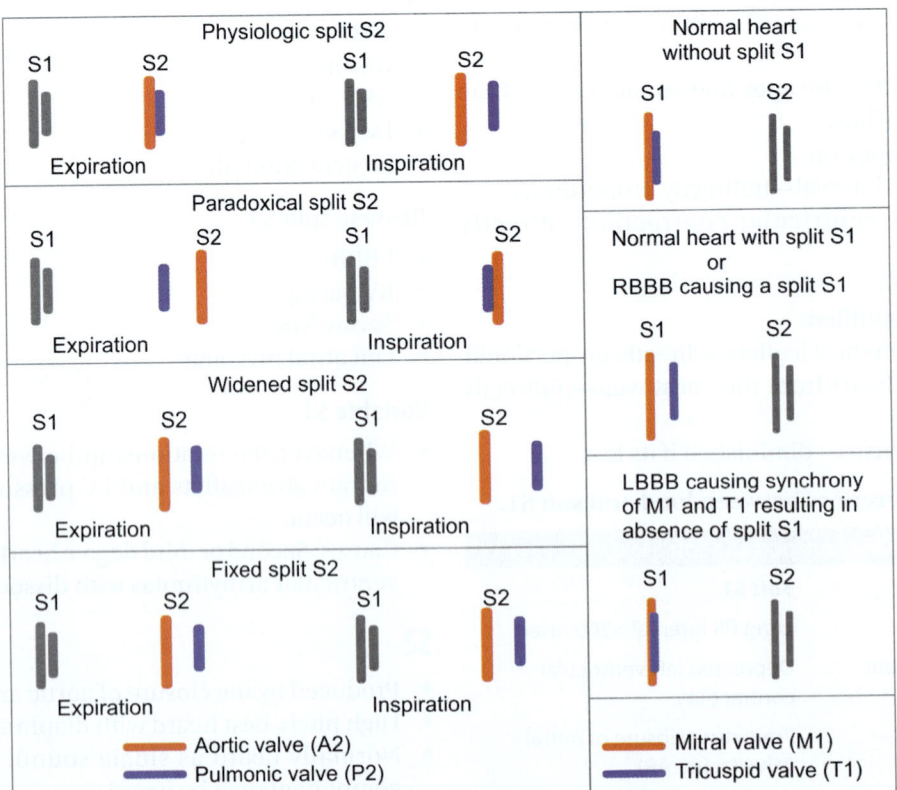

**Fig. 2.41:** Various characteristics of S2.

## S4

- Late diastolic sound corresponds to late ventricular filling with active atrial contraction
- Low intensity sound best heard with bell
- When arised from LV best heard at the apex with patient in left lateral decubitus position at the end of expiration
- When arised from RV best heard at the left lower sternal border or xiphoid with patient in supine position
- Never heard in atrial fibrillation

**Conditions associated are:**
- Ventricular hypertrophy
- IHD
- Ventricular aneurysm
- Hyperkinetic states

## MISCELLANEOUS

**Q. What are the signs of infective endocarditis?**

Signs of infective endocarditis (**Figs. 2.42A to F**):
- Fever
- Pallor
- Clubbing
- Splinter hemorrhages under nail beds
- Mucosal petechiae
- Janeway lesions
- Osler's nodes
- Roth spots on fundus.

**Q. What is the criteria for diagnosing Marfan syndrome?**

Refer **Table 2.59**.

**Table 2.59:** The revised Ghent criteria.

| | |
|---|---|
| In absence of family history: Aortic root dilatation/dissection + ectopia lentis = MFS Aortic root dilatation/dissection + FBN-1 mutation = MFS Aortic root dilatation/dissection + * systemic score >7 = MFS | |
| In presence of family history: Ectopia lentis + family history = MFS Systemic score >7 + family history of Marfan's = MFS Aortic root dilatation/dissection + family history = MFS | |
| ***Systemic score** | **Points** |
| Wrist and thumb sign | 3 |
| Pectus carinatum | 2 |
| Hindfoot deformity | 2 |
| Pneumothorax | 2 |
| Protrusio acetabula | 2 |
| Dural ectasia | 2 |
| Reduced upper segment to lower segment ratio and no severe scoliosis | 2 |
| Scoliosis or thoracolumbar kyphosis | 1 |

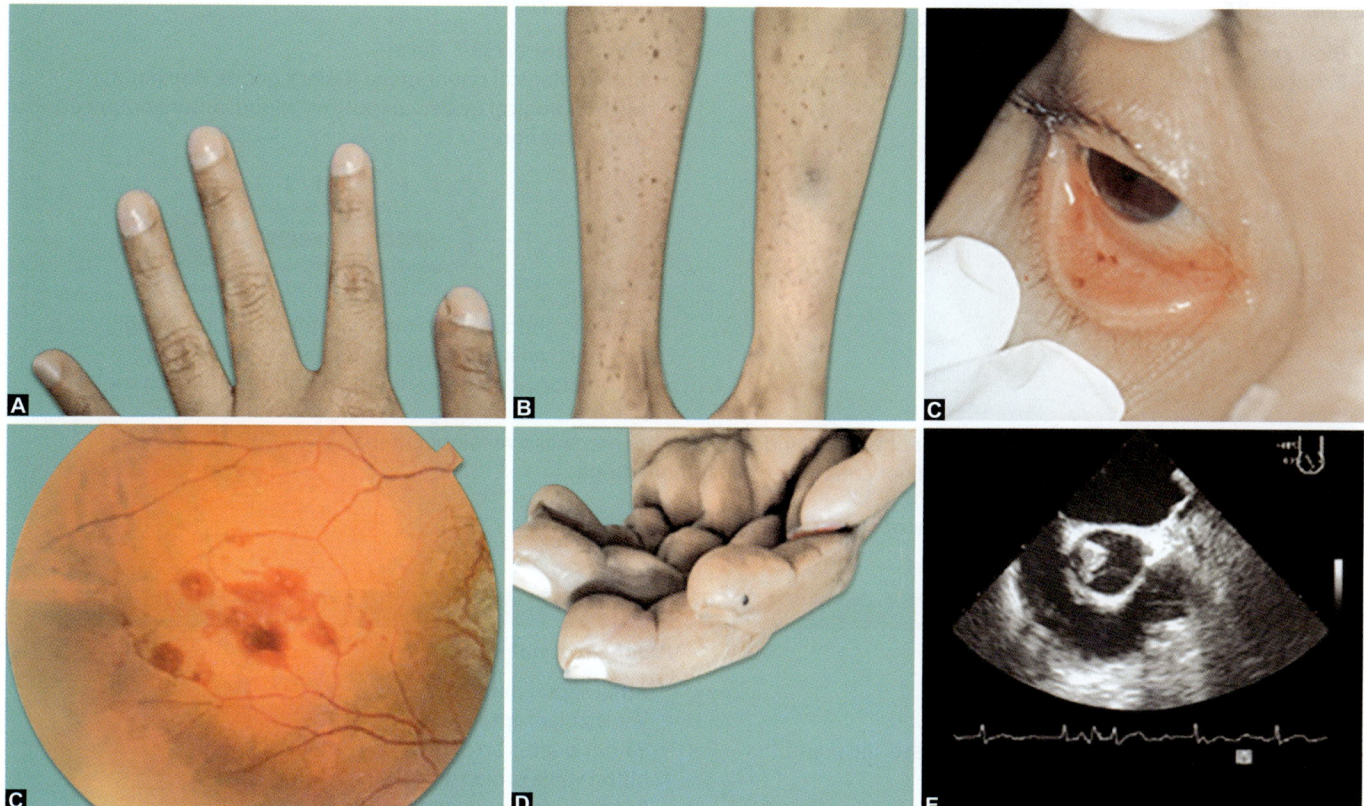

**Figs. 2.42A to F:** Signs of infective endocarditis: (A) Clubbing; (B) Petechiae; (C) Subconjunctival hemorrhage; (D) Roth spots; (E) Osler's nodes; (F) Echocardiography showing vegetation.

| | |
|---|---|
| Reduced elbow extension | 1 |
| Facial features (3/5) (dolichocephaly, enophthalmos, down- slanting palpebral fissures, malar hypoplasia, retrognathia | 1 |
| Skin striae | 1 |
| Myopia >3 diopters | 1 |

**Q. What are the signs of rheumatic fever?**
- Fever
- Arthritis
- Erythema marginatum
- Subcutaneous nodules
- Tachycardia.

**Q. What are the diagnostic criteria for acute rheumatic fever?**

Refer **Table 2.60**.

**Q. What are the diagnostic criteria for infective endocarditis?**

Refer **Table 2.61**.

**Table 2.60:** The modified Jones criteria (2015).

| Major criteria | Minor criteria |
|---|---|
| **LR populations** | |
| • Carditis—clinical and/or subclinical<br>• Arthritis—polyarthritis only<br>• Chorea<br>• Subcutaneous nodules<br>• Erythema marginatum | • Polyarthralgia<br>• Fever (≥38.5°C)<br>• ESR ≥60 mm/h and/or CRP ≥3.0 mg/dL<br>• Prolonged PR interval after accounting for age variability |
| **Moderate risk to HR populations** | |
| • Carditis—clinical and/or subclinical<br>• Arthritis—monoarthritis or polyarthritis, polyarthralgia<br>• Chorea<br>• Subcutaneous nodules<br>• Erythema marginatum | • Monoarthralgia<br>• Fever (≥38°C)<br>• ESR ≥30 mm/h and/or CRP ≥3.0 mg/dL<br>• Prolonged PR interval after accounting for age variability |

(CRP: C-reactive protein; ESR: erythrocyte sedimentation rate)

For all patient populations with evidence of preceding group A streptococcal infection. Diagnosis of initial ARF: 2 major manifestations or 1 major plus 2 minor manifestations.

**Table 2.61:** Modified Duke criteria for infective endocarditis.

| Major criteria | Minor criteria |
|---|---|
| **Mnemonic: BE** | **Mnemonic: TIMER** |
| • **B**lood culture positive >2 times 12 hours apart<br>• **E**chocardiographic evidence of endocardial involvement | • **T**emperature >38°C (fever)<br>• **I**mmunological phenomena (Osler's nodes, Roth spots)<br>• **M**icrobiological evidence (positive blood culture not meeting a major criterion)<br>• **E**mbolic phenomenon (arterial emboli, septic emboli, conjunctival hemorrhage and painless skin lesions)<br>• **R**isk factors (congenital heart condition or IV drug use) |

- **Definitive diagnosis:** Two major criteria or one major and three minor criteria or five minor criteria
- **Possible diagnosis:** One major and one minor criteria or three minor criteria

**Q. What are indications for prophylaxis of infective endocarditis?**

Refer **Table 2.62**.

**Table 2.62:** Prophylaxis of infective endocarditis.

| Prophylaxis indicated | Prophylaxis not indicated |
|---|---|
| • Prosthetic cardiac valves<br>• Previous infective endocarditis<br>• Unrepaired cyanotic congenital heart disease, including palliative shunts and conduits<br>• Completely repaired congenital heart defect with prosthetic material or device, during the first six months after the procedure | • Atrial septal defects<br>• Ventricular septal defects<br>• Patent ductus arteriosus<br>• Mitral valve prolapse<br>• Previous Kawasaki disease<br>• Hypertrophic cardiomyopathy |

| Prophylaxis indicated | Prophylaxis not indicated |
|---|---|
| • Repaired congenital heart disease with residual defects at the site or adjacent to the site of a prosthetic patch or prosthetic device (which inhibit endothelialization)<br>• Cardiac transplant recipients with cardiac valvulopathy<br>• Rheumatic heart disease if prosthetic valves or prosthetic material used in valve repair | • Previous coronary artery bypass graft surgery<br>• Cardiac pacemakers (intravascular and epicardial) and implanted defibrillators<br>• Bicuspid aortic valves<br>• Coarctation of the aorta<br>• Calcified aortic stenosis<br>• Pulmonic stenosis |

**Q. What is the regimen for infective endocarditis prophylaxis?**

Refer **Table 2.63**.

**Table 2.63:** Regimen for infective endocarditis prophylaxis.

| | |
|---|---|
| • Standard oral regimen<br>  – Amoxicillin: 2 g PO 1 h before procedure<br>• Inability to take oral medication<br>  – Ampicillin: 2 g IV or IM within 1 h before procedure<br>• Penicillin allergy<br>• Clarithromycin or azithromycin: 500 mg PO 1 h before procedure<br>• Cephalexin: 2 g PO 1 h before procedure<br>• Clindamycin: 600 mg PO 1 h before procedure | • Penicillin allergy, inability to take oral medication<br>• Cefazolin or ceftriaxone: 1 g IV or IM 30 min before procedure<br>• Clindamycin: 600 mg IV or IM 1 h before procedure |

**Q. What are the high-risk cardiac conditions during pregnancy?**

Refer **Table 2.64**.

**Table 2.64:** High-risk heart disease (HRHD) in pregnancy.

Preconception counseling and pregnancy risk stratification for all women with HRHD of child-bearing age

In women considering pregnancy: Switch to safer cardiac medications and emphasize importance of close monitoring

In women avoiding pregnancy: Discuss safe and effective contraception choices or termination in early pregnancy

| Valve disease | Complex congenital heart disease | Pulmonary hypertension | Aortopathy | Dilated cardiomyopathy |
|---|---|---|---|---|
| Pregnancy not advised in women with:<br>• Severe mitral and aortic valve disease<br>• Mechanical prosthetic valves if effective anticoagulation not possible | Pregnancy not advised in women with:<br>• Significant ventricular dysfunction<br>• Severe atrioventricular valve dysfunction<br>• Failing Fontan circulation<br>• $O_2$ saturation <85% | Pregnancy not advised for:<br>All women with established pulmonary arterial hypertension | Pregnancy not advised in some women with:<br>• Marfan syndrome (MFS)<br>• Bicuspid aortic valve (BAV)<br>• Turner syndrome<br>• Rapid growth of aortic diameter or family history of premature aortic dissection | Pregnancy not advised in women with:<br>• Left ventricular ejection fraction <40%<br>• History of peripartum cardiomyopathy |

| Valve disease | Complex congenital heart disease | Pulmonary hypertension | Aortopathy | Dilated cardiomyopathy |
|---|---|---|---|---|
| **Pregnancy management:**<br>✦ Close follow-up<br>✦ Drug therapy for heart failure or arrhythmias<br>✦ Balloon valvuloplasty or surgical valve replacement in refractory cases | **Pregnancy management:**<br>Close follow-up | **Pregnancy management:**<br>✦ Close follow-up<br>✦ Early institution of pulmonary vasodilators | **Pregnancy management:**<br>✦ Treat hypertension<br>✦ Beta-blockers to reduce heart rate<br>✦ Frequent echo assessment<br>✦ Surgery during pregnancy or after C-section if large increase in aortic dimension | **Pregnancy management:**<br>✦ Close follow-up<br>✦ Beta-blockers<br>✦ Diuretic agents for volume overload<br>✦ Vasodilators for hemodynamic and symptomatic<br>✦ improvement |
| **Delivery:**<br>✦ Vaginal delivery preferred<br>✦ C-section in case of fetal or maternal instability<br>✦ Early delivery for clinical and hemodynamic deterioration<br>✦ Consider hemodynamic monitoring during labor and delivery | **Delivery:**<br>✦ Vaginal delivery preferred<br>✦ C-section in case of fetal or maternal instability<br>✦ Consider hemodynamic monitoring during labor and delivery | **Delivery:**<br>✦ Vaginal delivery preferred<br>✦ C-section in case of fetal or maternal instability<br>✦ Timing of delivery depends on clinical condition and right ventricular function<br>✦ Early delivery advisable<br>✦ Diuresis after delivery to prevent RV volume overload<br>✦ Extended hospital stay after delivery | **Delivery:**<br>✦ C-section in cases of significant aortic dilation MFS >40 mm<br>✦ BAV >45 mm<br>✦ Turner: ASI >20 mm/m² | **Delivery:**<br>✦ Vaginal delivery preferred<br>✦ C-section in case of fetal or maternal instability<br>✦ Consider hemodynamic monitoring during labor and delivery<br>✦ Early delivery for clinical and hemodynamic deterioration |

**Q. What is dynamic auscultation?**

Refer **Figure 2.43**.

| | Venous return/preload | | Afterload | | Drugs | |
|---|---|---|---|---|---|---|
| | Increase<br>(Leg raise/squat) | Decrease<br>(Valsalva/standing) | Increase<br>(Handgrip) | Decrease<br>(Amyl nitrate) | Diuretic | ACEIs |
| MS, AS | ↑ | ↓ | ↓(AS)<br>Negligible effect in (MS) | ↑(AS) | Yes, but better<br>AS (replace)<br>MS (balloon) | ✗ |
| MR, AR | ↑ | ↓ | ↑ | ↓ | ✓ | ✓ |
| VSD | ↑ | ↓ | ↑ | ↓ | ✓ | ✓ |
| HOCM | ↓ | ↑ | ↓ | ↑ | ✗ | ✗ |
| MVP | ↓ | ↑ | ↓ | ↑ | ✗ | ✗ |

**Fig. 2.43:** Dynamic auscultation.

# Schematic Approach to Clinical Diagnosis in Cardiovascular System

| Cardiovascular system | | |
|---|---|---|
| **Pulse volume** | **Pulse regularity** | |
| | *Regular* | *Irregular* |
| High | AR | MR |
| Low | AS | MS |

| Precordium | | |
|---|---|---|
| **Parasternal pulsation/heave** | **Apical impulse** | |
| | *Localized* | *Diffuse* |
| Present | MS (tapping apex) | MR (hyperdynamic) |
| Absent | AS (heaving apex) | AR (hyperdynamic) |

**Q. Give examples of named murmurs.**

Refer **Table 2.65**.

| Table 2.65: Named murmurs. | |
|---|---|
| **Carey Coombs murmur** | Mid-diastolic murmur, in rheumatic fever |
| **Austin Flint murmur** | Mid-late diastolic murmur, in aortic regurgitation (AR) |
| **Graham-Steel murmur** | High pitched, diastolic, in pulmonary regurgitation |
| **Rytand's murmur** | Mid-diastolic atypical murmur, in complete heart block |
| **Docks murmur** | Diastolic murmur, left anterior descending (LAD) artery stenosis |
| **Mill wheel murmur** | Due to air in right ventricle (RV) cavity following cardiac catheterization |
| **Stills murmur** | Inferior aspect of lower left sternal border, systolic ejection sound, vibratory/musical quality in subaortic stenosis, small ventricular septal defect |
| **Gibson's murmur** | Continuous machinery murmur of patent ductus arteriosus (PDA) |
| **Key-Hodgkin murmur** | Diastolic murmur of aortic regurgitation. Hodgkin correlated this diastolic murmur with retroversion of the aortic valve leaflets, seen in syphilitic aortic regurgitation |
| **Cabot-Locke murmur** | Diastolic murmur heard best at the left sternal border. Heard in anemic patients. The murmur resolves with treatment of anemia |
| **Roger's murmur** | It is the loud pansystolic murmur which is heard maximally at the left sternal border in small ventricular septal defect (VSD) |
| **Pontains murmur** | Cervical venous hum in severe anemia |
| **Cole-Cecil murmur** | AR murmur in left axilla due to higher position of apex |
| **Cruveilhier-Baumgarten venous hum** | It is diagnostic of portal venous hypertension |

## Summary of Findings in Common Cardiovascular Diseases

| Findings | MS | MR | AS | AR | TR | ASD | VSD | PDA |
|---|---|---|---|---|---|---|---|---|
| Pulse | • Low volume<br>• Irregularly irregular (if associated with AF) | • High volume<br>• Irregularly irregular (if associated with AF) | • Low volume<br>• Pulsus parvus et tardus<br>• Anacrotic pulse<br>• Apicocarotid delay—severe AS | • High volume, **Collapsing pulse**<br>• Water hammer pulse<br>• Pulsus bisferiens | Normal | • Normal<br>• Irregularly irregular (if associated with AF) | High volume | High volume, collapsing |
| Blood pressure | • Low BP<br>• Mean of 3 readings to be taken if atrial fibrillation is present | • Wide pulse pressure<br>• Mean of 3 readings to be taken if atrial fibrillation is present | • Low BP<br>• Systolic decapitation<br>**Coanda effect:**<br>Right upper limb BP >left upper limb BP (supravalvular AS) | • Wide pulse pressure<br>• **Hills sign**— lower limb BP<br>• >20 mm of upper limb BP | Normal | Normal | Wide pulse pressure | Wide pulse pressure |
| JVP | • Raised in heart failure<br>• **Prominent a waves**— pulmonary hypertension without atrial fibrillation<br>• **Absence of a wave**—atrial fibrillation<br>• Prominent v waves (c-v waves) and rapid y descent<br>• → tricuspid regurgitation | • Raised in heart failure<br>• **Prominent a waves**— pulmonary hypertension without atrial fibrillation<br>• **Absence of a wave**—atrial fibrillation<br>• Prominent v waves (c-v waves) and rapid y descent<br>• → tricuspid regurgitation | • Usually normal<br>• Raised in heart failure<br>• Rarely prominent a wave—Bernheim effect | • Usually normal<br>• Raised in heart failure | • Raised with most prominent 'giant' v wave in the jugular venous pulse (a **c-v wave** replaces the normal x descent)<br>• **Earlobe pulsations** (Lancisi's sign) | "M" pattern— a and v waves have equal height, a wave becomes taller when pulmonary hypertension develops or associated mitral stenosis (MS) | Raised in heart failure | Raised in heart failure |
| Apex | **Tapping** apex | **Hyperdynamic** Down and out apex | Heaving | **Hyperdynamic** Down and out apex | Normal | Normal | Mild displaced down and out | Hyperdynamic: Down and out apex |
| Parasternal heave | Present (RVH or left atrial enlargement) | Present (RVH or left atrial enlargement) | No | No | | Present | Present | +/− |
| Thrills | Diastolic thrill at apex | Systolic thrill at apex in acute or severe MR | Systolic thrill over the aortic and carotid area | Diastolic thrill in aortic/neoaortic area | Systolic thrill in left lower sternal edge | Nil | Left 4–5 ICS parasternal area | Continuous thrill at the upper-left sternal edge |

# SECTION 2: Cardiovascular System

| Findings | | MS | MR | AS | AR | TR | ASD | VSD | PDA |
|---|---|---|---|---|---|---|---|---|---|
| Heart sounds | S1 | Loud | Soft | Normal | Soft | Soft | Loud | Soft | Loud |
| | S2 | Loud P2 (pulmonary hypertension) Narrow split (pulmonary hypertension) | Loud P2 (pulmonary hypertension) Narrow split (pulmonary hypertension) | Soft A2 (valvular AS) Loud A2 (bicuspid aortic valve) Paradoxical split (severe AS) | Normal tambour A2 in syphilitic AR | Loud P2 with narrow split (pulmonary hypertension) | P2 loud Wide fixed split | P2 loud | P2 loud paradoxical split |
| | S3 | RVS3 (present in failure) | RV/LVS3 (present in failure) | LVS3 in failure | LVS3 in severe AR | RVS3 | RVS3 | +/− | +/− |
| | S4 | Never | Present in acute MR | Present Indicates severe AS | +/− | — | RVS4 (Eisenmenger's) | RVS4 (Eisenmenger's) | RVS4 (Eisenmenger's) |
| | Others | Opening snap | OS in 10% | AEC in bicuspid aortic valve | — | — | PEC (Eisenmenger's) | PEC (Eisenmenger's) | PEC (Eisenmenger's) |
| Murmurs | | • MDM at mitral area<br>• PSM at tricuspid area<br>• ESM at pulmonary area<br>• EDM (Graham Steel) at pulmonary area | • PSM in mitral area radiation to axilla/base<br>• Flow MDM at mitral area<br>• PSM at tricuspid area<br>• ESM at pulmonary area<br>• EDM (Graham Steel) at pulmonary area | • ESM in aortic area conducting to carotid<br>• Systolic murmur at mitral area (Gallavardin phenomenon) | • EDM in aortic/ neoaortic area<br>• Flow ESM in aortic area<br>• MDM at mitral area (Austin Flint)<br>• Diastolic murmur in left axilla (Cole-Cecil murmur) | Blowing PSM: At the lower-left sternal border that is increased during inspiration and reduced during expiration (de-Carvallo's sign) | • ESM in pulmonary area and MDM in tricuspid area. Once Eisenmenger's in pulmonary area and PSM in tricuspid area | PSM heard best at the left sternal edge (3rd, 4th and 5th intercostal space) | • Continuous harsh "machinery-like"/Gibson's murmur heard with late systolic accentuation in the first left intercostal space below the clavicle |
| Other features | | Palpable P2 (diastolic shock) | Palpable P2 (diastolic shock) | — | Peripheral signs | Pulsatile liver | Precordial bulge | Aortic insufficiency in approximately 5% | Differential cyanosis and clubbing develops |

(AR: aortic regurgitation; AS: aortic stenosis; ASD: atrial septal defect; ESM: ejection-systolic murmur; EDM: early diastolic murmur; MDM: mid-diastolic murmur; MR: mitral regurgitation; MS: mitral stenosis; PS: pulmonary stenosis; PDA: patent ductus arteriosus; PSM: pansystolic murmur; TR: tricuspid regurgitation; VSD: ventricular septal defect)

## CARDIAC MURMURS—TIMING WITH OTHER CARDIAC EVENTS

Refer **Figure 2.44**.

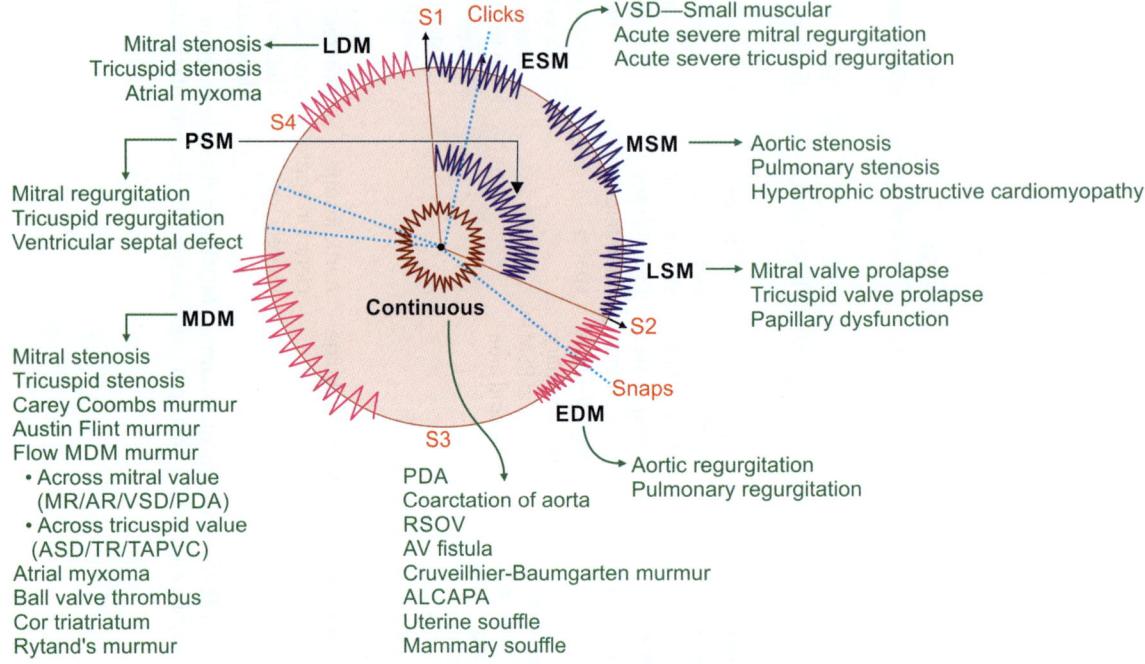

Fig. 2.44: Timing of cardiac murmurs and pictorial representation on the diagram of cardiac cycle.

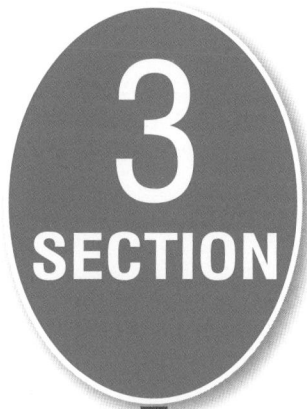

# SECTION 3: Gastrointestinal System

## Section Outline

- ◆ Case Sheet Format
- ◆ Diagnosis Format
- ◆ Sample Case Sheet and Discussion
  - Cirrhosis
  - Hepatomegaly
  - Splenomegaly
  - Ascites

# Case Sheet Format

## HISTORY TAKING

Name:
Age:
Sex:
Residence:
Occupation:

### Chief complaints
1. _____ × days
2. _____ × days
3. _____ × days

History of presenting illness

### Abdominal distension
- Duration
- Onset
- Progression
- Aggravating factors
- Relieving factors
- Associated symptoms
- Is it preceded by pedal edema or followed by it?

### Pedal edema:
- Duration
- Onset
- Progression
- Aggravating factors
- Relieving factors
- Is it preceded by facial puffiness or followed by it?

### Abdominal pain:
- Onset
- Site
- Type of pain
- Radiation
- Aggravating factors
- Relieving factors
- Associated symptoms

### Nausea and vomiting:
- Episodes
- Contents
- Blood tinged or not
- How many hours after consumption of food associated with pain abdomen?
- Conditions with nausea and vomiting but not associated with pain abdomen:
  - Metabolic
  - Neurologic
  - Drug, induced
  - Psychogenic

### Other symptoms:
- Heart burn, flatulence, and waterbrash
- Hematemesis and melena
- Dysphagia
- Constipation and diarrhea

### Altered bowel habit:
- Stool color
- Stool odor
- Stool frequency
- Blood tinged or melena

**Jaundice**—itching and high, colored urine

### Other symptoms:
- Fever
- Weight loss
- Pain in oral cavity
- Halitosis
- Hiccups
- Other relevant history

### Past history
- Asthma
- Chronic obstructive airway disease
- Tuberculosis
- History of contact with tuberculosis
- Diabetes mellitus (DM)
- Hypertension (HTN)
- Ischemic heart disease (IHD)
- Seizure disorder

### Family history
Draw a three generations pedigree chart

### Personal history
- Bowel habits
- Bladder habits
- Appetite
- Loss of weight
- Occupational exposure
- Sleep
- Dietary habits and taboo
- Food allergies
- Smoking index or pack years
- Alcohol history

### Menstrual and obstetric history
- GPLA
- Age of menarche
- Menopause at
- Flow—ameno/oligo/menorrhagia

**Summarize**
**Differential diagnosis:**
1.
2.
3.

## GENERAL EXAMINATION

**Patient**
- Conscious
- Coherent
- Cooperative
- Obeying commands

**Body mass index (BMI)**
- Weight (kg)/height$^2$ (meters)
- Grading according to WHO for Southeast Asian countries

**Vitals**
- **Pulse**
  - Rate:
  - Rhythm:
  - Volume:
  - Character:
  - Vessel wall thickening:
  - Radioradial delay and radiofemoral delay:
  - Peripheral pulses:
- **Blood pressure**
- **Respiratory rate**
  - Regular/irregular
  - Abdominothoracic/thoracoabdominal
  - Usage of accessory muscles:
- **Jugular venous pressure**
  - cm of blood above sternal angle (+ 5 cm water from right atrium)
- **Jugular venous pulse**
  - Waveform (describe waves)

**On physical examination**
- Pallor:
- Icterus:
- Cyanosis:
- Clubbing:
- Lymphadenopathy:
- Edema:

**Other Head-to-Toe Signs of Liver Cell Failure**
1. Alopecia
2. Fetor hepaticus
3. Jaundice
4. Parotid swelling
5. Gynecomastia
6. Testicular atrophy
7. Loss of secondary sexual characters
8. Spider nevi
9. Palmar erythema
10. Dupuytren's contracture
11. Asterixis
12. Xanthelasma
13. Signs of chronic cholestasis (scratch marks due to pruritus).

## SYSTEMIC EXAMINATION

The order of examination of abdomen is preferably done—Inspection → Auscultation → Palpation → Percussion (as the auscultatory findings might change post palpation and percussion).

**Inspection**
- Shape/distension (localized/generalized) and flanks (free/full)
- Skin over the abdomen
- Symmetry
- Umbilicus
- Movement of corresponding quadrants with respiration
- Dilated veins
- Visible mass
- Visible pulsations
- Visible peristalsis
- Scars or sinuses
- Divarication of recti

**Palpation**
- Superficial palpation
  - Warmth
  - Tenderness
  - Guarding
  - Rigidity
- Deep palpation
  - Liver
    - Size
    - Shape
    - Border or edge
    - Surface
    - Tenderness
    - Consistency
    - Movement with respiration
    - Pulsation
  - Spleen
    - Location
    - Size
    - Shape
    - Consistency
    - Surface
    - Edge
    - Tenderness
    - Movement with respiration
  - Gallbladder
  - Other palpable mass

- Bimanual palpation
  - Kidneys
    - Location
    - Size
    - Shape
    - Consistency
    - Surface
    - Edge
    - Tenderness
    - Movement with respiration
- Dipping method (in case of large ascites)
- Hernia orifices
- Direction of flow in veins (if dilated veins present)
- Abdominal girth measurement
- Spinoumbilical distance
- Xiphisternum to umbilicus distance (x) in cm
- Umbilicus to pubic symphysis distance in cm (y)
  - Ratio of x/y

**Percussion**
- Liver
- Spleen
- Traube's space
- Fluid
  - Shifting dullness
  - Fluid thrill
  - Puddle sign

**Auscultation**
- Bowel sounds
- Succussion splash
- Bruit
- Venous hum
- Friction rub

**Examination of**
- Scrotum
- Spine
- Supraclavicular fossa

**Per Rectal Examination**

**Per Vaginal Examination**

# Diagnosis Format

## CIRRHOSIS/LIVER DISEASE

- Acute hepatitis <4 weeks
  **or**
  Subacute hepatitis
  **or**
  Chronic (cirrhosis/hepatitis >6 months)
  **or**
  Acute on chronic liver disease (ACLD)
- Compensated or decompensated
- Possible etiology—alcohol/post-viral/toxin/nonalcoholic steatohepatitis (NASH)
- With complications—portal hypertension with or without gastrointestinal (GI) bleed/hepatic encephalopathy (preferable to mention stage)/spontaneous bacterial peritonitis/hepatocellular carcinoma/hepatorenal syndrome/others.

**Example:** Decompensated chronic liver disease—cirrhosis secondary to alcohol, with portal hypertension, with upper gastrointestinal (UGI) bleed, patient in stage 2 hepatic encephalopathy with no evidence of spontaneous bacterial peritonitis or other complications.

# Sample Case Sheet and Discussion

## Case 1: Cirrhosis

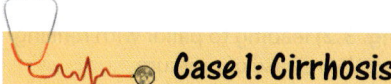

### Brief History
A 45-year-old male presented with following chief complaints:
- Distension of abdomen for 6 months
- Abdominal discomfort and a sense of heaviness for 6 months
- Scanty micturition for 1½ months
- Weakness, malaise, loss of appetite for 1½ months.

### History of Present Illness
- The patient states that he was reasonably well about 6 months back. Since then, he has been suffering from gradual swelling of his abdomen which has increased progressively over the last few days.
- It is not associated with abdominal pain, but there is discomfort and sense of heaviness. He also complains of scanty micturition, generalized weakness, malaise and loss of appetite for 1½ months.
- There is no history of hematemesis or loss of consciousness. There is history of passing dark colored stools whenever he is constipated.
- The patient does not give any history of fever, shortness of breath or cough, puffiness of the face, joint pain, skin rash, pigmentation, etc. His bowel habit and sleep pattern are normal.

### History of Past Illness
He suffered from jaundice 3 years back that lasted for about 5 months and then subsided. At that time, he took some herbal medications. There is no history of any injection, infusion, blood transfusion, IV drug abuse or sharing of needles.

### Personal History
He is a government service holder. He smokes about 20–30 sticks of cigarettes per day for the last 25 years. There is no history of taking alcohol. Wife says he is irritable and excessively sleepy in the day for the last 2 weeks.

### Family History
His parents are alive and in good health. His wife and two children are good health. There is no history of similar illness in his family.

### Drug and Treatment History
Patient is on tablet lasix, aldactone, pantoprazole, ursocol and B complex.

### General Examination
- The patient is ill-looking, emaciated, conscious and oriented.
- Face—hollowed temporal fossa, pinched up nose, malar prominence, muddy complexion of the skin, shallow and dry face with icteric conjunctiva
- Pallor present, angular cheilitis present
- Generalized pigmentation is present. There are few ecchymoses in upper limbs.
- Pitting pedal edema—present.
- Multiple spider angiomas are present over the upper part of chest and back.
- There is leukonychia (fingers and toes) and palmar erythema.
- Gynecomastia present.
- No koilonychia or cyanosis.
- No lymphadenopathy or thyromegaly.
- Dupuytren's contracture and flapping tremor are absent.

Vital signs: Pulse—88/min. BP—110/75 mm Hg. Temperature—99°F. Respiratory rate—18/min.

### Systemic Examination Abdomen
*Inspection*
- The abdomen is distended, flanks are full
- Umbilicus—everted
- Visible superficial veins with normal flow (away from umbilicus)
- There is no visible peristalsis, no scar mark.

*Palpation*
- No tenderness
- Liver—not palpable.
- Spleen is palpable, 4 cm from the left costal margin in anterior axillary line towards the right iliac fossa. The surface is smooth, firm in consistency, nontender.
- Testes—both testes are atrophied.
- Fluid thrill present.

Percussion: Shifting dullness present. Auscultation: No abnormality detected.

### Examination of Other Systems
*Nervous system*
Constructional apraxia present, no flaps, reflexes normal respiratory system (RS), cardiovascular system (CVS)—NAD.

*Provisional diagnosis*
Chronic decompensated parenchymal liver disease—cirrhosis with portal hypertension probably of etiology with ascites with features of hepatic encephalopathy and coagulopathy.
- It is not associated with abdominal pain, but there is discomfort and sense of heaviness. He also complains of scanty micturition, generalized weakness, malaise and loss of appetite for 1½ months.
- There is no history of hematemesis or loss of consciousness. There is history of passing dark colored stools whenever he is constipated.
- The patient does not give any history of fever, shortness of breath or cough, puffiness of the face, joint pain, skin rash, pigmentation, etc. His bowel habit and sleep pattern are normal.

## DISCUSSION

**Q. What are the gastrointestinal causes of clubbing?**

Biliary cirrhosis, ulcerative colitis, Crohn's disease, gastrointestinal tract (GIT) malignancy.

**Q. What is the evidence for portal hypertension clinically?**

Splenomegaly is the clinical evidence for portal hypertension in a case of cirrhosis liver. Other evidences are paraxiphoid umbilical hum and caput medusae which indicate intrahepatic portal hypertension.

**Q. What are the signs in favor of chronic liver disease?**
- Spider angiomata, sparse axillary hair, ascites, Dupuytren's contracture, gynecomastia.
- Signs in favor of alcohol etiology in cirrhosis patients
- Dupuytren's contracture.
- Parotid swelling.
- Alcohol peripheral neuropathy.

**Q. Consuming how much alcohol/day is associated with increased risk of developing alcoholic liver disease (ALD)?**

Consumption of 60–80 g alcohol/day in males for 10 years and 20–40 g alcohol/day for 10 years in females increases the risk of ALD.

**Q. What is spider angiomata and how many spider are significant?**

**Spider nevi (Table 3.1)**

**Table 3.1:** Spider nevi (spider telangiectasia; vascular spiders; spiderangiomas; arterial spiders, and nevus araneus).

| | |
|---|---|
| **Description** | ◆ Consists of a central arteriole from which numerous small vessels radiate peripherally-resembling spider's legs. Whole spider disappears when central arteriole is compressed with a pinhead. When compression is released filling occurs from center to periphery<br>◆ Spider angioma has three features: A body, legs, and surrounding erythema.<br>◆ Spider nevi may also be associated with numerous small vessels scattered randomly through the skin on the upper arms (**paper money skin**) |
| **Pathophysiology** | Due to arteriolar changes induced by hyperestrogenism |
| **Location** | ◆ Usually found only in the necklace area, i.e., above the nipples, territory drained by the superior vena cava, such as: head and neck, upper limbs, front and back of upper chest<br>◆ Rare below the diaphragm (possibly due to higher vasomotor gradient) |
| **Size** | Vary from pinhead to 0.5 mm in diameter |
| **Clinical demonstration** | Applying pressure over the body of spiders with a glass slide (diascopy) (**Fig. 3.1**), or pin head (**Fig. 3.2**) leading to pallor with refilling following the release of pressure |
| **Significance** | They are a strong indicator of liver disease but can be found in other conditions |
| **Causes** | **Liver disorders**<br>◆ Viral hepatitis<br>◆ Alcoholic hepatitis<br>◆ Hepatocellular carcinoma<br>◆ Treatment with sorafenib<br><br>**Others**<br>◆ Third trimester of pregnancy<br>◆ Rheumatoid arthritis<br>◆ Thyrotoxicosis<br>◆ Also normally seen in 2% of healthy population<br>◆ Oral contraceptives also can cause<br><br>Venous star, Campbell de Morgan spots, petechiae, insect/mosquito bites and hereditary hemorrhagic telangiectasias (Osler-Weber-Rendu syndrome) |
| **Differential diagnosis** | ◆ Differentiating features of venous star<br>  – Blood flows from the periphery of the star centrally and thence into the collecting vein; the direction of flow is the exact opposite of that in the arterial spider<br>  – The pattern, shape and size are much more variable than in the arterial spider.<br>  – Color frequently is blue<br>◆ Are common on the dorsum of the feet, around the ankle and the lower legs both front and back, and above the knee on the medial aspect of the thigh<br>◆ Histologically they are dilated veins |
| **Clinical significance in liver disease** | ◆ Spider nevi correspond with a higher risk of mortality among patients with the alcoholic liver disease. They also suggest a high likelihood of esophageal varices and are indicative of the extent of hepatic fibrosis.<br>◆ No of spider naevi significant is if more than 5<br>◆ Sudden disappearance of spider naevi may indicate an ongoing gastrointestinal bleed<br>◆ Size more 15 mm: 80% chances of variceal bleed<br>◆ *Florid spider telangiectasia, gynecomastia, and parotid enlargement are most common in* **alcoholic hepatitis**<br>◆ *Florid spiders and new onset clubbing in a patient with cirrhosis indicates* **hepatopulmonary syndrome** |

# SECTION 3: Gastrointestinal System

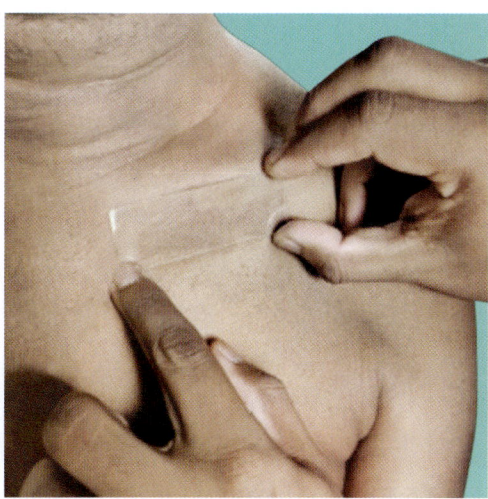

**Fig. 3.1:** Demonstration of spider nevi (glass slide method).

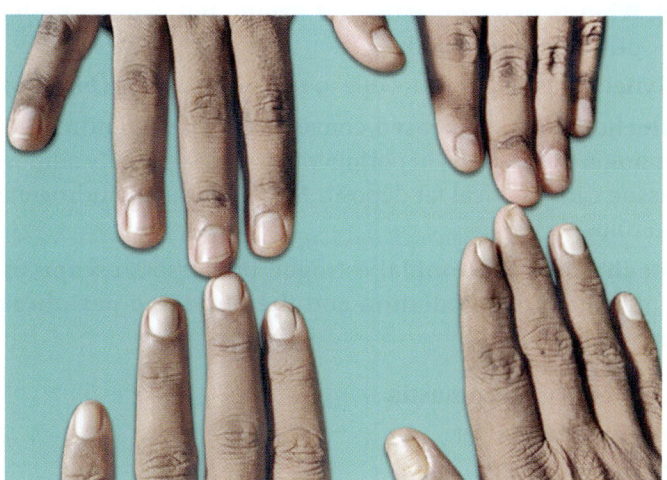

**Fig. 3.3:** Leukonychia—compare with nails of normal person (preferably hands to be placed side by side).

- Clubbing is present in primary biliary cirrhosis or hepatoma.

**Q. Clubbing is common in which type of cirrhosis?**

Clubbing is more common in biliary causes of cirrhosis.

**Q. What is Dupuytren's contracture and name some conditions associated with it?**

### Dupuytren's contracture (Fig. 3.4)

- Fibrosis of palmar aponeurosis is probably caused by local microvascular ischemia.
- Platelet and fibroblast-derived growth factors promote fibrosis
- Flexion contracture of the finger especially ring and little fingers
- Sign of alcoholism
- **Other causes:** Diabetes mellitus, rheumatoid arthritis, and manual labor (workers exposed to repetitive handling tasks or vibration)

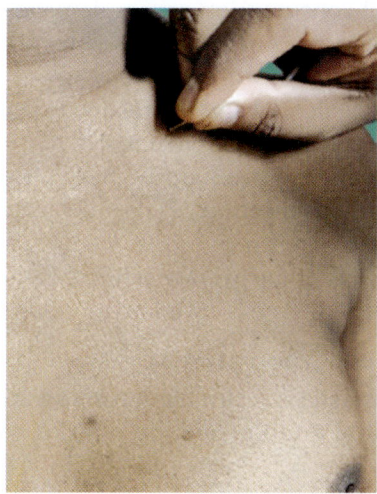

**Fig. 3.2:** Demonstration of spider nevi (pin head method).

**Q. What is palmar erythema?**

- Palmar erythema is reddening of the palms involving thenar and hypothenar eminences sparing the central portions of the palm.
- Involves thenar and hypothenar eminence, distal pads of fingers, circumungual areas on dorsum of fingers
- Central part of palm is clear
- Represents collection of A-V anastomosis
- Steroid estrogen precursors blamed
- Can occur in RA, pregnancy and OCP use

**Q. What nail changes are seen in chronic liver disease?**

### Leukonychia (Fig. 3.3)

- White (Terry's) chalky and brittle nails, proximal 2/3—white, distal 1/3—red
- **Muehrcke's nails:** Characterized by transverse white lines that disappear on applying pressure and these lines do not move with growth of nail.

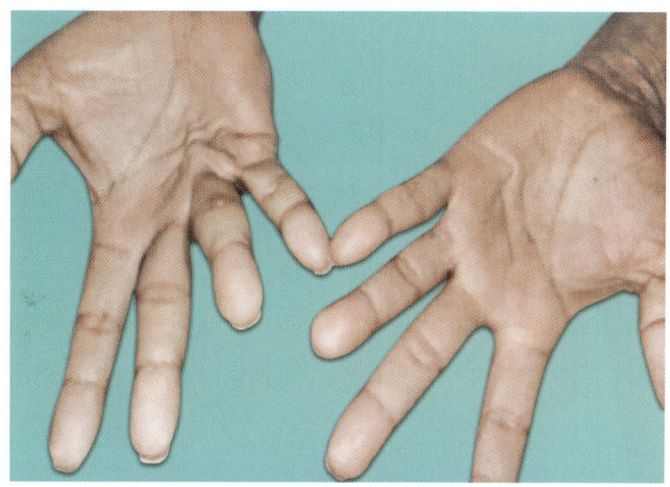

**Fig. 3.4:** Dupuytren's contracture.

**Q. What is gynecomastia and briefly tell causes, pathophysiology behind it?**

**Gynecomastia:** It occurs due to two mechanisms **(Fig. 3.5)**:

**Mechanism 1:** Increased conversion of weak androgenic steroids to estrogens in peripheral tissues especially adipose tissue causing local fat deposit. Alcohol induces androgenic steroids.

**Mechanism 2:** Steroidal estrogen precursors escape the enterohepatic circulation and then undergo peripheral conversion.

**Causes of gynecomastia**
- Cirrhosis of liver
- Drugs:
  - Spironolactone
  - Cimetidine
  - Digoxin
  - Ketoconazole
  - Estrogens
  - Isoniazid/antiandrogens
- Physiological (puberty/aging)
- Klinefelter's syndrome
- Hypogonadism
- Tumor:
  - Testes
  - Lung
  - **Examination (Fig. 3.6):** Appear as palpable nodule (2 cm or greater, subareolar).
  - **Microscopy:** Proliferation of glandular tissue of breast.

**Q. What is fetor hepaticus?**
- Established reason is mercaptans
- Mercaptans are thiols (sulfur-containing compounds) formed due to gut metabolism
- Newer evidence points to **dimethyl sulfide** as the reason for fetor hepaticus.

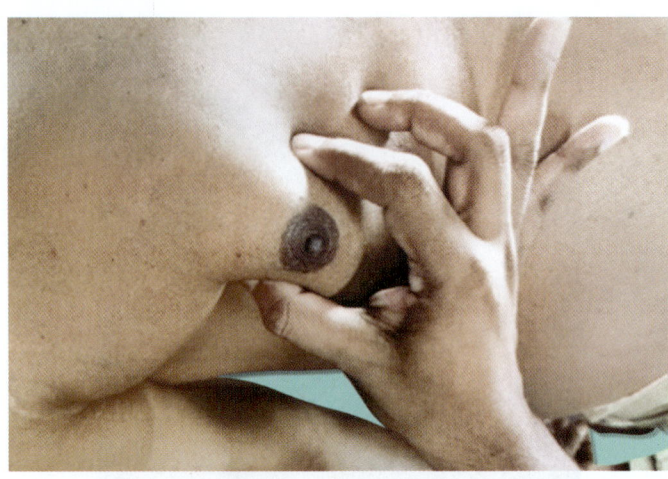

**Fig. 3.6:** Palpation breast bud in gynecomastia.

**Q. What is the mechanism of testicular atrophy?**
- High alcohol consumption causes damage to the Leydig cells and there by causes decreased testosterone levels **(Fig. 3.7)**.
- Direct effect of alcohol and not related to estrogen effect.
- Characteristic in alcoholic cirrhosis.
- Also occurs in hemochromatosis.
- Loss of testicular sensation
- Orchidometer
- The dimensions of the average adult testicle is 4.5 × 3.5 × 2.5 cm and the volume is 15–25 mL.

**Q. What is pseudogynecomastia?**

Pseudogynecomastia is accumulation of subareolar fat tissue without palpable nodule. Seen in obesity and Cushing's syndrome.

**Q. When to suspect hepatoma in cirrhosis patients?**

In patients with previously compensated cirrhosis who develop decompensation such as ascites, encephalopathy, jaundice, or variceal bleeding.

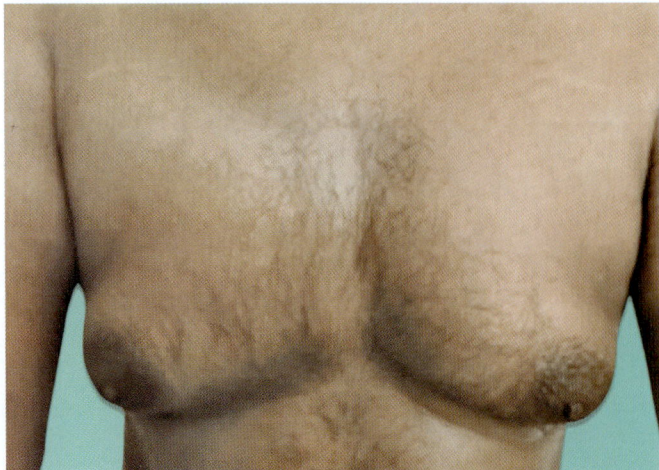

**Fig. 3.5:** Gynecomastia.

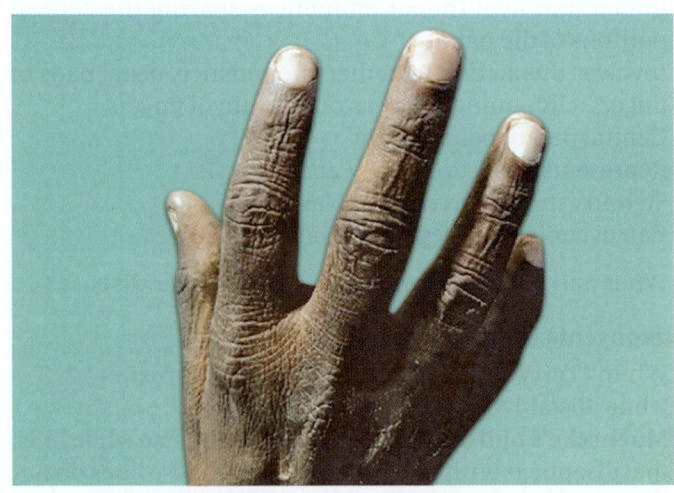

**Fig. 3.7:** White nails.

- Palpable mass in the upper abdomen.
- Mild to moderate upper abdominal pain
- Fever may develop in association with central tumor necrosis
- Intraperitoneal bleeding due to tumor rupture.
- Bone pain or dyspnea due to metastases
- A bruit heard over the liver.

### Q. What is the typical presentation of a primary biliary cirrhosis?

The typical patient is a middle-aged woman with a complaint of fatigue or pruritus. Other symptoms include right upper quadrant abdominal pain, anorexia, and jaundice. Fatigue, although relatively nonspecific, is considered to be the most disabling symptom by many patients, and it worsens in some patients as the disease progresses. Pruritus may occur at any point, early or late, in the course of the disease, or intermittently throughout the course. Pruritus generally is intermittent during the day and is most troublesome in the evening and at night.

**Symptoms and signs of primary biliary cirrhosis at presentation (Table 3.2)**

**Table 3.2:** Signs and symptoms of PBC.

| Symptoms or signs | Frequency (%) |
|---|---|
| Fatigue | 21–85 |
| Pruritus | 19–55 |
| Hyperpigmentation | 25 |
| Hepatomegaly | 25 |
| Splenomegaly | 15 |
| Xanthelasma | 10 |
| Jaundice | 3–10 |
| Right upper quadrant pain | 8 |
| None | 25–61 |

### Q. What is the morphological classification of cirrhosis?

**Figure 3.8** shows the morphological classification of cirrhosis.

## AUTOIMMUNE HEPATITIS

### Q. What are the clinical features of autoimmune hepatitis?

Refer **Table 3.3**.

**Table 3.3:** Clinical features of autoimmune hepatitis.

| Clinical features | Occurrence (%) |
|---|---|
| **Symptoms** | |
| Fatigue | 86 |
| Jaundice | 77 |
| Upper abdominal discomfort | 48 |
| Pruritus (mild) | 36 |
| None (at presentation) | 25–34 |

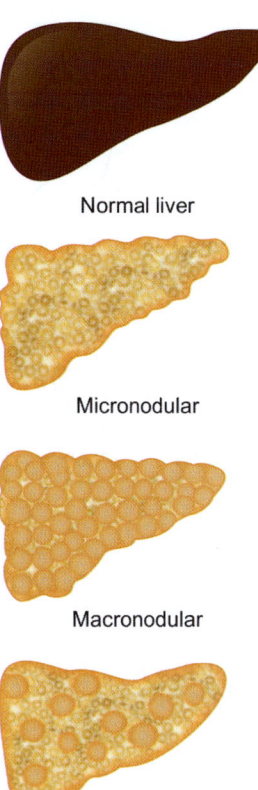

**Fig. 3.8:** Morphological classification of cirrhosis.

| Clinical features | Occurrence (%) |
|---|---|
| Anorexia | 30 |
| Myalgias | 30 |
| Diarrhea | 28 |
| Cushingoid features | 19 |
| Fever (≥40°C) | 18 |
| **Physical findings** | |
| Hepatomegaly | 78 |
| Jaundice | 69 |
| Spider angiomata | 58 |
| Concurrent immune disease | ≤38 |
| Splenomegaly | ≥32 |
| None | <25 |
| Ascites | 20 |
| Encephalopathy | 14 |

### Q. What is constructional apraxia?

Refer **Figures 3.9 and 3.10**.

Inability to reproduce simple designs with blocks or matches. Number connection tests may be used serially to assess progress.

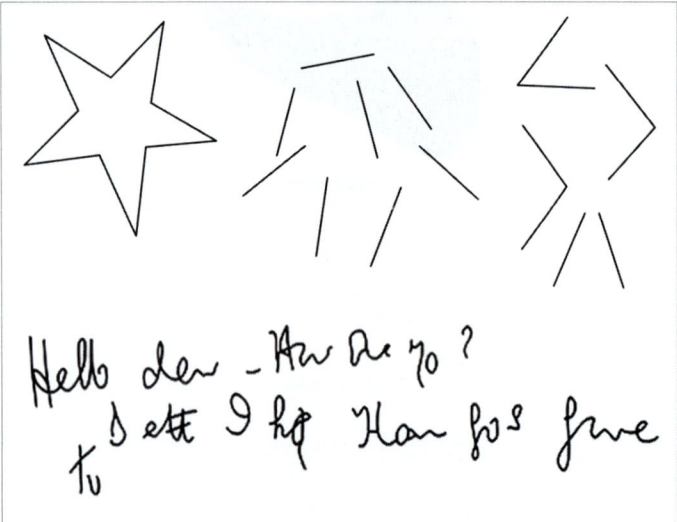

**Fig. 3.9:** Focal disorders in chronic portal-systemic encephalopathy elicited in patients with full consciousness and minimal intellectual defect, in the absence of gross tremor or visual disorder. Above: constructional apraxia. Below: writing difficulty. 'Hello dear. How are you? Better I hope. That goes for me too'.

**Fig. 3.10:** The reitan number connection test.

### Q. Define apraxia and classify?

Inability to carry out on request a high level, familiar and purposeful motor act in absence of any weakness, sensory loss, or other deficit involving the affected part. There are many varieties of apraxia. The ones seen most often are ideomotor, buccofacial, constructional, and dressing apraxia.

In ideomotor (motor) apraxia, the patient is unable to perform a complex command (e.g., salute, wave goodbye, snap the fingers, make a fist, show how to hitch-hike) with the involved extremity. In ideomotor apraxia, there may be a disconnection between the language or visual centers that understand the command and the motor areas tasked with carrying it out.

In ideational (conceptual) apraxia, the patient is able to carry out individual components of a complex motor act, but she cannot perform the entire sequence properly. Ideational apraxia may occur with damage to the left posterior temporoparietal junction or in patients with generalized cognitive impairment.

Constructional or dressing apraxia may occur with parietal lobe lesions that interfere with the patient's ability to comprehend spatial relationships.

### Q. How do you stage hepatic encephalopathy?

Refer **Table 3.4**.

| Table 3.4: Clinical grades of hepatic encephalopathy. | |
|---|---|
| **Clinical grade** | **Clinical sign** |
| Grade I | Mild confusion, euphoria, anxiety or depression |
| | Shortened attention span |
| | Slowing of ability to perform mental tasks (addition/subtraction) |
| | Reversal of sleep rhythm |
| Grade II | Drowsiness, lethargy, gross deficits in ability to perform mental tasks |
| | Obvious personality changes |
| | Inappropriate behavior |
| | Intermittent disorientation of time (and place) |
| | Lack of sphincter control |
| Grade III | Somnolent but rousable |
| | Persistent disorientation of time and place |
| | Pronounced confusion |
| | Unable to perform mental tasks |
| Grade IV | Coma with (IVa) or without (IVb) response to painful stimuli. |

### Q. Briefly explain how will you demonstrate hepatojugular reflux?

- Position the patient with his trunk initially around 45° from the horizontal, and observe the jugular pulsations during quiet breathing. Alter the position as needed to identify the highest angle of elevation at which these pulsations can be seen. This is the baseline venous pressure. (You will be searching for a 3-cm rise in venous pressure. Accordingly, if the jugular vein is too short to demonstrate such a rise, you may have to crank up the head of the bed so that the vein rises 3 cm on the vertical).

- Apply your hand to the right upper quadrant or the middle of the abdomen. It is not necessary to press over the liver to produce the phenomenon. (In fact, if there is tenderness, you should not press in that area because you do not wish the patient to guard, perform a Valsalva maneuver, or interrupt his normal breathing pattern in any way.)
- Press down, maintaining a pressure of 35 mm Hg. (You can practice over a semi-inflated blood pressure cuff or place the blood pressure cuff over the abdomen to be sure that sufficient pressure is applied.)
- Instruct the patient to continue to breathe normally through his mouth. Do not attempt to measure the venous pressure for at least 10 seconds to allow both respiratory artifacts and tensing of the abdominal muscles to subside (each alters jugular venous pressure). The best time to take another venous pressure measurement is at 1 minute of pressure. This should be used as the gold standard in ambiguous cases for reasons given in the section "For the Attending."
- A venous pressure rise of more than 3 cm is abnormal and hepatojugular reflux (or "abdominojugular reflux" as some now prefer) is said to be present, assuming of course that pain or performance of a Valsalva maneuver has not produced a false positive.
- Watch for an abrupt drop in jugular venous pressure as the abdominal pressure is relieved. The sudden fall is generally easier to perceive than the gradual rise.

## Q. What are the causes of drug-induced liver injury?

- **Acute hepatocellular injury:** Numerous drugs such as isoniazid, rifampicin, methyl dopa, telithromycin, ketoconazole, diclofenac
- **Mononucleosis:** Sulfonamides, phenytoin, dapsone
- **Fulminant hepatitis:** Paracetamol (acetaminophen)
- **Bland cholestasis:** Anabolic/androgenic steroids, ciclosporin
- **Cholestatic hepatitis:** Chlorpromazine, erythromycin, amoxicillin—clavulanate, clarithromycin
- **Chronic hepatitis:** Methotrexate, lisinopril, trazodone, uracil
- **Autoimmune hepatitis:** Nitrofurantoin, minocycline, methyldopa, oxyphenisatin
- **Macrovesicular hepatitis:** Corticosteroids, methotrexate, asparaginase, alcohol, halothane
- **Microvesicular hepatitis:** Valproic acid, tetracyclines, cocaine, amiodarone
- **Steatohepatitis:** Amiodarone, griseofulvin, perhexilline maleate
- **Cirrhosis:** Methotrexate, amiodarone
- **Granulomatous hepatitis:** Allopurinol, rosiglitazone, sulfonamide, phenylbutazone, quinidine
- **Primary biliary cirrhosis:** Chlorpromazine, erythromycin, amoxicillin—clavulanate, haloperidol
- **Peliosis hepatic:** Anabolic steroids, oral contraceptives
- **Portal vein thrombosis:** Oral contraceptives
- **Sinusoidal obstructive syndrome:** Pyrrolizidine alkaloids, adriamycin, floxuridine, oncotherapy
- **Nodular transformation:** Anabolic and contraceptive steroids
- **Adenoma:** Anabolic and contraceptive steroids
- **Hepatocellular carcinoma:** Thorotrast, anabolic and contraceptive steroids
- **Cholangiocarcinoma:** Thorotrast
- **Angiosarcoma:** Vinyl chloride, inorganic arsenicals.

## Q. What histological findings are seen in alcoholic liver disease?

The histologic features of alcohol-induced hepatic injury include steatosis (fatty change), lobular hepatitis, periportal fibrosis, Mallory bodies, nuclear vacuolation, bile ductal proliferation, and fibrosis or cirrhosis. Development of large-droplet (macrovesicular) steatosis (fatty liver) is the earliest and most common manifestation of ALD.

## Q. How to investigate a case of cirrhosis?

Occupation, age, sex, domicile.

**Clinical history**
- Fatigue and weight loss
- Anorexia and flatulent dyspepsia
- Abdominal pain
- Jaundice.
- Itching.
- Color of urine and feces
- Swelling of legs or abdomen
- **Hemorrhage:** Nose, gums, skin, alimentary tract
- Loss of libido; menstrual history
- **Past health:** Jaundice, hepatitis, drugs ingested, blood transfusion
- **Social:** Alcohol consumption
- **Family history:** Liver disease, autoimmune disease

**Examination**
- Nutrition, fever, fetor hepaticus, jaundice, pigmentation, purpura, finger clubbing, white nails, vascular spiders, palmar erythema, gynecomastia, testicular atrophy, distribution of body hair, parotid enlargement, Dupuytren's contracture, blood pressure
- **Abdomen:** Ascites, abdominal wall veins, liver, spleen, peripheral edema
- **Neurological changes:** Mental functions, stupor, tremor

**Investigations**
- **Hematology:** Hemoglobin, leukocyte and platelet count, prothrombin time (INR)
- **Serum biochemistry:**
  - Bilirubin
  - Transaminase
  - Alkaline phosphatase
  - γ-glutamyl transpeptidase
  - Albumin and globulin
  - Immunoglobulins
  - Transferrin saturation and serum ferritin
  - Serum ceruloplasmin and copper
  - α-1-antitrypsin phenotype
- **If ascites present:**
  - Serum sodium, potassium, bicarbonate, chloride, urea and creatinine levels
  - Weigh daily
  - 224 hours urine volume and sodium excretion
- **Serum immunological:**
  - Smooth muscle, mitochondrial, nuclear, LKM1 antibodies, and ANCA
  - Hepatitis B antigen (HBsAg), anti-HCV (other markers of hepatitis)
  - α-fetoprotein
- **Endoscopy**
- **Hepatic ultrasound, CT or MRI scan**
- **Needle liver biopsy if blood coagulation permits**
- **EEG if neuropsychiatric changes**

**Q. What are purpura, petechiae and ecchymoses?**

Purpurae are discoloration of skin or mucus membrane due to extravasation of red blood cells. Petechiae are small purpuric lesions up to 2 mm in size whereas ecchymoses are larger (>2 mm) extravasations of blood. They do not blanch on pressure. Extravasated blood is broken down into various other pigments derived from hem in 2–3 weeks. This accounts for the characteristic color changes (purple, orange, brown, blue and green) which occur in purpuric lesions.

**Q. Name the conditions where portal hypertension is present without dilated veins.**

Dilated veins around the umbilicus (caput medusae) are a feature of **intrahepatic** portal hypertension. Here, some blood from the left branch of portal vein may be deviated via paraumbilical veins to the umbilicus where it reaches the veins of the caval system. These are absent in **extrahepatic** portal hypertension where dilated veins may appear in the left flank.

**Q. What are the causes of extrahepatic portal hypertension?**

Extrahepatic portal vein obstruction-usually due to thrombosis.

Important causes are:
- Infections—more common in children following spread of infection from umbilical vein. Other causes are acute appendicitis, peritonitis, biliary infections.
- Hypercoagulable states like myeloproliferative disorders, deficiency of protein C, S or antithrombin 3 or the presence of prothrombin gene mutation.
- Invasion and compression usually by hepatocellular carcinoma or carcinoma of pancreas.
- Post-splenectomy

Cirrhotic patients can develop portal vein thrombosis usually due to invasion by hepatocellular carcinoma.

**Q. What are the causes of cirrhosis with enlarged liver?**
- Hemochromatosis
- Primary biliary cirrhosis
- Primary sclerosing cholangitis
- Hepatocellular carcinoma in a cirrhotic liver
- Nonalcoholic steatohepatitis
- Cardiac cirrhosis
- Budd-Chiari syndrome
- Storage diseases of liver

**Q. What is fulminant hepatic failure?**

Fulminant hepatic failure is said to be present when the time interval between jaundice and hepatic encephalopathy is less than 2 weeks in patients without pre-existing liver disease. It is also characterized by coagulopathy. When the onset of hepatic encephalopathy is after 2 weeks it's called as subfulminant hepatic failure **(Table 3.5)**.

**Table 3.5:** Types of acute liver failure.

| Types | Interval: Jaundice to encephalopathy |
|---|---|
| Hyperacute | <7 days |
| Acute | 8–28 days |
| Subacute | 29 days to 12 weeks |

The following features help to differentiate acute liver failure from acute on chronic disease **(Table 3.6)**.

**Table 3.6:** Acute liver failure versus acute on chronic liver failure.

| Clinical features | Acute | Acute on chronic |
|---|---|---|
| Nutrition | Good | Poor |
| Liver | ± | + Hard |
| Spleen | ± | + Hard |
| Spider naevi | Absent | ++ |

**Q. What is Gauchers disease and name the enzyme deficiency associated with Gauchers disease?**

This is a rare autosomal recessive disease. It is the most common lysosomal storage disorder. It is due to the deficiency of lysosomal **acid beta glucosidase** leading to the accumulation of glucosylceramide, derived from membrane glycosphingolipids in the reticuloendothelial system throughout the body, particularly in the liver, bone marrow and spleen.

There are three types depending on the type of mutations affecting the structural gene for acid beta glucosidase on chromosome 1:
1. **Type 1 (adult, chronic, non-neuronopathic):** Mildest and most common form. It occurs rarely in all ethnic groups but most common in Ashkenazi jews. The central nervous system is spared.
2. **Type 2 (infantile, acute, neuronopathic)—rare:** In addition to the visceral involvement there is massive, fatal neurological involvement with death in infancy.
3. **Type 3 (juvenile, subacute, neuronopathic):** Rare. There is gradual, heterogeneous neurological involvement.

The characteristic Gaucher cell (oval or polygonal in shape with pale cytoplasm with 2 or more peripherally placed hyperchromatic nuclei) accumulate in the perisinusoidal space and can form large aggregates associated with fibrosis which can be severe enough to resemble cirrhosis.

Treatment is by enzyme replacement therapy.

### Q. What skin, nail, hand manifestations are seen in chronic liver disease?

- Spider nevi (telangiectatic superficial blood vessels with central feeding vessel)
- Clubbing of hands (especially biliary cirrhosis and hepatocellular carcinoma)
- Leukonychia
- Palmar erythema (blotchy appearance over the thenar and hypothenar eminence)
- Bruising
- Dupuytren's contracture (sign of alcoholism)
- Scratch marks (cholestatic jaundice)
- Pyoderma gangrenosa: Associated inflammatory bowel diseases (IBD) PBC or autoimmune cirrhosis.

### Q. When does the abdominal bruit become significant?

Abdominal bruit becomes significant when it lateralizes to one side. Bruit will have both systolic and diastolic components and it suggests turbulent blood flow of partial arterial occlusion or arterial insufficiency.

Bruits confined to systole are relatively common and do not necessarily signify occlusive disease. Prolonged bruits are significant.

### Q. Where does the paraumbilical vein drain into?

The paraumbilical vein drain into left portal vein.

### Q. Briefly explain the anatomy of portal vein.

The portal vein begins at the level of the second lumbar vertebra and is formed from the convergence of the superior mesenteric and splenic veins. It lies anterior to the inferior vena cava and posterior to the neck of the pancreas. It lies obliquely to the right and ascends behind the first part of the duodenum, the common bile duct and gastroduodenal artery. At this point it is directly anterior to the inferior vena cava. It enters the right border of the lesser omentum, and ascends anterior to the epiploic foramen to reach the right end of the porta hepatis. It then divides into right and left main branches which accompany the corresponding branches of the hepatic artery into the liver. In the lesser omentum it lies posterior to both the common bile duct and hepatic artery. It is surrounded by the hepatic nerve plexus and accompanied by many lymph vessels and some lymph nodes. The right branch usually receives the cystic vein and then enters the right lobe. It usually forms an anterior division supplying segments V and VIII and a posterior division supplying segments VI and VII. The anterior division may give a branch to segment I. The left branch has a longer extra parenchymal course and tends to lie slightly more horizontal than the right branch but is often of smaller caliber. It gives off branches to segments I (caudate), II, III and IV (quadrate). As it enters the left lobe it is joined by paraumbilical veins and the ligamentum teres, which contains the functionless and partly obliterated left umbilical vein. It is connected to the inferior vena cava by the ligamentum venosum, a vestige of the obliterated ductus venosus. The small extrahepatic section of the left branch, from which the branches to segments II, III and IV arise, is a persistent part of the left umbilical vein.

The portal vein receives many branches including the splenic, superior mesenteric, left gastric, right gastric, paraumbilical and cystic veins. Portal venous blood is one route through which hepatic metastases from gastrointestinal primary malignancies may spread. Blood within the portal vein flows at such a rate that streaming may occur so that the blood from the splenic vein tends to remain on the left side of the portal bloodstream and drain preferentially to the left main branch. The clinical evidence to support this is very limited since colorectal cancer metastases commonly occur in the right lobe.

The following are common sites of portosystemic shunts:
- Between the left gastric and lower esophageal veins (portal) and the lower branches of the esophageal veins draining into the azygos and accessory hemiazygos veins (systemic). Enlargement of these anastomoses may result in the formation of varices, either esophageal or gastric. These may give rise to potentially fatal torrential bleeding.
- Between the superior rectal veins (portal) and the middle and inferior rectal veins draining into the internal iliac and pudendal veins (systemic). The dilated veins may be seen on the rectal wall, but rarely give rise to troublesome bleeding and are not a cause for internal hemorrhoids.
- Between persistent tributaries of the left branch of the portal vein running in the ligamentum teres and the periumbilical branches of the superior and inferior epigastric veins (systemic), forming the so-called 'caput medusae'.
- Between intraparenchymal branches of the right branch of the portal vein lying in liver tissue exposed in the 'bare

area' and retroperitoneal veins draining into the lumbar, azygos and hemiazygos veins.
- Between omental and colonic veins (portal) and retroperitoneal veins (systemic) in the region of the hepatic and splenic flexure.
- Rarely, between a patent ductus venosus connected to the left branch of the portal vein and the inferior vena cava.

**Q. What is venous hum and where will you look for venous hum?**

It is a continuous, low-pitched, soft murmur that may become louder with inspiration and diminish when more pressure is applied to the stethoscope. Typically, it is heard between xiphisternum and the umbilicus in cases of portal hypertension. It may radiate to chest or over to the liver.

Large volumes of blood flowing in the umbilical or paraumbilical veins in the falciform ligament are responsible. These channel blood from the left portal vein to the epigastric or internal mammary veins in the abdominal wall. A venous hum may occasionally be heard over the large vessels such as inferior mesenteric vein or after portocaval shunting. Sometimes a thrill is detectable over the site of maximum intensity of the hum. The Cruveilhier-Baumgarten syndrome is the association of a venous hum at the umbilicus and dilated abdominal wall veins. It is almost always due to cirrhosis of liver. It occurs when patients have a patent umbilical vein, which allow portosystemic shunting at this site. The presence of a venous hum or of prominent central abdominal veins suggest that the site of portal obstruction is intrahepatic rather than in the portal vein itself.

**Q. What are the cardinal features of IVC obstruction?**
- Dilated veins on the flanks and back.
- Cyanosis and edema of the legs appear, dilated varicose veins involve the legs, abdominal wall and even the thorax.
- Veins of the lower abdominal wall, which normally fill from above downwards, fill from below upwards.

**Q. What are the evidence of hepatic encephalopathy?**
- Flapping tremor—asterixis
- Disturbed consciousness
- Inversion of sleep rhythm
- Personality changes like childishness and irritability
- Constructional apraxia—inability to reproduce simple designs with blocks
- Intellectual deterioration elicited easily by number connection test.
- Monotonous slow and slurred speech.
- Exaggerated deep tendon reflexes.
- Increased muscle tone
- Sustained ankle clonus often associated with rigidity.
- Flexor plantar response
- Extensor plantar in deep stupor or coma
- Hyperventilation and hyperpyrexia may be terminal.

**Q. Name the staging criteria for hepatic encephalopathy and how will you grade hepatic encephalopathy?**

**West Haven criteria (Table 3.7)**

| Table 3.7: Grading of hepatic encephalopathy. | | |
|---|---|---|
| **Clinical stage** | **Impairment of intellectual function** | **Impairment of neuromuscular function** |
| Subclinical | Normal examination findings, but work or driving may be impaired | Subtle changes on psychometric or number connection tests |
| Stage 1 | Impaired attention, irritability, depression, or personality change | Tremor, incoordination, apraxia |
| Stage 2 | Drowsiness, behavioral changes, poor memory and computation, sleep disorders | Asterixis, slowed or slurred speech, ataxia |
| Stage 3 | Confusion and disorientation, somnolence, amnesia | Hypoactive reflexes, nystagmus, clonus, and muscular rigidity |
| Stage 4 | Stupor and coma | Dilated pupils and decerebrate posturing; oculocephalic ("doll's eye") reflex; absence of response to stimuli in advanced stages |

**Q. How will you test for constructional apraxia?**
- Number connection test **(Fig. 3.11)**
- Digit symbol test **(Fig. 3.12)**
- Serial dotting **(Fig. 3.13)**
- Line tracing test **(Fig. 3.14)**.
- Subjects are asked to join the numbers in sequence as quickly as possible. The time taken to complete the task is recorded.
- To be more informative, time taken should be compared with normal values of same age group.

**Digit symbol test**
- Subjects are asked to insert symbols in the blank squares below the numbers using the key provided.
- The exercise is timed and the number correctly completed in 90 seconds recorded.

**Serial dotting**

Subjects are asked to place a dot in the center of each circle and to complete the page as quickly as possible. The time taken to complete the task is recorded.

**Line tracing test**
- Subjects are asked to trace a line between the two guidelines as quickly and accurately as possible without moving the paper.
- The time taken to complete the task and the number of errors made are recorded.

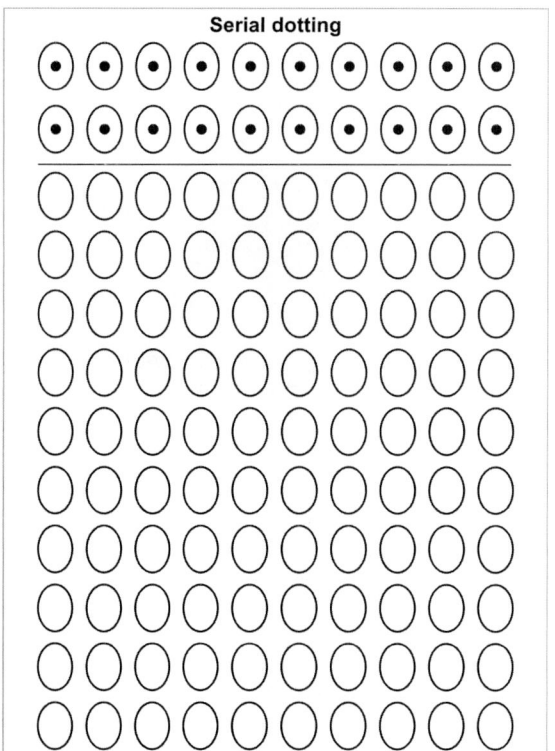

**Fig. 3.11:** Number connection test.

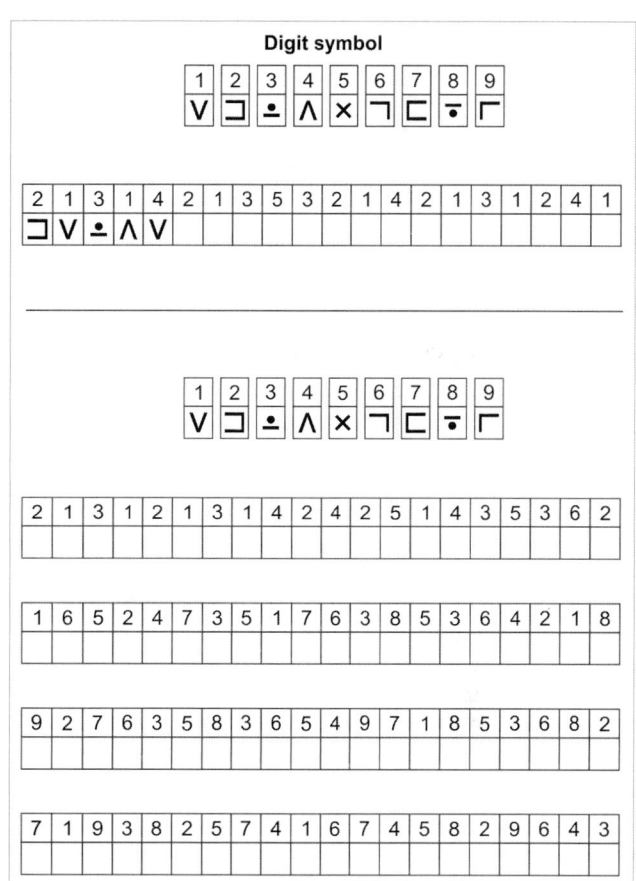

**Fig. 3.12:** Digit symbol test.

**Fig. 3.13:** Serial dotting.

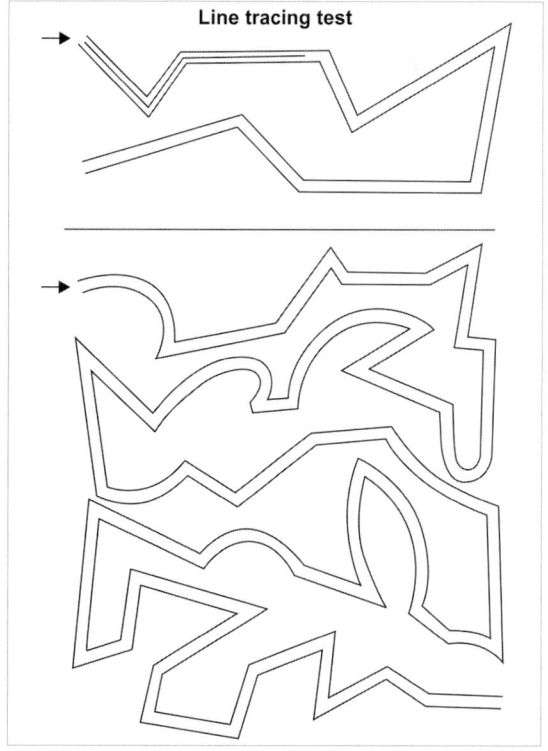

**Fig. 3.14:** Line tracing test.

This battery, which has been called the psychometric hepatic encephalopathy score (PHES), assesses the required domains of attention, visual perception and executive abilities; it is easily applied and has been shown to have a **_high specificity for the diagnosis of hepatic encephalopathy._**

### Q. What is the significance of cervical venous hum?

Heard as a continuous humming sound over prominent veins seen in the root of neck in supraclavicular region.
- Venous hum indicates that there is hyperkinetic circulation most commonly chronic compensated anemia.

**Characteristics of venous hum**
- Soft and low-pitched
- Often continuous with diastolic accentuation
- Best heard in sitting or erect position with the bell of the stethoscope
- Best audible in inspiration
- Disappears in pressing the bell of the stethoscope and with Valsalva maneuver.

### Q. What is a venous nevus?

Venous nevus is a vascular malformation that occurs due to a mutation during the postzygotic embryogenesis phase. These lesions never cross the midline.

These should be differentiated from other vascular malformations that are not categorized as nevi.

**Examples:** Varicose veins associated with Klippel-Trenaunay syndrome, deep vein anomalies of Parkes-Weber syndrome, multiple lesions of the blue rubber nevus syndrome.

### Q. What is the triad of portal hypertension?
- Splenomegaly—definite evidence of portal hypertension
- Ascites
- Dilated abdominal wall veins/varices.

### Q. How do you rule out chronic Budd-Chiari in this patient?

Patients with Budd-Chiari syndrome will have an absent hepatojugular reflux.

### Q. What are the noncardiac causes of raised JVP?
- Innominate vein thrombosis
- Superior vena cava (SVC) obstruction
- Chronic obstructive pulmonary disease (COPD)
- Massive right sided pleural effusion
- Pulmonary embolism
- Ascites
- Pregnancy
- Renal disease
- Excess IV fluids

### Q. How to know the site of obstruction in SVC by assessing JVP?

The rise in JVP is greater when the site of obstruction is near the junction with azygous and proximal to the opening of azygous **(Figs. 3.15 to 3.17)**.

### Q. What is the significance of the flow of veins from bottom to top?

In intrahepatic portal hypertension, blood from the left branch of the portal vein is deviated via the paraumbilical veins to the umbilicus from where it reaches the caval veins. In extrahepatic portal obstruction dilated veins appear on the flanks.

In IVC obstruction the flow of blood through the collaterals is from top to bottom to reach the superior vena caval system.

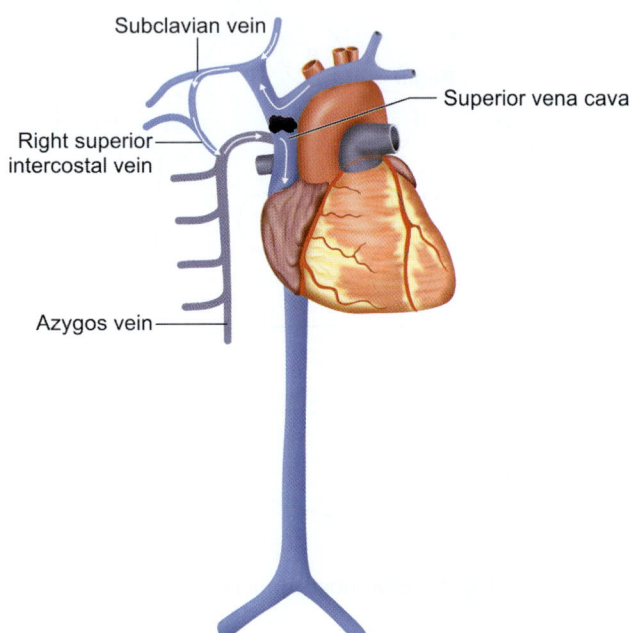

**Fig. 3.15:** Obstruction of SVC proximal to the opening of azygous vein.

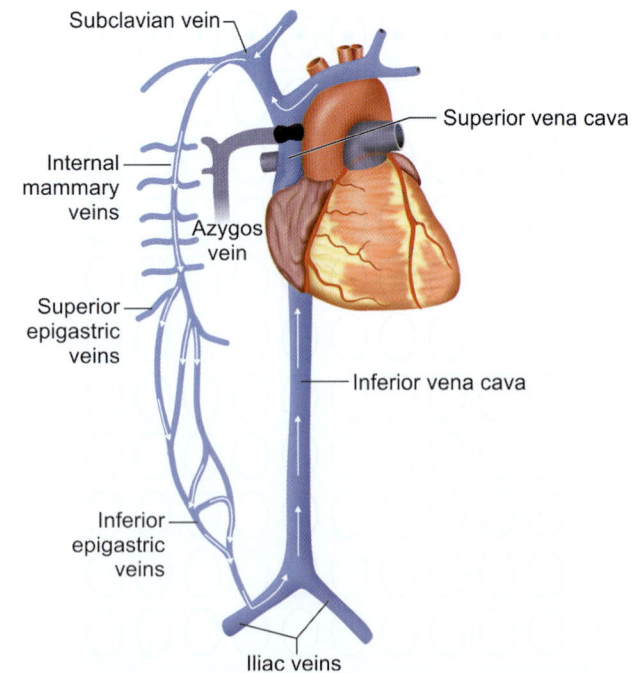

**Fig. 3.16:** Obstruction of SVC at junction with azygous.

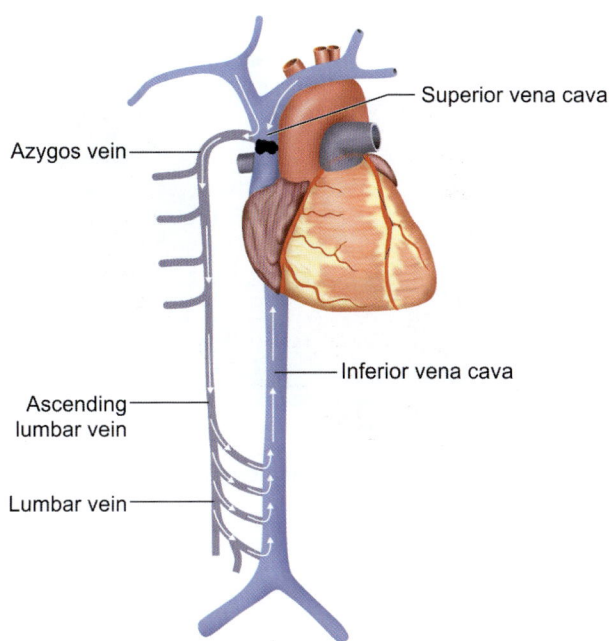

**Fig. 3.17:** Obstruction of SVC distal to opening of azygous vein.

Hence if collateral veins are present and the flow of veins is from bottom to top, it is highly suggestive of IVC obstruction **(Figs. 3.18A to C)**.

Sometime tense ascites may lead to functional obstruction of the IVC and cause difficulty in interpretation.

**Q. How do you classify portal hypertension?**

Portal hypertension can be classified into two types **(Fig. 3.19)**:

1. **Presinusoidal:**
    - Extrahepatic: Blocked portal vein and increased splenic flow. Examples: splenic vein and portal vein thrombosis, idiopathic tropical splenomegaly, IVC thrombosis, hepatic vein thrombosis, constrictive pericarditis, Budd-Chiari
    - Intrahepatic: Portal zone infiltrates, toxic and hepatoportal sclerosis. Examples: Schistosomiasis, early primary biliary cirrhosis, sarcoidosis
2. **Hepatic:**
    - Sinusoidal: Cirrhosis, cytotoxic drugs, acute alcoholic hepatitis
    - Postsinusoidal: Veno-occlusive disease, alcoholic central hyaline sclerosis.

**Posthepatic**
- Budd-Chiari syndrome
- Constrictive pericarditis
- Inferior vena caval obstruction
- Right-sided heart failure
- Severe tricuspid regurgitation

**Intrahepatic presinusoidal**
- Idiopathic portal hypertension
- PBC
- Sarcoidosis
- Schistosomiasis

**Sinusoidal**
- Alcoholic cirrhosis
- Alcoholic hepatitis
- Cryptogenic cirrhosis
- Postnecrotic cirrhosis

**Postsinusoidal**
- Sinusoidal obstruction syndrome

**Prehepatic**
- Portal vein thrombosis
- Splenic vein thrombosis

**Fig. 3.19:** Classification of portal hypertension.

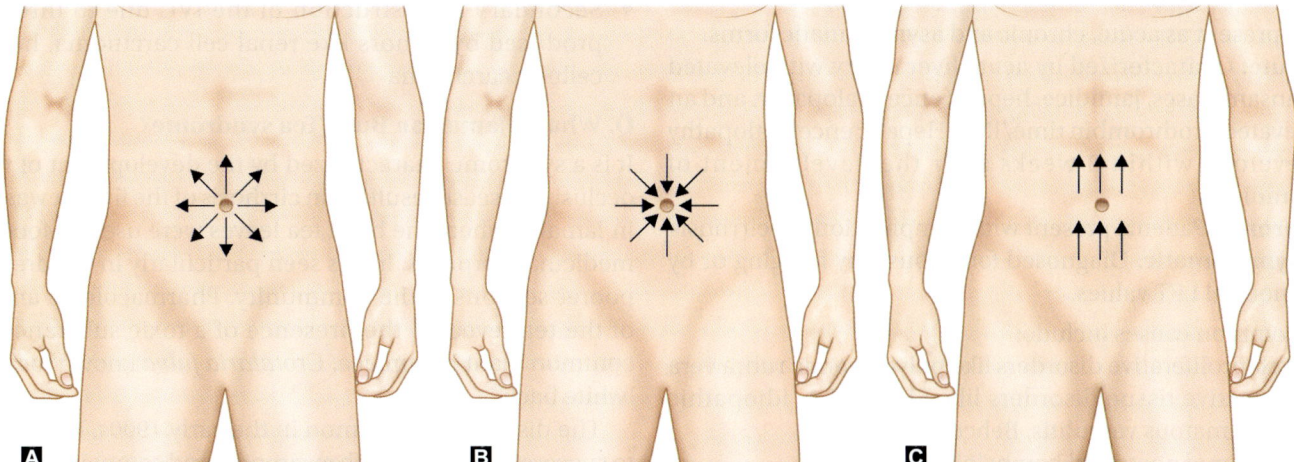

**Figs. 3.18A to C:** Direction: (A) Portal hypertension; (B) Portal vein thrombosis; (C) IVC obstruction.

**Q. What is the sine qua non of portal hypertension?**
Splenomegaly.

**Q. What are the clinical signs of IVC obstruction?** Cyanosis and edema of the legs.

Varicosities of the lower limbs and varicocele of the testes. Large dilated tortuous veins over the abdomen and chest.

Filling of the veins of the lower abdominal wall from bottom to top hematuria, albuminuria and casts if the renal vein is involved. Venous ulcer in the lower limbs due to stasis.

**Q. What are the differences between hepatic and prehepatic portal hypertension?**
Refer **Table 3.8**.

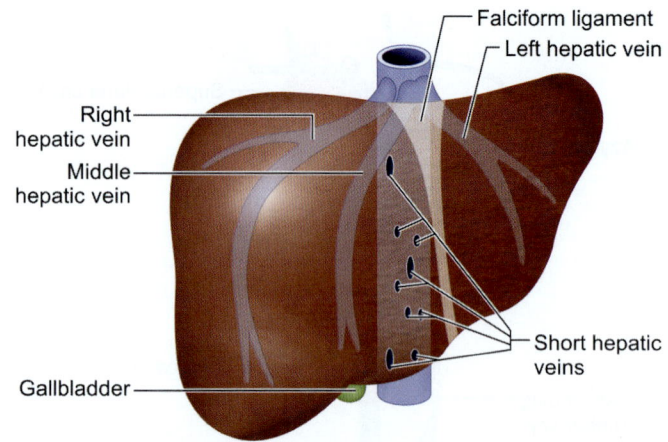

Fig. 3.20: Figure showing the anatomy of the hepatic veins.

| Table 3.8: Hepatic versus prehepatic portal hypertension. | | |
|---|---|---|
| *Clinical features* | *Hepatic* | *Prehepatic* |
| Ascites | Persistent and late | Transient and early |
| Sings of liver cell failure | Present | Absent |
| Dilated veins | Periumbilical dilated veins | Dilated veins over the flank |
| Venous hum | Present | Absent |
| Size of liver | Usually shrunken | Liver is normal |
| Causes | Cirrhosis, tumors of the liver, alcoholic hepatitis | Thrombosis of the splenic vein, portal vein thrombosis, IVC obstruction |

**Q. What are the causes and clinical features of Budd-Chiari syndrome?**

It is a syndrome which consists of hepatomegaly, abdominal pain, ascites and hepatic histology showing zone 3 sinusoidal distension and pooling. It is caused due obstruction of the hepatic vein at any site from the efferent vein of the acinus to the entry of the IVC. Other causes of obstruction like pericardial disease, cardiac disease and veno-occlusive disease have to be ruled out before a diagnosis of Budd- Chiari can be made **(Figs. 3.20 and 3.21)**.

It can present as acute, chronic and asymptomatic forms.
- **Acute:** Characterized by acute liver injury with elevated transaminases, jaundice, hepatic encephalopathy, and an elevated prothrombin time/INR. Hepatic encephalopathy develops within 8 weeks after the development of jaundice.
- **Chronic:** Patients present with complications of cirrhosis
- **Asymptomatic:** Diagnosed fortuitously by imaging or by abnormal LFT values.

The common causes include:
- Myeloproliferative disorders like polycythemia rubra vera
- Connective tissue disorders like SLE, APLA, idiopathic granulomatous vasculitis, Behcet's
- Paroxysmal nocturnal hemoglobinuria
- Protein C and protein S deficiency

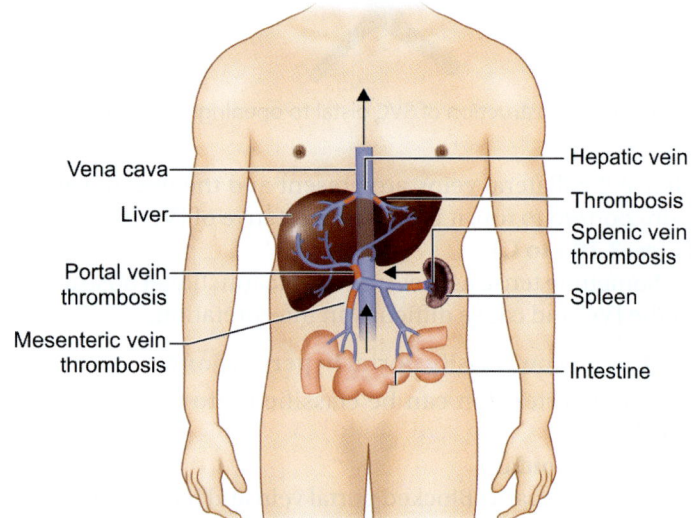

Fig. 3.21: Budd-Chiari syndrome.

- Antithrombin III deficiency
- Drugs—oral contraceptives
- Secondary to obstruction of the IVC due to thrombus produced by tumors like renal cell carcinoma, hepatocellular carcinoma

**Q. What is Jamaican Bush Tea syndrome?**

It is a syndrome characterized by the development of veno-occlusive disease resulting in cirrhosis of the liver. It was seen in Jamaica where the bush tea leaves were used as food and medicinal purposes. It was seen particularly in children and poorer sections of the community. Pharmacologic analysis of the tea revealed the presence of a toxic substance in a common plant in Jamaica, *Crotalaria fulva* known locally as 'white back'.

The disease was common in the early 1900s. By 1960 due to successful public health awareness and campaigning, there was a dramatic fall in the number of cases.

Internationally, it was recognized as the first cause of veno-occlusive disease leading to cirrhosis of the liver. It is rare to see the syndrome nowadays.

### Q. Define acute liver failure.

Acute liver failure is defined as the rapid progressive deterioration in liver function, specifically coagulopathy and mental status changes (encephalopathy) in a patient without known prior liver disease.

### Q. What are the clinical features of acute liver failure?

- Hepatomegaly
- Fatigue/malaise
- Lethargy
- Anorexia
- Nausea and/or vomiting
- Right upper quadrant pain
- Pruritus
- Jaundice
- Abdominal distension from ascites

### Q. What are the features of cholestatic jaundice?

- Deep jaundice with greenish hue
- Scratch marks (pruritis—as bile salts saponify the fat surrounding the free nerve endings)
- Bradycardia
- Xanthelasmas on the eyelids **(Fig. 3.22)** and xanthomas over tendons due to lipid deposit
- Palpable gallbladder in carcinoma head of pancreas
- Large hard irregular liver in malignancy
- Late features: Secondary biliary cirrhosis and signs of liver cell failure.

### Q. What is Courvoiser's law?

In the presence of jaundice, a palpable nontender gallbladder is unlikely due to gallstones.

In obstruction of common bile duct due to a stone, the gallbladder as a rule is impalpable (no distension). This is because the gallbladder is already shriveled, fibrotic and nondistensible and hence will not be palpable.

In obstruction from other causes (carcinoma head of pancreas) distension of gallbladder is common and hence gallbladder may be palpable.

### Q. What are the exceptions to Courvoisier's law?

- **Double impaction:** Stones, simultaneously occluding the cystic duct and distal common bile duct
- Pancreatic calculus obstructing the ampulla of Vater
- Oriental cholangiohepatitis
- Periampullary carcinoma in the patients with cholecystectomy
- Mirizzi syndrome—common hepatic duct obstruction caused by an extrinsic compression from an impacted stone in the cystic duct or Hartmann's pouch of gallbladder

### Q. What are the ultrasound features of portal hypertension?

- **Liver size:** <10 cm
- **Hepatic vein:** 11 mm
- **Portal vein:** 12 mm
- **Spleen:** >13 cm

### Q. What are the ultrasound features of chronic portal hypertension?

Intrahepatic portal cavernoma **(Fig. 3.23)**—occurs when the native portal vein is thrombosed, and myriads of collateral channels develop in the porta hepatis to bypass the occlusion. Cavernous transformation results from recanalization of the portal venous thrombus as well as dilatation of paracholedochal veins in an effort to bypass the portal venous obstruction.

In cirrhosis, cavernous transformation of the portal vein is rare because stasis of portal venous flow prevents the formation of collateral channels in and around the portal venous thrombus.

### Q. What is Murphy sign?

It is seen in acute cholecystitis, ask the patient to breath in deeply, and now try to palpate the gallbladder in sitting position. There is tenderness and catch in the breath at the height of inspiration with a mass felt there.

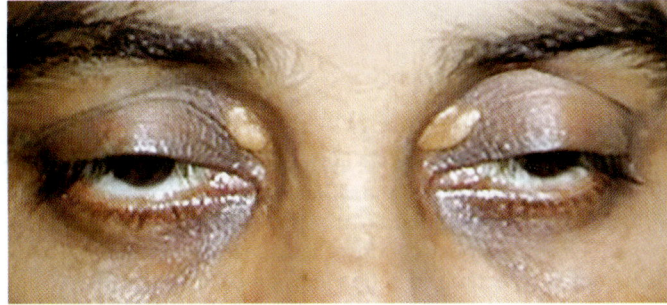

**Fig. 3.22:** Xanthelasmas around the eyes.

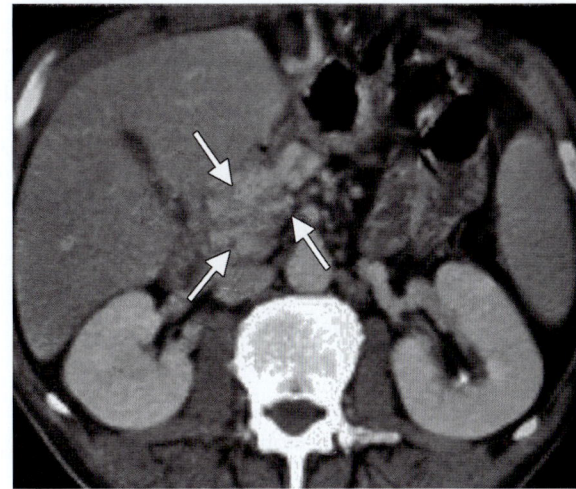

**Fig. 3.23:** CECT axial section reveals cavernoma formation in the extrahepatic portal vein marked by arrow heads.

**Q. What differentials will you consider when a CLD patient with ascites develops fever?**
- Spontaneous bacterial peritonitis
- Pneumonia, UTI, endocarditis, lymphangitis
- Hepatocellular carcinoma

**Q. What to look for in the hands in liver disease?**
- Leukonychia—hypoalbuminemia
- Knuckle pigmentation—hemochromatosis, Addison's disease
- Dupuytren's contracture and palmar erythema—alcoholic liver disease
- Clubbing—primary biliary cirrhosis.

**Q. If it is stomach carcinoma, what else to be looked for?**
- Virchows node (Troisier's sign)
- Jaundice—due to metastasis to liver
  - Or involvement of porta hepatis

**Q. Why are there dilated veins on the anterior wall of abdomen?**

This is suggestive of either portal hypertension or IVC obstruction due to massive ascites. Look for veins below the umbilicus and check the direction of flow. If the flow is away from the umbilicus suggestive of portal hypertension. If it is towards the umbilicus, due to IVC obstruction.

**Q. Define cirrhosis.**

Cirrhosis is the end stage of any chronic liver disease.

It is a diffuse process (entire liver is involved) characterized by fibrosis and conversion of normal architecture to structurally abnormal regenerating nodules of liver cells. **Table 3.9** summarizes types of cirrhosis.

**Table 3.9:** Types of cirrhosis.

| Micronodular cirrhosis | Macronodular cirrhosis | Mixed cirrhosis |
|---|---|---|
| • Also called Laennec's cirrhosis<br>• Regular and small regenerating nodules of <3 mm diameter<br>• Uniform thin regular fibrous connective tissue septa<br>• Involvement of every lobule of whole liver<br>• Alcoholic cirrhosis, biliary cirrhosis, venous occlusion | • Regenerating, irregular, coarse nodules of variable size, usually of >3 mm diameter<br>• Fibrous connective tissue is broad and variable in thickness<br>• Liver surface grossly distorted<br>• Increased risk of developing hepatocellular carcinoma<br>• Most common cause is postnecrotic cirrhosis (chronic viral hepatitis) | • Features of both micro and macronodular cirrhosis |

The three main morphologic characteristics of cirrhosis are:
1. Fibrosis
2. Regenerating nodules
3. Loss of architecture of the entire liver

Factor affecting liver cirrhosis is summarized in **Table 3.10** and main causes of cirrhosis are discussed in **Box 3.1**.

**Q. Why is it a decompensated cirrhosis?**

The symptom triad of decompensated cirrhosis:
- Abdominal distension (ascites)
- **Internal/external bleeding:** Varices/portal hypertension

**Table 3.10:** Factors affecting liver cirrhosis.

| | |
|---|---|
| Quantity of alcohol and gender | • **Males:** 40–80 g/day—fatty liver, >160 g/day—hepatitis, cirrhosis; >14 drinks/week—causes damage<br>• **Females:** >20 g/day or >7 drinks/week—causes damage |
| Coinfections | Moderate alcohol consumption but chronic infection with hepatitis B, C accelerates development of cirrhosis |
| Genetics | Patatin-like phospholipase domain-containing protein 3 (PNPLA3) is associated with alcoholic cirrhosis |
| Fatty liver | Co-existence of obesity and NASH are risk factors for development of cirrhosis in alcoholics |

**Box 3.1:** Main causes of cirrhosis.

- Alcohol (most common causes)
- Chronic viral hepatitis (most common cause)
  - Hepatitis B
  - Hepatitis C
  - Delta hepatitis (hepatitis D) + hepatitis B
- Nonalcoholic steatohepatitis (NASH) or nonalcoholic fatty liver disease (NAFLD) (earlier was considered as cryptogenic cirrhosis)
- Biliary cirrhosis
  - Primary biliary cholangitis
  - Secondary biliary cirrhosis
  - Primary sclerosing cholangitis
  - Autoimmune cholangiopathy, IgG4 cholangiopathy
- Autoimmune hepatitis
- Budd-Chiari syndrome
- Intrahepatic or extrahepatic biliary obstruction: Recurrent biliary obstruction (e.g., gallstones)
- Inherited metabolic liver disease
  - Hemochromatosis
  - Wilson's disease
  - $\alpha_1$ antitrypsin deficiency
  - Cystic fibrosis
  - Glycogen storage disease
- **Drug-induced cirrhosis:** For example, methotrexate, methyldopa, isoniazid, phenylbutazone, sulfonamides
- **Others:** Indian childhood cirrhosis, cardiac cirrhosis, chronic venous outflow obstruction, celiac disease. Hereditary hemotelangiectaria, infection [e.g., brucellosis, syphilis, echinococcosis, porphyria, idiopathic adulthood ductopenia (Carolia disease)]

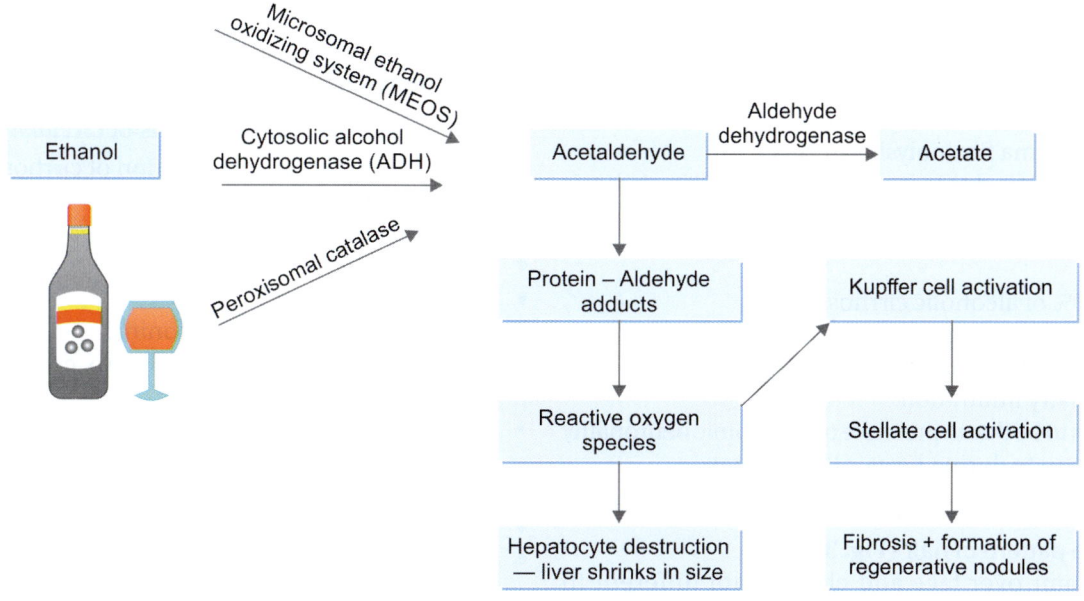

**Fig. 3.24:** Pathogenesis of alcoholic cirrhosis.

- Behavioral/mental changes—Encephalopathy
  Other decompensations:
- Jaundice
- Hepatocellular carcinoma (HCC)
  Pathogenesis of alcoholic cirrhosis is given in **Figure 3.24**.

**Q. What is the ophthalmic sign of liver cell failure?**

Bitot's spots **(Fig. 3.25)**
- Caused due to vitamin A deficiency as a consequence of malabsorption due to decreased fat content in bile.
- Rare in cirrhosis among adults irrespective of etiology.
- It is a sign of liver cell failure.

**Q. What is Kayser-Fleischer (KF) ring?**
- Named after Bernhard Kayser and Bruno Fleischer
- Copper deposited in Descemet's membrane.
- First appears at 12 o'clock position then at 6 o'clock position, then encircles completely.
- About 85–100% of patients with neurological and/or psychiatric manifestations of Wilson's disease but only 33–86% of patients with hepatic disease and 0–59% of asymptomatic patients.

- Slit lamp examination is mandatory to make a diagnosis of KF rings particularly in the early stages unless the rings are visible to the naked eye in conditions of severe copper overload.
- Also seen in other liver diseases such as primary biliary cirrhosis, neonatal hepatitis, and cryptogenic cirrhosis.
- Or elevated copper for other reasons such as in multiple myeloma, pulmonary carcinoma, benign monoclonal gammopathies, chronic lymphocytic leukemia, or even oral contraceptive use.
- After the initiation of treatment, the Kayser-Fleischer ring disappears in 85–90% of cases.

Differences between KF ring and Arcus is discussed in **Table 3.11**.

| Table 3.11: KF rings versus arcus. | | |
|---|---|---|
| **Features** | **KF ring** | **Arcus** |
| Naked eye examination | May be seen | Not seen |
| Site of the ring | Superior/interior/circumferential | Always circumferential |
| Color | Golden brown | Yellowish green |
| Texture | Granular | Homogenous |
| Layer of cornea involved | Descemet's membrane | Peripheral stroma |
| Relation to bilirubin level | Absent | Present |
| Response to chelation therapy | Improved | Not applicable |

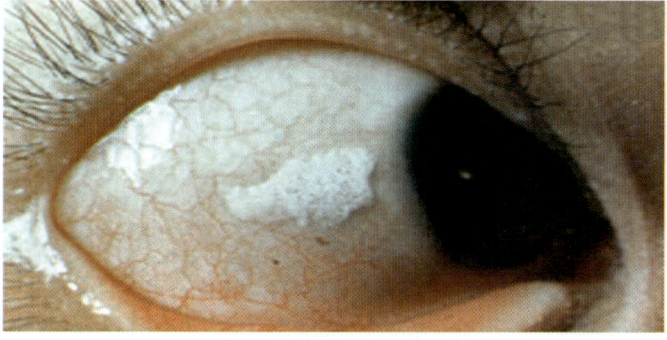

**Fig. 3.25:** Bitot's spot.

### Q. Why cirrhosis patients are prone for increased risk of bleeding?
- Often thought due to decreased coagulation factors
- May occur due to thrombocytopenia
- Increase in plasma fibrinolysins in cirrhosis
- Dysfibrinogenemia due to increased sialic acid in cirrhosis

### Q. Why does parotid enlargement seen in alcoholic cirrhosis?
- Occurs in 50% of alcoholic cirrhosis
- Painless and soft enlargement
- Earlier thought due to hypersecretory parotid
- Edema and fatty infiltration
- Now appears to be due to presence of autonomic neuropathy
- Size can fluctuate during heavy alcohol intake

### Q. Why is there a loss of facial/chest hair in cirrhosis?
- Loss of male pattern of hair (Fig. 3.26)
- Density of hair over face and chest is not different in cirrhosis compared to controls
- Asians by nature have sparse chest hair
- Clinical significance is questionable
- Scalp hair usually spared

### Q. What are the causes of jaundice in a cirrhosis patient?
- Mostly due to progressive hepatocellular injury
- Can be due to hypersplenism related to hemolysis
- Can be due to obstruction by gallstones (increase on account of hemolysis) or pancreatitis
- Hepatoma
- Superadded acute injury

### Q. What are the causes of acute decompensation in a chronic liver disease patient?
- Superadded hepatitis
- Sepsis including SBP
- Malignant transformation
- GI bleed
- Renal failure
- Cardiac failure
- Noncompliance

### Q. Enumerate the complications of cirrhosis.
Figure 3.27 shows the complication of cirrhosis.
- Portal hypertension
- Esophageal varices (Fig. 3.28) and gastropathy.
- Splenomegaly
- Edema and ascites.
- Spontaneous bacterial peritonitis.
- Bruising and bleeding. Due to coagulopathy and thrombocytopenia
- **Jaundice:** It is rare and can be seen with obstructive causes, hepatoma, or superadded hepatitis.
- Hepatic encephalopathy.
- Hepatocellular carcinoma
- Insulin resistance and type 2 diabetes. Diabetes mellitus is seen in 15–30% of patients with cirrhosis
- Immune system dysfunction
- Hepatorenal and hepatopulmonary syndromes
- Hepatic hydrothorax
- Portopulmonary hypertension
- Cirrhotic cardiomyopathy
- Hepatic osteodystrophy
- Hepatic neuropathy
- Hepatic myelopathy.

### Q. What are the causes of anemia in cirrhosis?
It can be due to various causes:
- Acute and chronic blood loss from varices
- Nutritional deficiency of vitamin B12 and folate
- Hypersplenism
- Bone marrow suppression by alcohol
- Hemolysis
- **Zieve's syndrome:** Alcohol-induced hemolytic anemia with hypercholesterolemia.

### Q. What is asterixis?
Refer **Table 3.12**.

| Table 3.12: Causes of asterixis. | |
|---|---|
| *Bilateral asterixis* | *Unilateral asterixis* |
| **Metabolic:** Liver failure, azotemia, respiratory failure | **Focal brain lesions at:** |
| **Sedatives:** Benzodiazepines, barbiturates | • Thalamus<br>• Corona radiata<br>• Anterior cerebral artery territory |
| **Anticonvulsants:** Phenytoin (phenytoin flap), carbamazepine, valproic acid, gabapentin | • Primary motor cortex<br>• Parietal lobe |
| **Antipsychotics:** Ceftazidime | • Cerebellum |
| **Others:** Metoclopramide | • Midbrain |
| **Dyselectrolytemia:** Hypomagnesemia, hypokalemia | • Pons |
| **Bilateral structural brain lesions** | |

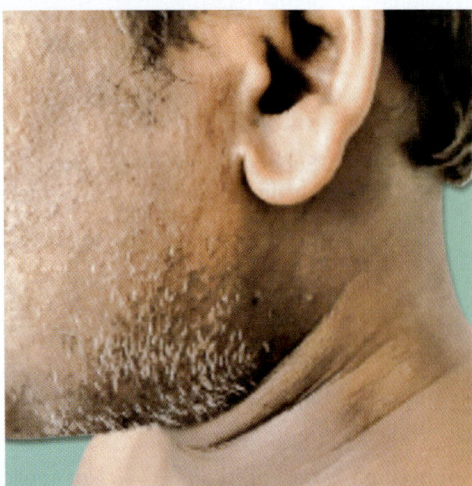

**Fig. 3.26:** Diminished facial hair with parotid enlargement.

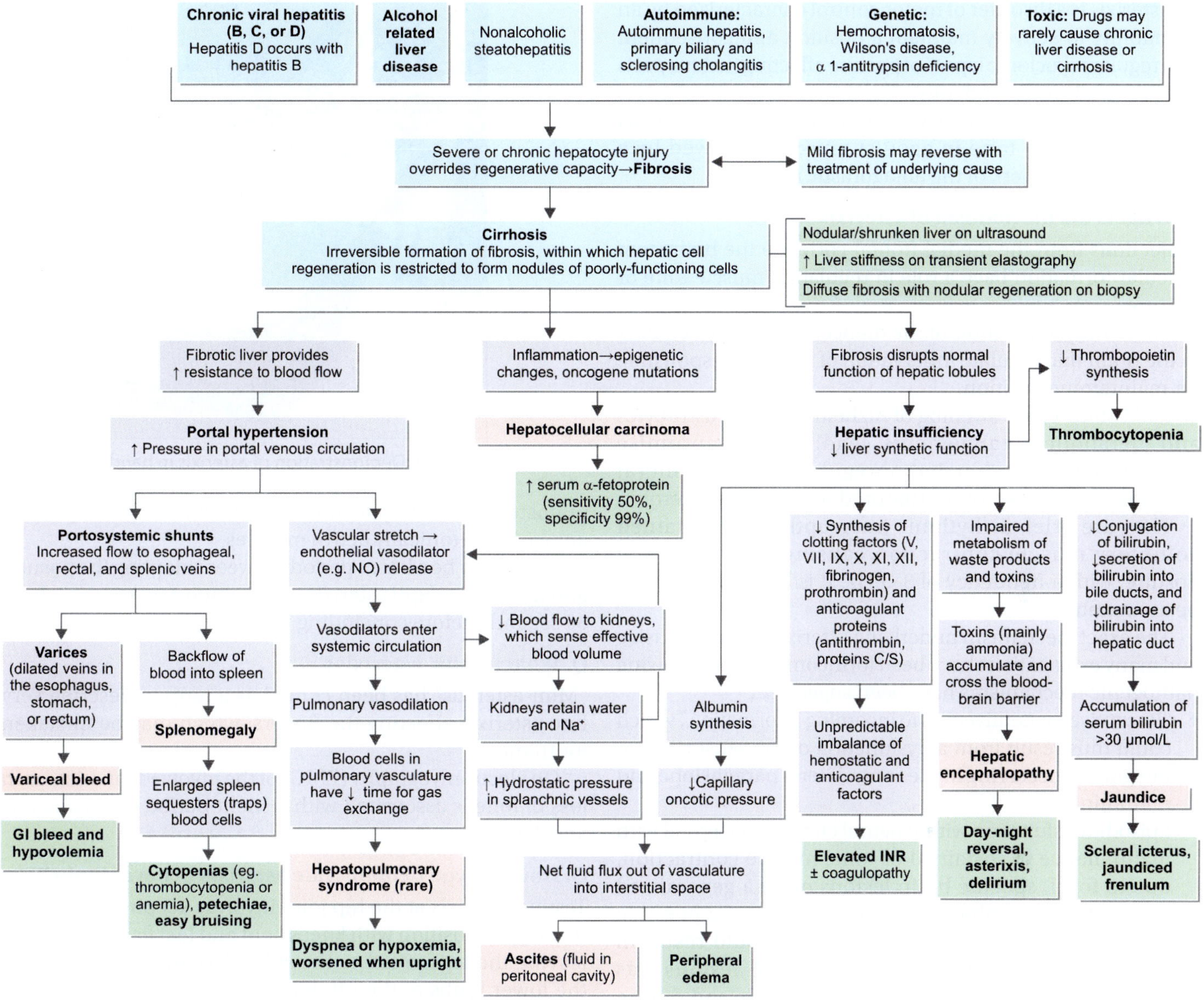

**Fig. 3.27:** Complications of cirrhosis.

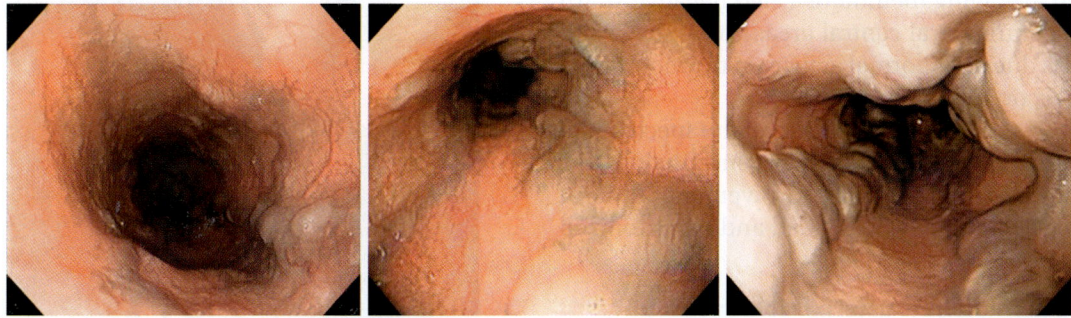

**Fig. 3.28:** Endoscopy view of esophageal varices (grade I, II, and III).

- Asterixis is a disorder of motor control characterized by an inability to actively maintain a position and consequent irregular myoclonic lapses of posture affecting various parts of the body independently.
- It is a type of negative myoclonus characterized by a brief loss of muscle tone in agonist muscles followed by a compensatory jerk of the antagonistic muscles.

### Q. What is the mechanism of asterixis?

Projections from the medial frontal cortex to the brainstem reticular formation have a role in regulating muscle tone or posture.

There is dysregulation of the diencephalic motor centers in the brain that regulate innervation of muscles responsible for maintaining position.

Fluid shifts cause swelling of Alzheimer type II astrocytes and metabolic derangements, leading to compromise in the blood–brain barrier, upregulation of peripheral benzodiazepine receptor, and the production of neurosteroids.

They are brief, arrhythmic interruptions of sustained voluntary muscle contraction causing brief lapses of posture, with a frequency of 3–5 Hz. It is bilateral, but may be asymmetric.

The exact mechanism underlying asterixis remains elusive and many explanations have been forthcoming. The following pathogenic mechanisms have been suggested:
- "Receptive inattentiveness to incoming information", which could thus result from a dysfunction of the sensorimotor integration occurring in the contralateral parietal lobe and midbrain.
- Episodic dysfunction within neural circuits concerned with maintenance of sustained or tonic muscle contraction, due to focal, specific brain lesions or by a generalized neurochemical imbalance. The existence of a possible neural subsystem whose dysfunction could result in asterixis rather than "nonspecific" CNS lesions was hypothesized. Drowsiness in normal people and diffuse CNS lesions can also produce asterixis, perhaps by their effects on alerting or arousal mechanisms rather than by nonspecific CNS actions.
- Electrophysiological evaluation of asterixis using silent period locked averaging method revealed negative sharp waves in the contralateral central area. It was suggested that asterixis is due to abnormal activity in the motor field in the cerebral cortex.
- Recently, mini-asterixis which is a part of the spectrum of the gross flapping tremor seen in hepatic encephalopathy, was proposed as being due to the involvement of motor cortex causing a pathologically slowed and synchronized motor cortical wave.

### Q. How will you demonstrate asterixis in upper limb?

Asterixis is tested by extending the arms, dorsiflexing the wrists, and spreading the fingers to observe for the "flap" at the wrist **(Fig. 3.29)**. The flap is due to irregular myoclonic lapses of posture caused by involuntary 50–200 ms silent periods appearing in tonically active muscles.

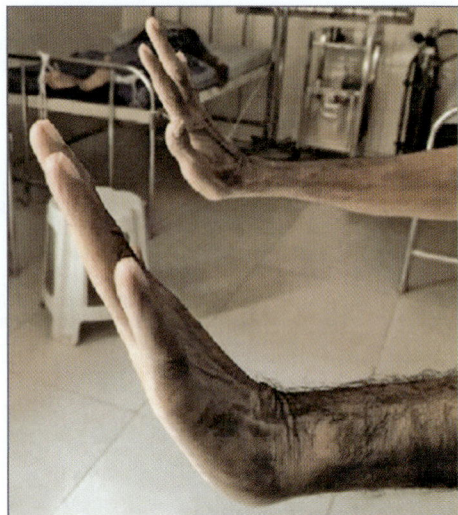

**Fig. 3.29:** Demonstration of asterixis in hands.

There may be a latent period between adopting the posture and the beginning of asterixis, so it is important to wait at least 30 seconds before concluding the test.

### Q. What is mini-asterixis?

"Mini-asterixis" has been coined as a term to describe very fine asterixis affecting the fingers, which may be mistaken for tremor.

On electromyography (EMG) of the involved muscles, each loss of tone is associated with a silent period of between 50 and 200 ms.

### Q. How will you demonstrate asterixis in lower limbs?

Testing asterixis at the hip joint involves keeping the patient in a supine position with knees bent and feet flat on the table, leaving the legs to fall to the sides. Negative myoclonus of the lower limbs at the hip joints repetitively occurs and is appreciated by looking at the knees **(Fig. 3.30)**.

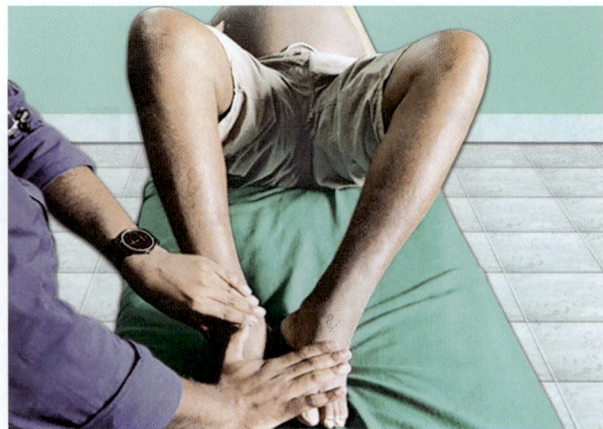

**Fig. 3.30:** Demonstration of flapping tremors in legs—on leaving the legs to fall apart a negative myoclonus can be noticed by observing the knee.

**Q. Name the other methods to elicit asterixis.**

- Request the patient to squeeze the doctor's hand or the doctor's extended fingers. Patients who are unable to maintain a posture usually are unable to maintain a steady squeeze.
- Have the patient squeeze a semi-inflated blood pressure cuff with instructions to maintain the reading. The readings bounce dramatically in patients with asterixis.

**Q. What are the signs pointing to the different etiologies of cirrhosis?**

Table 3.13 summarizes signs pointing the etiology of cirrhosis.

**Table 3.13:** Signs pointing the etiology of cirrhosis.

| Signs | Etiology of cirrhosis |
|---|---|
| Parotid enlargement, Dupuytren's contracture | Alcohol |
| Tattoo marks, jaundice | Hepatitis B/C |
| Metabolic syndrome | NASH |
| Xanthoma, xanthelasma, obstructive jaundice | Primary biliary cirrhosis |
| Skin hyperpigmentation, organomegaly, diabetes | Hemochromatosis |
| Emphysema and cirrhosis | Alpha-1 antitrypsin deficiency |
| Long-standing heart failure | Cardiac cirrhosis |
| Tender liver with absent abdominojugular reflux | Budd–Chiari syndrome |
| Arthritis, skin changes, nephritis | Autoimmune |
| Deforming arthritis on treatment | Methotrexate induced |
| Kayser–Fleischer (KF) ring on cornea | Wilson's disease |

**Q. What is hepatorenal syndrome?**

Hepatorenal syndrome is a severe life-threatening complication occurring in cirrhotic patients with ascites, and it is characterized by the development of renal failure in the absence of any identifiable renal pathology. It is a functional disturbance in the renal function rather than a structural defect.

**Q. What are the diagnostic criteria for hepatorenal syndrome?**

Refer **Box 3.2**.

**Box 3.2:** Diagnostic criteria for hepatorenal syndrome (HRS).

**All of the following must be present for the diagnosis of HRS:**
- Cirrhosis with ascites
- Serum creatinine >1.5 mg/dL
- No improvement of serum creatinine (decrease to a level of 1.5 mg/dL or less) after at least 2 days of diuretic withdrawal and volume expansion with albumin
- Absence of shock
- No current or recent treatment with nephrotoxic drugs
- Absence of parenchymal kidney disease as indicated by proteinuria >500 mg/day, microhematuria (>50 red blood cells per high power field), and/or abnormal renal ultrasonography

**Q. What are the types of HRS?**

Refer **Table 3.14**.

**Table 3.14:** Types of hepatorenal syndromes (HRS).

| Acute kidney injury (AKI) type of HRS (HRS-AKI) Type 1 hepatorenal syndrome | Non-AKI type of HRS (HRS-NAKI) Type 2 hepatorenal syndrome |
|---|---|
| • It is characterized by progressive oliguria, a rapid rise of the serum creatinine to above 2.5 mg/dL and has a very poor prognosis<br>• Usually precipitated by spontaneous bacterial peritonitis<br>• Without treatment, median survival is less than 1 month and almost all patients die within 10 weeks after the onset of renal failure | • It is characterized by a reduction in glomerular filtration, moderate and stable increase in serum creatinine (>1.5 mg/dL), but it is fairly stable and has a better prognosis than type 1 HRS<br>• Usually occurs in patients with refractory ascites (resistant to diuretics)<br>• Median survival is 3–6 months |

**Q. What are the precipitating factors of hepatorenal syndrome?**

Refer **Box 3.3**.

**Box 3.3:** Precipitating factors for hepatorenal syndrome.

- Gastrointestinal bleeding
- Aggressive paracentesis
- Diuretic therapy
- Sepsis including spontaneous bacterial peritonitis
- Diarrhea

**Q. What are the types of hepatic encephalopathy?**

Refer **Figure 3.31**.

**Q. What are the sites of portosystemic anastomosis?**

**Figure 3.32** shows sites of portosystemic anastomosis in cirrhosis.

**Q. How do you classify portal hypertension?**

**Figure 3.33** shows the classification of portal hypertension according to site of vascular obstruction.

**Q. What are the causes of hepatosplenomegaly/splenomegaly with ascites?**

- Cirrhosis of liver with portal hypertension
- Lymphomas
- Systemic lupus erythematosus
- Disseminated tuberculosis
- Acute leukemias

**Q. What is metabolic dysfunction-associated fatty liver disease?**

Metabolic dysfunction-associated fatty liver disease (MAFLD) is a novel concept proposed in 2020 aiming to replace the term NAFLD (nonalcoholic fatty liver disease). Unlike NAFLD,

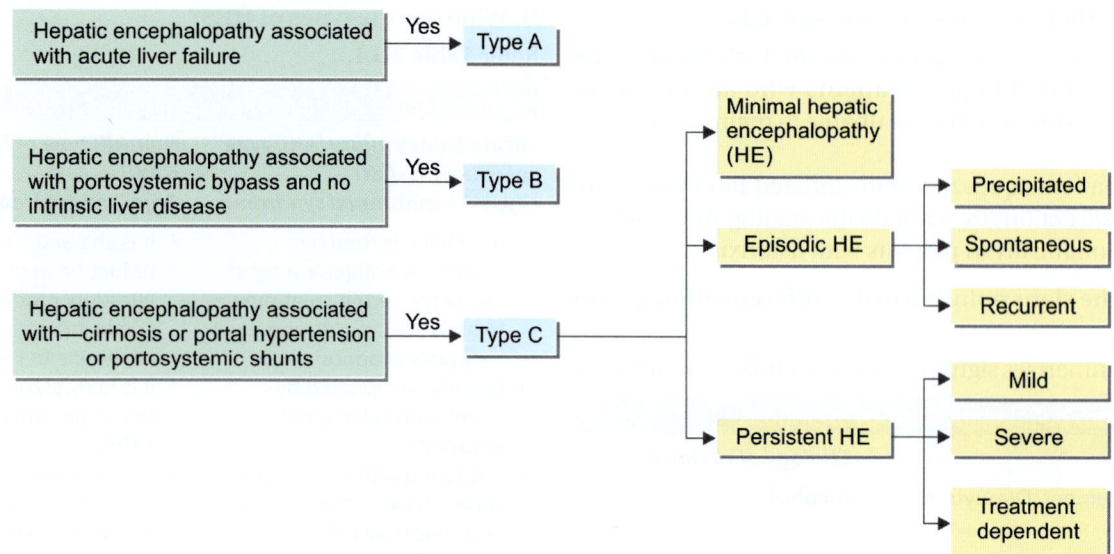

Fig. 3.31: Types of hepatic encephalopathy.

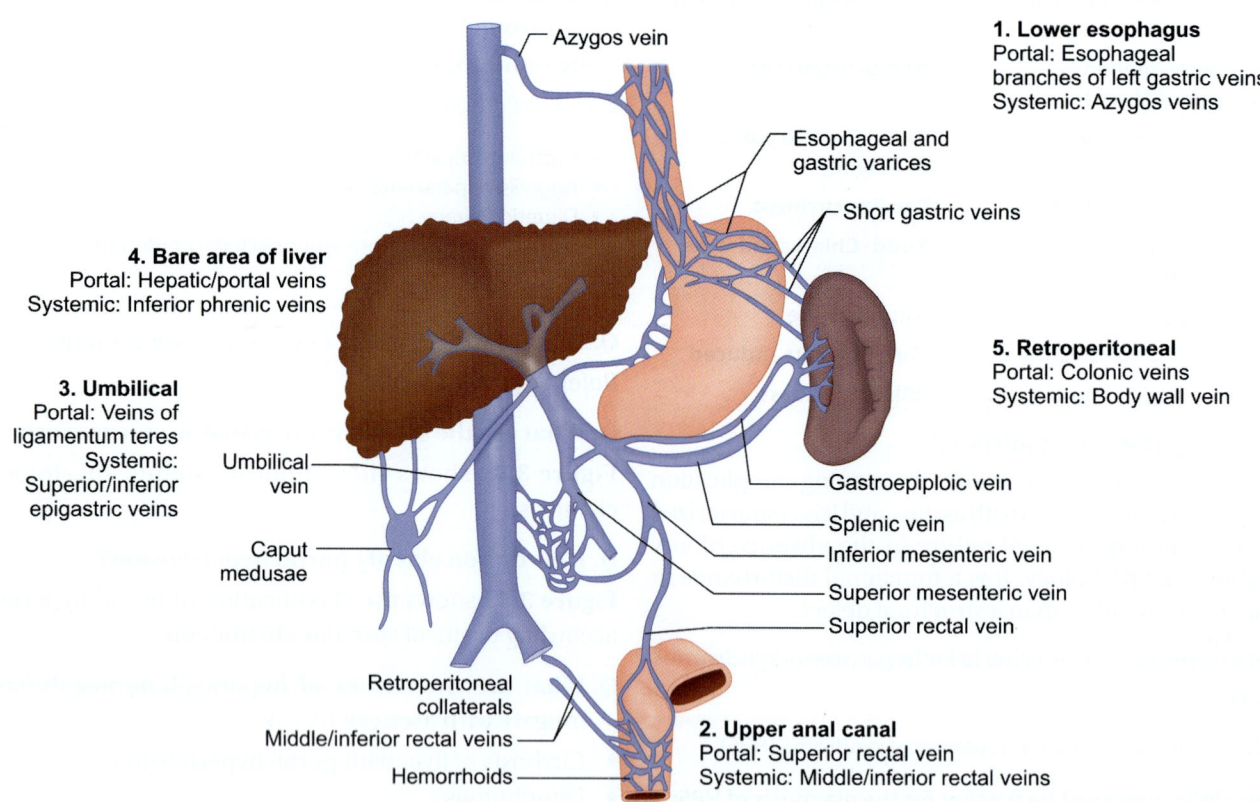

Fig. 3.32: Sites of portosystemic anastomosis in cirrhosis.

MAFLD does not require the exclusion of other etiologies of liver disease, such as excessive alcohol consumption or viral hepatitis **(Fig. 3.34)**.

MAFLD is diagnosed in patients when they have both hepatic steatosis and any of the following three metabolic conditions: overweight/obesity, diabetes mellitus, or evidence of metabolic dysregulation (MD) in lean individuals.

According to MAFLD definition, MD in this study was defined as the presence of at least two of the following criteria:

- Waist circumference ≥102 cm in men and 88 cm in women.
- Prediabetes [glycated hemoglobin (HbA1c) of 5.7–6.4%, or fasting plasma glucose (FPG) of 5.6–6.9 mmol/L, or 2-hour post-load glucose levels of 7.8–11.0 mmol/L].

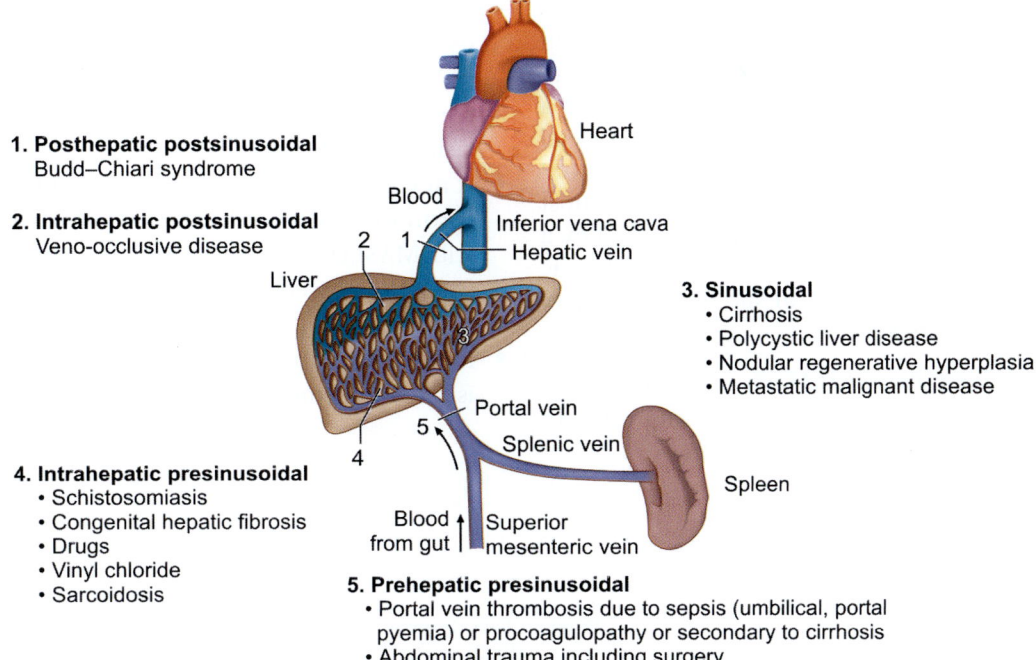

**Fig. 3.33:** Classification of portal hypertension according to site of vascular obstruction.

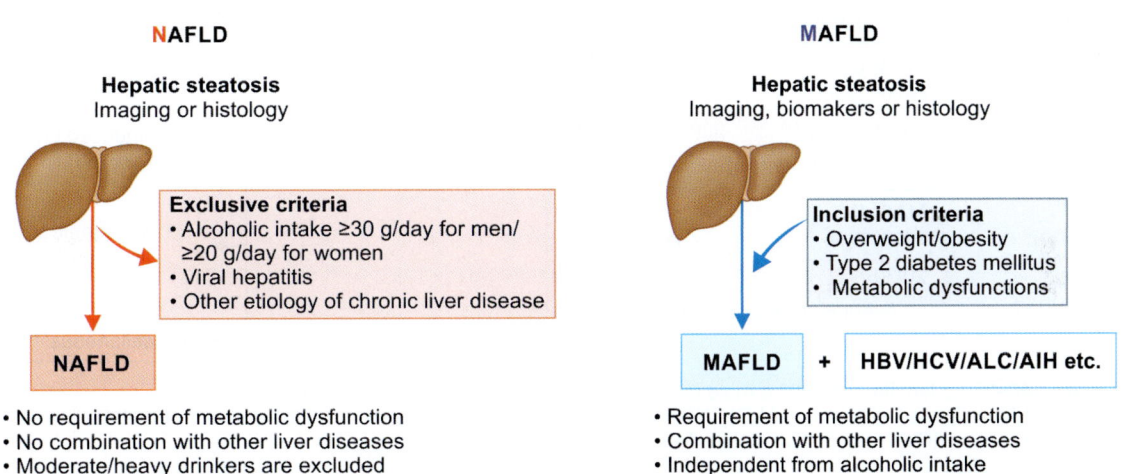

**Fig. 3.34:** Nonalcoholic fatty liver disease (NAFLD) versus metabolic (dysfunction)-associated fatty liver disease (MAFLD).

- Blood pressure ≥130/85 mm Hg or under antihypertension therapy.
- High-density lipoprotein cholesterol (HDLC) <1.0 mmol/L for males and <1.3 mmol/L for females.
- Triglyceride (TG) ≥1.70 mmol/L or specific drug treatment.
- Homeostasis model assessment-insulin resistance (HOMA-IR) score ≥2.5
- Hypersensitive C-reactive protein (hs-CRP) level >2 mg/L. MAFLD must be evaluated as a multisystemic disease affecting many extrahepatic organs.

The disease burden extends beyond liver-related complications, underlining the importance of multidisciplinary screening and disease management.

Moreover, patients with MAFLD should also be examined for CVD and cardiovascular risk. Further, treatment of dyslipidemia, T2DM, and hypertension is recommended to decrease the risk of cardiovascular and kidney diseases.

Importantly, the high rate of co-existing CVD, CKD, OSA, hypothyroidism, osteoporosis, and PCOS indicates that MAFLD patients should be evaluated for these extrahepatic diseases.

**Q. What is sinistral, or left-sided, portal hypertension?**

Sinistral portal hypertension (SPH) is also known as splenoportal, left-sided, segmental, regional, localized, compartmental or lineal portal hypertension.

It is a rare entity, accounting for less than 5% of all patients with portal hypertension, and results from splenic vein thrombosis or occlusion, with patent extrahepatic portal vein.

In fact, the name sinistral portal hypertension is a misnomer since portal pressure is usually within the normal range in these cases.

It is characterized by localized portal hypertension, most commonly due to obstruction of the splenic vein (SV) by a pancreatic pathology (acute or chronic pancreatitis, pancreatic pseudocysts, and malignancies) and/or subsequent surgery resulting in venous hypertension.

**Q. What is steatotic liver disease (SLD)?**

- Steatotic liver disease (SLD) is overarching term to encompass the various etiologies of steatosis.
- Non-alcoholic fatty liver disease (NAFLD) is metabolic dysfunction-associated steatotic liver disease (MASLD). MASLD encompasses patients who have hepatic steatosis and have at least one of five cardiometabolic risk factors.
- A new category, outside pure MASLD, termed MetALD (pronunciation: Met A-L-D) is used to describe those with MASLD who consume greater amounts of alcohol per week (140 g/week and 210 g/week for females and males respectively).
- Metabolic dysfunction-associated steatohepatitis (MASH) is the replacement term for NASH.

## Steatotic Liver Disease Sub-classification

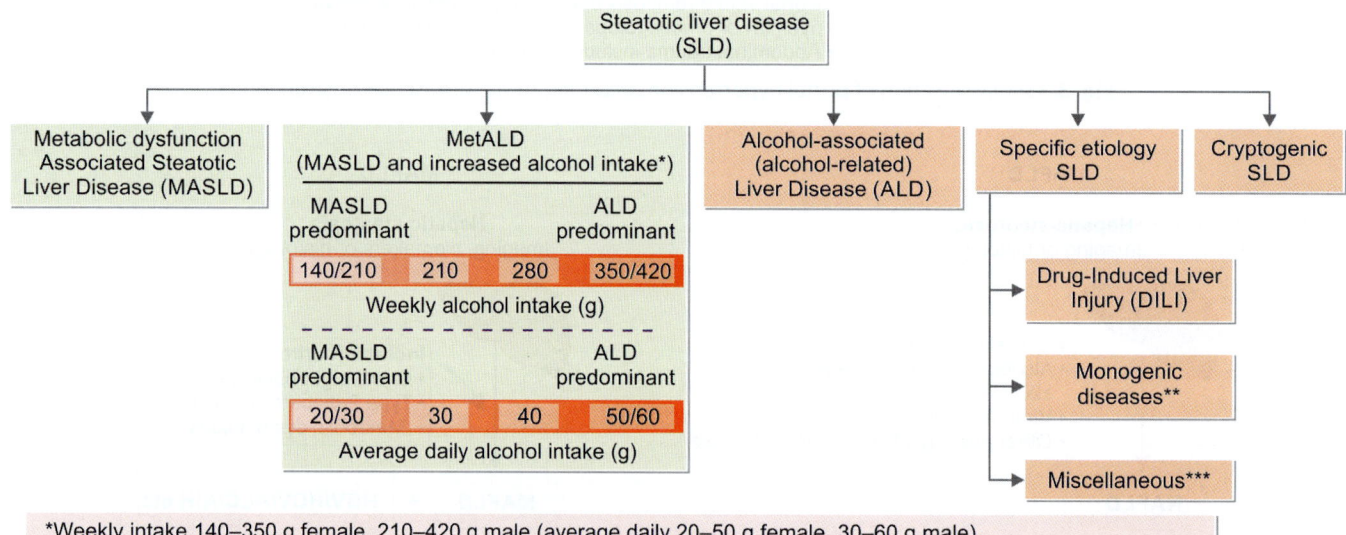

*Weekly intake 140–350 g female, 210–420 g male (average daily 20–50 g female, 30–60 g male)
**e.g., Lysosomal Acid Lipase Deficiency (LALD), Wilson disease, hypobetalipoproteinemia, inborn errors of metabolism
***e.g., Hepatitis C virus (HCV), malnutrition, celiac disease

## MASLD Diagnostic Criteria

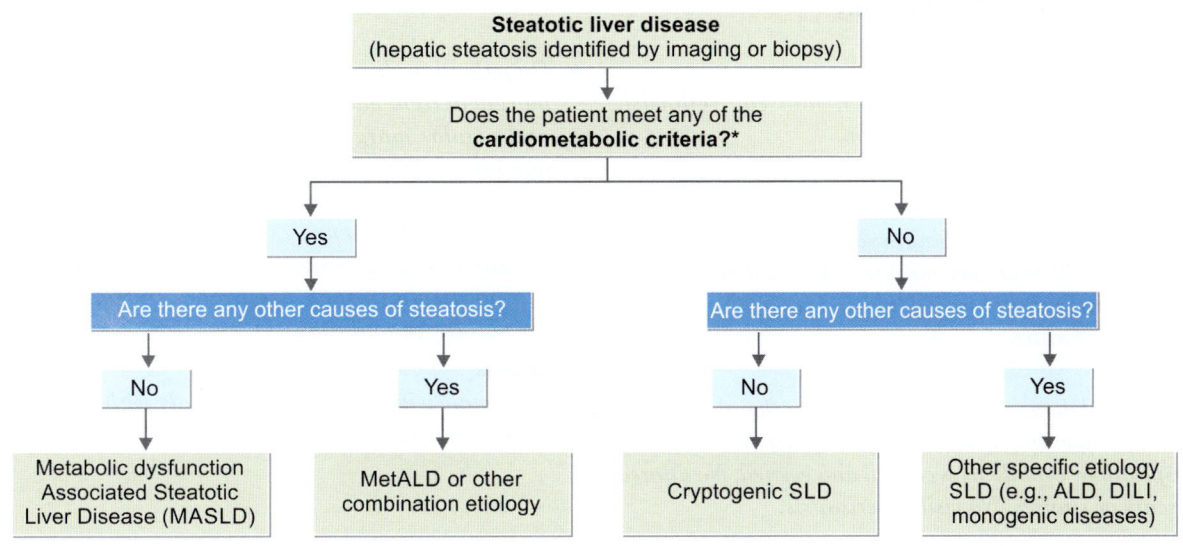

---

### *Cardiometabolic criteria

| Adult criteria | Pediatric criteria |
|---|---|
| **At least 1 out of 5:** | **At least 1 out of 5:** |
| ☐ BMI ≥25 kg/m² [23 Asia] **OR** WC >94 cm (M) 80 cm (F) **OR** ethnicity adjusted | ☐ BMI ≥85th percentile for age/sex (BMI z score ≥ +1) **OR** WC >95th percentile **OR** ethnicity adjusted |
| ☐ Fasting serum glucose ≥5.6 mmol/L [100 mg/dL] **OR** 2-hour post-load glucose levels ≥7.8 mmol/L [≥140 mg/dL] **OR** HbA1c ≥5.7% [39 mmol/L] **OR** type 2 diabetes **OR** treatment for type 2 diabetes | ☐ Fasting serum glucose ≥5.6 mmol/L [≥100 mg/dL] **OR** serum glucose ≥11.1 mmol/L [≥200 mg/dL] **OR** 2-hour post-load glucose levels ≥7.8 mmol [140 mg/dL] **OR** HbA1c ≥5.7% [39 mmol/L] **OR** already diagnosed/treated type 2 diabetes **OR** treatment for type 2 diabetes |
| ☐ Blood pressure ≥130/85 mm Hg **OR** specific antihypertensive drug treatment | ☐ Blood pressure age <13 years, BP ≥95th percentile **OR** ≥130/80 mm Hg (whichever is lower age ≥13years, 130/85 mm Hg **OR** specific antihypertensive drug treatment |
| ☐ Plasma triglycerides ≥1.70 mmol/L [150 mg/dL] **OR** lipid lowering treatment | ☐ Plasma triglycerides <10 years, ≥1.15 mmol/L [≥100 mg/dL]; age ≥10years, ≥1.70 mmol/L [≥150 mg/dL] **OR** lipid lowering treatment |
| ☐ Plasma HDL-cholesterol ≤1.0 mmol/L [40 mg/dL] (M) and ≥1.3 mmol/L [50 mg/dL] (F) **OR** lipid lowering treatment | ☐ Plasma HDL-cholesterol ≤1.0 mmol/L [≤40 mg/dL] **OR** lipid lowering treatment |

## Case 2: Hepatomegaly

*Brief History*
A young female with history of fever, nausea, yellowish discoloration of urine of 7 days duration.

*Examination*
- Patient is well-built and nourished with BMI of 21.0
- Has icterus. No Pallor, clubbing, cyanosis, pedal edema.
- Pulse rate of 120 beats per minute, RR of 20 breaths per minute and temperature of 101°F, BP 110/70. No signs of hepatocellular failure.

*Per Abdomen*
- Shape of the abdomen is normal, skin over the abdomen is normal, corresponding quadrants of abdomen move equally with respiration. Umbilicus is central and everted. No dilated veins, scars or sinuses. No visible peristalsis.
- On palpation, liver is enlarged 6 cm below the right costal margin at right midclavicular line, soft, tender with rounded and regular margin. It has a smooth surface and there is absence of pulsation rub or bruit. Spleen not palpable.
- No evidence of free fluid in the abdomen Tympanic note heard all over the abdomen.
- On auscultation, normal bowel sounds heard.
- Cardiovascular system, respiratory system, nervous system are within Normal limits.

*Diagnosis*
Young female with tender hepatomegaly with jaundice possible secondary to acute viral hepatitis.

## DISCUSSION

**Q. How do you asses liver span?**
Refer **Table 3.15**.

**Table 3.15:** Conditions associated by liver span.

| Liver span | Condition seen |
| --- | --- |
| Increased | Hepatomegaly |
| Decreased | Shrunken liver as in cirrhosis |

The liver span is the distance in centimeters between the upper border of the liver in the right midclavicular line, as determined by percussion (i.e., where lung resonance changes to liver dullness), and the lower border, as determined by either percussion or palpation.
- The upper border of the liver is assessed using a heavy percussion technique. Light percussion is used to locate the lower edge of the liver. Light percussion is required because heavy percussion may underestimate the lower extent of the liver border.
- The normal liver span is less than 13 cm.
- In midclavicular line: Normally 6–12 cm.
- In midsternal line (left lobe): Normally 4–8 cm.
- The clinical estimate of the liver span is usually an underestimation of the actual liver size by about 2–5 cm.
- There are several problems with predicting liver size by percussion.
- If ascites is present, the examiner can only speculate about the correct size of the liver.

A more common cause of overestimating liver size (false-positive measurement) is some form of chronic obstructive lung disease. This makes percussion of the upper border of the liver difficult.

## Description of Liver

Obesity in a patient can cause problems in both percussion and palpation. Distention of the colon may obscure the lower liver dullness. This may result in underestimating the size of the liver (false-negative measurement).

If the liver is enlarged and palpable, assess the following:
- **Location of the edge in cm below the costal margin in the midclavicular or anterior axillary line.**
- **Span (in cm)**
- **Tenderness** (tender/nontender)

**Q. What are the conditions in which liver is palpable but not enlarged?**
Refer **Table 3.16**.

**Table 3.16:** Conditions liver is palpable but not enlarged.

| False positive for enlarged liver | • Right sided pleural effusion<br>• Right lower lobe consolidation |
| --- | --- |

*Note:* In conditions like emphysema of the lung, the liver may be pushed down. The edge may be palpable, leading the examiner to believe that the patient has hepatomegaly when the real problem is a hyperinflated lung. Percussion will reveal that the upper border is lower than expected.

**Q. What are the causes of hepatomegaly?**
Refer **Figure 3.35**.

**Q. What are the causes of tender hepatomegaly and painless hepatomegaly?**
Refer **Table 3.17**.
- **Margins** (regular, irregular, rounded or sharp). In cancers the liver edge may be irregular **(Table 3.18)**.
- **Surface** (smooth, nodular) **(Table 3.19)**.

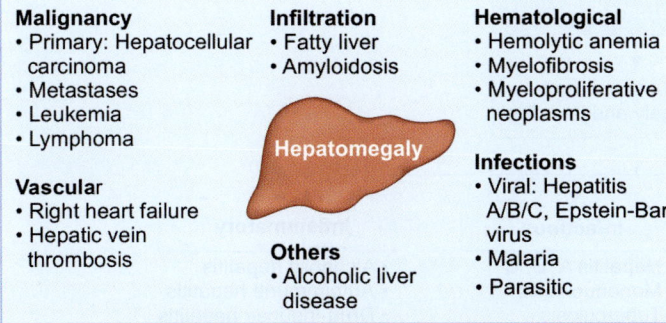

**Fig. 3.35:** Causes of hepatomegaly.

**Table 3.17:** Causes of tender hepatomegaly and painless hepatomegaly.

| Tender hepatomegaly | Painless hepatomegaly |
|---|---|
| ◆ Right heart failure<br>◆ Acute hepatitis (viral/alcoholic/drug induced)<br>◆ Liver abscess (amoebic/pyogenic)<br>◆ Hepatoma<br>◆ Infarcts<br>◆ Actinomycosis<br>◆ Acute Budd–Chiari syndrome | ◆ Fatty liver<br>◆ Infiltrative and storage disorders<br>◆ Malaria<br>◆ Leukemia<br>◆ Lymphoma |

**Table 3.18:** Margins of liver.

| Rounded | Infiltrative disorders |
|---|---|
| Sharp | Secondary metastases, acute hepatitis<br>Biliary obstruction<br>Chronic hepatitis |

**Table 3.19:** Surfaces of liver.

| Smooth | Malaria<br>Acute hepatitis<br>Infiltrative disorders, etc. |
|---|---|
| Nodular | Metastatic cancers<br>Hepatoma<br>Alcoholic cirrhosis (micronodular)<br>Posthepatic cirrhosis (macronodular) |

◆ **Consistency** (soft/firm/hard): In metastatic cancers and in obstructive jaundice, the liver is typically firm to hard.

### Q. What are the causes for pulsatile liver?

**Pulsatility** (pulsatile/not pulsatile): A pulsatile liver may be present in tricuspid regurgitation (systolic), tricuspid stenosis (diastolic), hepatocellular carcinoma, and hemangiomas.

### Q. What are the causes of false-positive measurement of liver?

Causes of hepatomegaly can be grossly grouped under the headings of infections, malignancies, infiltrative disorders, hematological disorders, and vascular disorders as shown in **Figure 3.35**. Massive hepatomegaly (>10 cm) seen with hepatoma.

### Caudate lobe (Fig. 3.36)

◆ Arises from the right lobe of the liver, on the posterosuperior surface
◆ Hypertrophy of caudate lobe is characteristic of hepatic outflow obstruction (Budd–Chiari syndrome).

### Riedel's lobe (Fig. 3.37)

◆ Congenital variant projecting from the right lobe of the liver
◆ May be mistaken for gallbladder or right kidney.

### Q. What are the types of hepatomegaly?

Types of hepatomegaly is shown in **Figure 3.38**.

### Q. What conditions a nonenlarged liver can be felt?

Normal liver can be felt, it is usually due to:
◆ Increased diaphragmatic descent
◆ Presence of a palpable caudate or Riedel's lobe
◆ Thin body habitus with a narrow thoracic cage

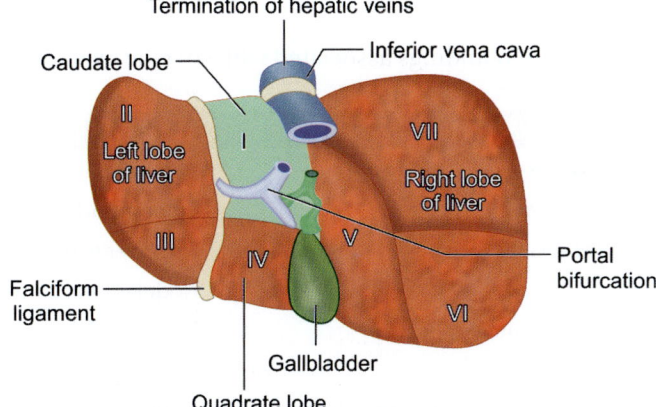

**Fig. 3.36:** Caudate lobe location and boundaries.

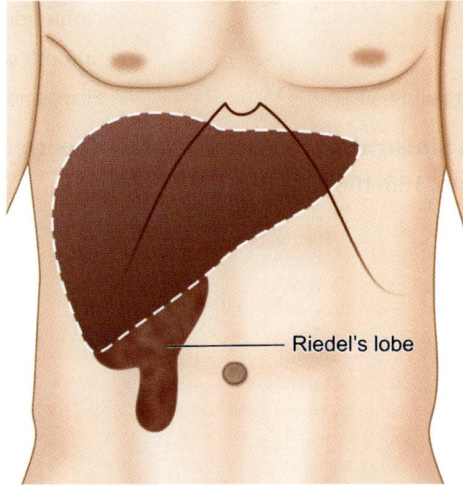

**Fig. 3.37:** Anomalous lobe of the liver projecting from right lobe.

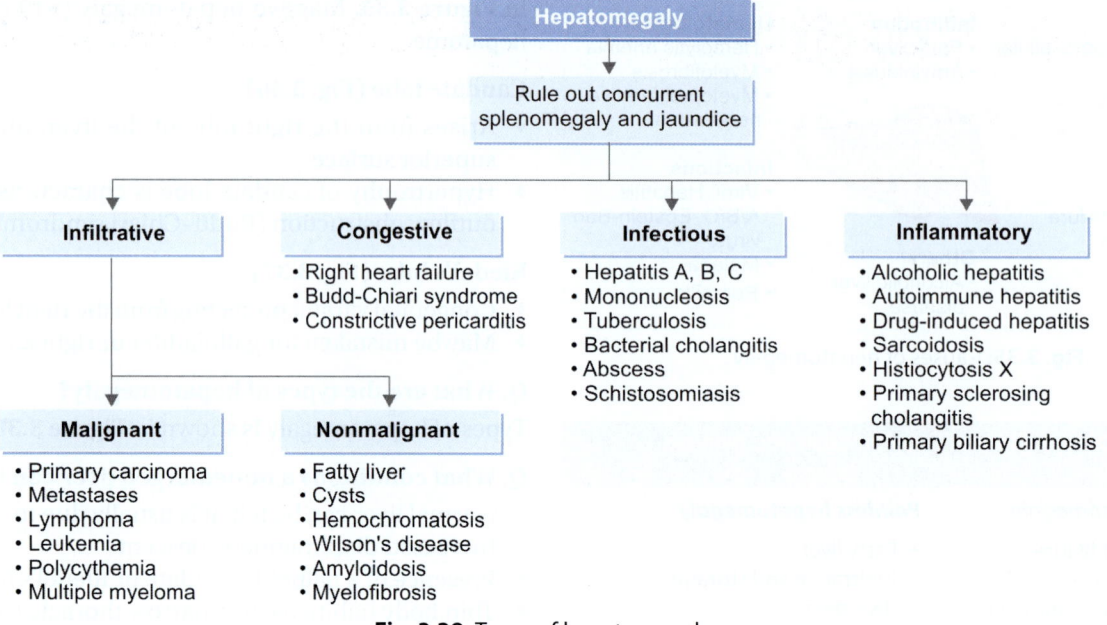

Fig. 3.38: Types of hepatomegaly.

- Presence of emphysema with an associated depressed diaphragm
- Visceroptosis.

Examination findings associated with specific liver diseases are discussed in **Table 3.20**.

| Table 3.20: Examination findings associated with specific liver diseases. | | |
|---|---|---|
| **Liver disease** | **Palpation** | **Size** |
| Acute hepatitis | Smooth surface tender | Enlarged |
| Chronic hepatitis | Firm liver edge | Enlarged, especially left lobe |
| | Nodules rare; tender | |
| Fulminant hepatitis | Tender surface | Shrinking size |
| Cirrhosis | Nontender, firm | Variable; late stages, liver decreases in size |
| Hepatocellular carcinoma (hepatoma) | Nodules, if present, large and hard | Moderate to massive enlargement |
| | Nontender | |
| Metastatic carcinoma | Large nodules | Enlarged |
| | Nontender | |
| Fatty liver | Smooth surface | Enlarged |
| Right heart failure | Firm, smooth, tender | Mild to massive enlargement |

**Q. What is Sinistral, or left-sided, portal hypertension?**

(*See* page no. 165-166)

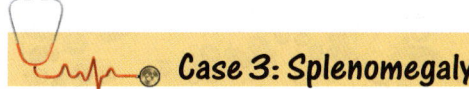

## Case 3: Splenomegaly

*Brief History*
A 45-year-old male with history of fatigue, early satiety and abdominal fullness of 4 months duration.

*General Physical Examination*
- Vitals: Pulse rate: 76/min, regular normal volume, character
- All peripheral pulses well felt
- Blood pressure: 130/80 mm Hg
- Respiratory rate: 20/min
- Afebrile
- Pallor+, no icterus/lymphadenopathy/ clubbing, minimal bilateral pitting pedal edema is present; no JVP or abdominojugular reflux
- Oral cavity: Coated tongue+
- Hands: Platynychia+ in both hands, Bouchard's nodes present in the proximal interphalangeal (PIP) joints
- Ecchymosis 2 × 2 cm present in the left cubital fossa
- No bony tenderness, no bleeding tendencies

*Per-abdominal Examination Inspection*
- All quadrants move equally with respiration
- No visible veins or scars
- Umbilicus inverted
- Hernial orifices intact palpation
- No superficial tenderness or rigidity/guarding.

*Deep Palpation*
Massive splenomegaly present 9 cm below the left costal margin in the splenoumbilical line, smooth surface, firm consistency, sharp margins, no palpable rub, or notch
- No other organomegaly
- No palpable mass per abdomen percussion
- No shifting dullness, no fluid thrill
- Liver span 15 cm in right midclavicular line auscultation
- Bowel sounds + 3–4/min; no bruit or venous hum
- No signs of liver cell failure
- No signs of hepatic encephalopathy

*Diagnosis*
Features of anemia with massive splenomegaly, possibilities:
- Chronic myeloid leukemia
- Chronic malaria
- Myelofibrosis

## DISCUSSION

**Q. How will you differentiate prehepatic, hepatic, posthepatic causes of portal hypertension?**
- Differentiate prehepatic, hepatic and posthepatic
- Causes of portal hypertension.

### Prehepatic causes
- Children may have growth retardation
- Bleeding from esophagogastric varices is the most common presentation.
- In those of neonatal origin, the first hemorrhage is at about the age of 4 years. The frequency increases between 10 and 15 years and decreases after puberty.
- Apart from frank bleeds, intermittent minor blood loss is probably common. This is diagnosed only if the patient is having repeated checks for fecal blood or iron deficiency anemia.
- **The spleen is always enlarged, and symptomless splenomegaly may be a presentation, particularly in children**.
- **Periumbilical veins are not seen but there may be dilated abdominal wall veins in the left flank.**
- **The liver is normal in size and consistency.**
- **Stigmata of hepatocellular disease, such as jaundice or vascular spiders, are absent.**
- With acute portal venous thrombosis, ascites is early and transient, subsiding as the collateral circulation develops.

### Hepatic causes
- The stigmata of cirrhosis include jaundice, vascular spiders and palmar erythema. Anemia, ascites and precoma may be present.
- In intrahepatic portal hypertension, some blood from the left branch of the portal vein may be deviated via paraumbilical veins to the umbilicus, whence it reaches veins of the caval system.
- Liver consistency, tenderness or nodularity should be recorded. A soft liver suggests extrahepatic portal venous obstruction. A firm liver supports cirrhosis.

### Posthepatic causes
- In the most acute form the picture is of an ill patient, often presenting with abdominal pain, vomiting, liver enlargement, ascites and mild icterus.
- If the hepatic venous occlusion is total, delirium and coma with hepatocellular failure and death occurs within a few days.
- In the more usual chronic form the patient presents with pain over an enlarged tender liver and ascites, developing over 1–6 months.
- Jaundice is mild or absent, unless zone 3 necrosis is marked.
- **Pressure over the liver may fail to fill the jugular vein (negative *abdominojugular reflux*).**
- **As portal hypertension increases, the spleen becomes palpable.**

- If the inferior vena cava is blocked, edema of the legs is gross and veins distend over the abdomen, flanks and back.

### Q. What are the peripheral smear findings you expect in CML?

Refer **Figure 3.39**.

In chronic phase, there is a marked granulocytic leukocytosis (generally >50 × 10⁹/L, range 20 to 500) dominated by the **entire spectrum of granulocytes** including rare myeloblasts and **an invariable basophilia**. Usually, <5% circulating blasts and <10% blasts and promyelocytes are noted, with the majority of cells being myelocytes, metamyelocytes, and band forms. There is a predominance of mature neutrophils but also an **increased percentage of myelocytes** (so-called myelocyte bulge). **Myeloblasts do not usually exceed 3% of the total WBC**. Many patients may also demonstrate **eosinophilia**. No significant dysgranulopoiesis is observed, although this may be seen later in the course of the disease. There may be an **absolute increase in the number of monocytes**, although they generally comprise <3% of total nucleated cells. **Platelets tend to be normal or increased in number** and occasionally may exceed 1 million/μL. There may **be mild anemia**.

Peripheral blood shows a characteristic leukoerythroblastic picture (immature granulocyte and erythrocyte precursors) with poikilocytosis, especially teardrop cells, nRBCs and elliptocytes. Platelets have a dysplastic morphology (giant, agranular). In the fibrotic stage, we will get pancytopenia **(Fig. 3.40)**.

### Q. What is the natural course of iron deficiency anemia?

When it is not a result of major blood loss, iron deficiency is the end result of a long period of negative iron balance. As the total body iron level begins to fall, a characteristic sequence of events ensues. **First, the iron stores in the hepatocytes and the macrophages of the liver, spleen, and bone marrow are depleted**.

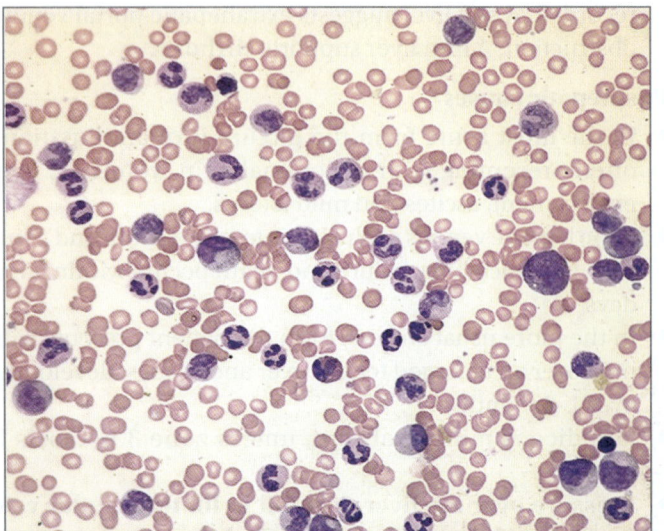

**Fig. 3.39:** Peripheral blood smear shows a marked leukocytosis with left-shift and basophilia.

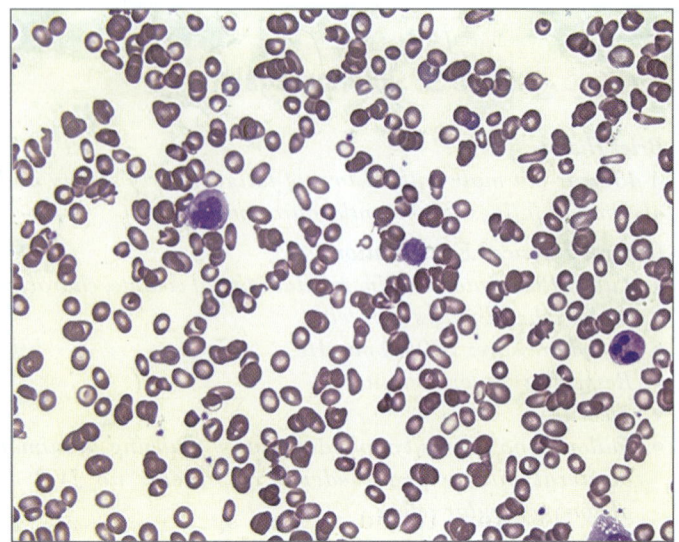

**Fig. 3.40:** Peripheral smear showing myelofibrosis.

Once stores are gone, **plasma iron content decreases**, and the **supply of iron to marrow becomes inadequate for normal hemoglobin production**. Consequently, the amount of free erythrocyte protoporphyrin increases, production of microcytic erythrocytes begins, and the blood hemoglobin level decreases, eventually reaching abnormal levels.

### Q. What are the stages of iron deficiency?

**This progression corresponds to three recognized stages:**

**Stage 1: Depletion of iron stores**—the first stage, also called prelatent iron deficiency or iron depletion, represents a **reduction in iron stores without reduced serum iron levels**. This stage is usually detected by a low serum ferritin measurement. Latent iron deficiency is said to exist when iron stores are exhausted, but the blood hemoglobin level remains higher than the lower limit of normal.

**Stage 2: Iron deficiency without anemia**—in this second stage, certain biochemical abnormalities of iron-limited erythropoiesis may be detected, including reduced transferrin saturation, increased TIBC, increased free erythrocyte protoporphyrin, increased zinc protoporphyrin, and increased serum TFRC. Other findings include subnormal urinary iron excretion after deferoxamine injection and decreased tissue cytochrome oxidase levels. **The mean corpuscular volume usually remains within normal limits, but a few microcytes may be detected on a blood smear**. Many patients report generalized fatigue or malaise, even though they are not yet anemic.

**Stage 3: Iron deficiency anemia**—finally, in the third stage, **the blood hemoglobin concentration falls below the lower limit of normal, and iron deficiency anemia is apparent**. Iron-containing enzymes, such as the cytochromes, also reach abnormally low levels during this period. **Epithelial manifestations of iron deficiency occur very late in iron deprivation**. This progression forms the basis for the stages of iron deficiency outlined in. It has been confirmed by experiments in which normal volunteers gradually were depleted of iron by phlebotomy.

**Q. What are the causes of platynychia?**
- Congenital
- Iron deficiency anemia.

**Q. Name the special stains used in the diagnosis of leukemias?**
- **Myeloperoxidase:** Primary granules of neutrophils and secondary granules of eosinophils contain myeloperoxidase.
- **Sudan black:** Positive staining of granulocytic cells and eosinophils, weak monocytic staining, and no staining of lymphocytes.
- **Toluidine blue:** Toluidine blue specifically marks basophils and mast cells by reacting with the acid mucopolysaccharides in the cell granules to form metachromatic complexes.
- **Periodic acid-Schiff (PAS):** This staining is seen in blasts of both acute lymphoblastic and acute myelogenous leukemias, although there is great variability between cases. Erythroleukemia demonstrate an intense diffuse cytoplasmic positivity with PAS, which may be helpful in diagnosis.
- **Acid phosphatase:** Acid phosphatase is found in all hematopoietic cells, but the highest levels are found in macrophages and osteoclasts. A localized dot like pattern is seen in many T lymphoblasts, but this staining pattern is not reliable. The tartrate-resistant acid phosphatase (TRAP) is an isoenzyme of acid phosphatase that is found in high levels in the cells of hairy cell leukemia and osteoclasts.
- **Leukocyte alkaline phosphatase:** Alkaline phosphatase activity is found in the cytoplasm of neutrophils, osteoblasts, vascular endothelial cells, and some lymphocytes. The alkaline phosphatase level of peripheral blood neutrophils is quantitated by the leukocyte alkaline phosphatase (LAP) score and is useful as a screening test to differentiate chronic myelogenous leukemia from leukemoid reactions and other myeloproliferative disorders.

**Q. How will you grade splenomegaly?**

**Figure 3.41** shows Hackett's grading system.

**Q. How will you grade splenomegaly based on the distance from the costal margin?**

Refer **Table 3.21**.

| Table 3.21: Based on distance from costal margin. | | |
|---|---|---|
| *Mild (tip) enlargement* | *Moderate enlargement* | *Severe (massive) enlargement* |
| **1-2 cm** (<3 cm) | **3–7 cm** (3–8 cm) between costal margin and umbilicus | **7+ cm** (>8 cm/>1,000 g) Beyond umbilicus crossing midline |

**Note:** Size of the spleen is measured from the left costal margin to the tip along the long axis of spleen.

**Q. What are the methods of examination of spleen?**
- **Inspection**
- **Palpation:**
  1. Classical method
  2. Bimanual method
     – In supine position
     – In right lateral position
  3. Hooking method
     – In supine position
     – In right lateral position
  4. Dipping method
- **Percussion**
  - Castell's method
  - Traube's space percussion
  - Nixon's method of percussion

**Q. What are the causes of splenomegaly?**

Refer **Table 3.22**.

**Q. What are the structures present in splenic hilum?**
- Gastrosplenic ligament-carrying the short gastric and left gastroepiploic vessels
- Splenicorenal ligament-carrying the splenic vessels and the tail of the pancreas.

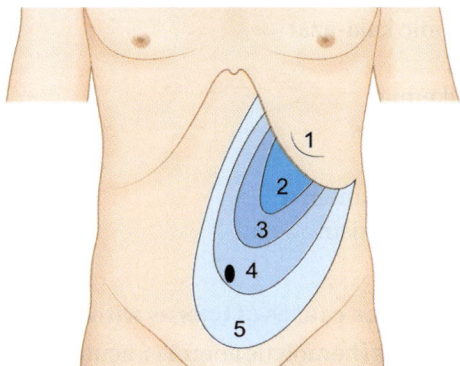

| Grade 0 | Normal impalpable spleen |
|---|---|
| Grade 1 | Spleen palpable only in deep inspiration |
| Grade 2 | Spleen palpable on midclavicular line half way between umbilicus and costal margin |
| Grade 3 | Spleen expands towards the umbilicus |
| Grade 4 | Spleen goes past the umbilicus |
| Grade 5 | Spleen expands towards public sumphysis |

**Fig. 3.41:** Hackett's grading of splenomegaly.

| Table 3.22: Causes of splenomegaly. | |
|---|---|
| **Mild splenomegaly** | |
| Acute infections | Infective endocarditis, enteric fever, infectious hepatitis, infectious mononucleosis, brucellosis, cytomegalovirus, toxoplasmosis |
| Chronic infections | Tuberculosis, syphilis, brucellosis, HIV |
| Parasitic infestations | Malaria, kala-azar, schistosomiasis |
| Inflammation | Rheumatoid arthritis, sarcoidosis, SLE |
| Others | Congestive cardiac failure, thalassemia minor |
| **Moderate splenomegaly** | |
| Neoplastic | Lymphomas, acute leukemias, CML, CLL |
| Non-neoplastic | Cirrhosis of liver (with portal hypertension), chronic hemolytic anemia, malaria, kala-azar, sarcoidosis, infectious mononucleosis, splenic abscess, amyloidosis, hemochromatosis, polycythemia vera |
| **Severe (massive) splenomegaly** | |
| Common causes | ✦ Chronic myeloid leukemia (Fig. 3.42)<br>✦ Myelofibrosis<br>✦ Kala-azar,<br>✦ Hairy cell leukemia<br>✦ Tropical malarial splenomegaly/hyperreactive Malarial splenomegaly,<br>✦ Portal hypertension (extrahepatic portal vein thrombosis),<br>✦ Thalassemia major |
| Uncommon causes | Lymphomas, Gaucher's disease, Niemann-Pick disease, splenic cysts, tumors of spleen, sarcoidosis, MAC infection in HIV |

### Q. What is the significance/importance of splenic notch?

The spleen develops as a thickening of the mesenchyme in the dorsal mesentery. In the earlier stages, the spleen consists of a number of mesenchymal masses that later fuse, but not completely. This is represented by the splenic notch which is present along *its anterior border.*

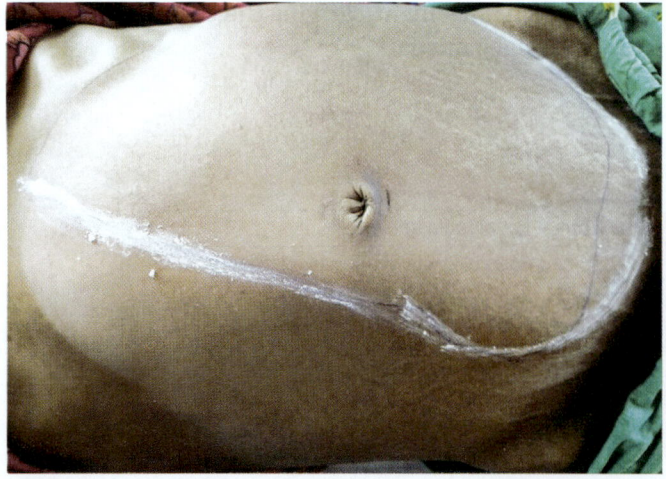

**Fig. 3.42:** Massive splenomegaly in chronic myeloid leukemia (CML).

### Q. What are the characteristics of a normal spleen?
Refer **Table 3.23**.

| Table 3.23: Characteristics of normal spleen. | |
|---|---|
| **Dimensions** | 12 cm length, 7 cm width<br>13 cm craniocaudal diameter |
| **Weight** | <250 g |
| **Location** | Along- 9th, 10th,11th ribs midaxillary line<br>Long axis along line of 10th rib. |
| **Extent** | **Anteriorly** (lower pole): Up to midaxillary line<br>**Posteriorly:** The superior angle of spleen is 4 cm lateral to D10 spine |
| **Margin** | There is a **notch** on the **inferolateral border**, and this may be palpated when the spleen is enlarged |

### Q. Clinically, how will you differentiate between spleen and left kidney?
Refer **Table 3.24**.

| Table 3.24: Differences between spleen and left kidney. | | |
|---|---|---|
| **Characteristics** | *Spleen* | *Left kidney* |
| Location | Left hypochondrium | Left lumbar |
| Direction of enlargement | Towards RIF | Towards left hypochondrium and LIF |
| Movement with respiration | + | – |
| Insinuation between left costal margin and organ | Not possible | Possible |
| Bimanual palpation | – | + |
| Ballotability | – | + |
| Crossing midline | Can cross midline | Never cross midline |
| Notch | + | – |
| Band of colonic resonance | – | + |

### Q. What are the causes of pallor with splenomegaly?
- Malaria
- Chronic kala-azar
- SBE
- Leukemia
- Lymphomas
- Cirrhosis
- Hemolytic anemia
- Hypersplenism
- CTDs

### Q. Name some causes of icterus with splenomegaly.
- Hemolysis (hemolytic anemias, acute malaria, lymphoma)
- Budd-Chiari syndrome (hepatic vein obstruction)
- Chronic liver disease

**Q. What differentials do you consider in a patient with fever and splenomegaly?**
- **Infections:** Malaria, kala-azar, enteric fever, SBE, miliary TB, acute viral hepatitis
- **Neoplasm:** Acute leukemias, CML, lymphoma
- Collagen vascular diseases

**Q. Name some conditions in which splenomegaly is associated with hemorrhagic spots?**
- Acute leukemia
- SBE
- SLE
- Acute leukemia
- Blast crisis of CML or CLL

**Q. Name the cause of splenomegaly with lymphadenopathy.**
- **Autoimmune disorders:** Felty's syndrome, SLE, sarcoidosis, AOSD
- **Infection:** Infectious mononucleosis, AIDS, toxoplasmosis, CMV, disseminated TB
- **Neoplasm:** Lymphomas and leukemias

**Q. Name some causes of tender spleen.**
- Splenic rupture
- SBE
- Infarct
- Abscess
- Tumors

**Q. What are other general examination findings in a patient with splenomegaly you should look for?**
- **Suffused conjunctiva:** Polycythemia vera
- **Clubbing:** SBE
- **Fundoscopy:** Roth spots (SBE), choroidal tubercle (miliary TB)
- **Pharyngitis:** EBV infection
- **Macroglossia, jugular vein distension or periorbital edema:** Amyloidosis

**Box 3.4:** Tropical splenomegaly syndrome or hyperactive malarial splenomegaly (HMS).

**Major diagnostic criteria:**
*Plasmodium falciparum*
- Gross splenomegaly in older children and adults
- High antibody levels for *Plasmodium falciparum*
- Elevated serum IgM (at least 2 standard deviations above the mean of the population)
- Clinical and immunological response to long-term appropriate therapy

**Minor diagnostic criteria**
- Hepatics sinusoidal lymphocytosis (80% of cases)
- Normal cellular and humoral immune responses to antigenic challenge, included PHA
- Hypersplenism
- Lymphocyte proliferation (in some populations)
- Occurrence within families, tribes

- **Mongoloid facies:** Thalassemia
- **Butterfly rash:** SLE
- **Janeway lesion:** SBE
- **New or changing murmurs:** SBE
- **Digital ischemia/gangrene or thrombosis:** Essential thrombocytosis
- **Joint deformities:** RA, Felty's syndrome, SLE
- **Lower extremity edema:** Amyloidosis

**Q. What is tropical splenomegaly syndrome?**

Tropical splenomegaly syndrome or hyperactive malarial splenomegaly (HMS) is elaborated in **Box 3.4**.

**Q. How do you treat HMS?**

Antimalarials clear the antigenic stimulus caused by repeated malarial infections and helps the immune system to return to normal. The selection of antimalarial depends upon the local sensitivity pattern. Chloroquine weekly or proguanil daily have been found to be effective. Pyrimethamine may be an alternative to the above medications.

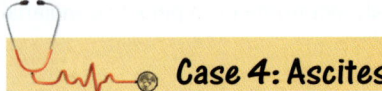

## Case 4: Ascites

*Brief History*
A 30-year-male, presents with complains of distension of abdomen—1 month duration.

*Examination*
Patient is moderately built, poor nourishment.
- Weight: 45.5 kg
- Height: 170 cm
- BMI: 15.7 kg/m$^2$
- Temporal fossa hollowing and loss of buccal pad of fat.
- Multiple hypopigmented macules (tinea versicolor) present over the trunk and back.
- BP: 120/80 mm of mercury in right arm supine position (no postural drop).
- PR: 108/min regular, normal volume, no specific character, all peripheral pulses well felt.
- Temperature: 98.6°F
- RR: 30/min predominantly thoracic.
- Pallor seen. Multiple inguinal lymph nodes maximum measuring 1 × 1 cm in size, nontender, no matting, mobile with normal overlying skin.
- Clubbing (grade II) seen in right index and ring finger.
- Bilateral pitting pedal edema seen up to shin of tibia.
- No icterus. No other signs of liver cell failure.

*Systemic Examination Gastrointestinal Tract*
Oral cavity
- Hyperpigmentation seen over the hard palate and the tongue.
- Poor oral hygiene.
- Per abdomen examination:
- Abdomen is distended, with dilated veins (not tortuous) seen over the epigastrium.
- Umbilicus is everted.
- Organs could not be palpated.
- Shifting dullness present, no fluid thrill.

*Diagnosis*
Ascites is disproportionate to pedal edema (ascites precox).

*Differential Diagnosis*
- Tuberculous ascites
- GI malignancy
- Constrictive pericarditis.
- Restrictive cardiomyopathy.

## DISCUSSION

**Q. What is the minimum amount of fluid required to elicit shifting dullness?**

More than 1,000 mL of fluid should be present to elicit shifting dullness.

**Q. What is the minimum amount of fluid required to elicit fluid thrill?**
- \>2,000 mL of fluid should be present to elicit fluid thrill
- Over 1,500 mL of fluid must collect in the peritoneal cavity before its presence can be detected by physical examination: because of the large size of the abdominal cavity and its many recesses.

**Q. What are the clinical signs of ascites?**
- Horseshoe dullness (**Fig. 3.43A**)
- Shifting dullness (**Fig. 3.43C**)
- Puddle sign (**Fig. 3.43E**)
- Fullness of flank (**Fig. 3.43B**)
- Fluid thrill/fluid wave (**Fig. 3.43D**)

**Q. What is Puddle sign?**

It can detect even ascites as low as 120 mL. Patient is asked to lie in prone position for 5 minutes, followed by knee elbow position. Place the diaphragm of the stethoscope on the most dependent part of the abdomen. Repeatedly flick one flank lightly. Diaphragm is gradually moved to the opposite flank. A marked change in the intensity and character of percussion note indicates the presence of fluid **(Fig. 3.43E)**

**Q. What are the grades of ascites?**
Refer **Table 3.25**.

| Table 3.25: Grading of ascites. | |
|---|---|
| **Severity** | |
| Grade 1 (mild) | Not clinically evident, diagnosed on ultrasound |
| Grade 2 (moderate) | Proportionate sensible abdominal distension |
| Grade 3 (severe) | Noticeable tense distension of abdomen |
| Uncomplicated | Not infected or associated with HRS |
| Refractory | Cannot be mobilized, early recurrence after LVP, not prevented satisfactorily with medical treatment (after 1 week) |
| Diuretic-resistant | No response to intensive diuretic treatment |
| Diuretic-intractable | Drug-induced adverse effects preclude diuretic treatment |

**Q. What are the theories/hypothesis of ascites?**

**"Volume deficiency" hypothesis**

According to this classic hypothesis, ascites is a result of increased hydrostatic pressure within the hepatic and splanchnic circulation, induced by portal hypertension.

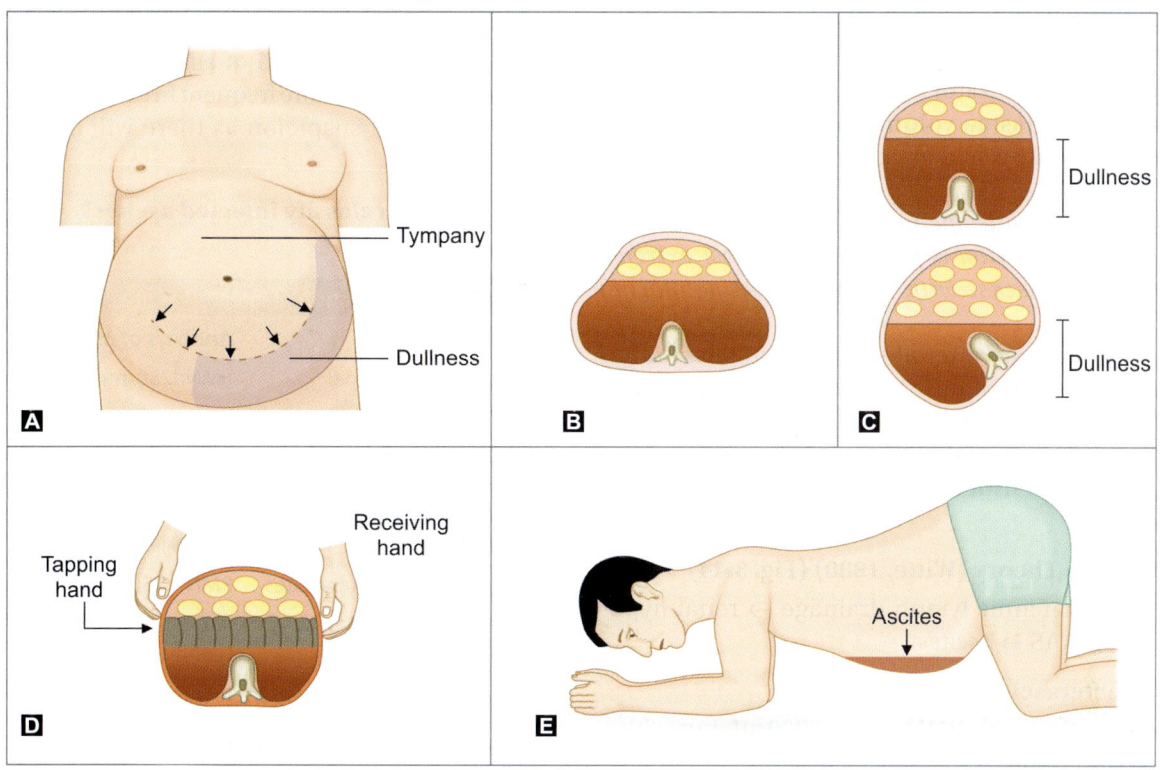

**Figs. 3.43A to E:** Clinical signs of ascites: (A) Horseshoe dullness; (B) Fullness (bulging) of flank; (C) Shifting dullness; (D) Fluid thrill/fluid wave; (E) Puddle sign.

Impairment of the Starling-balance leads to movement of fluids from intravascular compartment to the interstitial space.

The accumulation of fluid is compensated initially by an increased lymphatic outflow via thoracic duct into the systemic circulation. If, however, with increasing portal hypertension the lymphatic system is overburdened, fluid crosses into peritoneal cavity, and the intravascular volume decreases. The decrease in intravascular volume results in hypovolemia (secondary underfilling) which activates neurohormonal regulatory mechanisms resulting in compensatory renal sodium retention. Since the retained fluid continuously flows into the peritoneal cavity a vicious circle develops with ongoing stimulation of Na+ retaining mechanisms. However, this classic hypothesis is not able to explain the systemic hemodynamic changes observed in patients with liver cirrhosis, and nowadays is mainly of historical importance.

### "Overflow" hypothesis (Libermann, 1970)

This hypothesis assumes that the expansion of intravascular volume is the crucial event in the pathogenesis of ascites formation. Failure to escape from mineralocorticoid action in compensated cirrhosis is considered a major argument supporting the overflow theory of ascites. Portal hypertension combined with hypervolemia are then assumed to lead to an "overflow" of fluid into peritoneal cavity.

Liver cirrhosis → ↑renal Na+ retention → hypervolemia → ascites

However, experimental and clinical data do not support this hypothesis. Failure to escape from mineralocorticoids is uncommon in patients with compensated cirrhosis, is related to an inadequate expansion of effective plasma volume due to the accumulation of ascites, and occurs in patients with marked peripheral arteriolar vasodilation. Thus, the arterial system is not "overfilled", and increased renal sodium retention in the preascitic stage due to vasodilation and does not lead to intravascular hypervolemia.

### Underfilling (S Sherlock,1963)/peripheral arterial vasodilation (Schrier, 1988)" hypothesis

Primary arterial vasodilation with decreased effective arterial volume currently is considered to be the initiating and perpetuating event that results in increased renal sodium and water retention. The cause of peripheral and splanchnic vasodilation is not completely understood. Potential factor are an impaired clearance, portosystemic shunts, or an increased synthesis of vasodilators such as NO, substance P, CGRP, glucagon, adrenomedullin and prostacyclin. As a reaction to primary arterial vasodilation with decreased effective arterial volume, cardiovascular and renal receptors are activated that, via neurohormonal mechanism, result in increased renal retention of sodium and water. The compensatory increase (normalization) in plasma volume prevents the development of ascites. If these compensatory mechanisms succeed in normalizing effectively circulatory homeostasis, the activity of sodium retaining systems and renal sodium excretion normalize again—cirrhosis remains compensated. If, however, the compensatory systems are not sufficient to restore effective plasma volume, activation of sodium retaining systems persists and ongoing Na$^+$ retention results in ascites formation.

*The hepatorenal syndrome with systemic vasodilation and renal vasoconstriction is probably the most extreme manifestation of a disease with reduced effective plasma volume.*

The theory of primary arterial vasodilation best unifies the numerous hemodynamic alterations observed in patients with liver cirrhosis and ascites. The preferential accumulation of fluid within the abdominal cavity is explained by splanchnic vasodilation seen in portal hypertension.

**Lymph Imbalance Theory (Witte, 1980) (Fig. 3.44)**

Impedance in splanchnic lymph drainage → renal hypoperfusion and ↑ RAAS → ascites.

### Q. What are bacterascites?

Ascitic fluid infection with PMN count <250/μL but with a positive bacterial culture is called bacterascites.

### Q. What are classification of peritonitis?

Refer **Table 3.26**.
- Culture-negative neutrocytic ascites
- Monomicrobial non-neutrocytic bacterascites
- Polymicrobial bacterascites
- Secondary bacterial peritonitis
- Spontaneous bacterial peritonitis

### Q. What is spontaneous bacterial peritonitis?

- Spontaneous infection of ascitic fluid occurs in 8% of cirrhotic patients more frequent in decompensated disease.
- High index of suspicion as there will be subtle clinical features.

### Q. How will you classify infected ascites?

Refer **Table 3.26**.

**Table 3.26:** Classification of infected ascites.

| Category | Analysis of ascites |
|---|---|
| Spontaneous bacterial peritonitis | PMN $^3$250/mm$^3$, one pathogen |
| Culture-negative neutrocytic ascites | PMN $^3$250/mm$^3$, negative culture |
| Secondary bacterial peritonitis | PMN $^3$250/mm$^3$, usually several pathogens |
| Monomicrobial bacterascites | PMN <250/mm$^3$, one pathogen |
| Polymicrobial bacterascites | PMN <250/mm$^3$, several pathogens |

(PMN: polymorphonuclear granulocytes)

### Q. What are the clinical features of SBP?

- Suspect in Grade B and C cirrhosis with ascites
- Clinical features may be absent and WBC count normal
- Ascetic protein <1 g/dL
- Usually monomicrobial and gram negative
- Blood culture borne and positive in 80%
- Start antibiotics if ascites TC >250 mm polymorphs
- 50% die
- 69% recur in one year

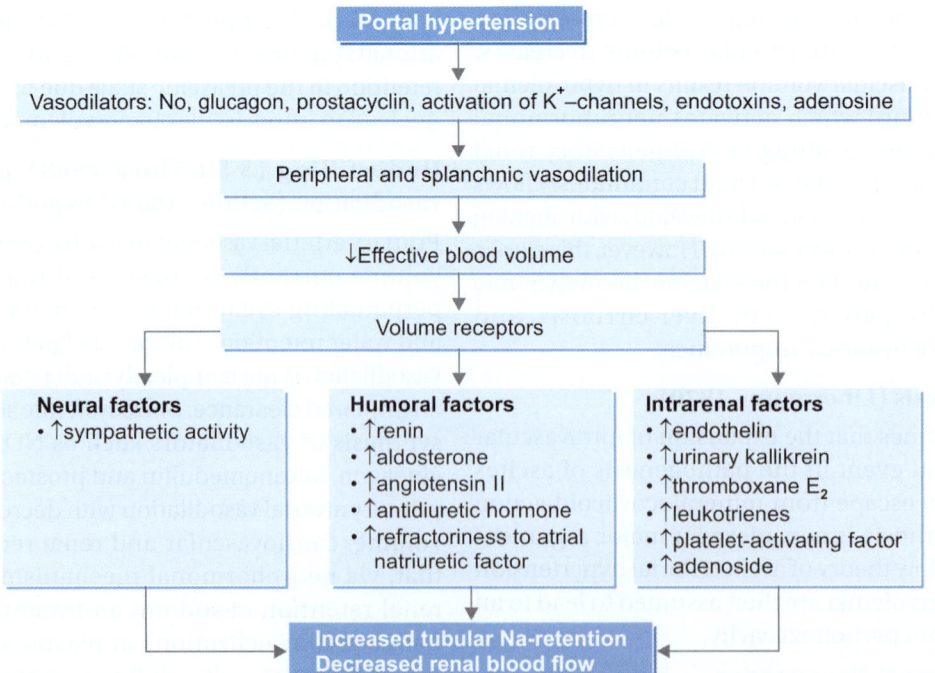

**Fig. 3.44:** Theories of ascites formation.

**Q. What is the pathophysiology of SBP?**

Cirrhotic patients there will be bacterial overgrowth, defective bactericidal activity and small intestinal dysmotility which in turn leads to increased rate of bacterial translocation across intestinal wall into mesenteric lymph nodes thereby causing SBP.

**Most common:** *E. coli* or Group D streptococci.

**Q. How will you treat SBP?**

**Antibiotic treatment**
- **Antibiotic regimen**
  - For community acquired SBP, a third generation cephalosporin, such as cefotaxime 2 g IV q8h or ceftriaxone 2 g IV daily, is recommended.
  - Other regimens for penicillin-allergic patients:
    – Ofloxacin 400 mg orally (PO) q12h
    – Levofloxacin 750 mg IV q24h
    – Ciprofloxacin 400 mg IV q12h
  - For suspected nosocomial SBP, a broader coverage is more appropriate (e.g., piperacillin-tazobactam or a carbapenem)
- **Duration of therapy:** A short-courses of treatment (five-day) for SBP are effective. Only patients who grow an unusual organism (e.g., *Pseudomonas, Enterobacteriaceae*), an organism resistant to standard antibiotic therapy, or an organism routinely associated with endocarditis (e.g., *Staphylococcus aureus* or viridians group streptococci) are initially considered for longer treatment.

**Q. What are the prophylactic measures to be taken to prevent SBP?**

**General measures:**
- **Diuretic therapy:** Diuresis concentrates ascitic fluid, thereby raising ascitic fluid opsonic activity, which may help prevent SBP.
- Early recognition and aggressive treatment of localized infections (e.g., cystitis and cellulitis). This can help to prevent bacteremia and SBP.
- Restricting use of proton pump inhibitors (PPIs).
  - PPI use has been shown to be associated with an increased risk of SBP in some studies. These should only be given to patients who have clear indications for their use.

**Prophylactic antibiotic:**
- Antibiotic prophylaxis to prevent SBP is recommended for patients at high risk of developing SBP and is associated with a decreased risk of bacterial infection and mortality.
- Indications and appropriate regimens are:
  - Patients with cirrhosis and gastrointestinal bleeding.
    – A *seven-day* course of antibiotic is recommended.
    – Ceftriaxone 1g IV per day. Can switch to oral antibiotics once bleeding is stopped and patient is able to eat. Oral regimen include, ciprofloxacin 500 mg BD OR trimethoprim-sulfamethoxazole (TMP-SMX) one double-strength BD, OR norfloxacin 400 mg BD.
  - Patients who have had one or more episodes of SBP.
    – Long-term daily prophylaxis with any of the following regimen trimethoprim-sulfamethoxazole (one double-strength daily) OR ciprofloxacin 500 mg/d or norfloxacin 400 mg/d.
  - Patients with cirrhosis and ascites if the ascitic fluid protein is <1.5 g/dL along with either impaired renal function (a creatinine ≥1.2 mg/dL, a BUN level ≥25 mg/dL or a serum Na ≤130 mEq/L) or liver failure (a Child-Pugh score ≥9 and a bilirubin ≥3 mg/dL).
    – Long-term use of norfloxacin 400 mg/d, OR TMP-SMX one double-strength per day.

**Q. What is monomicrobial non-neutrocytic bacterascites?**
- A positive ascitic fluid culture for a single organism.
- An ascitic fluid PMN count lower than 250 cells/mm$^3$ (0.25 × 10$^9$/L), and
- No evidence of an intra-abdominal surgically treatable source of infection.

**Q. What is culture-negative neutrocytic ascites?**
- The ascitic fluid culture grows no bacteria
- The ascitic fluid PMN count is 250 cells/mm$^3$ or greater
- No antibiotics have been given (not even a single dose)
- No other explanation for an elevated ascitic PMN count (e.g., hemorrhage into ascites, peritoneal carcinomatosis, tuberculosis, or pancreatitis) can be identified.

This variant of ascitic fluid infection seldom is diagnosed when sensitive culture methods are used.

**Q. What are the diagnostic criteria for SBP?**
- The ascitic fluid culture is positive (usually for multiple organisms).
- PMN count is 250 cells/mm$^3$ (0.25 × 10$^9$/L) or greater
- An intra-abdominal surgically treatable primary source of infection (e.g., perforated intestine, perinephric abscess) has been identified.

The importance of distinguishing this variant from spontaneous bacterial peritonitis is that secondary peritonitis usually requires emergency surgical intervention.

**Q. What are polymicrobial bacterascites?**
- Multiple organisms are seen on Gram stain or cultured from the ascitic fluid
- The PMN count is lower than 250 cells/mm$^3$

This diagnosis should be suspected when the paracentesis is traumatic. Polymicrobial bacterascites is essentially diagnostic of intestinal perforation by the paracentesis needle **(Fig. 3.45)**.

**Q. What are the causes of oral hyperpigmentation?**
- Addison's disease
- Peutz-Jeghers syndrome
- Malignant melanoma

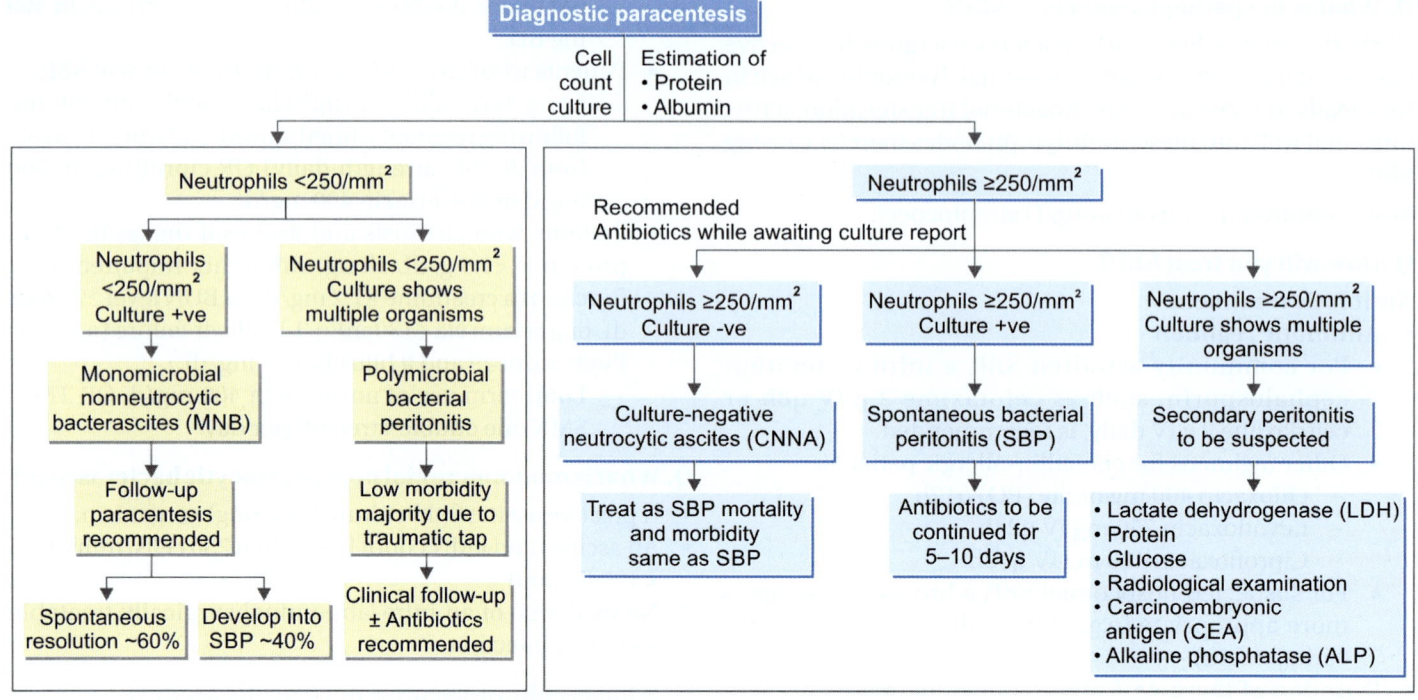

**Fig. 3.45:** Findings in diagnostic paracentesis.

- **Heavy metals:** Lead, lead, bismuth
- Oral contraceptives, minocycline, phenothiazines.

**Q. Peripheral signs of constrictive pericarditis.**

1. Pulsus paradoxus
2. Friedrich's sign—prominent Y descent.
3. Pericardial knock.

**Q. What are the differences between constrictive pericarditis, tamponade and restrictive cardiomyopathy?**

Refer **Table 3.27**.

**Q. How does tuberculosis causes ascites?**

- **Peritonitis:** The peritoneum constitutes a common site for extrapulmonary TB, usually due to the reactivation of

| Characteristic | Tamponade | Constrictive pericarditis | Restrictive cardiomyopathy | RVMI |
|---|---|---|---|---|
| **Clinical** | | | | |
| Pulsus paradoxus | Common | Usually absent | Rare | Rare |
| Jugular veins | | | | |
| Prominent y descent | Absent | Usually present | Rare | Rare |
| Prominent x descent | Present | Usually present | Present | Rare |
| Kussmaul's sign | Absent | Present | Present | Present |
| Third heart sound | Absent | Absent | Rare | May be present |
| Pericardial knock | Absent | Often present | Absent | Absent |
| **Electrocardiogram** | | | | |
| Low ECG voltage | May be present | May be present | May be present | Absent |
| Electrical alternans | May be present | Absent | Absent | Absent |
| **Echocardiography** | | | | |
| Thickened pericardium | Absent | Present | Absent | Absent |
| Pericardial calcification | Absent | Often present | Absent | Absent |
| Pericardial effusion | Present | Absent | Absent | Absent |

Table 3.27: Differences between constrictive pericarditis, tamponade and restrictive cardiomyopathy.

| Characteristic | Tamponade | Constrictive pericarditis | Restrictive cardiomyopathy | RVMI |
|---|---|---|---|---|
| RV size | Usually small | Usually normal | Usually normal | Enlarged |
| Myocardial thickness | Normal | Normal | Usually increased | Normal |
| Right atrial collapse and RVDC | Present | Absent | Absent | Absent |
| Increased early filling, ↑ mitral flow velocity | Absent | Present | Present | May be present |
| Exaggerated respiratory variation in flow velocity | Present | Present | Absent | Absent |
| CT/MRI | | | | |
| Thickened/calcific pericardium | Absent | Present | Absent | Absent |
| Cardiac catheterization | | | | |
| Equalization of diastolic pressures | Usually present | Usually present | Usually absent | Absent or present |
| Cardiac biopsy helpful? | No | No | Sometimes | No |

latent foci established after hematogenous dissemination from a primary lung infection.
- Constrictive pericarditis.
- Disseminated tuberculosis in immunocompromised
- Spread from genitourinary tuberculosis.

### Q. What is ascites praecox and in which conditions is it seen?

An abnormal accumulation of fluid with peritoneal cavity before the generalized edema.

**It is seen in following conditions:** Constrictive pericarditis, congestive cardiac failure with predominate right sided pathology like organic tricuspid valve stenosis or regurgitation and right ventricular endomyocardial fibrosis.

Other causes where there is predominant ascites with no pedal edema are tuberculous peritonitis, peritoneal carcinomatosis, acute Budd Chiari syndrome, and pancreatic malignancy.

### Q. What is the mechanism of ascites precox?

Ascites precox is classically reported in constrictive pericarditis. The reason why ascites precedes edema legs is long been speculative. Now we have evidence, the pericardial pathology, has a direct effect on the hepatic venous morphology. There can be a selective, partial constrictor effect on at least one of the hepatic vein as it enters the right atrium. In fact, the entry point of hepatic vein is delicately close to IVC/RA junction. Anatomical constriction has a mechanical effect on the hepatic venous drainage and subsequently alters the hepatic function. Segmental hepatic dysfunction is thought to ooze out the ascitic fluid from the surface of liver. Ultimately severe raise of hepatic venous pressure results in congestive hepatomegaly and could result in now obsolete, cardiac cirrhosis.

### Q. What is chylous ascites?

Has a milky or creamy appearance due to lymph in the abdominal cavity. Its triglyceride concentration exceeds that of plasma. The underlying mechanisms for the formation of chylous ascites are related to disruption of the lymphatic system. Traumatic injury or obstruction by tumors, especially malignant lymphomas are the most frequent causes. Chylous ascites is seen in 0.5–1% of patients with liver cirrhosis.

**Ascitic fluid**
- Milky or creamy
- High fat (triglycerides >1,000 mg/dL) content.
- Sudan III staining demonstrates fat globules.

### Q. What are the mechanisms of formation of chylous ascites?

- Leakage from the dilated subserosal lymphatics into the peritoneal cavity,
- Exudation of lymph through the walls of massively dilated retroperitoneal lymphatics, which leak fluid through a fistula into the peritoneal cavity (i.e., congenital lymphangiectasia).
- Thoracic duct obstruction from trauma or tumor with resulting dilated retroperitoneal lymphatic vessels with consequent direct leakage of chyle through a lymphoperitoneal fistula.

In liver cirrhosis, chylous ascites may develop as a result of increased hydrostatic pressure within the splanchnic lymphatics, with their consequent disruption.

### Q. What is Meigs' syndrome?

- Pleural effusion is most commonly right-sided, may be exudate or transudate. Approximately 70% of pleural effusions are right-sided, 15% left-sided, and 15% are bilateral
- Ascites
- The tumor is a benign fibroma or a fibroma-like tumor of the ovary (such as thecoma and granulosa cell tumors).
- Both ascites and pleural effusion resolve following excision of the pelvic tumor. Meigs' syndrome accounts for about 1% of ovarian tumors.

Other benign cysts of the ovary (such as struma ovarii, mucinous cystadenoma and teratomas), leiomyoma of the uterus, and secondary metastatic tumors to ovary if associated with hydrothorax are referred to as 'Pseudo-Meigs' syndrome.

### Q. What are the causes of ascites?
Refer **Box 3.5**.

**Box 3.5:** Causes of ascites.

- **Hepatic source**
  - Cirrhosis (~80%)
  - Acute liver failure
  - Alcoholic hepatitis
  - Hepatic vein thrombosis (Budd-Chiari syndrome)
- Heart failure (3%). It is usually associated with pulmonary hypertension.
- Malignancy-related ascites (10%)
  - Peritoneal carcinomatosis
  - Massive liver metastasis (causing portal hypertension)
- Peritoneal infection (e.g., peritoneal tuberculosis)
- **Other**
  - Other peritoneal disease (e.g., peritoneal dialysis), peritoneal carcinomatosis, ventriculoperitoneal shunt.
  - Obstetrics/gynecology: Endometriosis, abdominal pregnancy, ovarian hyperstimulation syndrome
  - Portal vein thrombosis
  - Nephrotic syndrome
  - Bowel perforation
  - Pancreatitis
  - Myxedema
  - Hemodialysis-associated ascites
- **Mixed (5%)**
- Ascites that results from combination of 2 or more causes, e.g., cirrhosis plus 1 other cause such as peritoneal carcinomatosis

### Q. What is SAAG?
- **Serum albumin: Ascitic fluid albumin (Table 3.28 and Fig. 3.46)**
- Gives a clue about portal hydrostatic pressure
- It is the best single test for classifying ascites into portal hypertensive (SAAG >1.1 g/dL) and nonportal hypertensive (SAAG <1.1 g/dL) causes.
- It correlates directly with portal pressure.
- The accuracy is approximately 97%.

**Table 3.28:** Causes of ascites based on serum-ascites albumin gradient.

| High gradient (≥1.1 g/dL) | Low gradient (<1.1 g/dL) |
|---|---|
| ◆ Cirrhosis | ◆ Peritoneal carcinomatosis |
| ◆ Alcoholic hepatitis | ◆ Tuberculous peritonitis |
| ◆ Cardiac failure | ◆ Pancreatic ascites |
| ◆ Massive liver metastases | ◆ Biliary ascites |
| ◆ Fulminant hepatic failure | ◆ Nephrotic syndrome |
| ◆ Budd-Chiari syndrome | ◆ Serositis |
| ◆ Veno-occlusive disease | ◆ Bowel infarction |
| ◆ Portal vein thrombosis | ◆ Bowel perforation |
| ◆ Fatty liver of pregnancy | |
| ◆ Myxedema | |

### Q. Can SAAG be elevated in non-PHT causes?
SAAG, the ascitic fluid to serum bilirubin concentration ratio, the protein and cholesterol levels and the number of leukocytes and differential are useful in determining the cause of ascites. They allow for classifying ascites into a transudate or an exudate and give hints to a possible malignant etiology or to a bacterial peritonitis **(Tables 3.29 and 3.30)**.

### Q. What are the drawbacks of SAAG?

**Falsely low SAAG**
- Arterial hypotension (decrease portal pressure)
- If serum albumin less than 1.1 g/dL.

**Falsely high SAAG**
Lipid, chylous ascites.

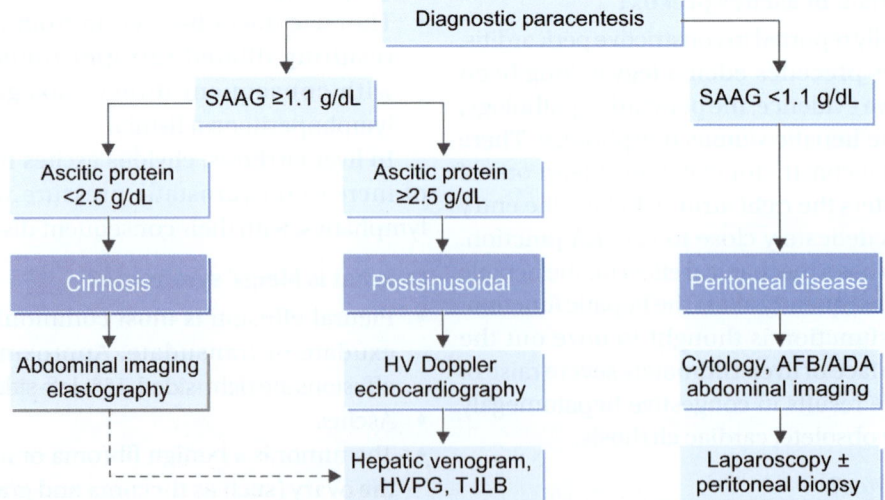

**Fig. 3.46:** Findings in diagnostic paracentesis.
(ADA: adenosine deaminase; AFB: acid fast bacterium; HV: hepatic venous; SAAG: serum-ascites albumin gradient; TJLB: transjugular liver biopsy)

**Table 3.29:** SAAG findings in different forms of ascites.

| | SAAG | Ascites protein |
|---|---|---|
| **Main etiological factors of ascites** | | |
| Cirrhosis or alcoholic hepatitis | High | Low |
| Congestive heart failure | High | High |
| Peritoneal malignancy | Low | High |
| Peritoneal tuberculosis | Low | High |
| **Other etiologies of cirrhosis (account for <2% of all cases)** | | |
| Massive hepatic metastases | High | Low |
| Nodular regenerative hyperplasia | High | Low |
| Fulminant liver failure | High | Low? |
| Budd-Chiari syndrome (late) | High | Low |
| Budd-Chiari syndrome (early) | High | High |
| Constrictive pericarditis | High | High |

**Table 3.30:** Biochemical findings in different forms of ascites.

| Ascitic fluid | Portal ascites | Malignant ascites | Infectious ascites |
|---|---|---|---|
| **Protein (g%)** | <3 (transudate) | >3 (exudate) | >3 (exudate) |
| Serum albumin (g/dL) | >1.1 | <1.1 | <1.1 |
| Ascitic albumin (g/dL) | | | |
| Leukocytes/mm$^3$ | <500 | >50 | >1,000 (neutrophils) |
| Serum LDH: | <1.4 | >1.4 | >1.4 |
| Ascitic LDH | | | |
| pH | >7.45 | <7.45 | <7.31 |
| Lactate (mmol/L) | | <4.5 | >4.5 |
| Cholesterol (mg/dL) | | >48 | |
| Serum glucose: | | <1 | >1 |
| Ascites glucose | | | |
| Tumor markers | – | + | – |
| Bacterial culture | – | – | +$^a$ |
| Cytology | – | + | – |

$^a$Ascitic mycobacterial cultures are 50% sensitive.

### Q. What is corrected SAAG?
- Corrected SAAG = Uncorrected SAAG × 0.16 × (Serum globulin + 2.5)
- Serum hyperglobulinemia (Serum globulin >5 g/dL).

### Q. Can you get exudative ascites in portal hypertension?
- Cardiac ascites
- Acute Budd-Chiari syndrome
  - High protein in ascitic fluid >2.5: Heart failure and Budd-Chiari syndrome
  - Low protein in ascitic fluid <2.5: Liver cirrhosis

### Q. How will you manage a case of ascites?
**Diagnostic paracentesis** typically to characterize the fluid origin, and whether it is sterile, infectious and/or malignant **(Fig. 3.47)**.

### Q. What are the indications for diagnostic paracentesis?
- Any new onset of ascites.
- Testing of ascitic fluid in a patient with preexisting ascites who is admitted to the hospital, regardless of the reason for admission.
- Any patient with cirrhosis and ascites who has signs of clinical deterioration, e.g., GI bleeding (is a high-risk time for infection), fever, abdominal pain/tenderness, hepatic encephalopathy, hypotension, peripheral leukocytosis, worsening renal function, or metabolic acidosis.
- Clinical suspicion for spontaneous bacterial peritonitis.

### Q. How will you manage a case of uncomplicated ascites?
The goals of therapy in patients with ascites are to minimize ascitic fluid volume and decrease peripheral edema, without causing intravascular volume depletion **(Fig. 3.48)**.

The rate at which fluid can safely be removed in cirrhosis depends upon the presence or absence of peripheral edema.
- In patients with peripheral edema, fluid mobilization can be rapid (maximum weight loss of 1 kg per day) without detectable intravascular volume depletion.
- In patients with ascites without edema, the recommended maximum weight loss is 0.5 kg per day.

More rapid fluid removal with diuretics can lead to plasma volume depletion and azotemia. If more rapid fluid removal is required, an initial large-volume paracentesis (LVP) should be performed.

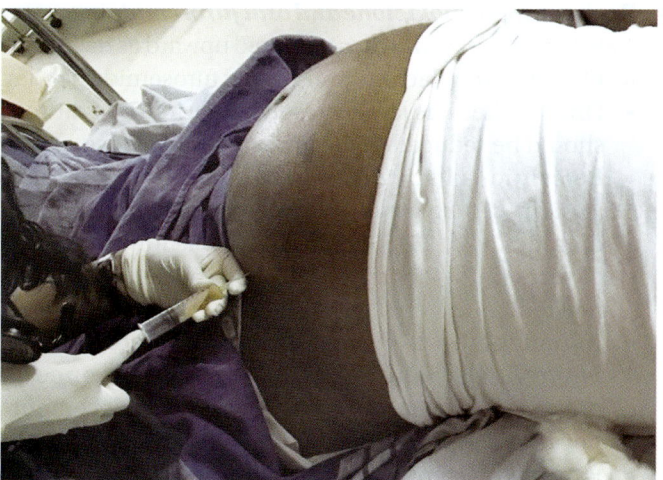

**Fig. 3.47:** Ascitic tap.

# SECTION 3: Gastrointestinal System

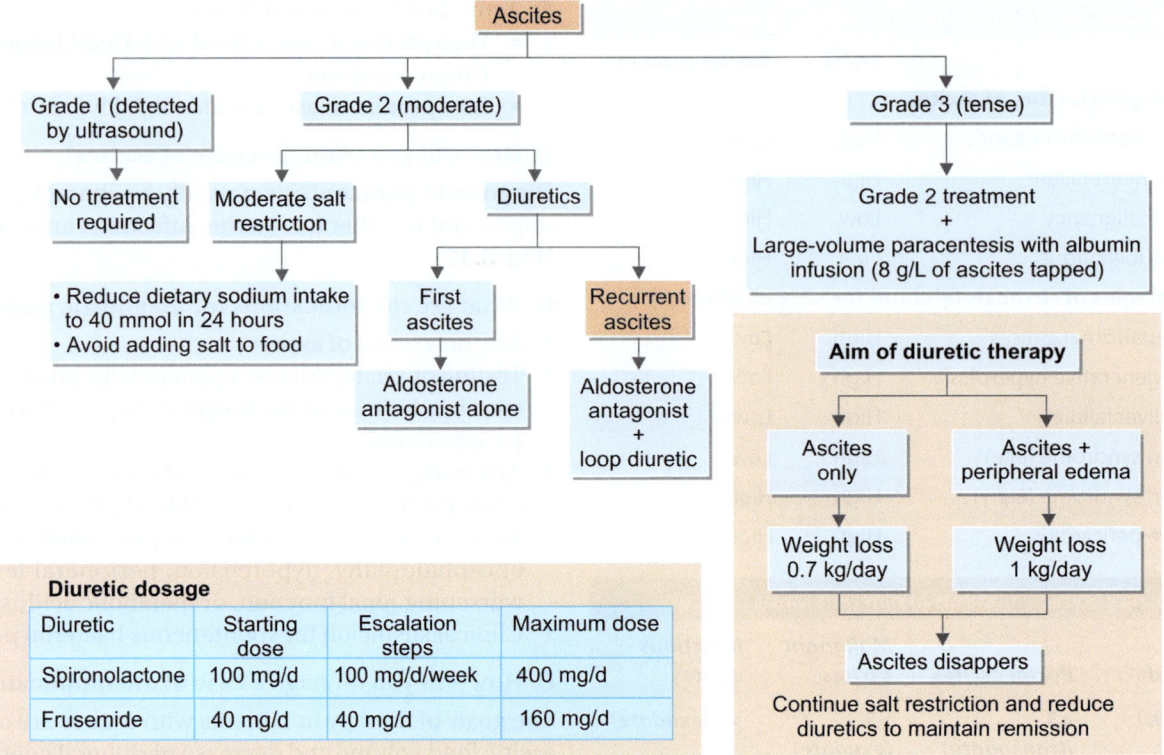

**Fig. 3.48:** Management protocol of ascites.

**Fluid removal**
- Cirrhotic ascites can be mobilized in approximately 90% of patients.
- The initial step involves dietary *sodium restriction* to <2 g per day (≤90 mmol/day)
- **Diuretics:**
  - **Indications to initiate diuretics**
    - Clinically apparent (grade 2–3) ascites
    - Absence of frank persistent hepatic encephalopathy, active GI bleeding, AKI
    - Absence of ascitic complications, such as bacterial peritonitis.
- **Regimen:** *Spironolactone and oral furosemide* in a ratio of 100:40 mg per day, with doses titrated upward as needed (up to 400 mg spironolactone and 160 mg furosemide per day).
  - Once ascites has largely resolved, the dose of diuretics should be reduced to the lowest effective dose.
  - Be cautious in *small-volume ascites, small patients (weight <50 kg) and elderly*. Start with *lower dose* of diuretics, e.g., 25–50 mg of spironolactone and 20 mg of furosemide per day. This can be titrated upward if needed.
  - In patients with *hypokalemia*, start *spironolactone monotherapy* and only add furosemide once the potassium normalizes and potassium replacement is no longer needed.
  - Furosemide should be stopped if severe hypokalemia occurs (<3 mmol/L).
- Antimineralocorticoids should be stopped if severe hyperkalemia occurs (>6 mmol/L).

**Q. What are the indications for therapeutic paracentesis?**
- Tense ascites: Tense ascites may increase intra-abdominal pressure and cause a compartment syndrome. Such patients may not respond well to diuresis, due to renal dysfunction as well.
- Massive ascites in the absence of peripheral edema.
- Refractory ascites
- Symptomatic hydrothorax.
- Active variceal bleeding or those at high risk of variceal hemorrhage.
- Exudative ascites or those disorders that are not responsive to diuretic treatment, e.g., peritoneal carcinomatosis, hepatic vein thrombosis.

**Q. What is large volume paracentesis?**
If the patient has tense ascites or if the patient or the clinician is in a hurry to decompress the abdomen, a 5 L paracentesis is more rapid than diuretic therapy. Removal of less than 5 liters of fluid does not appear to have hemodynamic consequences, and post-paracentesis albumin infusion does not appear to be necessary.

For LVP, **albumin** (6–8 g per liter of fluid removed) can be administered.
- A meta-analysis demonstrated a survival advantage with albumin infusion after paracentesis involving mean volumes of 5.5–15.9 L

### Q. What is complicated ascites?

Ascites is complicated when it is refractory, infected or associated with hepatorenal syndrome.

### Q. What is diuretic resistant ascites and how will you manage it?

It is considered to be present if at least one of the following criteria is fulfilled in the absence of therapy with a NSAID or other nephrotoxic medications.

- An inability to mobilize ascites (manifested by weight loss <0.8 kg over 4 days) despite confirmed adherence to the dietary sodium restriction and the administration of maximum tolerable doses of oral diuretics.
- Reappearance of grade 2 or 3 ascites within 4 weeks of initial mobilization
- The development of diuretic-induced complications such as progressive azotemia, hepatic encephalopathy, or progressive electrolyte imbalances.

**Management**

- Stop medications that decrease systemic blood pressure (and thus renal perfusion), such as beta blockers, angiotensin converting enzyme inhibitors (ACEIs), and angiotensin receptor II blockers (ARBs).
- Stop nephrotoxins and NSAIDs.
- Continue sodium restriction and diuretics.
- Consider discontinuing diuretics when urinary Na excretion is < 30 mEq/d.
- Large volume paracentesis followed by albumin administration.
- Consider trans jugular intrahepatic portosystemic stent shunt (TIPS) placement in the appropriate patients.
- Slow low-dose continuous albumin, furosemide with or without terlipressin SIFA(T) infusion.

### Q. What is alfa pump?

- The automated low-flow ascites pump (alfa pump®) is a subcutaneously-implanted novel battery-driven device that pumps ascitic fluid from the peritoneal cavity into the urinary bladder. Ascites can therefore be aspirated in a time- and volume-controlled mode and evacuated by urination.
- Liver transplantation.

## EXAMINATION OF TONGUE

**Q. Describe the characteristics of tongue.**

Tongue is a muscular organ in the oral cavity that is covered with moist pink tissue called mucosa. Examination of tongue is a routine part of general physical examination, as well as cranial nerve examination. tongue acts as a mirror of our body and lesions of tongue might be the first sign or symptom of an underlying systemic disease. Unfortunately lesions of Tongue are often overlooked by primary care physicians. So knowledge about the lesions of the tongue and associated systemic diseases is very important.

First of all, it is important to know about the characteristics of a healthy tongue.

**Characteristics of a healthy tongue:**
- **Color:** Tongue should be pinkish to slightly reddish color on the dorsal side and the ventral surface may be a little bluish in color add have some visible vasculature.
- **Texture:** Surface of the tongue is slightly rough in nature, due to the presence of papillae. It should not have any ulcers, furrows. Ventral surface of the tongue is smooth in nature.
- **Size:** The tongue should be fit comfortably within the oral cavity with the tip of the tongue against the lower incisors.

**Q. What are the changes in color?**
- **Pale tongue**—seen in severe anemia **(Fig. 3.49)**
- **Blotting paper like pallor with pigmented margins**— seen in hookworm infestation (Ancylostoma duodenale)
- **White tongue:**
  - Oral candidiasis (oral thrush) **(Fig. 3.50)**
  - Oral lichen planus (white lace like pattern)
  - Leukoplakia
  - Hairy leukoplakia **(Fig. 3.51)**
  - Syphilis
- **Red color/beefy red tongue (Fig. 3.52)**—vitamin $B_{12}$ deficiency.

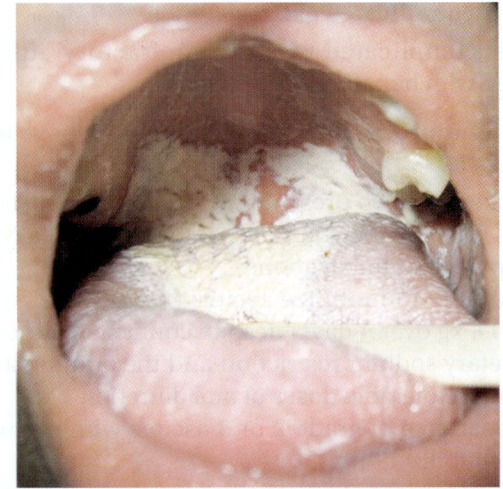

Fig. 3.50: Oral candidiasis.

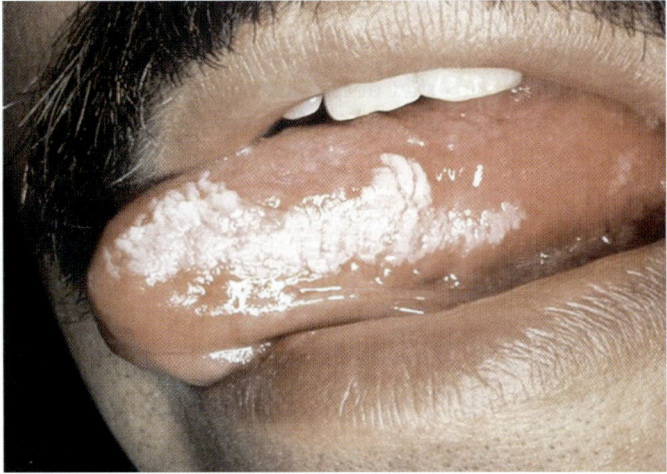

Fig. 3.51: Hairy leukoplakia.

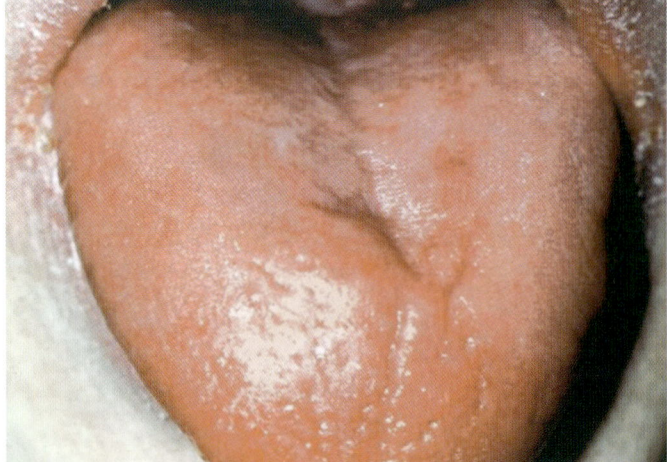

Fig. 3.52: Beefy red tongue.

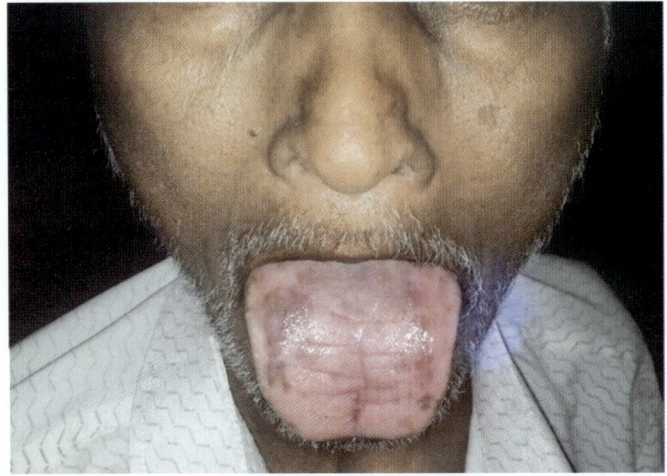

Fig. 3.49: Pale tongue in anemia.

- **Magenta red color (Fig. 3.53)**—riboflavin deficiency
- **Hairy leukoplakia :** Hairy leukoplakia is characterized by irregular white patches usually on the side/margins of the tongue but may be present anywhere on the tongue. Hairy

- **Magenta red color (Fig. 3.53)**—riboflavin deficiency
- **Hairy leukoplakia :** Hairy leukoplakia is characterized by irregular white patches usually on the side/margins of the tongue but may be present anywhere on the tongue. Hairy leukoplakia differs from oral candidiasis in which the white patch occurs commonly on the dorsal surface of the tongue which can be easily rubbed off and responds very well to antifungal therapy. Hairy leukoplakia is commonly seen in people with HIV/immunocompromised state, Ebstein-Barr virus (EBV).
- **Blue-colored tongue (Fig. 3.54)**—central cyanosis, methemoglobinemia/sulphemoglobinemia, etc.
- **Bluish red color or purple color tongue**—polycythemia.
- **Slate-blue tongue**—seen in hemochromatosis
- **Black color (Fig. 3.55):**
  - Addison disease
  - Nelson's syndrome
  - Peutz-Jeghers syndrome
  - Fungal infection (actinomycosis)
  - Malabsorption
  - Poor oral hygiene

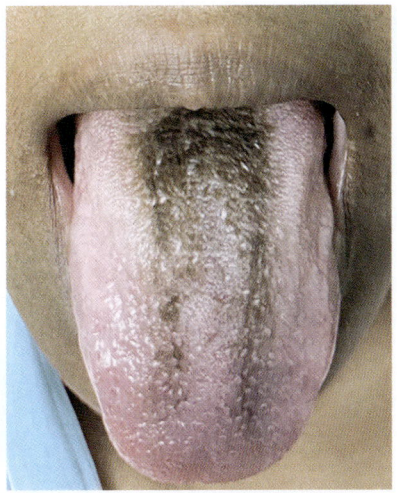

**Fig. 3.55:** Black-colored tongue.

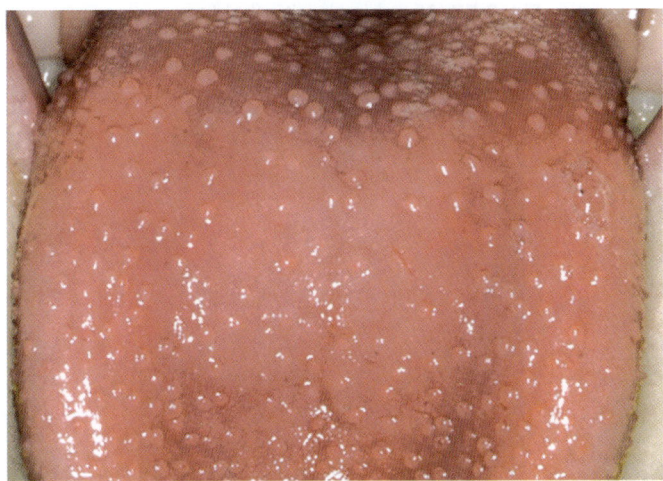

**Fig. 3.56:** Strawberry tongue.

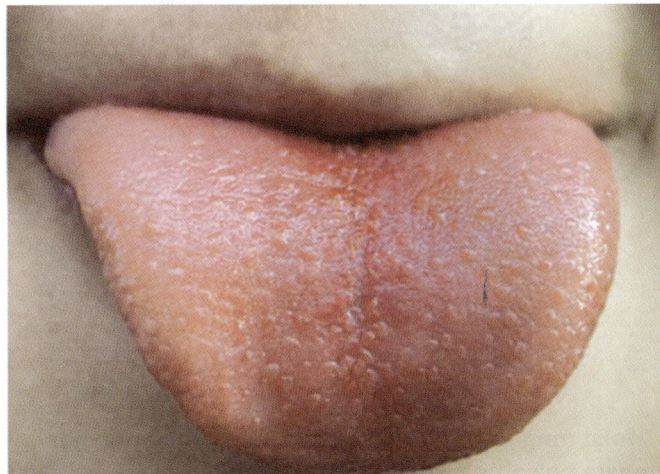

**Fig. 3.53:** Magenta red color tongue.

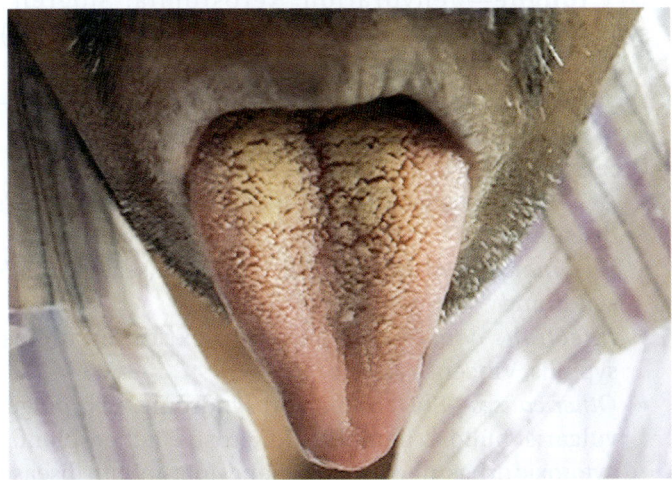

**Fig. 3.54:** Blue-colored tongue.

- Smoking
- Iron, bismuth, opium
- Drugs—linezolid, etc.
- **Yellow color**—jaundice, can also be seen in nitric acid or hydrochloric acid poisoning, etc.
- **Brownish**—chronic kidney disease (uremia).
- **Strawberry tongue (Fig. 3.56)**—scarlet fever, toxic shock syndrome, Kawasaki disease.
- **Raspberry tongue**—early stages of scarlet fever.

**Q. What are the changes in surface texture?**

- **Bald tongue (atrophic glossitis) (Fig. 3.57)**—seen in vitamin $B_{12}$ deficiency, iron deficiency, celiac disease, tropical sprue, pellagra.
- **Geographic tongue (Fig. 3.58)**—also known as benign migratory glossitis or wandering rash of the tongue. On the dorsum of the tongue, loss of filiform papillae leads to a red patchy depapillated area with circumferential white polycyclic borders, giving the appearance of a map. These lesions can change location, size, pattern very rapidly and so the name

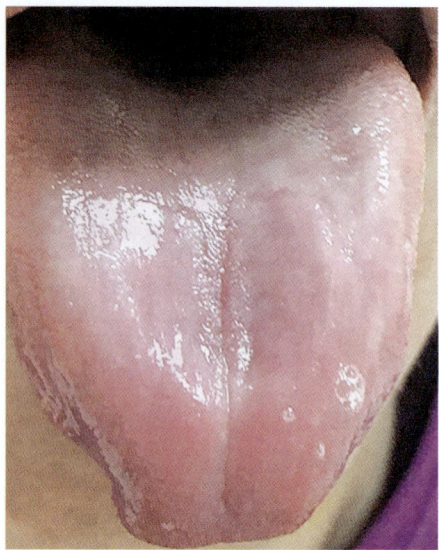

Fig. 3.57: Atrophic glossitis (bald tongue).

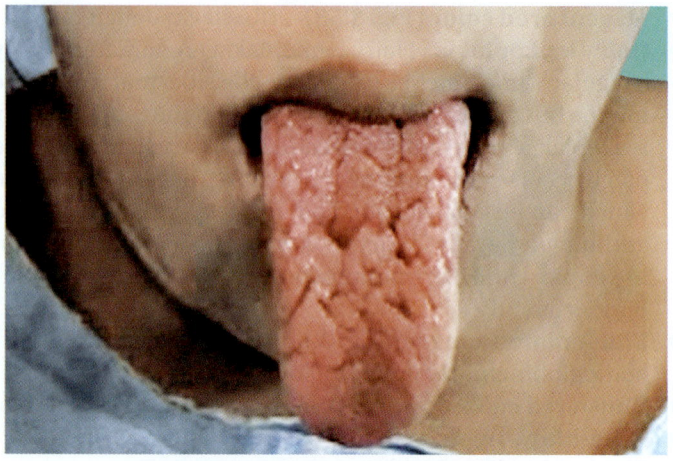

Fig. 3.59: Fissured tongue (scrotal tongue).

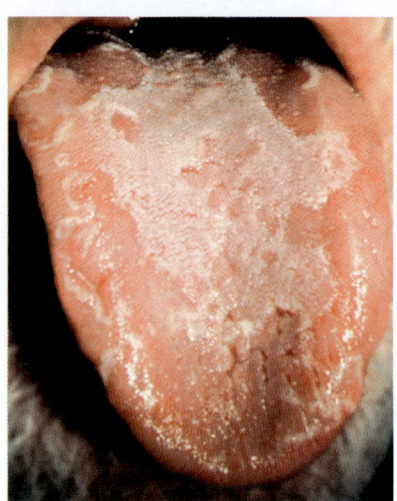

Fig. 3.58: Geographic tongue.

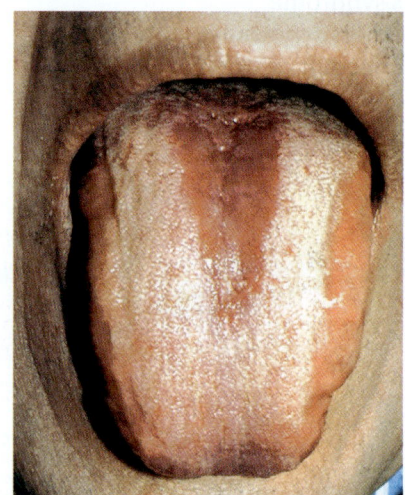

Fig. 3.60: Median rhomboid glossitis.

migratory glossitis. This condition is frequently associated with atopic individuals, psoriasis, reactive arthritis, etc.
- **Fissured tongue (Fig. 3.59)**—also known as scrotal tongue, fissured tongue, lingua plicata, etc. Seen in Melkersson-Rosenthal syndrome, Down syndrome, Cowden syndrome, etc.
- **Median rhomboid glossitis (Fig. 3.60)**—also known as central papillary atrophy of the tongue. It is an uncommon benign condition presenting as a red depapillated area usually rhomboid in shape on the dorsum of the tongue in the midline, anterior to the foramen cecum. It is considered as a form of chronic atrophic candidiasis. It is associated with smoking use of corticosteroid sprays or inhalers, and in immunodeficiency conditions.
- **Bite marks with hematomas**—accidental bites during convulsions, etc.

- **Moist tongue**—sialorrhea, heavy metal and organophosphate poisoning, parkinsonism, gastroesophageal reflux disease.
- **Dry tongue**—dehydration, xerostomia, Sjögren's syndrome, anticholinergic drug therapy (atropinization), mouth breathing, etc.
- **Dry red tongue with atrophy of papillae and fissures**—seen in Sjogren's syndrome **(Fig. 3.61)**.
- **Ulcers:**
  - *GIT causes*—celiac disease, ulcerative colitis, Crohn's disease
  - *Rheumatological causes*—SLE, Behçet's disease, Reiter's syndrome
  - *Infectious causes*—herpes simplex, tuberculosis, syphilis, Vincent's angina, etc.
  - *Other causes*—Steven Johnson syndrome, pemphigus vulgaris, bullous pemphigoid, erosive lichen planus, cytotoxic drugs, neutropenia, hand-foot-mouth disease, etc.

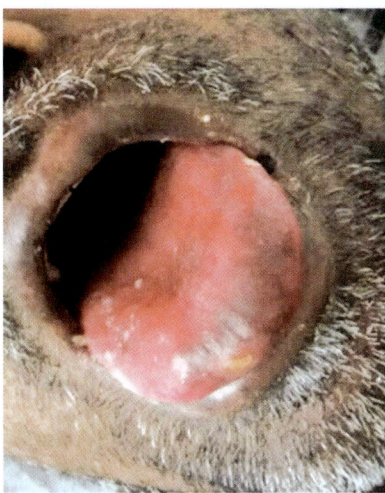

**Fig. 3.61:** Dry red tongue.

- *Single ulcer*—tuberculosis, syphilis, malignancy.
- *Multiple ulcers*—herpes, aphthous ulcers, pemphigus, chickenpox **(Fig. 3.62)**
- *Recurrent ulcers*:
  - Behçet's disease
  - Pemphigus
  - Lichen planus
  - Neutropenia
  - SLE
  - Celiac disease and Crohn's disease.
- *Traumatic ulcers*—margins of the tongue in epilepsy
- *Whooping cough*—ulcer of frenulum of the tongue (sublingual ulcer).
- *Tubercular ulcer*—usually single painful ulcer and tends to occur at the tip of the tongue.
- *Syphilis*:
  - Primary syphilis—single painless indurated ulcer with lymphadenopathy.
  - Secondary syphilis—"snail track" ulcers with grayish slough and lymphadenopathy
  - Tertiary syphilis—midline punched out ulcers.

**Q. What are the changes in the size?**

- ♦ **Macroglossia**—seen in:
  - Amyloidosis
  - Downs syndrome
  - Beckwith-Wiedemann syndrome
  - Acromegaly
  - Hypothyroidism
  - Cretinism
  - Myxedema mucopolysaccharidoses (Hurlers syndrome)
  - Glycogen storage disorders (von Gierke's disease), congenital AV malformations between lingual artery and vein
  - Angioedema
  - Lymphangioma
  - Tumor infiltration
  - NSAIDs
  - Angiotensin-converting enzyme inhibitors, etc.
- ♦ **Microglossia**:
  - Smith-Lemli-Opitz syndrome
  - Freeman-Sheldon syndrome
  - Hanhart syndrome
  - Ankyloglossia (tongue tie)
  - Atrophic glossitis pseudobulbar palsy (small pointed compact looking tongue)
  - Facial hemiatrophy
  - Myasthenia gravis (triple longitudinal furrowing)
- ♦ **Glossoptosis**—posterior displacement of the tongue into the pharynx. It is seen in Pierre-Robins syndrome.

**Q. What are the changes in movements of tongue?**

- ♦ **Tremors of the tongue**—Parkinson's disease, thyrotoxicosis, delirium tremens, bulbar palsy, alcohol withdrawal, etc.
- ♦ **Jack in the box (Lizard tongue)**—rheumatic chorea
- ♦ **Chewing tongue**—seen in athetosis
- ♦ **Fasciculations**—motor neuron disease
- ♦ **Deviation of tongue**—tongue deviates to the affected side in 12th nerve lesion.
- ♦ **Flaccid tongue with fasciculations**—seen in bulbar palsy.
- ♦ **Spastic tongue without fasciculations**—seen in pseudobulbar palsy.

**Q. Enumerate the miscellaneous conditions of tongue.**

- ♦ **Gorlin's tongue sign**—seen in Ehler-Danlos syndrome, etc.
- ♦ **Trombone tongue**–general paresis of insane (GPI).
- ♦ **Angry looking tongue**—enteric fever
- ♦ **Mushroom like tongue**—corrosive poisoning.
- ♦ **Cobblestone tongue**
- ♦ **Crocodile tongue**
- ♦ **Alligator tongue**

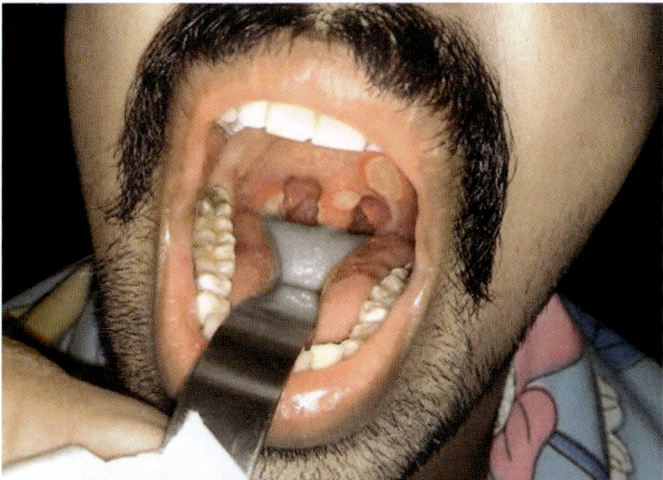

**Fig. 3.62:** Multiple ulcers.

## SECTION 7: Gastrointestinal System

- Secondary syphilis—"snail track" ulcers with grayish slough and lymphadenopathy
- Tertiary syphilis—midline punched out ulcers.

**Q. What are the changes in the size?**

- **Macroglossia**—seen in:
  - Amyloidosis
  - Down syndrome
  - Beckwith-Wiedemann syndrome
  - Acromegaly
  - Hypothyroidism
  - Cretinism
  - Mucopolysaccharidoses (Hurler's syndrome)
  - Glycogen storage disorders (Pompe's disease)
  - congenital AV malformations between lingual artery and vein
  - Angioedema
  - Lymphangioma
  - Tumor infiltration
  - AL amyloidosis
  - Hamartoma—involving mucous membrane, muscles, vessels
  - Mouth-ear-hand syndrome
  - Freeman-Sheldon syndrome
  - Kabuki syndrome
  - Ankyloglossia (tongue tie)
- **Atrophic glossitis**, pseudobulbar palsy (mean protrusion cannot lick tongue).
- Facial hemiatrophy
- Absent tongue (total or partial lingual hypoplasia)
- Cyclopia—is seen due to failure of the tongue to develop. It is seen in 13 to 18 gene syndrome.

**Q. What are the changes in movements of tongue?**

- **Tremors of the tongue**—Parkinson's disease, thyrotoxicosis, Delirium tremens, bulbar palsy, alcohol withdrawal, etc.
- **Jack in the box (Lizard tongue)**—rheumatic chorea
- **Chewing tongue**—seen in athetosis
- **Fasciculations**—motor neuron disease
- **Deviation of tongue**—tongue deviates to the affected side in 12th nerve lesion.
- **Flaccid tongue with fasciculations**—seen in bulbar palsy
- **Spastic tongue without fasciculations**—seen in pseudobulbar palsy.

**Q. Enumerate the miscellaneous conditions of tongue.**

- Gorlin's tongue sign—seen in Ehlers-Danlos syndrome, etc.
- **Trombone tongue**—general paresis of insane (GPI)
- **Angry looking tongue**—enteric fever
- **Mushroom like tongue**—corrosive poisoning.
- **Cobblestone tongue**
- Crocodile tongue
- Alligator tongue

Fig. 7.61: Hairy red tongue

- **Single ulcer**—tuberculosis, syphilis, malignancy
- Multiple ulcers—aphthous ulcers (Fig. 7.62), pemphigus, stomatitis (Fig. 7.62).
  - Recurrent ulcers
  - Behcet's disease
  - Pemphigus
  - Lichen planus
  - Stomatitis
  - SLE
- Celiac disease and Crohn's disease.
- Aphthous ulcers—tiny ulcers over the tongue in early days.
- Erythema migrans—several red patches of the tongue with hyperemia.
- Hepes zoster—usually single painful lesion and it seen over pole to occur in the floor of the tongue.
- Syphilis
- Primary syphilis—single painless but raised ulcer with lymphadenopathy

Fig. 7.62: Multiple ulcers

# SECTION 4
# Nervous System

## Section Outline

- ◆ Case Sheet Format
- ◆ Sample Case Sheet and Discussion
  - Stroke
  - Spinal Cord Diseases
  - Peripheral Neuropathy
  - Guillain-Barré Syndrome
  - Ataxia
  - Parkinson's Disease
  - Muscle Disease
  - Motor Neuron Disease
  - Movement Disorders

# Case Sheet Format

## HISTORY TAKING

Name:

Age:

Sex:

Residence:

Occupation:

**Chief complaints**

1. _____ × days
2. _____ × days
3. _____ × days

**History of presenting illness:**

## HIGHER MENTAL FUNCTION

**Altered state of consciousness:**
- Onset
- Any seizures and blackouts
- Any fall/injuries
- Any ear or nose bleed
- Fever
- Any ear pain or discharge
- Drug history
- Any addictions.

**Mental state and cognition:**
- Changes in the memory
- State of alertness and drowsiness
- Changes in the mood and affect (loss of spontaneity)
- Language changes
- Loss of spatial orientation
- Diminished ability to carry out routine activities of daily living.

**Other higher mental functions:**
- Speech difficulty
- Difficulty to recognize people or objects
- Inappropriate crying or laughter
- Lack of interest
- Social disinhibition
- Delusions/hallucinations.

## CRANIAL NERVE DYSFUNCTION

**Ask about:**
- Loss of vision, smell, and taste
- Alteration in facial feeling
- Double vision/visual symptoms
- Problems with swallowing and chewing
- Speech alterations
- Vertigo/hearing abnormalities
- Hoarseness of voice, dysphagia, nasal regurgitation, and nasal intonation of speech
- Pain/difficulty in neck movements.

**Example**

*Left lower motor neuron (LMN) 7th nerve palsy: History of retro-auricular pain followed by abrupt onset deviation of angle of mouth to right with slurring of speech and difficulty in left eye closure with history of hyperacusis.*

## MOTOR DYSFUNCTION

### Weakness

**Distribution of weakness:**
- Is it symmetrical/asymmetric:
- Paresis or plegia:
- Limbs involved: Ipsilateral or contralateral:
- Patterned weakness.

**Example**

*Right middle cerebral artery (MCA) territory embolic infarct: History of sudden onset, complete loss of power in left upper limb and lower limb. Weakness maximum at onset and nonprogressive.*

**Onset and progression:**

*Acute, subacute, or chronic.*

**Progression of the weakness:**
- *Ascending weakness or descending weakness*
- *Ellsberg phenomenon*
- *Variation throughout the day*
- *Muscles/limb(s) involved.*

| | |
|---|---|
| **Proximal upper limb—shoulder/arm** | Difficulties in combing hair, reaching for high objects, winging of scapula |
| **Distal upper limb—forearm/hand** | Finger/wrist drop, poor hand grip, cannot open jar, difficulty in buttoning/unbuttoning |
| **Proximal lower limb—pelvic/thigh** | Cannot rise from chair or squatting position, waddling gait |
| **Distal upper limbs—leg/foot** | Difficulty in gripping *chappals*, cannot walk on heels/toes foot drop |
| **Neck muscles** | Dropped head/broken neck |
| **Trunk** | Inability to roll on the bed |

### Example
*Guillain–Barré syndrome (GBS):* History of preceding gastrointestinal (GI) infection followed by acute onset difficulty in getting up from squatting position, difficulty walking, progressing to involve upper limbs (difficulty combing hair), and neck muscle weakness. No sensory symptoms.

### Wasting/Loss of Muscle Bulk
- Wasting—present/absent
- Fasciculations—present/absent

### Stiffness of Limbs
- Stiffness—present/absent
- Heaviness—present/absent

### Gait Abnormalities
- Limp or dragging foot
- Scissoring/circumduction.

### Involuntary Movements
- Type
- Symmetrical/asymmetrical
- Part of the body involved
- Present at rest
- Functional disability.

## SENSORY DYSFUNCTION
- Numbness/loss of feeling
- Altered feeling:
  - Paresthesia
  - Dysesthesias (tingling and pin-needles)
  - Spontaneous pain
- Pattern of sensory loss.

## CEREBELLAR HISTORY
- Swaying to one side
- Tremors while reaching objects
- Lack of coordination of activities
- Overshooting acts
- Abnormal involuntary eye movements (oscillopsia/nystagmus).

## HISTORY SUGGESTING MENINGITIS/RAISED INTRACRANIAL PRESSURE
- Headache
- Neck pain
- Projectile vomiting
- Blurring of vision
- Seizures
- Photophobia.

## HISTORY SUGGESTING AUTONOMIC DYSFUNCTION
- Dryness of skin
- Palpitations
- Perspiration
- Syncopal attacks/postural giddiness
- Bladder dysfunction:
  - Urinary retention
  - Loss of awareness of bladder control
  - Frequency, urgency
  - Urge/overflow incontinence.

## REVIEW OF COMMON NEUROLOGICAL SYMPTOMS

### Headaches
- Onset and duration of headache
- Location of headache, unilateral versus bilateral
- Severity
- Frequency
- Radiation
- Quality of headache (dull and diffuse)
- Types:
  a. Continuous
  b. Pulsating
  c. Stabbing
  d. Sharp
  e. Throbbing
  f. Dull
  g. Thunderclap
- Alleviating factors
- Triggers for the headache/aggravating factors
- Temporal association (headache not worse in mornings)
- Association with nausea/vomiting/tearing of eyes/redness of eyes
- Vision changes before or during headache
- Precipitating factors:
  - Stress
  - Menses
  - Allergens
  - Sleep deprivation
  - Coughing
  - Straining
  - Bending forwards
- Associated motor/sensory symptoms—weakness, numbness, and tingling in upper or lower extremities
- Photophobia/phonophobia
- Systemic symptoms—weight loss, low energy, and anorexia
- Fever and neck stiffness
- History of head trauma
- History of migraine
- Family history of migraines
- Effect on daily activities

- Use of oral contraceptive pills
- Caffeine intake
- Smoking and alcohol history.

**Example**

*Classical migraine: Visual aura followed by insidious onset, unilateral, severe pulsating type of heading lasting for >4 hours associated with nausea and photophobia. Repeated such attacks every month with history of some identifiable precipitating factors and a positive family history of migraine.*

## Seizures

- Onset and duration
- Frequency
- Factors which precipitate these episodes
- Injury sustained as a result of the seizure
- Postictal symptoms: Confusion
- Associated sensory deficits
- Associated motor deficits
- Associated cognitive deficits
- Muscle spasms
- Anatomical progression of motor involvement (e.g., Jacksonian March)
- Symptoms suggesting aura
- Associated incontinence
- Tongue biting and salivation
- Automatisms associated with these episodes
- History of head trauma
- Perinatal infection
- Drug history
- History of seizure disorder
- Family history of seizure disorders
- Effect on daily activities.

**Example**

*Generalized tonic-clonic seizure (GTCS): Abrupt onset tonic-clonic contraction of muscle associated with tongue bite and urinary incontinence. Patients generally regain consciousness within few minutes with postictal confusion and headache.*

**Past history:**

- Asthma
- Chronic obstructive airway disease
- Tuberculosis
- History of contact with tuberculosis
- Diabetes mellitus (DM)
- Hypertension (HTN)
- Ischemic heart disease (IHD)
- Seizure disorder and drugs used (in detail).

**Family history:**

(Draw pedigree chart representing three generations)

**Personal history:**

- Bowel habits
- Bladder habits
- Appetite
- Loss of weight
- Occupational exposure
- Sleep
- Dietary habits and taboo
- Food allergies
- Smoking (in smoking Index or Pack years)
- Alcohol history (_____grams of alcohol/day or_____units of alcohol/week).

**Menstrual and obstetric history:**

- G P L A
- Age of menarche
- Menopause at
- Flow—amenorrhea/oligorrhea/menorrhagia.

**Summarize:**

**Differential diagnosis:**

1.

2.

3.

# GENERAL EXAMINATION

## Patient

- Conscious
- Cooperative
- Obeying commands

## Body Mass Index (BMI)

- Wt (kg)/Ht (meters)
- Grading according to WHO for Southeast Asian countries.

## Vitals

- **Pulse**
  - Rate
  - Rhythm
  - Volume
  - Character
  - Vessel wall thickening
  - Radioradial delay and radiofemoral delay
  - Peripheral pulses
- **Carotid and vertebral bruit**
- **Blood pressure**
  - Right arm
  - Left arm
  - Leg—right/left
- **Respiratory rate**
  - Regular
  - Abdominothoracic (male) or thoracoabdominal (female)
  - Usage of accessory muscles

- **Jugular venous pulse**
  - Waveform
- **Jugular venous pressure**
  - cm of blood above sternal angle (+ 5 cm water)

## On Physical Examination

- Pallor
- Icterus
- Cyanosis
- Clubbing
- Lymphadenopathy
- Edema

## Others Head to Toe

- Nerve thickening
- Neurocutaneous markers
- External markers of atherosclerosis
- Signs of nutritional deficiency, alcoholism, etc.
- Any other general examination finding

# NERVOUS SYSTEM EXAMINATION

- Right/left handed person
- Education

# HIGHER MENTAL FUNCTIONS

- Consciousness—if impaired document using Glasgow coma scale
- Orientation to time/place/person
- Memory:
  - Immediate (repetition—30 seconds)
  - Recent (up to 5 minutes—recall)
  - Remote (>5 minutes)
- Intelligence
- Mood/emotion
- Concentration and calculation (subtract seven from 100)
- Speech:
  - Spontaneous speech—comprehension
  - Fluency
  - Repetition
  - Reading
  - Writing
  - Naming objects
  - Phonation
  - Aphasia
  - Dysarthria
- Apraxias—present/absent
- Hemineglect—present/absent
- Hallucinations and delusions—present/absent

| Cranial nerves | R | L |
|---|---|---|
| **Olfactory—I nerve:**<br>Sense of smell (peppermint, soap, coffee, lemon peel or vanilla)<br>*Both eyes shut, one nostril checked at a time<br>Appreciate smell ± identify it | | |

| Cranial nerves | R | L |
|---|---|---|
| **Optic—II nerve:**<br>Visual acuity (perception of light/hand movements and finger counting/Snellen's chart at 6 meters/Jaeger's chart at 14 inches)<br>Visual field (confrontation method/menace reflex)—mention defects, if any<br>Color vision (Ishihara's test)<br>Fundus | | |
| **Oculomotor, trochlear, abducens—III, IV, VI nerves:**<br>Eyelids (any ptosis)<br>Position of eyeballs at rest (any deviation, exophthalmos, enophthalmos)<br>Extraocular movements:<br>✦ Binocular movements<br>　– Saccadic:<br>　– Pursuit:<br>　– Reflex (Doll's eye, caloric stimulation)<br>✦ Uniocular movements<br>(#Comment on ophthalmoplegia, if present—supranuclear, internuclear, individual nerves, or muscles)<br>Pupil<br>✦ Size (in mm)<br>✦ Shape<br>✦ Reaction<br>✦ Direct light reflex<br>✦ Consensual light reflex<br>✦ Accommodation reflex<br>✦ Nystagmus<br>(Describe whether spontaneous or provoked/type—horizontal, vertical, rotatory, pendular) | | |
| **Trigeminal nerve—V nerve:**<br>✦ Sensory:<br>　– Touch<br>　– Pain<br>　– Temperature<br>　(To be checked on all three divisions around the jawline, on the cheek, and on the forehead)<br>✦ Motor:<br>　– Jaw deviation<br>　– Hollowing above and below zygoma<br>　– Clenching teeth (feel temporalis and masseter)<br>　– Open mouth against resistance<br>　– Side to side movement of jaw (pterygoid)<br>✦ Reflexes:<br>　– Corneal—present/absent (superficial reflex, 5th nerve afferent, 7th nerve efferent)<br>　– Jaw jerk—present/absent/exaggerated (deep reflex, afferent and efferent, both 5th nerve, center mid-pons) | | |

**Facial nerve—VII nerve:**
Facial asymmetry (look for absence of wrinkling, drooping of corner of mouth, obliteration of nasolabial fold, widened palpebral fissures)

| Cranial nerves | R | L |
|---|---|---|
| ♦ **Motor:** | | |
| – Frontalis (raise the eyebrows) | | |
| – Orbicularis oculi (shut the eyes tight) | | |
| – Buccinator (show teeth, smile, blow check, whistle) | | |
| – Orbicularis oris (close lips, pronounce labials "p","b","m") | | |
| – Platysma (pull down the corners of mouth) (## Look for Bell's phenomenon) | | |
| ♦ **Sensory:** | | |
| – Anterior 2/3rd tongue taste (sugar, lime, salt, quinine) | | |

**Lacrimation hyperacusis**—present/absent
**Emotional fibers checking**—emotions preserved or not

**Vestibulocochlear nerve—VIII nerve:**
The ability to hear the sound produced by rubbing the thumb and forefinger together is then tested for each ear at distances up to a few centimeters
♦ Rinne's test—air conduction/bone conduction (AC/BC)
♦ Weber's test—lateralized/centralized
♦ Caloric test [Irrigates one external auditory canal with cool (about 30°C) or warm (40°C) water. Normally, cool water in one ear produces nystagmus on the opposite side. Warm water produces it on the same side]

**Glossopharyngeal, vagus IX, X nerve:** Note the patient's ability to drink water and eat solid food and also see the character, volume and sound of the patient's voice.
♦ Position of uvula
♦ Movement of uvula on saying "ah"—any deviation
♦ Gag reflex—present/absent/exaggerated (taste over the posterior third of the tongue and can be tested)

**Spinal accessory—XI nerve:**
♦ Sternocleidomastoid (instruct the patient to rotate head against resistance applied to the side of the chin to tests the function of the opposite sternocleidomastoid muscle. To test both sternocleidomastoid muscles together, the patient flexes the head forward against resistance placed under the chin)
♦ Trapezius (shrugging a shoulder against resistance)

**Hypoglossal nerve—XII:**
Inspection (inside the mouth):
♦ Size of tongue
♦ Symmetry/any wasting
♦ Fasciculation (on protrusion)
♦ Deviation—side
♦ Tremors
♦ Palpation:
♦ Tone
♦ Power
♦ Speech

## MOTOR SYSTEM

### Attitude

♦ Upper limb
♦ Lower limb

### Bulk

♦ **Inspection:** Symmetry, generalized wasting comment on small muscle wasting, deformities, claw hand, foot drop, if any.

| Measurement in cm | R | L |
|---|---|---|
| Arm (10 cm above olecranon) | | |
| Forearm (10 cm below olecranon) | | |
| Thigh (18 cm above the superior border of patella) | | |
| Leg (10 cm below the tibial tuberosity) | | |

**Note:** Bilateral similar distance from fixed bony points till the maximum bulk of muscle.

### Tone

| | R | L |
|---|---|---|
| Upper limb | | |
| Lower limb | | |

**Note:** Comment whether normal, hypotonia or hypertonia (spasticity/rigidity).

### Power

Checked both isometric (resistance against movement) and isotonic (resistance at end of movement).

| 0 | Complete paralysis |
|---|---|
| 1 | A flicker of contraction only |
| 2 | Power detectable only when gravity is excluded by postural adjustment |
| 3 | Limb can be held against gravity but not resistance |
| 4 | Limb can be held against gravity and some resistance |
| 5 | Normal power |

| Muscle | R | L |
|---|---|---|

**Neck**
- **Flexors** (SCM, platysma, scalene, suprahyoid, infrahyoid, longus colli and capitis, rectus capitis)
- **Extensors** (trapezius and paravertebral muscles—splenius, erector spinae, transversospinalis, interspinal intertransverse)
  *Note:* Avoid active movement checking if cervical cord injury suspected

**Shoulder**
- **Abduction** (0–15°—supraspinatus, 15–90°—middle fibers of deltoid, above 90°—trapezius and serratus anterior)
- **Adduction** (pectoralis major, latissimus dorsi and teres major)

| Muscle | R | L |
|---|---|---|

- **Flexion** (biceps brachii (both heads), pectoralis major, anterior deltoid, and coracobrachialis)
- **Extension** (posterior deltoid, latissimus dorsi, and teres major)

**Elbow**
- Flexion (biceps brachii)
- Extension (triceps brachii)

**Wrist**
- Flexion (FCR, FCU)
- Extension (ECRL, ECRB, ECU)

**Hand grip** (long flexors)

Small muscles of hand

**Trunk** (rectus abdominis, transversus abdominis, oblique, pyramidalis)
- Elevation of head or leg in supine position
- Beevor's sign if present
- Abdominal binding to check for intercostal muscle weakness
- Intercostal binding to check for diaphragmatic weakness

**Hip**
- Flexion (iliopsoas)
- Extension (gluteus maximus)
- Abduction (gluteus medius and minimus, tensor fascia lata)
- Adduction (adductor longus, brevis, and magnus)

**Knee**
- Flexion (hamstrings)
- Extension (quadriceps)

**Ankle**
- Plantar flexion (gastrocnemius, soleus)
- Dorsiflexion (tibialis anterior)

**Small muscles of** foot, EHL if needed

# REFLEXES

| Superficial reflexes | R | L |
|---|---|---|

Corneal (cranial nerve V and VII)

**Abdominal:**
- Epigastric (T6–T9)
- Mid-abdominal (T9–T11)
- Hypogastric (T11–L1)

Cremasteric (L1, L2)

Anal reflex (S2, S3)

**Plantar:**
- Reflexogenic zone—S1
- Afferent nerve—tibial nerve
- SC segments—L4, L5, S1, S2

Chaddock's (lateral aspect of foot from below up), Gordon's (calf), Oppenheim's (anterior tibia), Schaffer's (Achilles tendon), Gonda's (press down 4th toe), Stransky's (adduct little toe), Bing's (pinprick on dorsolateral foot)

| Deep tendon reflexes | R | L |
|---|---|---|

Jaw jerk (afferent and efferent both 5th nerve and center mid-pons)

Biceps (C5, C6)

Brachioradial/supinator/radial periosteal (C5, C6)

Triceps (C6, C7, C8)

Knee jerk/quadriceps/patellar reflex (L2, L3, L4)

Ankle jerk (L5, S1, S2)

Clonus—present/absent
- Patellar
- Ankle

Latent reflexes (suggest pyramidal lesion if present unilaterally)
Tromner's/finger flexor reflex/Hoffmann's sign
Wartenberg's sign

By convention the deep tendon reflexes are graded as follows:
- 0 = no response; always abnormal
- 1+ = a slight but definitely present response; may or may not be normal
- 2+ = a brisk response; normal
- 3+ = a very brisk response; may or may not be normal
- 4+ = a tap elicits a repeating reflex (clonus); always abnormal

Please do reinforcement maneuvers before saying DTR's are absent

**Primitive reflexes**
- Glabellar tap
- Palmomental (both sides)
- Sucking
- Rooting
- Pout and snout
- Grasp

Involuntary movements (describe in detail)
Coordination (described later under cerebellum)

## SENSORY SYSTEM

| Primary sensation | R | L |
|---|---|---|
| Touch | | |
| Pain | | |
| Temperature | | |
| Vibration | | |
| Joint position sense<br>Any sensory level<br>Pattern of sensory loss<br>(graded/dissociative/crossed/hemi) | | |

| Cortical sensation (to be tested only in the presence of primary sensation intact) | R | L |
|---|---|---|
| Tactile localization (topognosis) | | |
| Two point discrimination | | |
| Stereognosis | | |
| Graphesthesia | | |
| Sensory extinction | | |

## ROMBERG'S TEST

### Cerebellar Signs

| Upper extremity | R | L |
|---|---|---|
| **Limb ataxia:**<br>• Outstretched arm test<br>• Finger nose test<br>• Nose-finger-nose test<br>• Finger-finger test | | |
| **Rapid alternating movements:**<br>• Rapid hand tapping<br>• Pronation-supination<br>• Thigh slapping | | |
| Pointing and past pointing | | |
| Writing (macrographia) | | |
| Rebound phenomenon (arm) | | |
| Tremors (intention) | | |

| Lower limbs | R | L |
|---|---|---|
| Heel knee test | | |
| Pendular knee jerk | | |
| Finger toe test | | |
| Rapid alternating movements—foot tapping | | |
| *General* | | |
| Titubation | | |
| Nystagmus | | |
| Tremors | | |

| Lower limbs | R | L |
|---|---|---|
| Hypotonia | | |
| Truncal ataxia | | |
| Tandem walking | | |
| Gait | | |

### Gait

- Base—wide or narrow
- Slow/rapid
- Falling to sides
- Look which part of foot touches ground first (toe/heel)
- How high foot lifted above ground?
- Hand swing
- Turning around
- Position of hip, sound produced while foot touches ground.

### Signs of Involvement of Autonomic Nervous System

- Dryness of skin/excessive sweating/spoon test
- Postural hypotension
- Heart rate—baseline, on respiration, on standing
- Palpable bladder
- Pupillary reactions
- Valsalva maneuver.

### Signs of Meningeal Irritation

- Neck stiffness
- Kernig's sign
- Brudzinski's sign—neck, leg, and pubis.

### Skull and Spine

- Deformities
- Tenderness
- Short neck.

## SOFT NEUROLOGICAL SIGNS

- ***Pyramidal drift*** describes a tendency for the hand to move upward and supinate if the hands are held outstretched in a pronated position (palms downward), or to pronate downward if the hands are held in supination.
- ***Cerebellar drift*** is generally upward with excessive rebound movements if the hand is suddenly displaced downward by the examiner.
- ***Parietal drift*** is an outward movement on displacing the ulnar border of the supinated hand.

## OTHER SYSTEMS

**Respiratory system**

- Inspection:
- Palpation:

- Percussion:
- Auscultation:

**Cardiovascular system:**
- Inspection:
- Palpation:
- Percussion:
- Auscultation:

**Gastrointestinal system:**
- Inspection:
- Palpation:
- Percussion:
- Auscultation:

# Sample Case Sheet and Discussion

## Case 1: Stroke

### Brief History
A A 40-year-old female named Mrs_____ hailing from_____ village, a coolie worker by occupation presented with:

### Presenting Complaints
- Sudden onset of weakness of right upper and lower limb since 20 days.
- Difficulty in speech since 20 days
- Deviation of angle of mouth to left since 20 days

### History of Presenting Illness
Patient was apparently normal 20 days back when she developed sudden onset weakness of right side involving both upper and lower limb equally, was also associated with deviation of angle of mouth to left side and loss of speech. Patient had one episode of loss of consciousness that lasted for approximately 5 minutes with no history of involuntary movements, tongue bite, up rolling of eyes, urinary or fecal incontinence. Patient was taken to a local hospital, advised for treatment in higher hospital, but was taken for Ayurvedic treatment and patient was at home for three days and was then shifted to Wenlock Hospital for further management where the patient stayed for 16 days. During her stay, patient feels there is improvement is weakness of the right side, improvement in her speech with minimal difficulty in speech.
- No history of convulsions
- No history of abnormal smell sensation.
- No history of difficulty in vision or double vision. No history of difficulty in chewing.
- No history of vertigo or difficulty in hearing or tinnitus.
- No history of nasal regurgitation.
- No history of hoarseness of voice or difficulty in swallowing. No history of involuntary movements.
- No history of decreased sensations or tingling or numbness. No history of head ache or vomiting.
- No history of swaying.
- No history of urinary retention or incontinence or diarrhea or constipation. No history of abnormal sweating.
- No history of fever.
- No history of neck pain.
- No complaints of chest pain, palpitations or dyspnea

### Past History
- No history of similar complaints in the past.
- No history of diabetes mellitus, hypertension, ischemic heart disease, asthma, seizures, prior transient ischemic attack, oral contraceptive usage.

### Personal History
- Patient consumes mixed diet. No bladder and bowel disturbances. No sleep disturbances.
- Appetite is normal.
- No history of any substance abuse, alcohol consumption.

### Family History
Not significant. Drug history: Not significant

### Marital History
- Married 10 years back, no history of any abortions Single male child aged 7 years.
- Last menstrual cycle —15th June 2018

### Summary
A 42-year-old female with no comorbidities presented with right-sided weakness, angle of deviation of mouth to left side and aphasia with no sensory and bladder involvement—left MCA infarct—embolic > thrombotic.

### General Examination
- Patient is conscious, cooperative and well oriented to time place and person. Moderately built, well nourished
- Length—1.55 meters.
- Weight—could not be assessed.
- Pallor present, no icterus, no cyanosis, no clubbing, no lymphadenopathy, no edema.
- PR=98/min irregularly irregular rhythm, varying volume, apex pulse deficit of 24 minutes, all peripheral pulses felt
- BP = Average of 100/70 mm Hg.
- No neurocutaneous markers, xanthelasmas, carotid/vertebral bruit.

### Nervous System Examination
- Right handed (by history), studied up to 7th standard Memory—immediate—normal
  - Recent—normal
  - Remote—normal
- Intelligence—normal
- No emotional lability
- Calculation—unable to assess
- Concentration—inattentive
- Speech—comprehension, repetition, naming, reading—normal fluency—labored speech
- Writing—unable to assess

### Cranial Nerve Examination

| Cranial nerve | Right | Left |
| --- | --- | --- |
| Olfactory nerve | Normal | Normal |
| Optic nerve | Normal | Normal |
| Visual acuity | Normal | Normal |

| Cranial nerve | Right | Left |
|---|---|---|
| Visual field | Normal | Normal |
| Color vision | Normal | Normal |
| Fundus 3rd, 4th, 6th nerves | Reactive to light | Reactive to light |
| Pupil | Present | Present |
| Light and accommodation reflex | Normal | Normal |
| Extraocular movements | Normal | Normal |
| Trigeminal nerve Sensory and motor functions | Normal | Normal |
| Corneal reflex | Present | Present |
| Facial nerve | Normal | Angle of mouth deviated to the left |
| Vestibulocochlear nerve | Normal | Normal |
| Glossopharyngeal and vagus nerve | Gag reflex present | Gag reflex present |
| Spinal accessory nerve | Could not be assessed | Normal |
| Hypoglossal nerve | Normal, no wasting or fasciculations | Normal, no wasting or fasiculations |

**Motor System**

*Attitude:*
- Upper limb—right side adducted at shoulder, extended at elbow and externally rotated.
- Lower limb—right side extended and externally rotated at hip joint and knee (R>L), plantar flexion.

| Bulk | Right | Left |
|---|---|---|
| Arm | 22 | 22 |
| Forearm | 18 | 18 |
| Thigh | 35 | 35 |
| Leg | 24 | 24 |

| Tone | Right | Left |
|---|---|---|
| Upper limb | Increased | Normal |
| Lower limb | Increased | Normal |
| Power | Right | Left |
| Upper limb | 0/5 | 5/5 |
| Lower limb | 0/5 | 5/5 |

No involuntary movements

*Reflexes*

| | Right | Left |
|---|---|---|
| Biceps | +++ | ++ |
| Triceps | +++ | ++ |
| Supinator | +++ | ++ |
| Knee | +++ | ++ |
| Ankle | Clonus | ++ |
| Plantar | Extensor | Flexor |

- Sensory system examination: Normal.
- Cerebellar signs: could not be assessed.
- Gait: Could not be assessed.
- Skull and spine: Normal

**Respiratory System**
- Trachea central
- Bilateral chest movements equal.
- Normal vesicular breath sounds heard bilaterally. No added sounds.

**Cardiovascular System**
- Examination Apex beat in left 5th intercostal space 1 cm medial to midclavicular line
- S1, S2 heard, no murmur

**Per Abdomen**
- Soft, non-tender, no organomegaly, no free fluid
- Bowel sounds present.

**Final Diagnosis**

Right-sided hemiparesis with right 7th cranial nerve UMN palsy, no sensory disturbances, no bladder and bowel disturbance, no signs of raised ICT, with atrial fibrillation, etiology being emboli leading to ischemia probably in the MCA territory.

## DISCUSSION

### Q. Define stroke.

A stroke (cerebrovascular accident is a vague term which should be avoided) is defined as a syndrome of rapid (abrupt) onset of a neurologic deficit that is attributable to a focal vascular cause.

**World Health Organization (WHO) definition:** Stroke is a "rapidly developing clinical signs of focal (or global) disturbance of cerebral function, with symptoms lasting for 24 hours or longer or leading to death, with no apparent cause other than of vascular origin".

### Q. How do you classify stroke?

Refer **Figure 4.1**.

### Q. What are the types of stroke?

1. **Progressing stroke (or stroke in evolution):** It is a stroke in which the focal neurological deficit worsens after the patient first presents. It may be due to increasing volume of infarction, secondary hemorrhage in the infarcted area, or increasing cerebral edema.
2. **Complete stroke:** Rapid onset with persistent focal neurological deficit which does not progress beyond 96 hours.

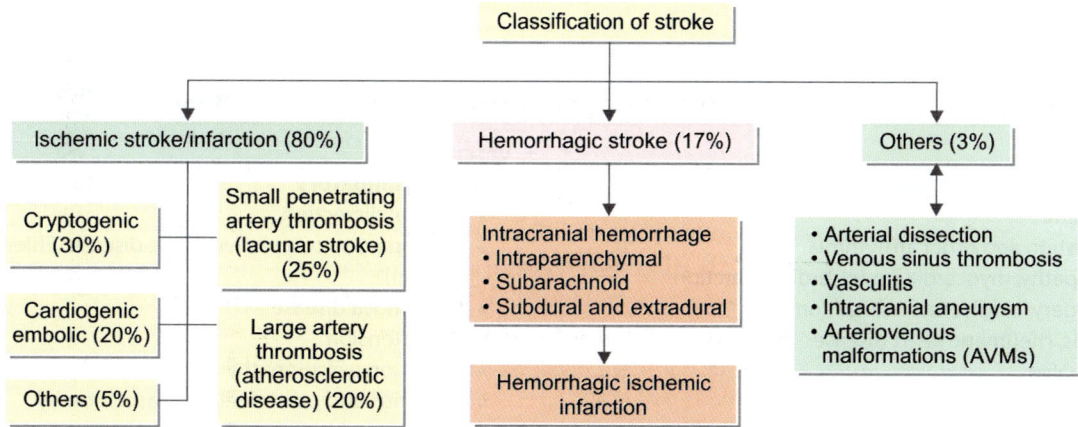

**Fig. 4.1:** Classification of stroke.

3. **Evolving stroke:** Gradual stepwise development of neurological deficits. Focal cerebral deficits that develop slowly (over weeks to months) are unlikely to be due to stroke and are more suggestive of tumor or inflammatory or degenerative disease.

### Q. Define RIND, TIA and stuttering hemiplegia?

Several terms are used to classify strokes mainly based on the duration and evolution of symptoms.

- **Transient ischemic attack (TIA):** Described later.
- **Reversible ischemic neurological deficit (RIND):** In some cases, deficits last for longer than 24 hours but resolve completely or almost completely within a few days.
- **Stuttering hemiplegia:** Internal carotid lesions are characterized by repeated episodes of TIA followed by fully evolved stroke.

### Q. What are the risk factors for stroke?

Refer **Table 4.1**.

**Table 4.1:** Risk factor for stroke.

***Risk factors in patients of all age groups***

***High-risk***

| | |
|---|---|
| • Hypertension (including isolated systolic) | • High cholesterol |
| • Smoking | • Obesity |
| • Diabetes mellitus | • Vasculitis: Systemic vasculitis [e.g., polyarteritis nodosa—PAN), granulomatosis with polyangiitis (Wegener's) etc.], primary CNS vasculitis |
| • Atrial fibrillation | |
| • Drugs: Cocaine, amphetamine | |
| • Dilated cardiomyopathy | • Meningitis (syphilis, tuberculosis, fungal, bacterial, zoster) |
| • Endocarditis | |

***Low-risk***

| | |
|---|---|
| • Migraine | • Recent myocardial infarction |
| • Oral contraceptives or alcohol | • Prosthetic valve |
| • Patent foramen ovale | • Sleep apnea |

***Additional risk factors that are more common in young patients***

***Hypercoagulable disorders***

| | |
|---|---|
| • Protein C and S deficiencies | • Sickle-cell anemia |
| | • Hyperhomocysteinemia |
| • Antithrombin III deficiency | • Thrombotic thrombocytopenic purpura |
| • Antiphospholipid antibody syndrome | • Arterial dissection |
| • Factor V Leiden mutation | • Infections (e.g., syphilis, HIV) |
| • Prothrombin G20210A heterozygous mutation | • Systemic malignancy |

(CNS: central nervous system; HIV: human immunodeficiency virus)

**Q. What are the causes for stroke in young?**
Refer **Table 4.2**.

**Table 4.2:** Causes for young stroke.

- **Cardiac**
  - Congenital heart disease, patent foramen ovale
  - Atrial myxoma
  - Atrial fibrillation and other arrhythmia
  - Cardiomyopathy, myocarditis, myocardial infarction
  - Cardiac surgery, cardiac catheterization
  - Endocarditis, rheumatic heart disease
  - Prosthetic valve
- **Hematologic**
  - Sickle cell disease, iron deficiency anemias, polycythemia vera
- **Hypercoagulable states**
  - Inherited prothrombotic states, protein C and S deficiency, antithrombin III deficiency, factor V Leidengene mutation, prothrombin gene mutation
  - Antiphospholipid antibody syndrome
  - Hyperhomocysteinemia
  - Myeloproliferative disorders (e.g., leukemia, lymphoma)
  - Pregnancy exposure to hormonal treatments, such as anabolic steroids and erythropoietin, nephrotic syndrome
- **Vascular**
  - **Noninflammatory**
    » Arterial dissection
    » Secondary to connective tissue disease (Ehlers-Danlos, Marfan)
    » Moyamoya disease
    » Hypertension
    » Radiation vasculopathy
    » Vasculitis and postinfectious vasculopathy
    » Migraine
    » Cerebral autosomal dominant arteriopathy with subcortical infarcts and leukoencephalopathy (CADASIL)
    » Fibromuscular dysplasia, Susac's syndrome, Sneddon's syndrome, Fabry's disease
- **Inflammatory**
  - Takayasu arteritis
  - Giant cell arteritis
  - Kawasaki disease
  - Polyarteritis nodosa
  - Human immunodeficiency virus (HIV)
  - Bacterial meningitis

**Illicit drug use:** Cocaine, amphetamine

**Q. List the differences between hemorrhagic, thrombotic, and embolic strokes.**
Refer **Table 4.3**.

**Table 4.3:** Differences between hemorrhagic, thrombotic, and embolic strokes.

| Feature | Hemorrhagic stroke (intra-cerebral or subarachnoid hemorrhage) | Ischemic stroke | |
| --- | --- | --- | --- |
| | | Thrombotic | Embolic |
| Time of onset of stroke | During activity | Suddenly and often during sleep or in the early morning (4 AM) | Any time (usually during activity) |
| Rapidity of onset and progression | Over minutes and hours | On waking up or over hours | Rapid within seconds deficit maximum at onset |
| Transient ischemic attacks (TIAs) | Absent | Precedes stroke | Precedes stroke |
| Vomiting | Recurrent | Absent or occasional | Absent or occasional |
| Headache | Severe and prominent | Mild or absent | Mild or absent |
| Early resolution (within minutes or days) | Unusual | Variable | Possible |
| Meningeal irritation | May be present | Absent | Absent |
| Carotid bruit and absence of pulse | Not observed | Highly supports the diagnosis | Possible |
| Valvular heart disease and atrial fibrillation | Not found | Unusual | Highly supports the diagnosis |
| CT scan findings | Hemorrhage | Early stage: Normal Later: Pale infarct | Early stage: Normal Later: Pale infarct |

## Q. Discuss the salient features of stroke based on site of lesion.

Refer **Table 4.4** and **Figures 4.2A to C**.

| Table 4.4: Localization of stroke. | |
|---|---|
| **Site of lesion** | **Predominant clinical features** |
| Cortex | • Monoplegia common (brachial—MCA territory; crural—ACA territory)<br>• Hemiplegia (may be present but never dense)<br>• Contralateral 7th cranial nerve palsy (UMN variant)<br>• Seizures<br>• Aphasias (in dominant hemisphere)<br>• Apraxias (in nondominant hemisphere) |
| Subcortical (usually secondary to hypoperfusion) | • Monoplegias common<br>• Transcortical aphasias common |
| Internal capsule lesion (Fig. 4.3) | • Contralateral hemiplegia (dense)<br>• Contralateral hemisensory loss<br>• 7th cranial nerve palsy (UMN variant)<br>• Homonymous hemianopia<br>• Broca's like aphasia (only site to have subcortical aphasia).<br>*Note: Most common etiology being ischemic and hence is territory specific. Since different parts of internal capsule has blood supply from different blood vessels, all the above-mentioned features may not be present at same time. However, if present, it suggests hemorrhage or tumor compressing internal capsule* |
| Brainstem lesion | Discussed in separate table |
| High cervical cord lesion (Brown-Sequard syndrome) | • Ipsilateral hemiplegia<br>• Ipsilateral loss of posterior column sensation<br>• Contralateral loss of pain and temperature sensation<br>• Usually no cranial nerve involvement |

(ACA: anterior cerebral artery; MCA: middle cerebral artery; UMN: upper motor neuron)

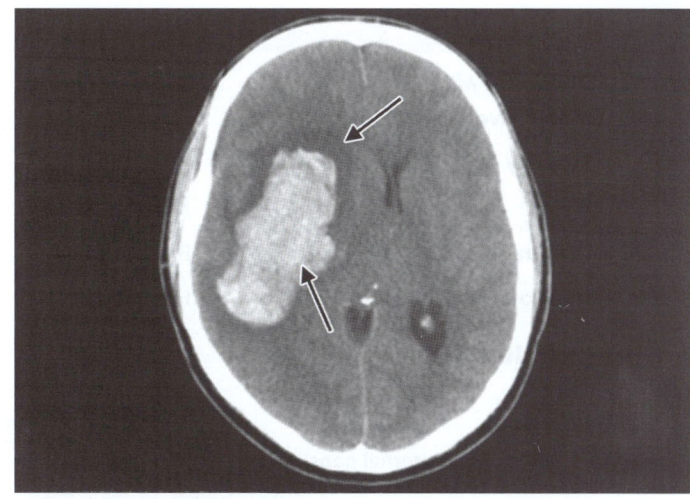

**Fig. 4.3:** CT showing hemorrhage in internal capsule.

## Q. What are the features of MCA stroke?

Refer **Table 4.5**.

| Table 4.5: Middle cerebral artery lesions and clinical features. | | | |
|---|---|---|---|
| **Internal carotid artery** | **Stem of MCA** | **M1 branch of MCA** | **M2 branches of MCA** |
| Both anterior cerebral artery (ACA) and middle cerebral artery (MCA) territory involved along with ophthalmic artery causing amaurosis fugax | • Global aphasia<br>• Dense hemiplegia (as internal capsule is also involved due to involvement of lenticulostriate branches of MCA) | • Global aphasia<br>• Internal capsule spared | • Superior division<br>• Inferior division (differences described below) |

## Q. What are features of M2 strokes?

Refer **Table 4.6**.

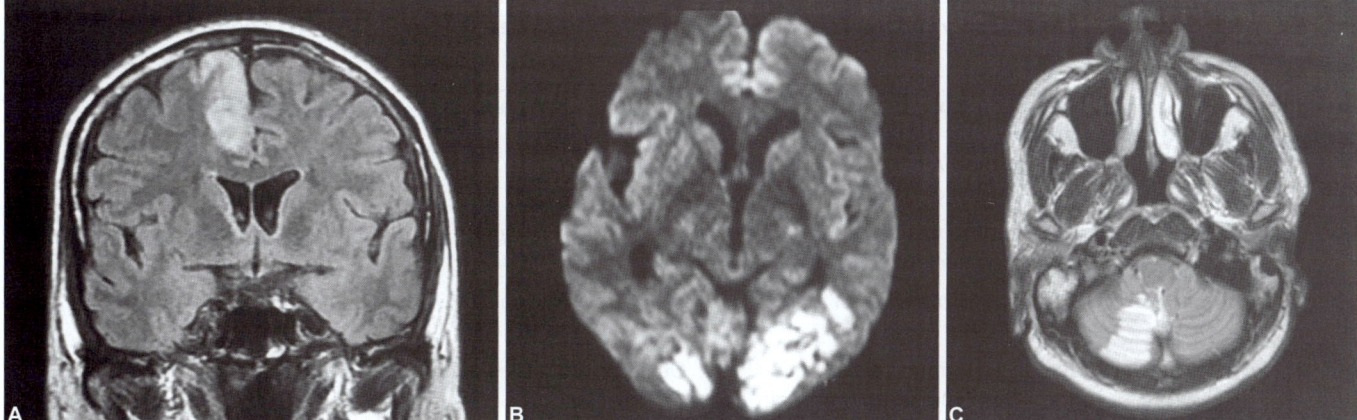

**Figs. 4.2A to C:** Neuroimaging in stroke: (A) Acute right anterior cerebral artery (ACA) infarct; (B) Acute bilateral posterior cerebral artery (PCA) infarct—Anton's syndrome; (C) Right lateral medullary syndrome.

| Table 4.6: M2 stroke. | | |
|---|---|---|
| **Division of M2** | **Superior division** | **Inferior division** |
| Motor involvement | Face, arm > leg | Nil |
| Sensory | Face, arm | Nil |
| Vision | Nil | Quadrantanopia |
| Language | Broca's aphasia | Wernicke's aphasia |
| Nondominant | Hemineglect | Constructional apraxia |

**Q. What is localization of hemiplegia?**

Refer **Figure 4.4**.

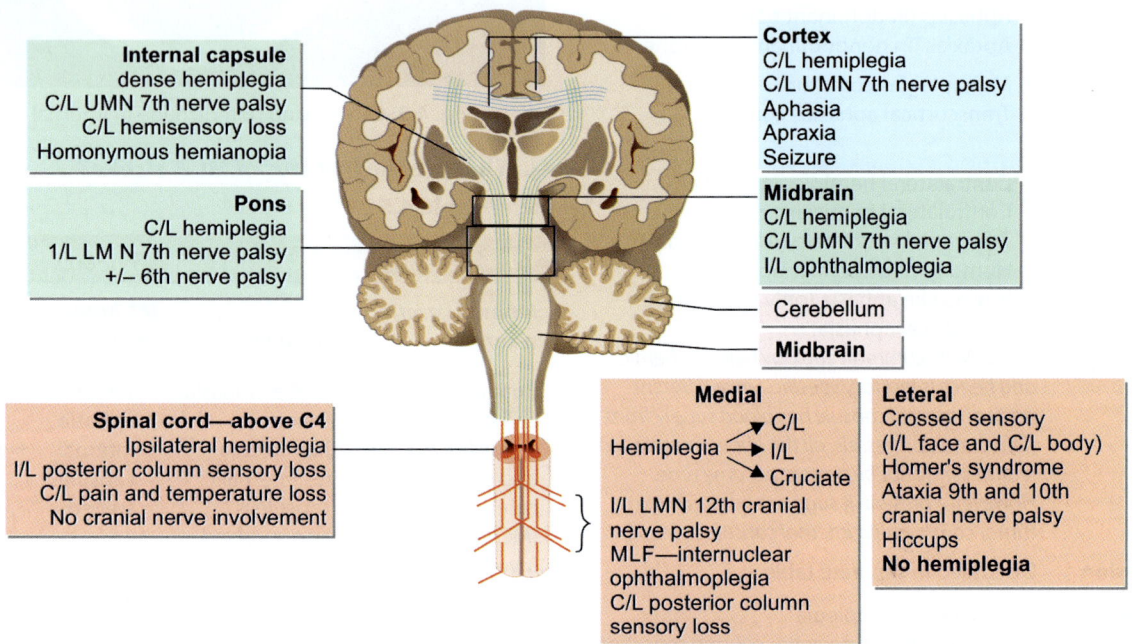

**Fig. 4.4:** Localization of hemiplegia.
(UMN: upper motor neuron; LMN: lower motor neuron; MLF: medial longitudinal fasciculus)

**Q. Discuss the features of brainstem syndromes based on location.**

Refer **Table 4.7 and Figures 4.5 to 4.12**.

| Table 4.7: Brainstem syndromes. | | | |
|---|---|---|---|
| **Site of lesion/syndrome** | **Blood supply and tracts involved** | **Ipsilateral features** | **Contralateral features** |
| **Midbrain** | | | |
| **Benedict's syndrome (Claude's + Weber)** | Interpeduncular branches of basilar artery, PCA—posterior cerebral artery (midbrain tegmentum—CN III fibers; red nucleus; CST; SCP) | Ipsilateral CN III palsy | Ataxia + Hyperkinesia and tremor ("rubral tremor") + Hemiparesis |
| **Claude's syndrome** | PCA (midbrain tegmentum—CN III fibers; red nucleus; SCP) | Ipsilateral CN III palsy | Ataxia + Tremor ("rubral tremor") |
| **Weber's syndrome** | Paramedian branches of the basilar artery, PCA | Ipsilateral CN III palsy | Hemiparesis |
| **Nothnagel syndrome** | Basilar penetrating artery, mesencephalic artery (midbrain tectum—ipsilateral or bilateral CN III) | Oculomotor palsies; ataxia | |

| Site of lesion/syndrome | Blood supply and tracts involved | Ipsilateral features | Contralateral features |
|---|---|---|---|
| **Parinaud syndrome** | Midbrain dorsum (quadrigeminal plate region; pretectum; periaqueductal gray matter) | Impaired gaze (Sunset sign); convergence retraction nystagmus; dilated pupils with light near dissociation, pseudo-ARP, Collier's sign (overactive LPS), pseudo-abducent palsy | |
| **Top of basilar artery syndrome** | + Midbrain<br>+ Thalamus<br>+ Portion of temporal and occipital lobe involved | + Behavioral abnormalities<br>+ Ocular finding<br>+ Visual defects<br>+ Pupillary abnormalities<br>+ Motor deficits | |
| **Artery of Percheron stroke** | Single thalamic perforating artery from the proximal PCA | + Altered sensorium<br>+ Vertical gaze palsy<br>+ Memory impairment | |
| **Pons** | | | |
| **Raymond syndrome** | Long circumferential branch of basilar artery (CN VI; CST) | 6th nerve palsy | Hemiparesis |
| **Millard-Gubler syndrome** | Basilar artery (CN VII; CST) | 7th nerve palsy (± Lateral rectus palsy) | Hemiparesis |
| **Foville's syndrome** | Basilar artery (CN VII; lateral gaze center, CST) | 7th nerve palsy +Ipsilateral Horizontal gaze palsy | Hemiparesis |
| **Pierre-Marie-Foix syndrome** | AICA | 6th + 7th nerve palsy Horner's syndrome + Ipsilateral Ataxia | Hemiparesis |
| **Medulla** | | | |
| **Wallenberg syndrome (lateral medullary syndrome)** | Vertebral artery > PICA (lateral medullary tegmentum—spinal tract of CN V and its nucleus; nucleus ambiguus; emerging fibers of CNs IX and X; LST; descending sympathetic fibers; vestibular nuclei; inferior cerebellar peduncle; afferent spinocerebellar tracts; lateral cuneate nucleus) | + Loss of pain and temperature of face<br>+ Ipsilateral decreased corneal reflex<br>+ Ipsilateral weakness of soft palate<br>+ Ipsilateral loss of gag reflex<br>+ Ipsilateral paralysis of vocal cord<br>+ Ipsilateral central Horner's syndrome<br>+ Nystagmus<br>+ Cerebellar ataxia of ipsilateral limbs<br>+ Lateropulsion<br>+ **Hiccups** | Loss of pain and temperature of body |
| **Dejerine syndrome (medial medullary syndrome)** | Vertebral > anterior spinal artery | Ipsilateral tongue weakness | Hemiparesis |
| **Avellis' syndrome** | Medullary tegmentum | Ipsilateral palatal and vocal cord weakness | Loss of pain and temperature |
| **Jackson's syndrome** | Medullary tegmentum | Ipsilateral flaccid paralysis of soft palate, pharynx, and larynx; flaccid weakness and atrophy of SCM and trapezius (partial), and of the tongue | |
| **Schmidt's** | Lower medullary tegmentum | Ipsilateral paralysis of soft palate, pharynx, and larynx; flaccid weakness and atrophy of SCM and trapezius (partial) | |

| Site of lesion/syndrome | Blood supply and tracts involved | Ipsilateral features | Contralateral features |
|---|---|---|---|
| Céstan-Chenais | Due to vertebral artery occlusion below origin of the PICA (nucleus ambiguus; ICP; sympathetics; CST; ML) | Ipsilateral weakness of soft palate, pharynx, and larynx; cerebellar ataxia; Horner's syndrome | Contralateral hemiparesis with loss of posterior column function |
| Internuclear ophthalmoplegia (INO) | MLF lesion in the midbrain | Ipsilateral adduction palsy | Contralateral gaze evoked nystagmus |
| Wall eyed bilateral internuclear ophthalmoplegia (WEBINO) | Bilateral MLF lesion in the brain | Bilateral adduction deficit and primary gaze position exotropia | |
| PCA syndromes | | | |
| Gerstmann syndrome | Parietal lobe | Inability to write (dysgraphia or agraphia), the loss of the ability to do mathematics (acalculia), the inability to identify one's own or another's fingers (finger agnosia), and inability to make the distinction between the right and left side of the body | |
| Anton syndrome | Bilateral occipital cortex involvement due to bilateral PCA infarct | Anton's syndrome describes the condition in which patients deny their blindness despite objective evidence of visual loss, and moreover confabulate to support their stance | Anosognosia (or lack of awareness of defect) and confabulation |
| Balint syndrome | Parieto-occipital lobes on both sides of the brain | Inability to perceive the visual field as a whole (simultanagnosia), difficulty in fixating the eyes (oculomotor apraxia), and inability to move the hand to a specific object by using vision (optic ataxia) | |

(CN: cranial nerve; CST: corticospinal tract; SCP: superior cerebellar peduncle; AICA: anterior inferior cerebellar artery; PICA: posterior inferior cerebellar artery; LST: lateral spinothalamic tract; SCM: sternocleidomastoid muscle; ICP: intracranial pressure; CST: corticospinal tract; ML: medial lemniscus; MLF: medial longitudinal fasciculus; PCA: posterior cerebral artery)

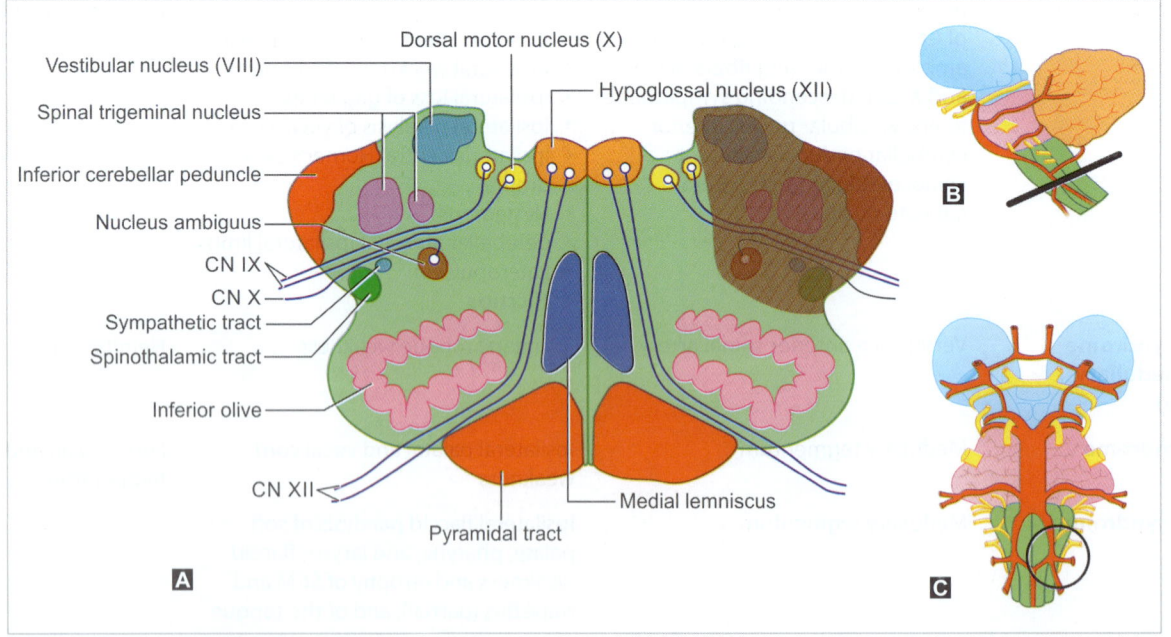

**Figs. 4.5A to C:** Lateral medullary syndrome.

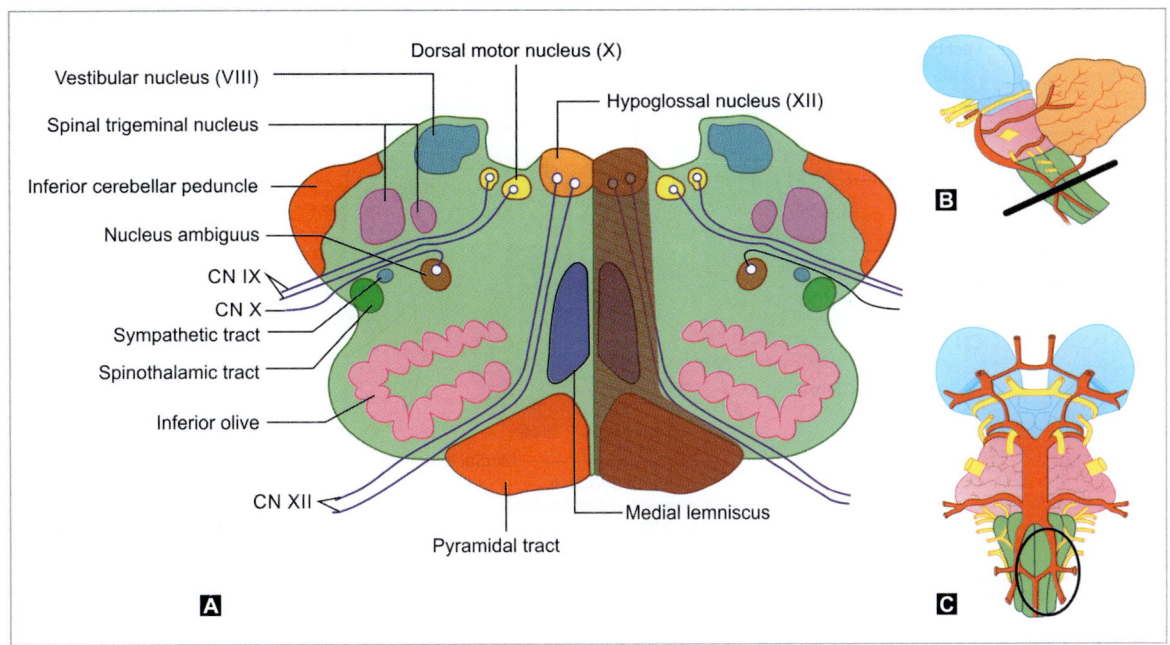

**Figs. 4.6A to C:** Medial medullary syndrome.

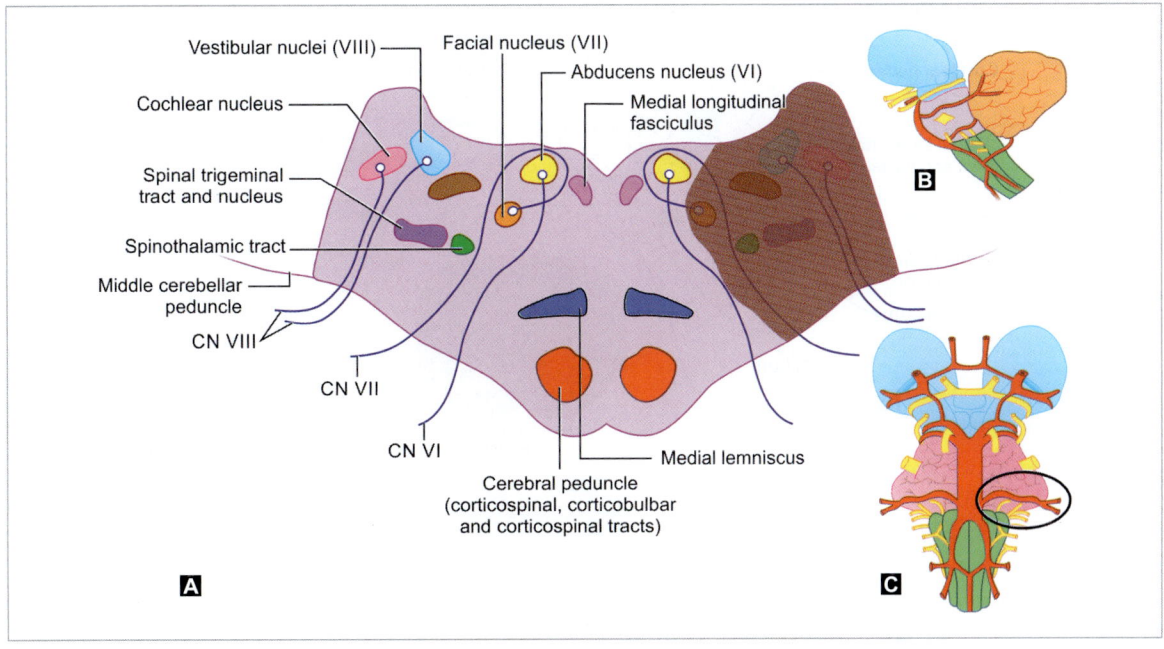

**Figs. 4.7A to C:** Lateral pontine syndrome.

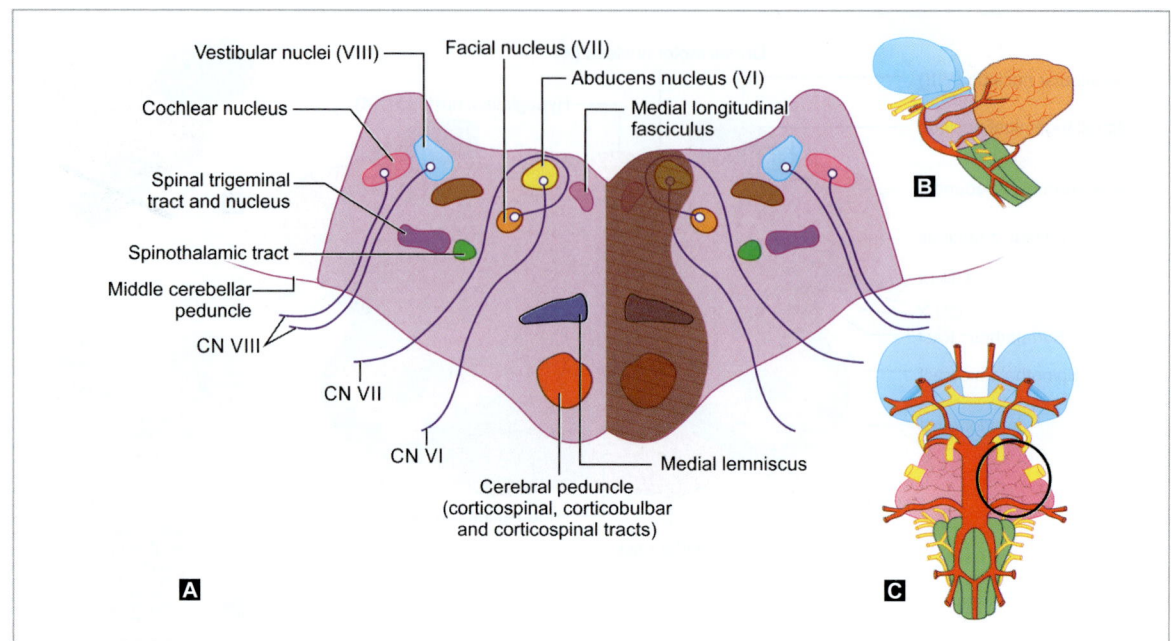

**Figs. 4.8A to C:** Medial pontine syndrome.

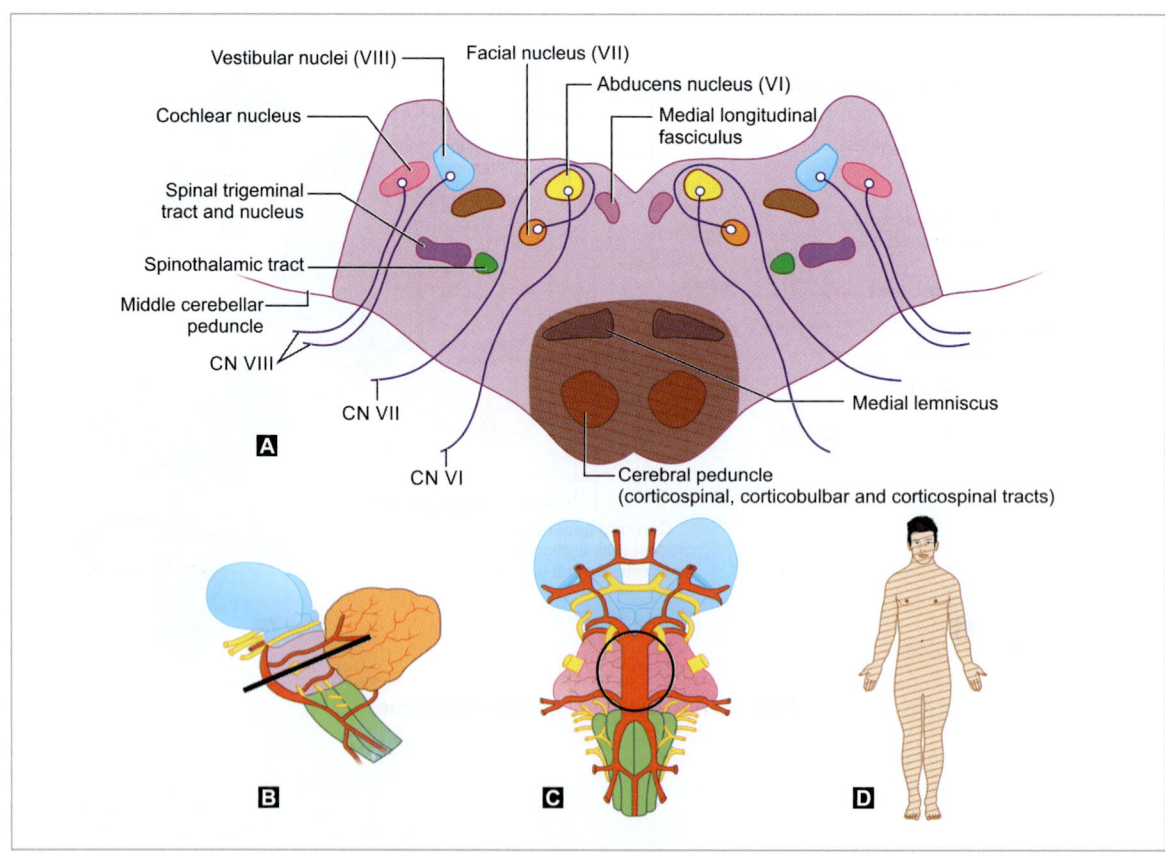

**Figs. 4.9A to D:** Ventral pontine syndrome.

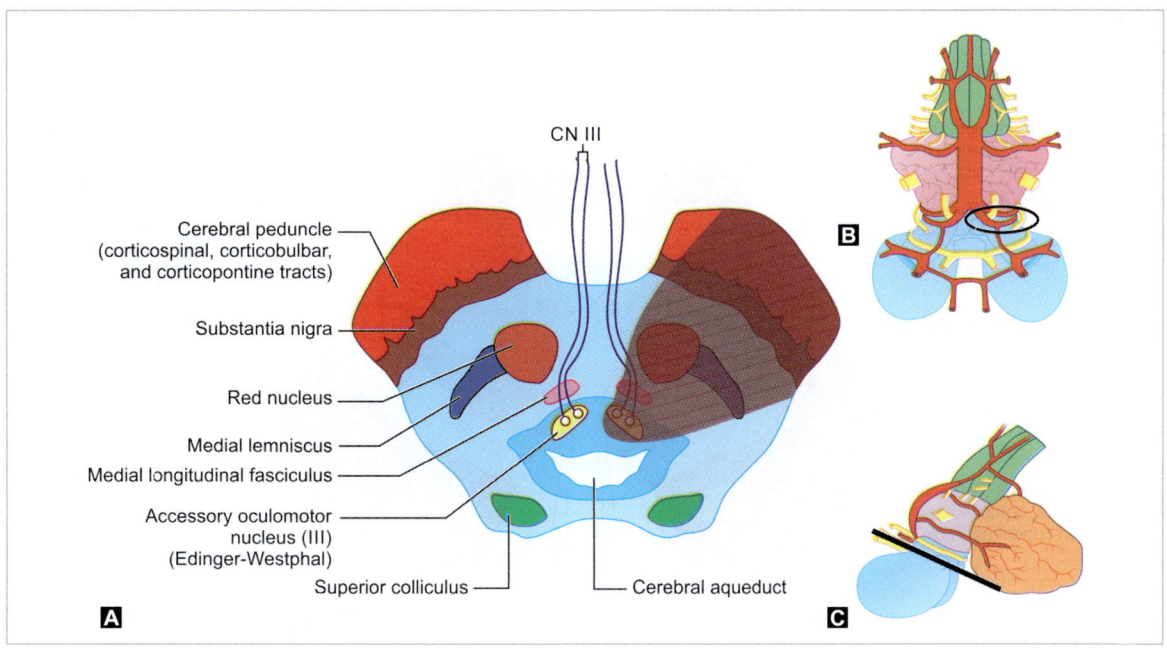

**Figs. 4.10A to C:** Lateral midbrain syndrome.

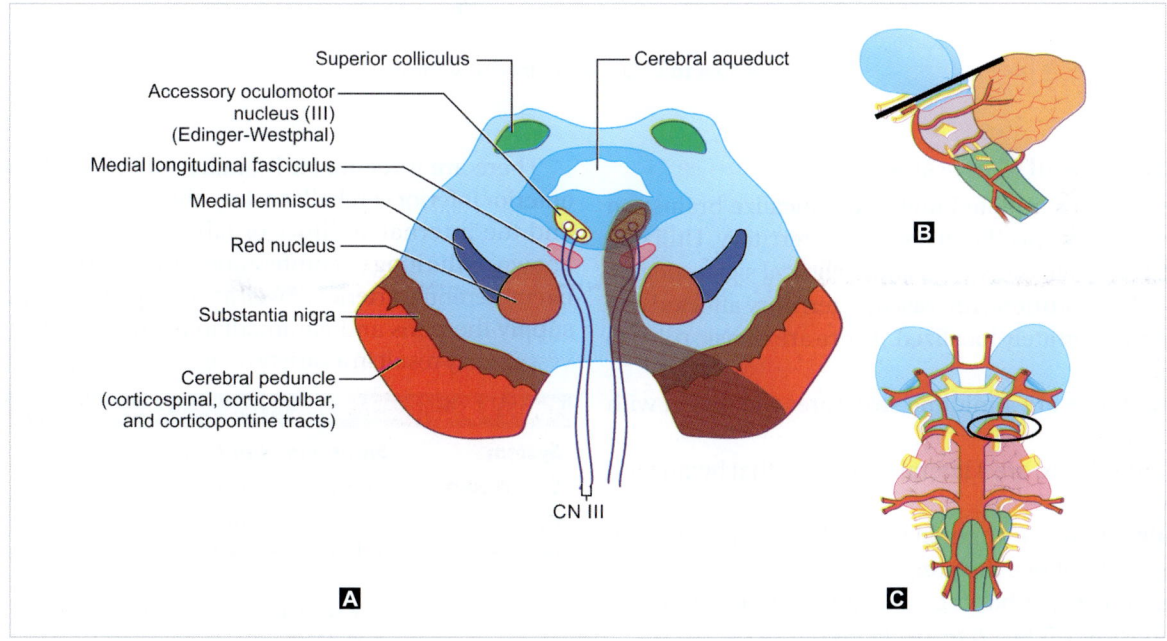

**Figs. 4.11A to C:** Medial midbrain syndrome.

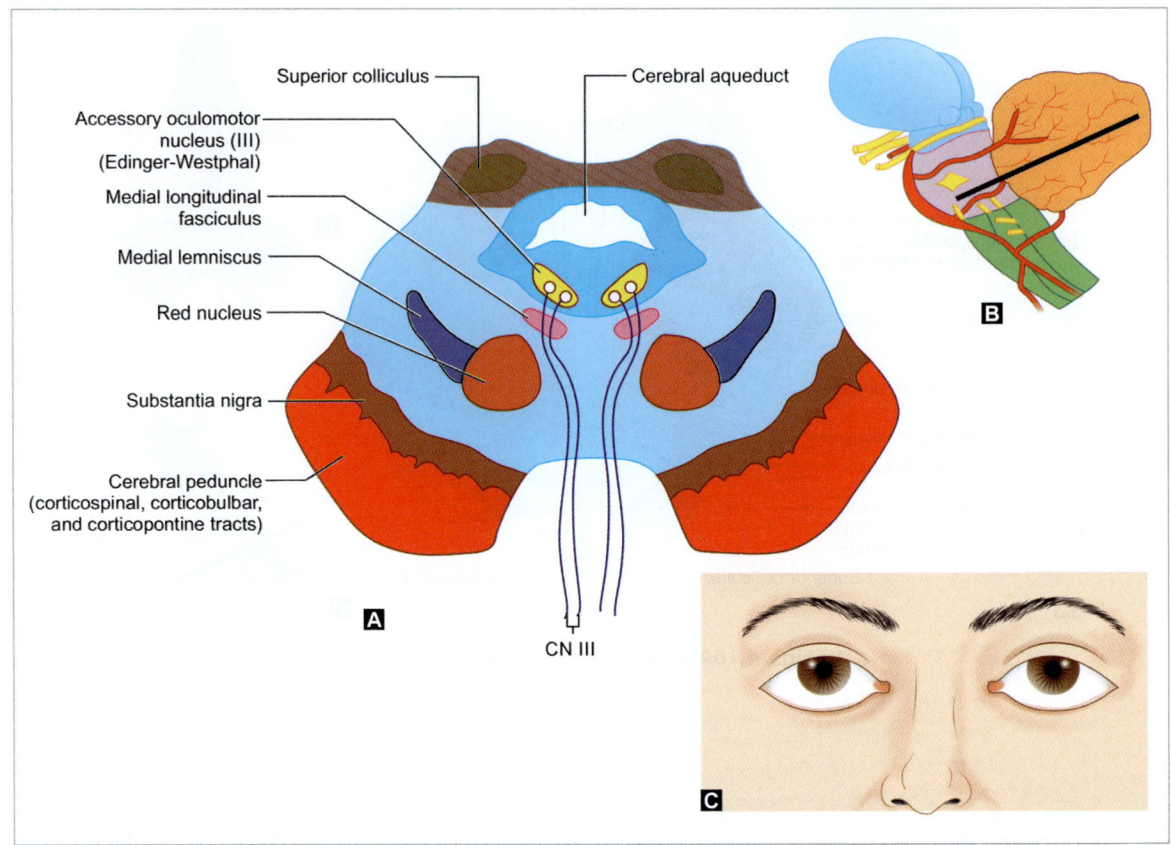

**Figs. 4.12A to C:** Dorsal midbrain syndrome.

### Q. What is the "rule of 4" in brainstem?

The "rule of 4" is a simplified method to localize brainstem vascular syndromes specific to a vascular territory. Utilizing the "rule of 4" as well as distinguishing clinical signs specific to each vascular syndrome, the vascular territory affected can be quickly and accurately localized. There are 4 basic rules to this schema

1. **First rule:** There are 4 midline structures that begin with the letter M.
2. **Second rule:** There are 4 lateral structures that begin with the letter S
3. **Third rule:** There are 4 cranial nerves below the pons, 4 in the pons, and 4 above the pons
    - Medulla: Glossopharyngeal, vagus, spinal accessory, hypoglossal (CN 9–12, respectively)
    - Pons: Trigeminal, abducens, facial, vestibulocochlear (CN 5–8, respectively)
    - Midbrain: Oculomotor, trochlear (CN 3–4, respectively)
4. **Fourth rule:** There are 4 midline cranial nerve motor nuclei
    - The nuclei of cranial nerves 3, 4, 6, and 12.

### Q. What are the clinical features of basilar artery ischemia?

The basilar artery is formed at the junction of the medulla with the pons by the merger of the two vertebral arteries.

There are three major branches of the basilar artery—the anterior inferior cerebellar artery, the superior cerebellar artery and the internal auditory or labyrinthine artery. These are known as the long circumferential arteries. There are also short circumferential arteries as well as small penetrating arteries that supply the pons and paramedian regions. Occlusion of these vessels may result in a variety of signs and symptom **(Table 4.8)**.

| Table 4.8: Clinical features of basilar artery ischemia. | |
|---|---|
| **System** | **Signs and symptoms** |
| Sensorium | Alterations of consciousness |
| Cranial nerves | • Pupil abnormalities<br>• III, IV and VI with dysconjugate gaze<br>• Horner's syndrome<br>• V with ipsilateral facial hypoalgesia<br>• Nystagmus<br>• VII with unilateral LMN facial paralysis<br>• Caloric and oculocephalic reflexes<br>• Vertigo<br>• IX and X with dysphagia, dysarthria |
| Motor | Quadriplegia or contralateral hemiplegia |
| Sensory | Contralateral limb hypoalgesia |
| Cerebellum | Ipsilateral or bilateral cerebellar abnormalities |
| Respiratory | Respiratory irregularities |
| Cardiac | Cardiac arrhythmias and erratic blood pressure |

**Q. What is anatomy of posterior cerebral artery (PCA)?**

Although the posterior cerebral arteries primarily supply the occipital cerebral hemispheres they usually arise from the posterior circulation. The posterior cerebral arteries arise as terminal branches of the basilar artery in 70% of individuals, from one basilar and the opposite carotid in 20–25% and directly from the carotid circulation in 5–10%. Both PCAs receive a posterior communicating vessel from the internal carotid artery and then arch posteriorly around the cerebral peduncles to the tentorial surface of the cerebrum. They supply the inferolateral and medial surfaces of the temporal lobe, the lateral and medial surfaces of the occipital lobe and the upper brainstem. Included in this area is the midbrain, visual cortex, cerebral peduncles, thalamus and splenium of the corpus callosum.

**Q. List the clinical features of PCA syndrome.**

Refer **Table 4.9**.

**Table 4.9:** Syndromes of PCA occlusions.

| | |
|---|---|
| Thalamoperforate branch occlusion | • Involuntary movement disorders<br>• Hemiataxia<br>• Intention tremor<br>• Weber's syndrome: Ipsilateral oculomotor palsy with contralateral hemiparesis<br>• Claude's or Benedict's syndrome: Ipsilateral oculomotor palsy with contralateral cerebellar ataxia |
| Thalamogeniculate branch occlusion (thalamic syndrome) | • Contralateral sensory loss<br>• Transient contralateral hemiparesis<br>• Contralateral mild involuntary movements<br>• Intense, persistent, burning pain |
| Cortical branch occlusion | • Contralateral homonymous hemianopsia<br>• Dominant hemisphere—alexia, memory impairment or anomia, especially for naming colors<br>• Non-dominant hemisphere—topographic disorientation (usually due to parietal damage)<br>• Prosopagnosia (failure to recognize faces) |
| Bilateral PCA occlusions | • Visual agnosia or cortical blindness (intact pupillary reflexes)<br>• Severe memory loss |

**Q. Define TIA.**

Transient ischemic attack (TIA) is characterized by a brief episode of neurological dysfunction (sudden loss of function) in which symptoms and signs resolve completely after a brief period within 24 hours (usually within 30 minutes).
- Transient ischemic attack is defined as a transient episode of neurologic dysfunction caused by focal brain, spinal cord, or retinal ischemia, without evidence of acute infarction on imaging. However, TIAs may herald a stroke.
- Newly proposed definition classifies those with new brain infarction as ischemic strokes regardless of whether symptoms persist.

**Clinical features:** Hemiparesis and aphasia are most common. Other features include amaurosis fugax (sudden transient loss of vision in one eye), hemisensory loss, hemianopic visual loss, diplopia, vertigo, vomiting, choking and dysarthria, ataxia, etc.

**Q. What is ABCD2 score?**

The ABCD2 score is very important for predicting subsequent risks of TIA or stroke. The ABCD2 score was derived from providing a more robust prediction standard. The ABCD2 score includes factors including age, blood pressure, clinical symptoms, duration, and diabetes.
- **A**ge: Older than 60 years (1 point)
- **B**lood pressure greater than or equal to 140/90 mm Hg on first evaluation or hypertension on treatment.
- **C**linical symptoms: A focal weakness with the spell (2 points) or speech impairment without weakness (1 point)
- **D**uration greater than 60 min (2 points), or 10–59 min (1 point)
- **D**iabetes mellitus (1 point).
- The 2-day risk of stroke was 0% for scores of 0 or 1, 1.3% for 2 or 3, 4.1% for 4 or 5, and 8.1% for 6 or 7.

**Q. What are the types of transient ischemic attack?**
- Large artery low-flow TIA—recurrent, short lasting episodes of stereotyped symptoms (shotgun TIA/thrombotic TIA)
- Embolic TIA—longer lasting less frequent episodes with varied symptoms, changing territories
- Lacunar TIA.

**Q. What are lacunar strokes? List the common lacunar stroke syndromes?**
- Small penetrating arterial branches of 200–800 μm in diameter, supply the deep brain parenchyma. Each of these small branches can be occluded either by atherothrombotic disease at its origin or by the development of occlusive vasculopathy—lipohyalinotic thickening (consequence of hypertension) **(Table 4.10)**. The lacunar stroke size varies from 3 mm to 20 mm in dimension.

**Table 4.10:** Signs and symptoms of lacunar stroke depending on location of lesion.

| Syndrome | Signs/symptoms | Localization | Vascular supply |
|---|---|---|---|
| Pure motor | Contralateral hemiparesis or hemiplegia. Affects face, arm and leg equally | Posterior limb of internal capsule Corona radiata—basis pontis | Lenticulostriate branches of the middle cerebral artery (MCA) or perforating arteries from basilar artery |

| Syndrome | Signs/symptoms | Localization | Vascular supply |
|---|---|---|---|
| Pure sensory | Contralateral hemisensory loss. Persistent or transient numbness and/or tingling on one side of the body | Ventral posterolateral (VPL) nucleus of thalamus | Lenticulostriate branches of MCA. Small thalamo-perforators of posterior cerebral artery (PCA) |
| Mixed sensorimotor | Contralateral weakness and numbness. Hemiparesis or hemiplegia with ipsilateral sensory impairment | Thalamus and adjacent posterior limb of internal capsule | Lenticulostriate branches of MCA |
| Dysarthria clumsy hand | Slurred speech and weakness of contralateral hand (fine motor) | Basis pontis | Basilar artery perforators |
| Ataxic hemiparesis | Combination of cerebellar and motor symptoms. Contralateral hemiparesis and ataxia out of proportion to weakness | Internal capsule—posterior limb Basis pontis Corona radiata | Lenticulostriate branches of MCA Perforating arteries of basilar artery |
| Hemiballismus/hemichorea | Contralesional limb flailing/dyskinesis | Subthalamic nucleus | Perforating arteries of anterior choroidal or posterior communicating artery (PCOM) |

**Q. Describe the blood supply to the brain.**
Refer **Figure 4.13**.

**Q. Describe the blood supply of the internal capsule.**
Refer **Figure 4.14**.

**Q. Define speech defects.**
Refer **Table 4.11**.

### Table 4.11: Types of speech defects.

| Phonation | It is defined as the production of vocal sounds without word formation; it is entirely a function of the larynx |
|---|---|
| Vocalization | It is the sound made by the vibration of the vocal folds, modified by working of the vocal tract |
| Speech (Fig. 4.16) | It consists of words which are articulate vocal sounds that symbolize and communicate ideas |
| Articulation | It is the enunciation of words and phrases; it is a function of organs and muscles innervated by the brainstem |
| Language (Fig. 4.15) | It is a mechanism for expressing thoughts and ideas as follows:<br>✦ By speech (auditory symbols)<br>✦ By writing (graphic symbols), or<br>✦ By gestures and pantomime (motor symbols)<br>✦ Language may be regarded as any means of expressing or communicating feeling or thought using a system of symbols.<br>✦ It is a function of the cerebral cortex |
| Aphasia | Aphasia is an acquired disorder with loss or defective language content of speech resulting from damage to the speech centers within the dominant (usually left in 97%) hemisphere |
| Paraphasia | Substitution in the components of speech, e.g., food for spoon |
| Neologism | Use of words which are nonexistent. Classically seen with Wernicke's aphasia |
| Jargon | Completely meaningless speech containing neologisms and paraphasias. Described in Wernicke's aphasia |
| Echolalia | Continuous repetition of heard words or sentences. Seen with transcortical sensory and transcortical mixed aphasias. |
| Alexia | It is the impairment of visual word recognition, in the context of intact auditory word recognition and writing ability |
| Agraphia | It is the inability to write, as a language disorder resulting from brain damage |
| Anomia | In this, word approximates the correct answer but it phonetically inaccurate (plentil for pencil)—phonemic paraphasia. When the patient cannot say the appropriate name when an object is shown but can point the object when the name is provided, it is known as one way or retrieval-based naming deficit |
| Mutism | Unable to speak or make sound |
| Aphonia | Unable to produce sound |
| Aphemia | Loss of speech |

**Q. What is the difference between aphasia and dysarthria?**
Refer **Table 4.12**.

### Table 4.12: Difference between aphasia and dysarthria.

| Aphasia | Dysarthria |
|---|---|
| Aphasia is a disorder of language | Dysarthria is a disorder of the motor production or articulation of speech |
| Usually due to cerebral dysfunction/lesions | Dysarthria is defective articulation of sounds or words of neurologic origin (usually brainstem) |
| Aphasia usually affects other language functions, such as reading and writing | In dysarthria, there are often other accompanying bulbar abnormalities, such as dysphagia |

SECTION 4: Nervous System

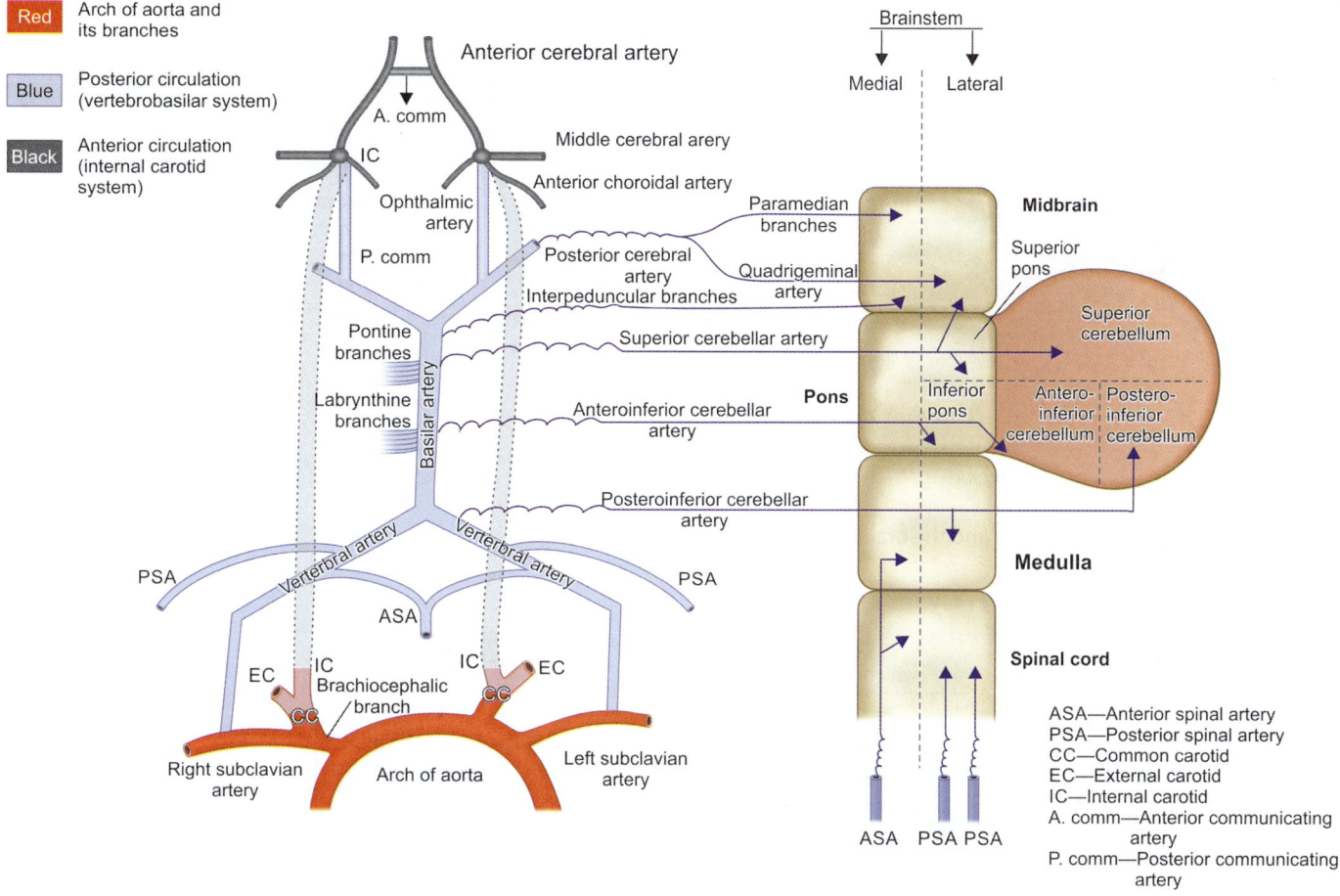

**Fig. 4.13:** Cerebrovascular system (a comprehensive diagram of arterial system).

**Fig. 4.14:** Blood supply of internal capsule.
(ACA: anterior cerebral artery; MCA: middle cerebral artery; PCA: posterior cerebral artery; AChA: anterior choroidal artery; IC: internal carotid artery (direct branches); P. Comm: posterior communicating artery)

# SECTION 4: Nervous System

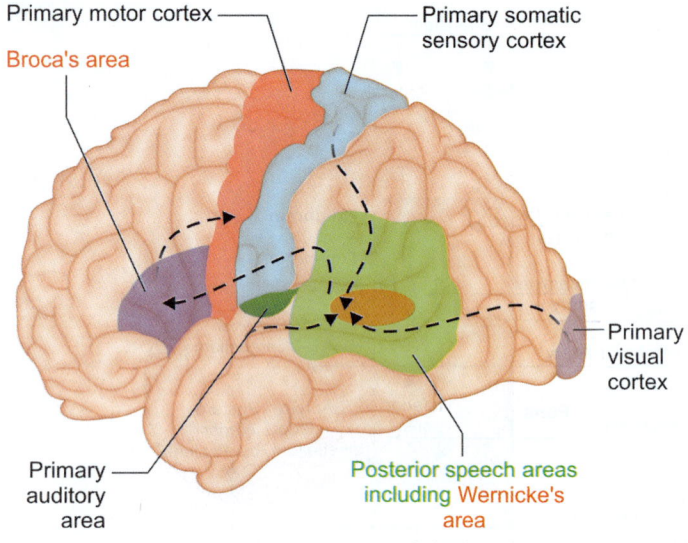

**Fig. 4.15:** Language and the brain.

## Q. What are the speech areas?

Refer **Table 4.13** and **Figure 4.16**.

| **Table 4.13:** Types of speech areas. | | |
|---|---|---|
| **Wernicke's area (area 22)** | **Arcuate fasciculus** | **Broca's area (area 44)** |
| Decoding of sounds into language information (comprehension) | Communication between the Broca's and Wernicke's area. Needed for speech repetition | Responsible for spontaneous speech output, i.e., fluency. Approximate number words produced per minute is 100/min for males and 150/min for females |

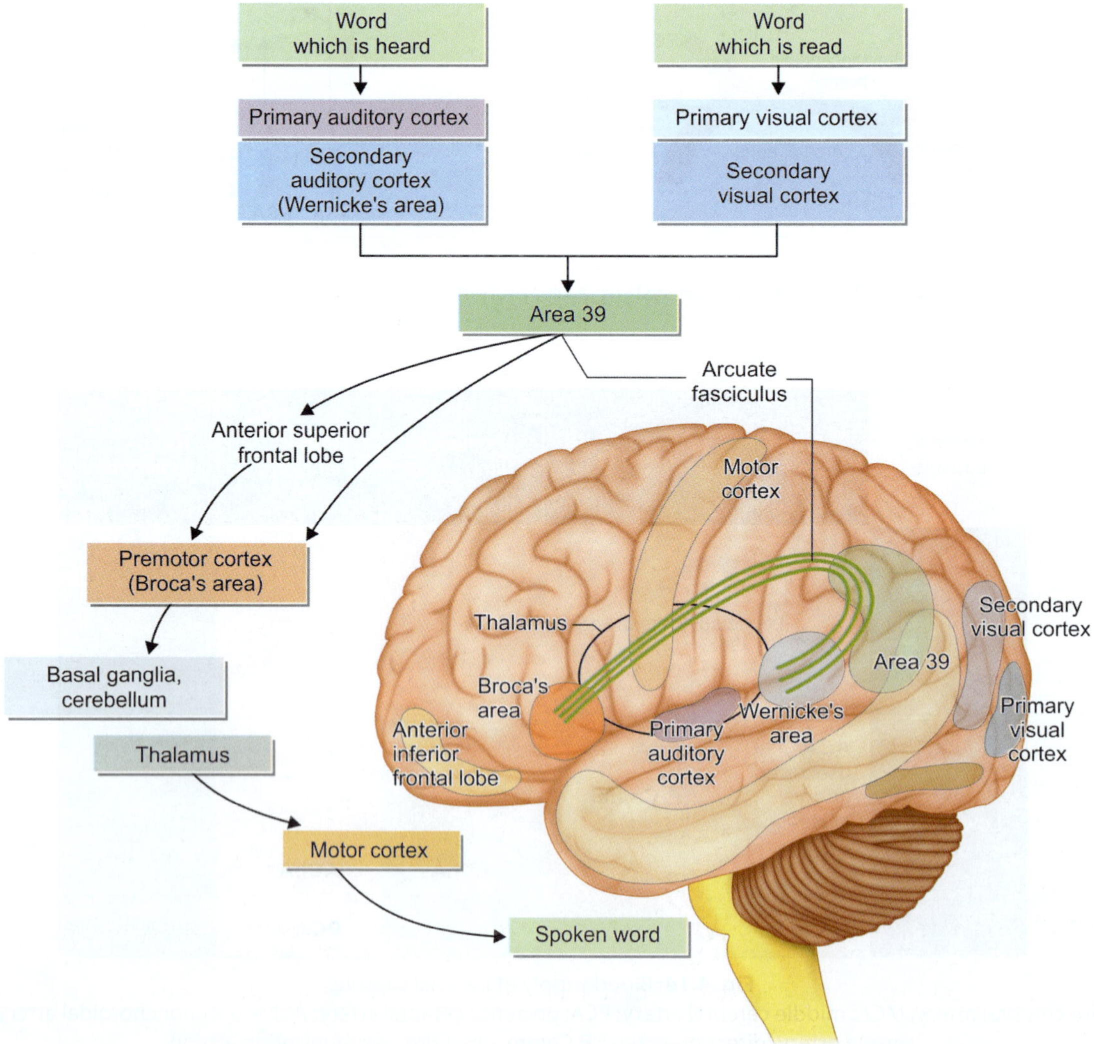

**Fig. 4.16:** Genesis of speech.

## Q. Define aphasia. What are the common types?

- Aphasia is an acquired disorder with loss or defective language content of speech resulting from damage to the speech centers within the dominant (usually left in 97%) hemisphere.
- A language disturbance occurring after a right hemisphere lesion in a right hander is known as crossed aphasia.
- It includes defect in or loss of the power of expression by speech, writing, or gestures or a defect in or loss of the ability to comprehend spoken or written language or to interpret gestures.
- Aphasia may be categorized according to whether the speech output is fluent or nonfluent.
- **Fluent aphasias** (receptive aphasias) are impairments.
- Mostly due to the input or reception of language with difficulties either in auditory verbal comprehension or in the repetition of words, phrases, or sentences spoken by others. For example, Wernicke's aphasia.
- **Nonfluent aphasias** (expressive aphasias) are difficulties in articulating with relatively good auditory, verbal comprehension. For example, Broca's aphasia..
- **Normal fluency** 100–150 words/min, sentence length >7 words.
- Reduced fluency in Broca's aphasia, transcortical motor, global aphasia, and primary progressive aphasia.

Types of aphasia are shown in Table 4.14.

**Table 4.14:** Types of aphasia.

| | Aphasia | Site of lesion | C | R | F |
|---|---|---|---|---|---|
| 1. | Wernicke's—sensory/receptive/posterior | Infarction of inferior division of middle cerebral artery | – | – | + |
| 2. | Broca's—motor/expressive/anterior | Infarction of superior frontal branch of middle cerebral artery | + | – | – |
| 3. | Conduction/arcuate | Arcuate fasciculus | + | – | + |
| 4. | Transcortical sensory | Posterior watershed zone | – | + | + |
| 5. | Transcortical motor | Anterior watershed zone | + | + | – |
| 6. | Isolation aphasia (mixed transcortical aphasia) | Both anterior and posterior watershed areas | – | + | – |
| 7. | Global aphasia | Dominant frontal, parietal and superior temporal lobe | – | – | – |
| | | | R | W | N |
| 8. | Alexia without agraphia | Occipitotemporal region | – | + | + |
| 9. | Alexia with agraphia | Left angular gyrus | – | – | + |
| 10. | Nominal/anomic/amnesic | Temporoparietal | + | + | – |

Note:
C—Comprehension R—Repetition F—Fluency
- C—Comprehension (requires intact Wernicke's and transcortical sensory area)
- R—Repetition (requires intact Wernicke's, arcuate fibers, and Broca's area)
- F—Fluency (requires intact Broca's and transcortical motor area)

Once the comprehension, repetition, and fluency are intact, we look for reading, writing, and naming disorders associated with reading, writing, and naming.

## Q. What are the domains of language?

- Lesions in the anterior limb of internal capsule/basal ganglia can produce Broca's like aphasia.
- Lesions in the thalamus can produce Wernicke's like aphasia.
- Most common type of aphasia seen in stroke: Broca's aphasia.
- Overall most common type of aphasia is anomic aphasia. Schematic representation of types of aphasia and approach to aphasia are shown in **Figure 4.17 and 4.18** respectively.
- Spontaneous speech/fluency
- Comprehension
- Repetition
- Reading
- Writing
- Naming

## Q. What is subcortical aphasia?

Damage to subcortical components of the language network (e.g., the striatum and thalamus of the left hemisphere) also can lead to aphasia. The resulting syndromes contain combinations of deficits in the various aspects of language but rarely fit the specific patterns. In a patient with a CVA, an anomic aphasia accompanied by dysarthria or a fluent aphasia with hemiparesis should raise the suspicion of a subcortical lesion site

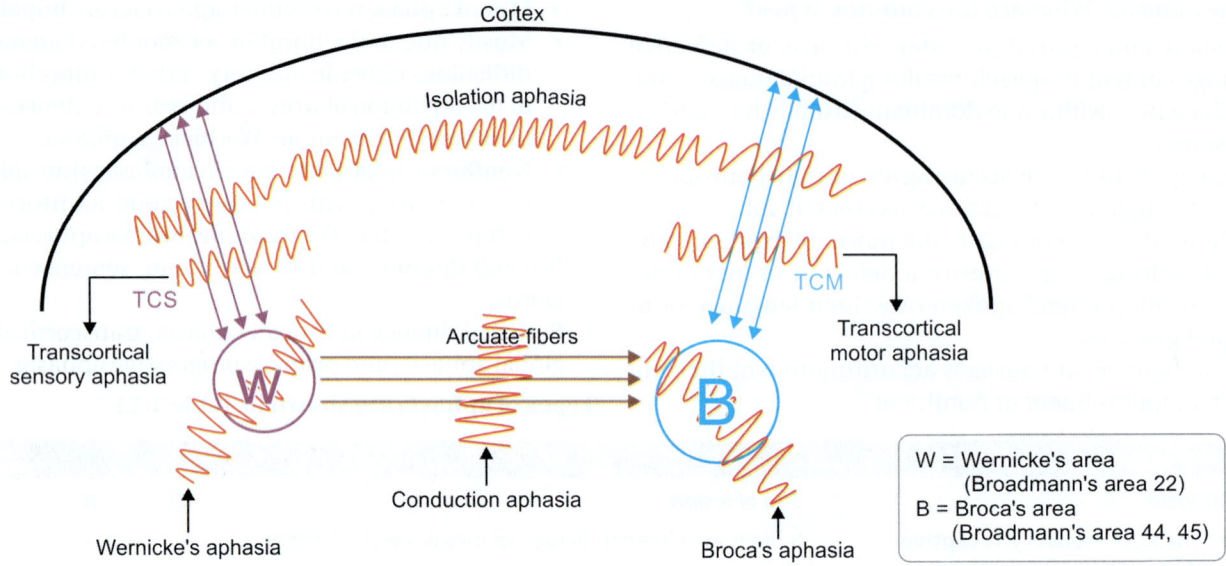

**Fig. 4.17:** Schematic representation of aphasias and associated lesions.

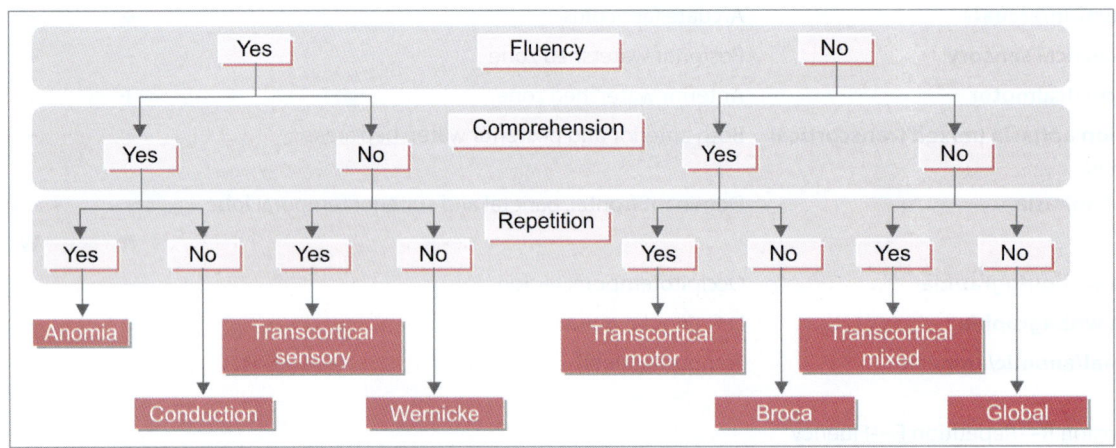

**Fig. 4.18:** Approach for aphasias.

### Q. What are the types of dysarthria?

**Production of sounds requires:**
- Normal respiration
- Muscles of articulation (labial, lingual, and palatal muscles)
- Phonation (by larynx)
- Resonance (by nasopharynx).

**Articulated sounds:**
- **Articulated labials** (b, p, m, and w) are formed principally by the lips.
- **Modified labials** (o and u, and to a lesser extent i, e, and a) are altered by lip contraction.
- **Labiodentals** (f and v) are formed by placing the teeth against the lower lip.
- **Linguals** are sounds formed with tongue action.
- **t, d, l, r, and n are tongue point, or alveolar sounds** formed by touching the tip of the tongue to the upper alveolar ridge. **S, z, sh, zh, ch, and j are dentals**, or tongue blade sounds. **To hear distorted linguals**, place the tip of your tongue against the back of your bottom teeth, hold it there and say "top dog," "go jump", and "train".
- **To hear distorted labials**, hold your upper lip between the thumb and forefinger of one hand and your bottom lip similarly with the other and say "my baby".
- **Gutturals** (velars, or tongue back sounds, such as k, g, and ng) are articulated between the back of the tongue and the soft palate.
- **Palatals** (German ch and g, and the French gn) are formed when the dorsum of the tongue approximates the hard palate.

**Table 4.15** shows the types of dysarthria.

**Table 4.15:** Types of dysarthrias.

| Types | Description | Cause |
|---|---|---|
| Flaccid (lingual, buccal, and guttural) | LMN weakness of facial, lingual, or pharyngeal muscles.<br>♦ **Facial paralysis** causes difficulty with labials, such as b, p, m, and w.<br>♦ **Tongue paralysis** affects a large number of sounds, particularly l, d, n, s, t, and x.<br>♦ **Palatal paralysis** produces a nasal twang in speech. | Cerebrovascular accidents (especially brainstem lesions) |
| Spastic (hot potato voice) | Strained, slurred hot potato-like voice | UMN weakness (bilateral), e.g., pseudobulbar palsy |
| Ataxic speech | ♦ *Scanning speech:* Undue separation of syllables (monosyllable speech)<br>♦ **Staccato speech:** Explosive type of speech with emphasis on syllables | Cerebellar diseases |
| Hypokinetic | Slow monotonous, low voice with inappropriate silence | Extrapyramidal (parkinsonism) |
| Hyperkinetic dysarthria | Distorted speech with continuous change in articulation | Chorea, athetosis, and dyskinesias |
| Myasthenic dysarthria | Voice is normal in the beginning but becomes weak as sentences progress | Myasthenia gravis |

## Q. What is Monro-Kellie hypothesis?

The Monro-Kellie doctrine, or hypothesis, is that the **sum of volumes of brain, CSF, and intracranial blood is constant**. An increase in one should cause a decrease in one or both of the remaining two. This hypothesis has substantial theoretical implications in increased intracranial pressure and in decreased CSF volume. Many of the MRI abnormalities seen in intracranial hypotension or CSF volume depletion can be explained by the Monro-Kellie hypothesis. These abnormalities include meningeal enhancement, subdural fluid collections, engorgement of cerebral venous sinuses, prominence of the spinal epidural venous plexus, and enlargement of the pituitary gland.

## Q. What is Cushing's reflex?

When intracranial pressure is increased, **the blood supply to RVLM (rostral ventrolateral medulla) neurons is compromised**, and the local hypoxia and hypercapnia increase their discharge. The **resultant rise in systemic arterial pressure (Cushing reflex)** tends to restore the blood flow to the medulla and over a considerable range, the blood pressure rise is proportional to the increase in intracranial pressure. The rise in blood pressure causes a **reflex decrease in heart rate** via the arterial baroreceptors. This is why bradycardia rather than tachycardia is characteristically seen in patients with increased intracranial pressure.

## Q. Discuss the pathogenesis of CNS tuberculosis.

♦ Central nervous system TB results from the hematogenous dissemination of *M. tuberculosis* to the brain with the formation of **small subpial or subependymal foci. These are called Rich foci**,
♦ The development of TBM requires rupture of a Rich focus with release of *M. tuberculosis* into the subarachnoid space. This heralds the onset of meningitis, which, if left untreated, will result in death in most cases.

Three processes produce the subsequent neurological pathology:

♦ **Granulomatous meningeal inflammation** with exudate and adhesion formation.
♦ An **obliterative vasculitis**, and an **encephalitis or myelitis.**
♦ Granulomas can coalesce to **form tuberculomas**, predominantly meningeal in origin, which can cause diverse clinical consequences dependent upon their anatomical location. Adhesions result from a dense basal meningeal exudate that contains lymphocytes, plasma cells, and macrophages, with increasing quantities of fibrin. **Adhesions can block the basal subarachnoid cisterns, obstruct the flow of CSF, and cause hydrocephalus;** they can also compromise cranial nerves, particularly II, III, IV, VI, and VII.
♦ An **obliterative vasculitis** of both large and small vessels can cause infarctions, which commonly occur in the territories of the proximal middle cerebral artery and the perforating vessels to the basal ganglia.
♦ The intensity of the basal inflammatory process extends into the parenchyma, resulting in **encephalitis**. Edema, occurring as a consequence, can be marked throughout both hemispheres and contributes to rising intracranial pressure and the global clinical neurological deficit.
♦ The pathogenesis of symptomatic, expanding, **intracranial tuberculomas** (that occur without meningitis) is more speculative. An ill-defined **'immunological' hypothesis that suggests localized upregulation of the cellular immune response to *M. tuberculosis* antigens within Rich foci has been proposed**. Evidence for this suggestion is scant, although the ability of corticosteroids to reduce the size of lesions, and the association between tuberculoma development in HIV-infected individuals and immune reconstitution with highly active retroviral therapy, is persuasive.

**Q. What are the neurological complications of tubercular meningitis?**

The neurological complications of TBM are legion and their nature and diversity can be predicted from the site of disease and the pathogenesis.

- Cranial nerve palsies are found in 30% at presentation, particularly of the IIIrd, VIth, and VIIth nerves.
- Mono- or hemiparesis occurs in 20%; paraparesis complicates 1–5% of cases.
- CSF obstruction leads to raised intracranial pressure, hydrocephalus, and reduced conscious level.
- Seizures are unusual in adults, but may be caused by hydrocephalus, tuberculoma, and hyponatremia.
- Hyponatremia affects more than 50% of patients with TBM and causes confusion and coma.
- A 'cerebral salt wasting syndrome' associated with TBM and attributed to a renal tubular defect.
- The syndrome of inappropriate antidiuretic hormone (SIADH) may cause some cases of TBM-associated hyponatremia, but reduced plasma volumes and persistent natriuresis despite normal concentrations of antidiuretic hormone (ADH) have been reported that suggest other mechanisms.
- TBM occurs with spinal involvement in 10% of cases and should always be considered in those presenting with root pain, with both spastic or flaccid paralysis, and loss of sphincter control.
- Vertebral TB (Pott's disease) accounts for 25% of cases and may be associated with a gibbus.
  - Extradural cord tuberculomas cause more than 60% of cases of non-osseous paraplegia, although tuberculomas can occur in any part of the cord
  - Tuberculous radiculomyelitis is a rare but well-reported accompaniment to TBM and is characterized by a subacute paraparesis, radicular pain, and bladder dysfunction.

**Q. What are the opportunistic CNS infections in HIV positive patients?**

- Toxoplasmosis
- Cryptococcosis
- Progressive multifocal leukoencephalopathy
- Cytomegalovirus
- Syphilis
- *Mycobacterium tuberculosis*
- HTLV-I infection
- Amebiasis

**Q. What are the clinical features of cryptococcal meningitis?**

- *C. neoformans* is the leading infectious cause of meningitis in patients with AIDS. It is the initial AIDS-defining illness in 2% of patients and generally occurs in patients with CD4+ T cell counts <100/L.
- **Most patients present with a picture of subacute meningoencephalitis with fever, nausea, vomiting, altered mental status, headache, and meningeal signs. The incidence of seizures and focal neurologic deficits is low**.
- In addition to meningitis, **patients may develop cryptococcomas and cranial nerve involvement**. The diagnosis of cryptococcal meningitis is made by identification of organisms in spinal fluid with India ink examination or by the detection of cryptococcal antigen. Blood cultures for fungus are often positive. A biopsy may be needed to make a diagnosis of CNS cryptococcoma. Symptoms may recur with initiation of cART as an immune reconstitution syndrome. **Other fungi that may cause meningitis in patients with HIV infection are *C. immitis* and *H. capsulatum*. Meningoencephalitis has also been reported due to *Acanthamoeba* or *Naegleria*.**

**Q. Can you get hemiplegia in subarachnoid hemorrhage?**

- **Vasospasm:** Narrowing of the arteries at the base of the brain following SAH causes symptomatic ischemia and infarction in 30% of patients and is the major cause of delayed morbidity and death. Signs of ischemia appear 4–14 days after the hemorrhage, most often at 7 days. The severity and distribution of vasospasm determine whether infarction will occur.
- Delayed vasospasm is believed to result from direct effects of clotted blood and its breakdown products on the arteries within the subarachnoid space. In general, the more blood that surrounds the arteries, the greater the chance of symptomatic vasospasm. Spasm of major arteries produces symptoms referable to the appropriate vascular territory. All of these focal symptoms may present abruptly, fluctuate, or develop over a few days. In most cases, focal spasm is preceded by a decline in mental status.

**Q. What are sentinel bleeds?**

Aneurysms can undergo small ruptures and leaks of blood into the subarachnoid space, so-called sentinel bleeds. Sudden unexplained headache at any location should raise suspicion of SAH and be investigated, because a major hemorrhage may be imminent.

**Q. What are paraneoplastic CNS syndromes?**

**Usually occur with cancer association:**
- Encephalomyelitis
- Limbic encephalitis
- Cerebellar degeneration (adults)
- Opsoclonus-myoclonus
- Subacute sensory neuronopathy
- Gastrointestinal paresis or pseudo-obstruction
- Dermatomyositis (adults)
- Lambert-Eaton myasthenic syndrome
- Cancer or melanoma associated retinopathy

**May occur with or without cancer association:**
- Brainstem encephalitis
- Stiff-person syndrome
- Necrotizing myelopathy

- Motor neuron disease
- Guillain-Barré syndrome
- Subacute and chronic mixed sensory-motor neuropathies
- Neuropathy associated with plasma cell dyscrasias and lymphoma
- Vasculitis of nerve
- Pure autonomic neuropathy
- Acute necrotizing myopathy
- Polymyositis
- Vasculitis of muscle
- Optic neuropathy
- BDUMP (bilateral diffuse uveal melanocytic proliferation)

### Q. What are the features of herpes simplex encephalitis?

- Herpes simplex encephalitis has a predilection for the temporal lobe and orbital frontal cortex, and **aphasia can be an early symptom**, along with headache, confusion, fever, and seizures. **Aphasia is often a permanent sequel in survivors of herpes encephalitis.**
- Fever and headache are consistent features of HSE.
- Onset of symptoms may be abrupt with focal or generalized seizures, or more protracted, with behavioral changes, an amnestic syndrome, aphasia, or other focal signs.
- The diagnosis of HSE should be considered in any febrile patient with an altered level of consciousness, with/without other focal neurological deficits. **The presence of hallucinations, particularly olfactory hallucinations**, should suggest the possibility of HSE. There is no pathognomonic set of clinical findings of HSE. **Focal signs, hemiparesis, hemisensory loss, ataxia, or focal seizures are seen in approximately one half of patients at presentation.**

### Q. What is the anatomy of trigeminal CN nucleus?

The trigeminal, or fifth cranial, nerve (CN V) is the largest and one of the most complex cranial nerves. It has a large sensory part and a much smaller motor part. The sensory component has three divisions—the first, or ophthalmic division (CN V1), the second or maxillary division (CN V2), and the third or mandibular division (CN V3). The motor and principal sensory nuclei are located in the midpons. The spinal tract and nucleus, which subserve pain and temperature, extend from the pons down into the upper cervical spinal cord. The mesencephalic root receives proprioceptive fibers. Trigeminal nuclear structures thus extend from the rostral midbrain to the rostral spinal cord. The sensory portion innervates the face, teeth, oral and nasal cavities, the scalp back to the vertex, the intracranial dura, and the cerebral vasculature, and provides proprioceptive information for muscles of mastication. Fibers subserving pain and temperature take a much more circuitous route to the thalamus. The spinal tract, or the descending root, of the trigeminal extends from the principal sensory nucleus down through the lower pons and medulla, into the spinal cord as far as C3, or even C4. The motor portion innervates the muscles of mastication.

### Q. What are the variants of multiple sclerosis?

- Relapsing/remitting MS (RRMS)
- Secondary progressive MS (SPMS)
- Primary progressive MS (PPMS)
- Progressive/relapsing MS (PRMS)

### Q. What are the causes of sudden loss of vision?

Sudden painless loss of vision sudden painful loss of vision.
- CRAO
- CRVO
- AION
- TIA (amaurosis fugax)
- Retinal detachment
- Vitreous hemorrhage

### Q. Where is the site of lesion for unilateral loss of vision?

Sudden painful loss of vision:
- Optic neuritis
- Acute glaucoma
- Trauma
- Endophthalmitis

Any lesion in the optic nerve up to optic chiasma. Lesions at optic chiasma can cause bitemporal/binasal hemianopia. Lesions beyond optic chiasma causes homonymous hemianopia.

### Q. What is clonus?

Clonus is a series of rhythmic involuntary muscular contractions induced by the sudden passive stretching of a muscle or tendon. It often accompanies the spasticity and hyperactive DTRs seen in corticospinal tract disease. Clonus occurs most frequently at the ankle, knee, and wrist, occasionally elsewhere. Ankle clonus consists of a series of rhythmic alternating flexions and extensions of the ankle. It is easiest to obtain if the examiner supports the leg, preferably with one hand under the knee or the calf, grasps the foot from below with the other hand, and quickly dorsiflexes the foot while maintaining slight pressure on the sole at the end of the movement. Clonus indicates hypertonia.

### Q. What is spasticity and rigidity?

The spasticity, or increase in tone, is most marked in the flexor and pronator muscles of the upper limb and the extensors of the lower, more apparent with an attempt to extend or supinate the muscles of the upper extremity or flex those of the lower.

Spasticity is due to lesions involving the corticospinal pathways. The hypertonicity to passive movements differs from that of rigidity because it is not uniform throughout the range of movement, and it varies with the speed of movement.

In spasticity only one group of muscles (either gravity or anti-gravity) have increased tone. While in rigidity both gravity and anti-gravity group of muscles have increased tone.

### Q. Discuss the anatomy of the internal capsule.

- **Location:**
  - The anterior limb separates the caudate nucleus and lenticular nucleus (putamen + globus pallidus)

- The posterior limb separates the thalamus and lenticular nucleus
♦ **Types of fibers:**
  - Anterior limb: Frontopontine fibers (frontal cortex to pons), thalamocortical fibers (thalamus to frontal lobe)
  - Genu (angle): Corticobulbar fibers (cortex to brainstem)
  - Posterior limb: Corticospinal fibers (posterior 2/3), sensory fibers (anterior 1/3)
♦ **Blood supply:**
  - Anterior limb: Lenticulostriate branches of middle cerebral artery and branch of anterior cerebral artery
  - Genu: Lenticulostriate branches of middle cerebral artery.
  - Posterior limb: Lenticulostriate branches of middle cerebral artery and anterior choroidal artery of internal carotid artery.

## Q. What is the location for vertebral artery bruit?
The bruit is heard anywhere between the line joining the tip of mastoid process and midpoint of clavicle. It should examined when suspecting posterior circulation stroke.

## Q. Why is superficial reflex lost in UMN lesion?
The superficial reflexes respond more slowly to the stimulus than do the stretch reflexes, their latency is longer, they fatigue more easily, and they are not as consistently present as tendon reflexes. The primary utility of superficial reflexes is that they are abolished by pyramidal tract lesions, which characteristically produce the combination of increased deep tendon reflexes and decreased or absent superficial reflexes. Pyramidal tracts have a facilitatory action upon the superficial reflexes and when corticospinal tracts are involved this facilitatory action is lost and hence there is absence of the superficial reflex.

## Q. What is frontal opercular syndrome?
Partial syndrome due to embolic occlusion of a single branch of MCA M2 affecting hand, or arm and hand, weakness alone (brachial syndrome) (or)

Facial weakness with nonfluent (Broca) aphasia, with/without arm weakness = frontal opercular syndrome

## Q. What are the causes for ptosis?
*Causes of ptosis*
♦ *Neurogenic ptosis* which includes oculomotor nerve palsy, Horner's syndrome, Marcus Gunn jaw winking syndrome, Third cranial nerve misdirection.
♦ *Myogenic ptosis* which includes myasthenia gravis, myotonic dystrophy, ocular myopathy, simple congenital ptosis, blepharophimosis syndrome.
♦ *Aponeurotic ptosis* which may be involutional or post-operative.
♦ *Mechanical ptosis* which occurs due to edema or tumors of the upper lid.
♦ *Neurotoxic ptosis* which is a classic symptom of envenomation by elapids, such as cobras, or kraits.

## Q. Which cardiac events are better appreciated using the bell of the stethoscope?
*3rd heart sound, 4th heart sound., mid-diastolic murmurs.* Bell of the stethoscope is the choice for low frequency sound. Firm pressure by the bell causes accentuation of lower frequency. Hence, it should be placed lightly on the skin.

## Q. Differences between bulbar and pseudobulbar palsy.
Refer **Table 4.16**.

## Q. What is agnosia?
Agnosia refers to the higher synthesis of sensory impulses, with the resulting perception, appreciation, and recognition of stimuli. Agnosia refers to the loss or impairment of the ability to know or recognize the meaning or import of a sensory stimulus, even though it has been perceived. Agnosia occurs in the absence of any impairment of cognition, attention, or alertness. The patients are not aphasic and do not have word-finding or a generalized naming impairment.

## Q. What is hallucination?
Subjective sensory perceptions in the absence of relevant external stimuli. The person may or may not recognize the experiences as false. Hallucinations may be auditory, visual, olfactory, gustatory, tactile/somatic (false perceptions associated with dreaming, falling asleep, and awakening are not classified as hallucinations). Hallucinations may occur in delirium, dementia (less commonly), post-traumatic stress disorder, schizophrenia, and alcoholism.

## Q. What is illusion?
Misinterpretations of real external stimuli. Illusions may occur in grief reactions, delirium, acute and post-traumatic stress disorders, and schizophrenia.

## Q. What is delusion?
False, fixed, personal beliefs that are not shared by other members of the person's culture or subculture. Delusions

**Table 4.16:** Differences between bulbar and pseudobulbar palsy.

| Bulbar palsy | Pseudobulbar palsy |
| --- | --- |
| LMN involvement of bulbar nerves | UMN involvement |
| Jaw jerk absent | Jaw jerk exaggerated |
| Not associated with long tract signs | Associated with bilateral long tract signs |
| Emotional lability absent | Emotional lability present |
| Atrophy and fasciculations of tongue | Tongue is SPASTIC |
| Present, e.g., motor neuron disease, botulism | For example, bilateral hemispheric medullary infarction, CADASIL |

and feelings of unreality or depersonalization are more often associated with psychotic disorders.

Delusions may also occur in delirium, severe mood disorders, and dementia.

### Q. What are clinical features of herniation?

Central transtentorial herniation denotes a symmetric downward movement of the thalamic medial structures through the tentorial opening with compression of the upper midbrain. Miotic pupils and drowsiness are the heralding signs.

Uncal transtentorial herniation refers to impaction of the anterior medial temporal gyrus (the uncus) into the tentorial opening just anterior to and adjacent to the midbrain. The uncus compresses the third nerve as it traverses the subarachnoid space, causing enlargement of the ipsilateral pupil (putatively because the fibers subserving parasympathetic pupillary function are located peripherally in the nerve).

### Q. What is Hutchinson's pupil?

The pupil is usually involved early and prominently with third nerve compression due to uncal herniation (Hutchinson pupil).

### Q. What is Adie pupil?

The patient presenting with Adie's tonic pupil is typically a young woman who suddenly notes a unilaterally enlarged pupil, with no other symptoms. The pupillary reaction to light may appear absent, although prolonged illumination may provoke a slow constriction. The reaction to near, although slow, is better preserved. Once constricted, the tonic pupil re-dilates very slowly when illumination is removed or the patient looks back at distance, often causing a transient reversal of the anisocoria. The pathology in Adie's pupil lies in the ciliary ganglion or short ciliary nerves, or both; its precise nature remains unknown. Holmes-Adie's syndrome is the association of the pupil abnormality with depressed or absent deep tendon reflexes.

### Q. What are the clinical features of Takayasu arteritis?

The generalized symptoms include malaise, fever, night sweats, arthralgias, anorexia, and weight loss, which may occur months before vessel involvement is apparent. These symptoms may merge into those related to vascular compromise and organ ischemia. Pulses are commonly absent in the involved vessels, particularly the subclavian artery. Hypertension occurs in 32–93% of patients and contributes to renal, cardiac, and cerebral injury.

### Q. Name neurocutaneous markers.

- Ash-leaf macules, shagreen patch, ungual fibroma, adenoma sebaceum, confetti lesions, poliosis—tuberous sclerosis
- Café au lait spots, subcutaneous neurofibroma, plexiform neurofibroma, axillary freckling—neurofibromatosis type 1
- Yellowish plaques or papules over neck, axilla, abdomen, inguinal decubital or popliteal areas—pseudoxanthoma elasticum
- Cutaneous telangiectasias on face lips hands and rarely on trunk and nasal mucosa—Osler-Weber-Rendu syndrome
- Port-wine nevus of face—Sturge-Weber syndrome
- Telangiectasias mainly involves sclera, earlobes and bridge of nose, hypertrichosis, gray hair, progeric changes, cutaneous granulomas—ataxia telangiectasias.
- Brittle, light colored twisted hair and trichorrhexis nodosa—kinky hair syndrome
- Tendon xanthomas—cerebrotendinous xanthomatosis
- Epidermal nevus—epidermal nevus syndrome
- Hypopigmented Whorls streaks and patches which follows Blaschko's lines, café-au-lait, cutis marmorata, aplasia cutis, nevus of Ota, nail dystrophy, trichorrhexis, focal hypertrichosis—hypomelanosis of Ito
- Dark to light brown nevus with satellite nevi over lower trunk and perineal area (swimming trunk nevus)—neurocutaneous melanosis retinal hemangioblastomas—VHL syndrome facial angiomas in trigeminal distribution—Wyburn-Mason syndrome sunlight sensitivity, freckling, atrophy xerosis, telangiectasias, actinic keratosis, angioma, keratoacanthoma, fibroma, malignant tumors—xeroderma pigmentosum.

### Q. What is the reason for pendular reflexes in cerebellar lesion?

Pendular reflexes are caused by muscle hypotonicity and the lack of normal checking of the reflex response.

### Q. Describe the speech in cerebellar dysfunction.

Cerebellar dysfunction causes a defect of articulatory coordination (scanning speech, ataxic dysarthria, or speech asynergy). There is a lack of smooth coordination of the tongue, lips, pharynx, and diaphragm. Ataxic speech is slow, slurred, irregular, labored, and jerky. Words are pronounced with irregular force and speed, with involuntary variations in loudness and pitch lending an explosive quality. There are unintentional pauses, which cause words and syllables to be erratically broken. Excessive separation of syllables and skipped sounds in words produce a disconnected, disjointed, faltering, staccato articulation (scanning speech).

### Q. How is consciousness maintained?

- Consciousness has two dimensions: Arousal and cognition.
- Arousal is a primitive function sustained by deep brainstem and medial thalamic structures.
- Cognitive functions require an intact cerebral cortex and major subcortical nuclei.
- In coma, stupor, and hypersomnia there is a lowering of consciousness; in confusion and delirium, there is a clouding of consciousness.

**The anatomy of consciousness:** The ascending reticular activating system is a system of fibers which arises from the reticular formation of the brainstem, primarily the paramedian tegmentum of the upper pons and midbrain, and projects to the paramedian, parafascicular, centromedian and intralaminar nuclei of the thalamus. Neurons in the reticular formation also receive collaterals from the ascending spinothalamic pathways and send projections diffusely to the entire cerebral cortex, so that sensory stimuli are involved not only with sensory perception but—through their connections with the RAS—with the maintenance of consciousness. The fibers in the RAS are cholinergic, adrenergic, dopaminergic, serotonergic, and histaminergic. Experimentally, stimulation of the RAS produces arousal, and destruction of the RAS produces coma. The hypothalamus is also important for consciousness; arousal can be produced by stimulation of the posterior hypothalamic region.

**Q. What are the features of lateral medullary syndrome?**
- Ipsilateral facial hypalgesia and thermoanesthesia (due to trigeminal spinal nucleus and tract involvement). Ipsilateral facial pain is common
- Contralateral trunk and extremity hypalgesia and thermoanesthesia (due to damage to the spinothalamic tract).
- Ipsilateral palatal, pharyngeal, and vocal cord paralysis with dysphagia and dysarthria (due to involvement of the nucleus ambiguus).
- Ipsilateral Horner syndrome (due to damage of the descending sympathetic fibers). Ipsilateral hypohidrosis of the body may occur, probably due to interruption of the mostly uncrossed excitatory sweating pathway, which descends from the hypothalamus through the tegmental area of the mesencephalon and pons and, more caudally, through the posterolateral area of the medulla to synapse with the sympathetic sudomotor neurons of the intermediolateral cell column of the spinal cord.
- Vertigo, nausea, and vomiting (due to involvement of the vestibular nuclei).
- Ipsilateral cerebellar signs and symptoms (due to involvement of the inferior cerebellar peduncle and cerebellum).
- Occasionally, hiccups (singultus) attributed to lesions of the dorsolateral region of the middle medulla and diplopia (perhaps secondary to involvement of the lower pons).

**Q. How do we differentiate stroke mechanism based on TIA?**
- TIAs in the same vascular territory are frequent precursors of thrombotic stroke, so their presence, especially when multiple, is virtually diagnostic of that stroke mechanism.
- Some evidence supports the notion that embolism is more likely to produce less frequent but longer attacks, whereas low flow states produce briefer but more frequent attacks. Shotgun-like repeated episodes of ischemia in the same vascular territory virtually always indicate a critical degree of vessel narrowing.
- Single but longer attacks are more often associated with an ulcerated plaque or another embolic source.

**Q. What are the causes for cerebral embolism?**
Refer **Box 4.1**.

**Q. What are the causes of recurrent fall?**
Refer **Box 4.2**.

**Q. What are the etiologies of cerebellar atxia?**
Refer **Table 4.17**.

**Q. Define pack-years.**
Average number of packs of cigarettes smoked per day multiplied by the total number of years of smoking.

**Q. Define the endocrine cause of ataxia—hypothyroidism.**
Occasional patients with hypothyroidism develop a mild gait ataxia in conjunction with their systemic symptoms. Thyroid function needs to be tested in patients with progressive ataxia because replacement treatment may improve the symptoms.

**Q. What are the risk factors for thrombosis?**
Refer **Table 4.18**.

**Q. What is crescendo TIA?**
Two or more attacks of TIA within 24 hours. It should be considered as a medical emergency.

**Q. What does 'stroke in evolution' indicate?**
It indicates thrombotic stroke.

**Q. How do you evaluate of thrombotic, hemorrhagic and embolic stroke from the history?**

**Thrombotic:** Most thrombotic strokes occur when the circulation is least active and most sluggish, e.g., during the night or during a nap with the deficit usually noticed on awakening.

It has a stuttering onset with an improvement in the deficit followed by a worsening and a second improvement **(Figs. 4.19A to C)**.

**Embolic:** The stroke which was maximum at the onset and not associated with head ache is most compatible with an embolic mechanism.

**Box 4.1:** Causes of cerebral embolism.

- **Cardiac origin**
  - Atrial fibrillation and other arrhythmias (with rheumatic, atherosclerotic, hypertensive, congenital, or syphilitic heart disease)
  - Myocardial infarction with mural thrombus
  - Acute and subacute bacterial endocarditis
  - Heart disease without arrhythmia or mural thrombus (mitral stenosis, myocarditis, etc.)
  - Complications of cardiac surgery
  - Valve prostheses
  - Nonbacterial thrombotic (marantic) endocardial vegetations
  - Prolapsed mitral valve
  - Paradoxical embolism with congenital heart disease (e.g., patent foramen ovale)
  - Myxoma
- **Noncardiac origin**
  - Atherosclerosis of aorta and carotid arteries (mural thrombus, atheromatous material)
  - From sites of dissection and/or fibromuscular dysplasia of carotid and vertebrobasilar arteries
  - Thrombus in pulmonary veins
  - Fat, tumor, or air
  - Complications of neck and thoracic surgery
  - Pelvic and lower extremity venous thrombosis in presence of right-to-left cardiac shunt
- **Undetermined origin**

**Box 4.2:** Causes of recurrent falls.

- Weakness
- Balance deficit
- Gait disorder
- Visual deficit
- Mobility limitation
- Cognitive impairment
- Impaired functional status
- Postural hypotension

**Table 4.17:** Etiology of cerebellar ataxia.

| Symmetric and progressive signs | | | Focal and ipsilateral cerebellar signs | | |
|---|---|---|---|---|---|
| *Acute (hours to days)* | *Subacute (days to weeks)* | *Chronic (months to years)* | *Acute (hours to days)* | *Subacute (days to weeks)* | *Chronic (months to years)* |
| Intoxication: Alcohol, lithium, phenytoin, barbiturates | Intoxication: Mercury, solvents, gasoline, glue; cytotoxic chemotherapeutic, hemotherapeutic drugs | Paraneoplastic syndrome Anti-gliadin antibody syndrome Hypothyroidism | Vascular: Cerebellar infarction, hemorrhage, or subdural hematoma Infectious: cerebellar abscess | Neoplastic: Cerebellar glioma or metastatic tumor Demyelinating: Multiple sclerosis | Stable gliosis secondary to vascular lesion or demyelinating plaque |
| Acute viral cerebellitis Postinfection syndrome | Alcoholic-nutritional (vitamin $B_1$ and $B_{12}$ deficiency) Lyme disease | Inherited diseases Tabes dorsalis Phenytoin toxicity Amiodarone | | AIDS-related multifocal leukoencephalopathy | Congenital lesion: Chiari or Dandy-Walker malformations |

**Hemorrhagic:** Gradual development of a progressive focal deficit accompanied by gradually developing symptoms of increased intracranial pressure (head ache, vomiting and decrease in the level of consciousness) suggest intracranial hemorrhage.

**Q. What are the fibers in the internal capsule?**
Refer **Figure 4.20**.

**Q. What are the various middle cerebral artery syndromes and their clinical features following occlusion at various levels?**
Refer **Figure 4.21**.

## SECTION 4: Nervous System

**Table 4.18:** Risk factors for thrombosis.

| Venous | Venous and Arterial |
|---|---|
| ◆ Inherited<br>  – Factor V Leiden<br>  – Prothrombin G20210A<br>  – Antithrombin deficiency<br>  – Protein C deficiency<br>  – Protein S deficiency<br>  – Elevated FVIII | ◆ Inherited<br>  – Homocystinuria<br>  – Dysfibrinogenemia<br>  – Mixed (inherited and acquired)<br>  – Hyperhomocysteinemia |
| ◆ Acquired<br>  – Age<br>  – Previous thrombosis<br>  – Immobilization<br>  – Major surgery<br>  – Pregnancy and puerperium<br>  – Hospitalization<br>  – Obesity<br>  – Infection<br>  – APC resistance, nongenetic<br>  – Smoking | ◆ Acquired<br>  – Malignancy<br>  – Antiphospholipid antibody syndrome<br>  – Hormonal therapy<br>  – Polycythemia vera<br>  – Essential thrombocythemia<br>  – Paroxysmal nocturnal hemoglobinuria<br>  – Thrombotic thrombocytopenic purpura<br>  – Heparin-induced thrombocytopenia<br>  – Disseminated intravascular coagulation |
| ◆ Unknown<br>  – Elevated factor II, IX, XI<br>  – Elevated TAFI levels<br>  – Low levels of TFPI | |

### Q. How to check for two point discrimination?

It is done using a two pronged instrument with blunt ends. Sharp ends will stimulate pain fibers instead of touch. Discrimination capacity is maximum in the palmar aspect of fingers especially 1st and 2nd fingers, where at a distance of <5 mm two point discrimination is possible. On the dorsum of foot even >5 cm is normal.

### Q. What are the features of ACA occlusion?

ACA occlusion is divided into proximal and distal Precommunal (A1)—ACA till anterior communicating artery. (A2)—distal to anterior communicating artery.

| A1 | A2 |
|---|---|
| ◆ Anterior limb of internal capsule<br>◆ Amygdala<br>◆ Anterior hypothalamus | ◆ Medial part of frontal lobe Paracentral lobule<br>◆ Medial part of sensory and motor cortex |

◆ A1 occlusion is mostly asymptomatic because of anterior communicating artery collateral supply.
◆ **A2 occlusion features:**
  - Contralateral monoplegia (lower limb >upper limb).
  - Cortical sensory loss over foot and leg.
  - Urinary incontinence (social inhibition of bladder is lost).
  - Contralateral grasp reflex, sucking reflex, Gegenhalten.

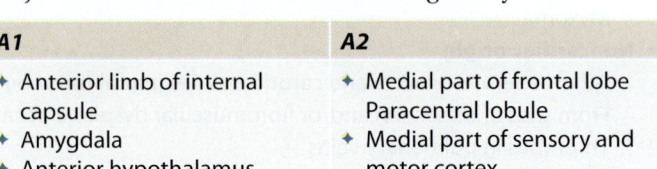

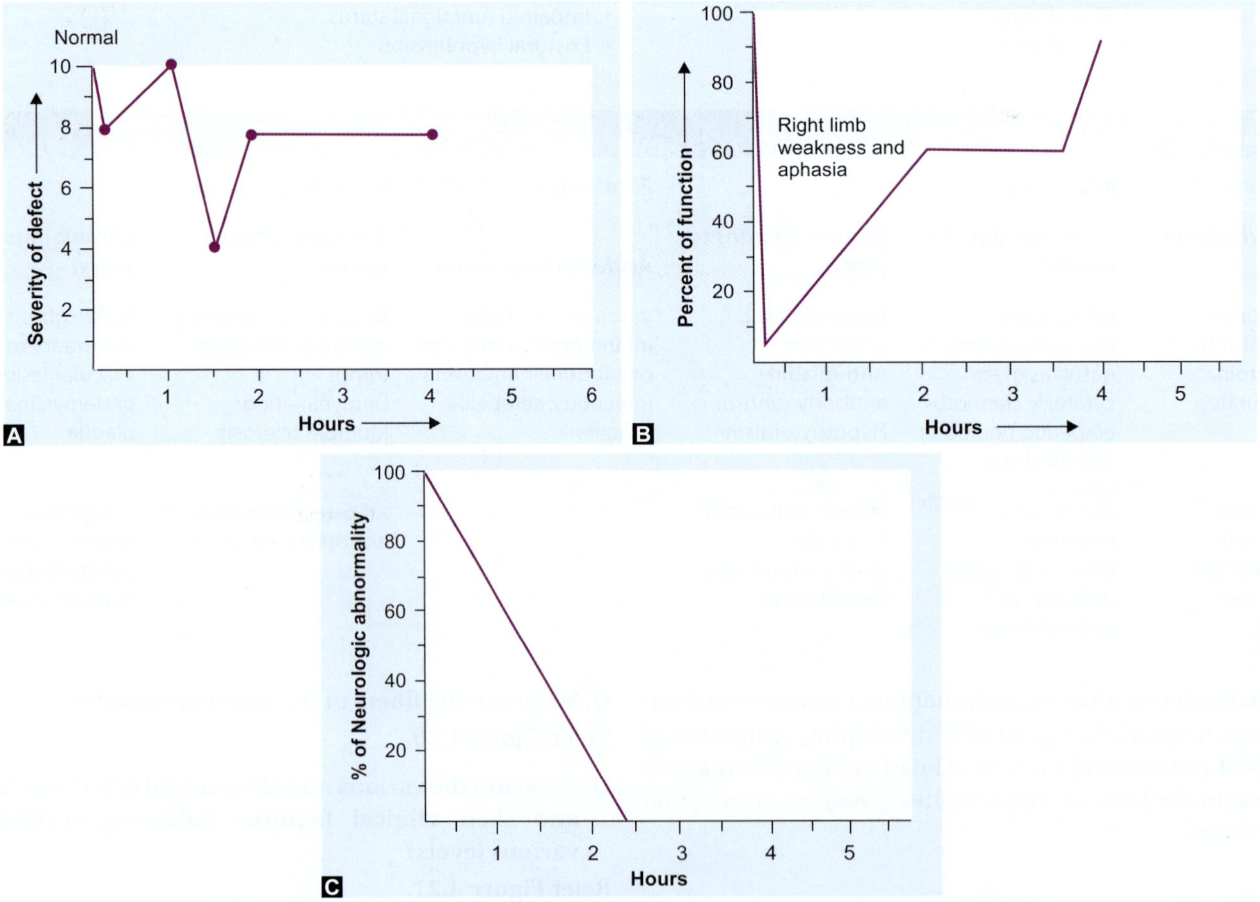

**Figs. 4.19A to C:** (A) Thrombotic stroke; (B) Hemorrhagic stroke; (C) Embolic stroke.

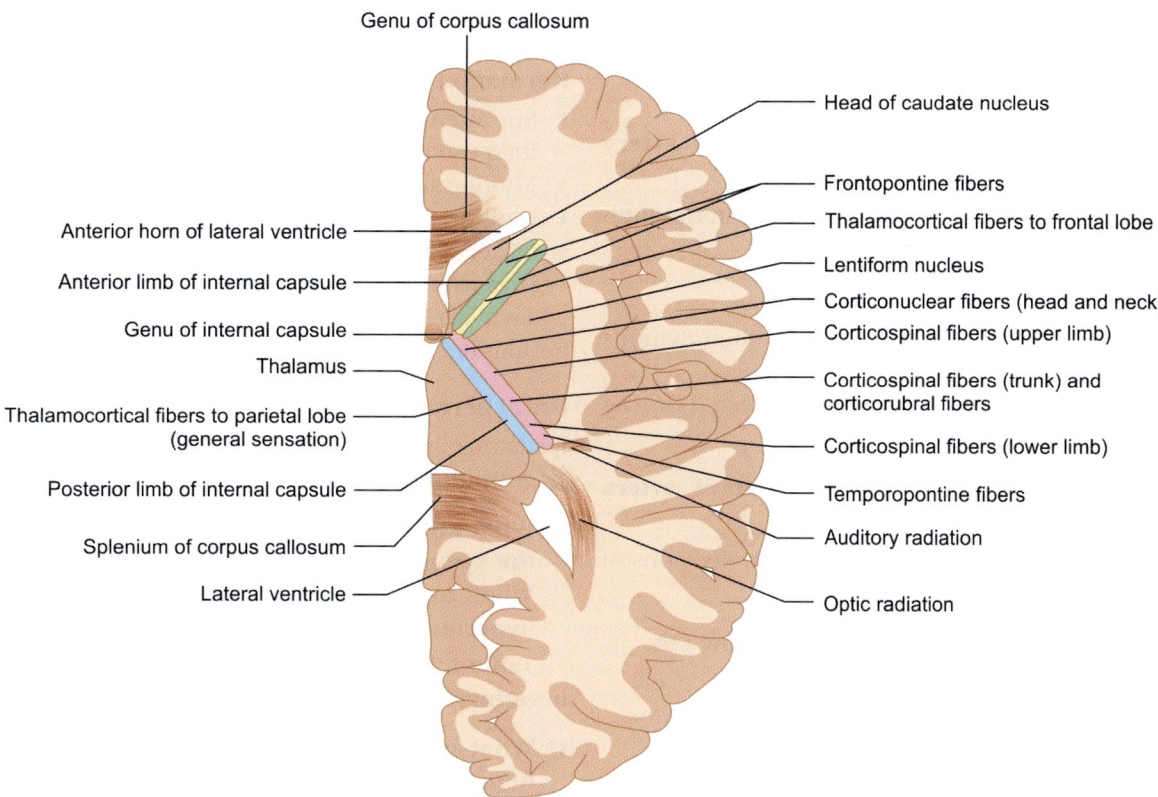

**Fig. 4.20:** Fibers in the internal capsule.

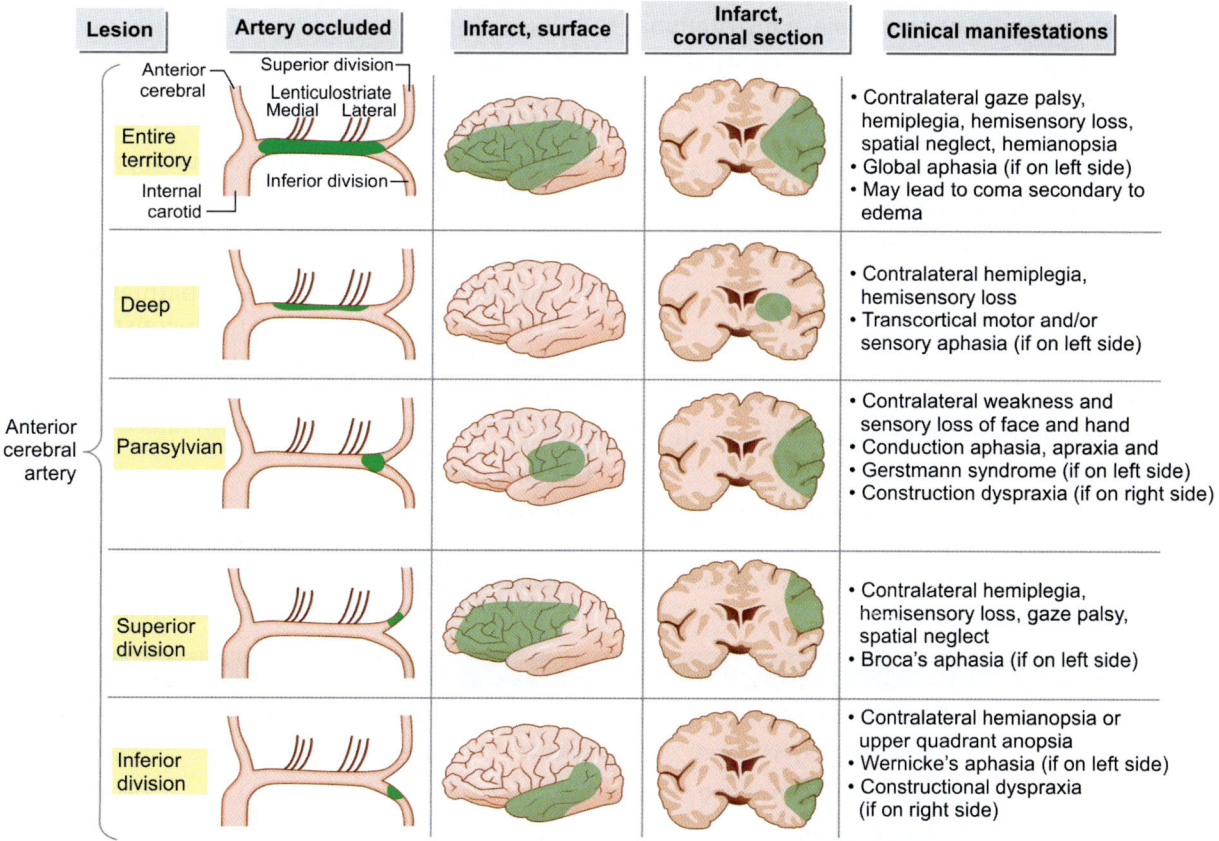

**Fig. 4.21:** Patterns of occlusion of the MCA and their anatomic correlates.

- Abulia, decreased spontaneity, intermittent interruption of activity (lack of attention).
- Gait apraxia.

### Q. What are the features of anterior choroidal artery occlusion?

Branch of internal carotid artery that supplies posterior limb of internal capsule and calcarine fibers.

**Clinical features**
- Contralateral hemiplegia, hemianesthesia, homonymous hemianopia.
- Stroke—MC cause is in situ thrombosis affected during iatrogenic aneurysmal clipping.

### Q. What are the features of middle cerebral artery occlusion?

MC cause of occlusion in proximal MCA/main divisions of MCA is emboli (artery to artery, cardiac).

**Atherosclerosis of proximal MCA causes low flow TIA.**
- Superior division—frontal and superior parietal cortex.
- Inferior division—inferior parietal and temporal cortex.

**Features of mainstem MCA occlusion (Table 4.19):**
- Contralateral hemiplegia, hemianesthesia, homonymous hemianopia, gaze preference to ipsilateral side, dysarthria, facial weakness, global aphasia (dominant hemisphere involvement), anosognosia, constructional apraxia, hemineglect (non-dominant hemisphere involvement).
- Frontal eye field supplied by MCA territory.
- Superior division occlusion causes contralateral hemiplegia, hemianesthesia, Broca's aphasia.
- Inferior division occlusion causes Wernicke's aphasia, no weakness.

### Q. What is meant by akinetic mutism?

**Akinetic mutism:**
- Lack of motor response in an awake individual.
- Lesion in supplementary motor areas responsible for initiating movement.
- Patient follows with eyes but does not initiate movements or obeys commands.
- Patients tone, postural reflexes (such as cold caloric stimulation) remain intact.

### Q. What are various types of herniation syndromes?

**Herniation syndromes:**
- Supratentorial mass lesions cause lateral displacement followed by downward displacement.
- Midline shift of >8 mm—impairment of consciousness.
- Midline shift of >11 mm—coma.
- Other clinical features—papilledema, Cushing's triad (hypertension, bradycardia, irregular respiration).

Two variants of supratentorial herniation—central herniation, uncal herniation.

**Uncal herniation:**
Ipsilateral 3rd nerve involvement followed by diencephalon stage, midbrain, pontine, medullary stage.

### Q. What are the causes of secondary hypertension? List the symptoms suggestive of secondary hypertension. What are the specific investigations of secondary hypertension?

Table 4.20 depicts the findings and specific investigations in various secondary hypertension.

### Q. What are the non-hypertensive causes of intracerebral hemorrhage?

- Vascular malformations
- Intracranial tumors
- Bleeding disorders, anticoagulants, and fibrinolytic treatment
- Cerebral amyloid angiopathy
- Granulomatous angiitis of central nervous system and other vasculitides.
- Sympathomimetic agents (including amphetamine and cocaine).
- Hemorrhagic infarction.
- Head trauma.
- Miscellaneous—other vasculopathies, e.g., moyamoya disease, reversible cerebral vasoconstriction syndrome, cerebral autosomal dominant arteriopathy with subcortical infarcts and leukoencephalopathy (rarely) and septic emboli/arteritis in the setting of infective endocarditis.

**Cocaine use**

The association of cocaine use to aneurysm growth is likely due to the transient increase of blood flow and BP.

Coarctation of aorta, pheochromocytoma, and cocaine use have been associated with intracranial aneurysm most

**Table 4.19:** Features of sites of herniation.

| Anatomic stage | Respiratory pattern | Pupils | Vestibulo-ocular reflexes | Motor response |
|---|---|---|---|---|
| Diencephalon | Regular or Cheyne Stokes | Small, reactive | Present | Localizes pain stimulus |
| Midbrain and upper pons | Cheyne Stokes breathing | Mid-position, fixed | Absent | Decerebrate |
| Lower pons and upper medulla | Ataxic breathing | Mid-position, fixed | Absent | No movements |
| Medulla | Irregular | Mid-position, fixed | Absent | No movements |

**Table 4.20:** Findings and specific investigations in various secondary hypertension.

| Findings | Disease suspected | Specific investigation |
|---|---|---|
| Paroxysmal | Pheochromocytoma | Urine VMA, |
| Hypertension, palpitations, headache, diaphoresis | | Metanephrine |
| Fatigue, weight gain, menstrual irregularities, diastolic hypertension | Hypothyroidism | Plasma serum TSH (thyroid stimulating horn) |
| Weight loss, tachycardia, tremors, heat intolerance, systolic hypertension | Hyperthyroidism | Serum TSH |
| Depression, muscle weakness, kidney stones, osteoporosis | Hyperparathyroidism | Serum calcium, PTH (parathormone) |
| Enlarged extremities | | |
| Headaches, fatigue, visual disturbances, enlarged tongue, | Acromegaly | GH (growth hormone) |
| Weight gain, muscle weakness, striae, obesity, amenorrhea, moon facies | Cushing's syndrome | Serum cortisol |
| Obesity, snoring, daytime somnolence | Obstructive sleep apnea (OSA) | Polysomnography |
| Enlarged palpable kidneys, family history positive | Autosomal dominant polycystic kidney disease (ADPKD) | Ultrasound abdomen |
| Proteinuria, elevated serum creatinine, edema, anemia | Chronic kidney disease (CKD) | Ultrasound |
| Abdominal/renal bruit | Reno vascular cause | MR angiogram |
| Fatigue, hypokalemia, hypernatremia | Aldosteronism | Plasma rennin to aldosterone ratio |

likely because of elevated blood pressures that occur under these conditions.

### Q. What are the common sites of hemorrhagic strokes?

Hypertensive intraparenchymal hemorrhage usually results from spontaneous rupture of a small penetrating artery deep in the brain.
- Basal ganglia especially putamen
- Thalamus
- Cerebellum
- Pons.
- Frontal and parietal lobes, cortical bleeds rare

### Q. What are the stages of hypertensive retinopathy?

Hypertensive retinopathy is referred to fundus changes occurring in patients suffering from systemic hypertension **(Figs. 4.22 and 4.23)**.

**Pathogenesis**

Three factors which play role in the pathogenesis of hypertensive retinopathy are:
- Vasoconstriction,
- Arteriosclerosis and
- Increased vascular permeability.

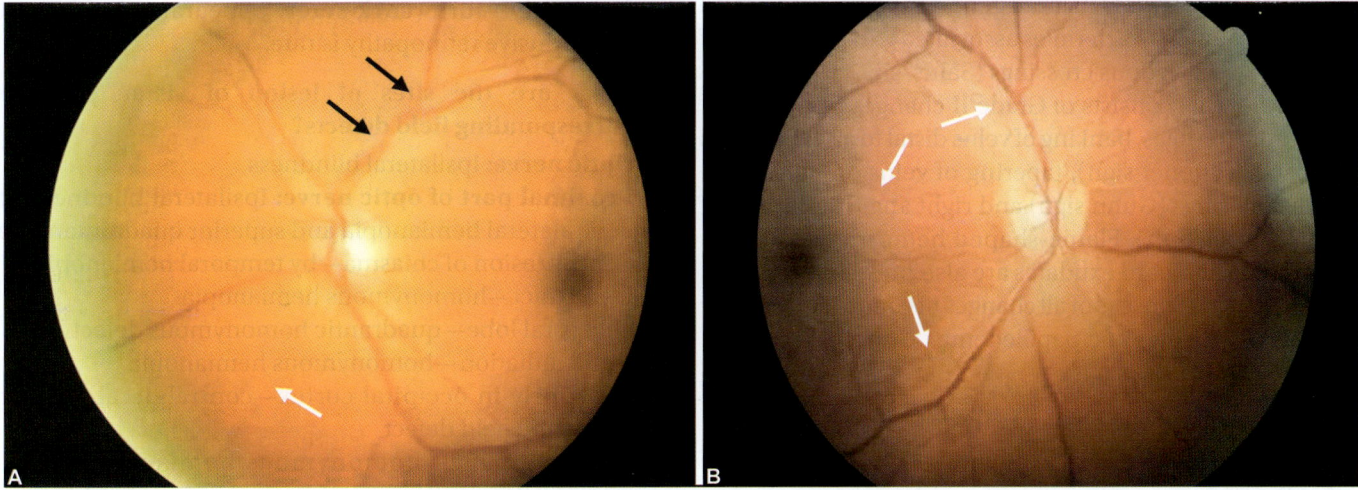

**Figs. 4.22A and B:** Mild hypertensive retinopathy.

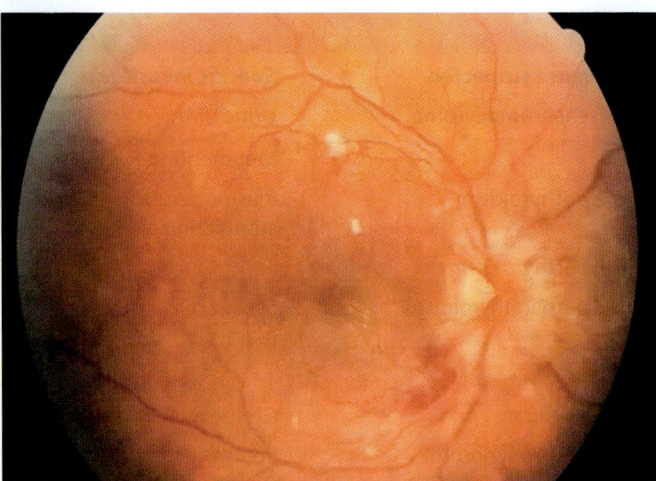

**Fig. 4.23:** Malignant hypertensive retinopathy.

- **Vasoconstriction:** Primary response of the retinal arterioles to raised blood pressure is narrowing (vasoconstriction) and is related to the *severity* of hypertension. It occurs in pure form in young individuals, but is affected by the pre-existing involutional sclerosis in older patients.
- **Arteriosclerotic changes,** which manifest as changes in arteriolar reflex and A-V nipping result from thickening of the vessel wall and are a reflection of the *duration* of hypertension. In older patients arteriosclerotic changes may pre-exist due to involutional sclerosis.
- **Increased vascular permeability** results from hypoxia and is responsible for hemorrhages exudates and focal retinal edema. **Grading of hypertensive retinopathy.**

**Q. How do you grade the hypertensive retinopathy?**

Keith and Wegner (1939) have classified hypertensive retinopathy changes into following four grades:
- **Grade I:** It consists of generalized arteriolar attenuation, particularly of small branches, with broadening of the arteriolar light reflex and vein concealment.
- **Grade II:** It comprises marked generalized narrowing and focal attenuation of arterioles associated with deflection of veins at arteriovenous crossings (Salus' sign).
- **Grade III:** This consists of Grade II changes plus copper-wiring of arterioles, banking of veins distal to arteriovenous crossings (Bonnet sign), tapering of veins on either side of the crossings (Gunn sign) and right angle deflection of veins (Salu's sign). Flame-shaped hemorrhages, cotton wool spots and hard exudates are also present.
- **Grade IV:** This consists of all changes of Grade III plus silver wiring of arterioles and papilledema.

**Q. If confrontation perimetry test of field of vision is not possible, what is the alternate test?**

In a non-cooperative patient, and in a patient who is unable to sit in the bed:
- Menace reflex to be done.
- Menace reflex a shiny object is moved from the periphery to the center and ascertain whether the patient is able to see it, or move your hand quickly towards patient's face and observe the reflex blinking of both eyes.
- Visual field examination is important to localize the lesion
- Frontoparietal location—patient will have hemiplegia and hemisensory syndrome, and if in dominant hemisphere, patient will have aphasia.
- In occipital hematomas patient will have homonymous visual defect.

**Q. What are the clinical signs of coarctation of aorta?**

**Basic bedside features of coarctation of aorta:**
- The upper extremity and thorax may be more developed in comparison to lower extremities.
- Upper extremity pulses are normal. Palpation of pulses may reveal radiofemoral delay (symmetrical reduction and delay of femoral pulses in comparison to radial pulses). All the pulses, such as radial, carotid, brachial, femoral, popliteal and arteria dorsalis pedis should be examined in details. Pulsation of arteria dorsalis pedis may be absent.
- Prominent suprasternal and carotid pulsation.
- Collateral pulsations are present (seen as well as felt) in axilla, trunk and infrascapular area (Suzman's sign). Suzman's sign (dilated, tortuous and pulsatile arteries) is best elicited when the patient stands and bends forward with arms hanging down at sides.
- Systemic hypertension (upper extremity high BP with low or normal BP in lower extremity).
- Bruit over the collaterals.
- **Left ventricular type of cardiac enlargement (heaving apical impulse):** A systolic murmur may be heard over the anterior chest and back. Continuous murmur may be present over collaterals.
- Clinical association bicuspid aortic valve, PDA, VSD, berry aneurysm, polycystic kidneys, Turner's syndrome.
- **Fundoscopy**—retinal arteries are tortuous with frequently—turn (**cork-screw** appearance). Curiously, hypertensive retinopathy is rare.

**Q. What are the sites of lesion of visual path and corresponding field defects?**
- **Optic nerve:** Ipsilateral blindness
- **Proximal part of optic nerve:** Ipsilateral blindness and contralateral hemianopia and superior quadrantanopia
- Central lesion of chiasma—by temporal hemianopia
- Optic tract—homonymous hemianopia
- Temporal lobe—quadrantic homonymous defect
- Optic radiation—homonymous hemianopia
- Anteriorly in occipital cortex—contralateral temporal crescentic field defect
- Occipital lobe—homonymous hemianopia usually sparring the macula.

**Figure 4.24** shows the optic tract lesion and its effects.

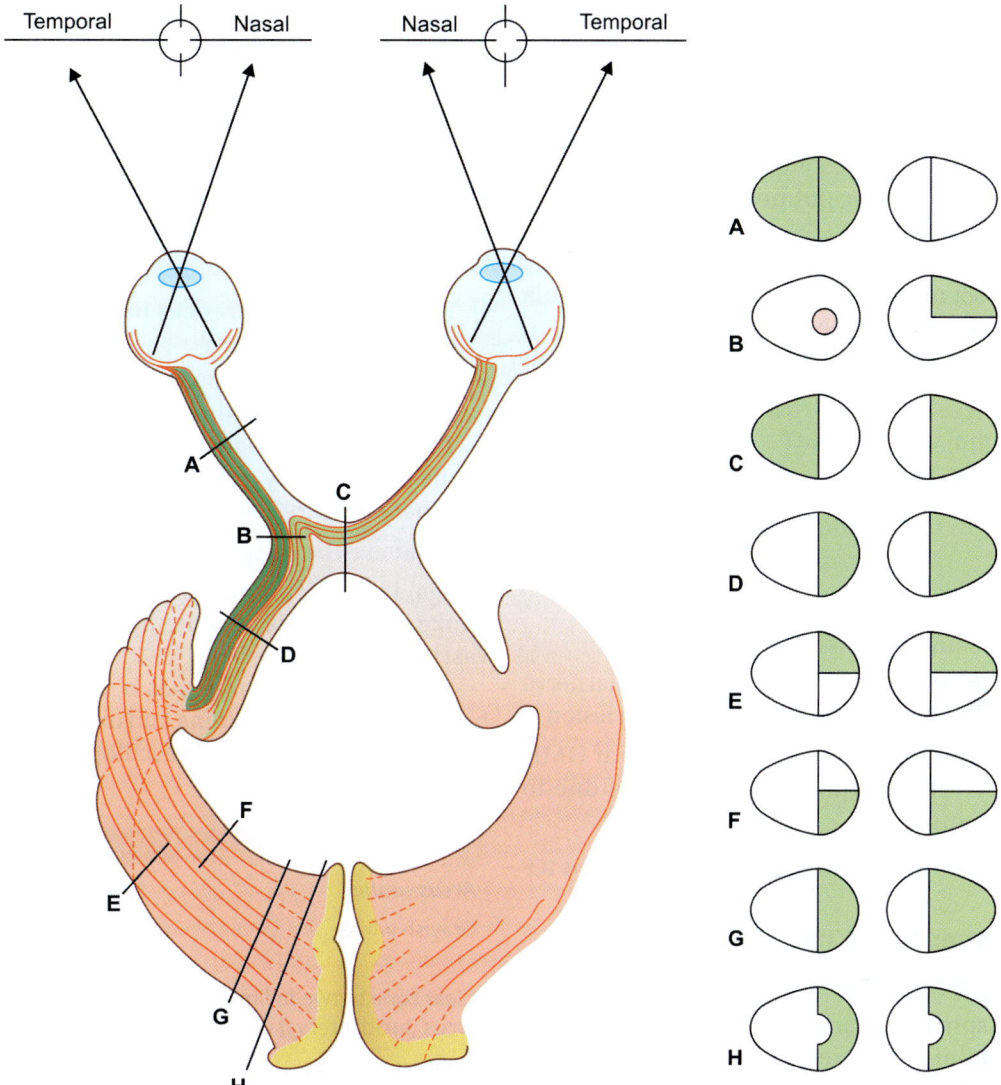

**Fig. 4.24:** Optic tract lesion and its effects.

### Q. What is Kernohan-Woltman sign?

Uncal transtentorial herniation refers to impaction of the anterior medial temporal gyrus (the uncus) into the tentorial opening just anterior to and adjacent to the midbrain. The uncus compresses the third nerve as the nerve traverses the subarachnoid space, causing enlargement of the ipsilateral pupil (the fibers sub-serving parasympathetic pupillary function are located peripherally in the nerve). The coma that follows is due to compression of the midbrain against the opposite tentorial edge by the displaced parahippocampal gyrus. Lateral displacement of the midbrain may compress the opposite cerebral peduncle against the tentorial edge, producing a Babinski sign and hemiparesis contralateral to the hemiparesis that resulted from the mass (the Kernohan-Woltman sign).

### Q. What are stroke mimickers?

- Multiple sclerosis
- Hemiplegic migraine
- Todd's palsy
- CNS abscess
- CNS tumor
- Drug toxicity—lithium, phenytoin, carbamazepine
- Hypertensive encephalopathy
- Hypoglycemia/hyperglycemia
- Psychogenic
- Wernicke's encephalopathy
- Head trauma

### Q. What are "stroke chameleons"?

- The converse of the "stroke mimic" is a presentation suggestive of another condition, which actually represents stroke. These would be "stroke chameleons." The recognition of a chameleon as stroke has implications for therapy and quality of care.
- The common chameleons were initially diagnosed as altered mental status (AMS), syncope, hypertensive

emergency, acute vertigo, systemic infection, and suspected acute coronary syndrome (ACS).

**Q. What is paradoxical embolism?**

Paradoxical embolism or venous thromboembolism transit from right to left sided cardiac chambers, may occur via interventricular, interatrial or pulmonary arteriovenous malformation.

The clinical diagnosis requires a venous source of embolism, an intracardiac defect or a pulmonary arteriovenous fistula and an evidence of arterial embolism.

The most common intracardiac shunt is a PFO. Patent foramen ovale.

**Q. What is the normal word output?**

100–115 words/minute.

**Q. What is the symptom specific for posterior circulation stroke?**

Ataxia.

**Q. What are crossed and uncrossed hemiplegia?**

**Crossed hemiplegia:** Presence of ipsilateral LMN cranial nerve palsy with contralateral hemiplegia due to brainstem lesion

**Uncrossed hemiplegia:** Presence of contralateral UMN cranial nerve palsy with contralateral hemiplegia due to lesions above the brainstem.

**Q. What are the differences between arcus senilis and KF ring?**

Refer **Figures 4.25A and B, and Table 4.21**.

**Q. What is the principle of Osler's maneuver?**

Inflate the cuff of sphygmomanometer above the systolic pressure, if the radial artery remains palpable the real blood pressure may be less than the one obtained through auscultation, this is called pseudohypertension from calcified hardened arteries.

**Q. Can malignancy produce stroke?**

**Yes, malignancy can lead to stroke via:**
- Hypercoagulability
- Non-bacterial thrombotic endocarditis
- Direct tumor compression of blood vessels
- Treatment related effects which potentiate stroke
- Tumor embolism

**Q. What is gag reflex involvement in acute stroke?**

Most stroke patients have transient absent gag reflex until the compensatory action of the opposite corticobulbar fibers take over.

**Q. What are the differences between large vessel infarcts and lacunar infarcts?**

- Lacunar infarcts are due to occlusion of small penetrating branches and measure
- They occur due to lipohyalinosis or microatheroma from the parent artery or hypoperfusion when there is stenosis of parent artery. Large vessel infarcts are atherothrombotic.

**Q. What are the drugs causing stroke?**

Drugs, in particular amphetamines, cocaine, may cause stroke on the basis of acute hypertension or drug-induced vasculopathy.

Phenylpropanolamine has been linked with intracranial hemorrhage, as has cocaine and methamphetamine, perhaps related to a drug-induced vasculopathy.

**Table 4.21:** Depicts the arcus senilis versus Kayser-Fleischer (KF).

| Arcus senilis | Kayser–Fleischer |
|---|---|
| Grayish white | Golden brown or greenish brown |
| Clear zone between limbus and arcus (lucid interval of Vogt) | No clear zone between limbus and KF |
| Appears as a ring | Appears first at upper pole |
| Always forms a complete ring | Can be an incomplete ring |
| Lipid deposits in mainly 2 layers of peripheral cornea stroma—one adjacent to bowman layer and another near Descemet's membrane | Cu deposited in the Descemet's membrane |

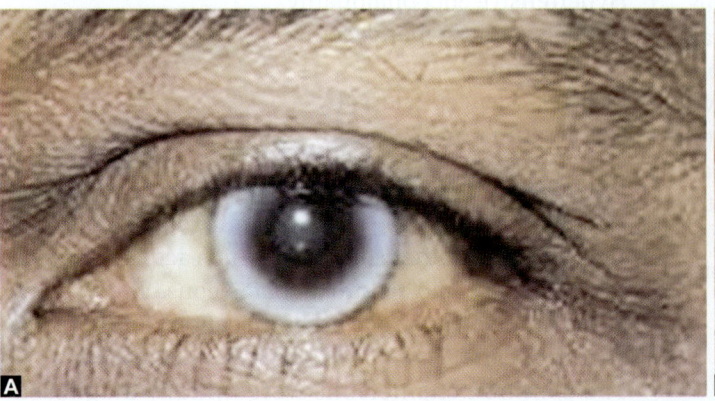
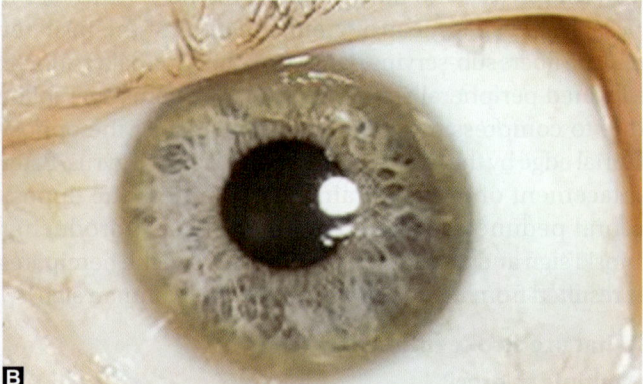

**Figs. 4.25A and B:** Arcus senilis and Kayser–Fleischer (KF) ring.

### Q. What are the effects of alcohol on the nervous system?

- **Acute intoxication:**
  - Euphoria (25–50 mg/dL)
  - Incoordination (50–100 mg/dL)
  - Ataxia (100–200 mg/dL)
  - Stupor (200–400 mg/dL)
  - Coma (400–900 mg/dL)
- Withdrawal syndrome
- Toxic amblyopia.
- Alcohol dementia—cerebral atrophy
- Wernicke-Korsakoff syndrome
- Marchiafava-Bignami syndrome
- **Cerebrovascular accident:**
  - Intracerebral bleed
  - Subarachnoid hemorrhage
  - Subdural hematoma
- Cerebellar degeneration.
- Central pontine myelinolysis
- Peripheral neuropathy
- Saturday night palsy—radial nerve
- Alcoholic hallucinosis
- Delirium tremens
- Depression, anxiety
- Alcohol blackouts
- SACD
- Indirect effects—falls and head injury, hypoglycemia, encephalopathy

### Q. What are the features of Wernicke's encephalopathy?

Alcoholic patients with chronic thiamine deficiency may have central nervous system (CNS) manifestations known as Wernicke's encephalopathy, which consists of:

- Horizontal nystagmus
- Ophthalmoplegia (due to weakness of one or more extraocular muscles)
- Cerebellar ataxia
- Mental impairment

When there is an additional loss of memory and a confabulatory psychosis, the syndrome is known as Wernicke-Korsakoff syndrome.

### Q. What are the features of beri-beri?

Prolonged thiamine deficiency causes beriberi, which is classically categorized as:

- Wet or dry although there is considerable overlap between the two categories.
- Wet beri-beri—primarily presents with cardiovascular symptoms (due to impaired myocardial energy metabolism and dysautonomia)
  - Can occur after 3 months of a thiamine-deficient diet.
  - **C/F:** Enlarged heart, tachycardia, high-output congestive heart failure, peripheral edema, and peripheral neuritis.
- Dry beri-beri—present with a symmetric peripheral neuropathy of the motor and sensory systems, with diminished reflexes.

### Q. What do you mean by delirium tremens?

Approximately 2% of alcoholics experience delirium tremens (DTs), where the withdrawal includes delirium (mental confusion, agitation, and fluctuating levels of consciousness) associated with a tremor and autonomic overactivity (e.g., marked increases in pulse, blood pressure, and respirations). The risks for seizures and DTs can be diminished by identifying and treating any underlying medical conditions early in the course of withdrawal.

### Q. What is Marchiafava-Bignami syndrome?

A rare idiopathic syndrome of dementia and seizures with degeneration of the corpus callosum (reported primarily in male Italian red wine drinkers) (Marchiafava-Bignami disease).

- **Course**:
  - Acute
  - Subacute
  - Chronic

**Clinical features:** Dementia, spasticity, dysarthria and inability to walk CT—lesions appear as hypodense areas in portions of corpus callosum.

**Treatment:** Aggressive nutritional supplementation along with reduction in drinking can prevent the development of the disease.

### Q. Define the criteria for diagnosing multiple sclerosis.

**McDonald criteria:** The McDonald criteria for the diagnosis of MS, as revised in 2017, apply primarily to patients who have a typical clinically isolated syndrome.

- Criteria are not intended for distinguishing MS from other neurologic conditions.
- The core requirement of the diagnosis is the objective demonstration of dissemination of central nervous system lesions in both space and time, based upon either clinical findings alone or a combination of clinical and MRI findings.
- The McDonald criteria can only be applied after careful clinical evaluation of the patient. Additional data needed to confirm the diagnosis of MS depend upon the clinical presentation:
  - Dissemination in space is demonstrated with MRI by one or more hyperintense T2 lesions that are characteristic of MS in at least two of four MS-typical regions of the central nervous system (periventricular, cortical or juxtacortical, infratentorial, and spinal cord) or by the development of an additional clinical attack implicating a different central nervous system site.
  - Dissemination in time is demonstrated with MRI by the simultaneous presence of gadolinium enhancing and nonenhancing lesions at any time, or a new hyperintense T2 and/or gadolinium enhancing lesion(s) on follow-up MRI, irrespective of its timing with reference to a baseline scan, or demonstration of cerebrospinal-fluid

specific oligoclonal bands, or by the development of an additional clinical attack.
- For patients with two or more clinical MS attacks who have objective clinical evidence of two or more lesions or objective clinical evidence of one lesion with reasonable historical evidence of a prior attack involving a lesion in a distinct anatomic location, no additional data are required to make the diagnosis of MS. Nevertheless, brain MRI should be done for all patients being evaluated for MS. For patients with insufficient clinical and MRI evidence to support the diagnosis of MS, and for patients with a presentation other than a typical clinically isolated syndrome or for patients with atypical features, spinal cord MRI and/or cerebrospinal fluid examination are suggested to confirm the diagnosis of MS.

Alternative diagnoses should be considered if MRI and other tests (e.g., cerebrospinal fluid) are negative.
- For patients with two or more attacks who have objective clinical evidence of one lesion, the criteria require additional evidence of dissemination in space.
- For patients with one attack who have objective clinical evidence of two or more lesions, the criteria require additional evidence of dissemination in time.
- For patients with one attack who have objective clinical evidence of one lesion, the criteria require additional evidence of dissemination in space and time.
- For patients who present with insidious neurological progression suggestive of primary progressive MS, the criteria require evidence of the one year of disease progression (retrospectively or prospectively determined), independent of clinical relapse, plus two of the three following criteria:
  - One or more hyperintense T2 lesions characteristic of MS in one or more of the periventricular, cortical or juxtacortical, or infratentorial areas.
  - Two or more hyperintense T2 lesions in the spinal cord.
  - Presence of cerebrospinal fluid-specific oligoclonal bands.

An MS attack (also called a relapse or exacerbation) is defined by the McDonald criteria as a monophasic clinical episode with patient-reported symptoms and objective findings typical of MS, reflecting a focal or multifocal.

The McDonald criteria assign diagnostic confidence as follows:
- The diagnosis of MS is given if the McDonald criteria are fulfilled and there is no better explanation for the clinical presentation.
- The diagnosis of possible MS is given if MS is suspected by virtue of a clinically isolated syndrome but the McDonald criteria are not completely met.

### Q. What are the causes of atrial fibrillation?
- Systemic hypertension
- Myocardial infarction
- Coronary artery disease
- Valvular heart disease
- Congenital heart disease
- An overactive thyroid gland (hyperthyroidism) or other metabolic imbalance
- Exposure to stimulants, such as medications, caffeine, tobacco or alcohol
- Sick sinus syndrome
- Lung diseases
- Previous heart surgery
- Viral infections
- Stress due to pneumonia, surgery or other illnesses
- Sleep apnea

### Q. What is lone atrial fibrillation?
Referred to patients with paroxysmal, persistent, or permanent AF who have no structural heart disease.
- In patients >60 years of age
- It identifies a group of individuals at lowest risk of complications associated with AF including embolization.

### Q. What is amaurosis fugax?
**Definition:** Amaurosis fugax refers to a transient ischemic attack of the retina. Interruption of blood flow to the retina for more than a few seconds results in transient monocular blindness, a term used interchangeably with amaurosis fugax.

**Clinical features:** Patients describe a rapid fading of vision like a curtain descending, sometimes affecting only a portion of the visual field.

**Pathogenesis:** Amaurosis fugax usually results from an embolus that becomes stuck within a retinal arteriole.
- Emboli are composed of cholesterol (Hollenhorst plaque), calcium, or platelet-fibrin debris. The most common source is an atherosclerotic plaque in the carotid artery or aorta.
- Ophthalmoscopy reveals zones of whitened, edematous retina following the distribution of branch retinal arterioles.
- Complete occlusion of the central retinal artery produces arrest of blood flow and a milky retina with a cherry-red fovea.
- Retinal arterial occlusion also occurs rarely in association with retinal migraine, lupus erythematosus, anticardiolipin antibodies, anticoagulant deficiency states (protein S, protein C, and antithrombin deficiency), pregnancy, IV drug abuse, blood dyscrasias, dysproteinemias, and temporal arteritis.

**Treatment:** Aspirin may be useful.

### Q. What is pseudotumor cerebri?
An elevated pressure, with normal cerebrospinal fluid, points by exclusion to the diagnosis of pseudotumor cerebri (idiopathic intracranial hypertension).

Young, female, and obese.

**Drugs causing pseudotumor cerebri:** Hypervitaminosis A
- Tetracyclines

- Amiodarone
- **Treatment:** Carbonic anhydrase inhibitor, such as acetazolamide lowers intracranial pressure by reducing the production of cerebrospinal fluid.

### Q. What are the causes of stroke in young?
Refer **Box 4.3.**

### Q. What is cerebral autosomal dominant arteriopathy with subcortical infarcts and leukoencephalopathy (CADASIL)?
Cerebral autosomal dominant arteriopathy with subcortical infarcts and leukoencephalopathy.
- Inherited disorder
- Onset 4th–5th decade
  - Presents as small-vessel strokes, progressive dementia, and extensive symmetric white matter changes often including the anterior temporal lobes visualized by MRI.
  - Approximately 40% of patients have migraine with aura, often manifest as transient motor or sensory deficits. Onset is usually in the fourth or fifth decade of life.
  - This autosomal dominant condition is caused by one of several mutations in Notch-3, a member of a highly conserved gene family characterized by epidermal growth factor repeats in its extracellular domain.
- Other monogenic ischemic stroke syndromes include cerebral autosomal recessive arteriopathy with subcortical infarcts and leukoencephalopathy (CARASIL) and hereditary endotheliopathy, retinopathy, nephropathy, and stroke (HERNS).

### Q. What are the causes of Bell's palsy?
- Acute inflammatory demyelinating polyneuropathy,
- Lyme disease
- Intratemporal facial nerve schwannomas within the facial canal
- Traumatic fractures of the temporal bone
- Occult skull-based neoplasms of the temporal bone
- Complicated otitis media with mastoiditis
- Gradenigo's syndrome results from inflammation of the petrous apex and causes facial nerve palsy in combination with trigeminal and abducens nerve
- Parotid neoplasms
- Surgical procedures
- Infiltration of facial skin cancers along facial motor nerve branches
- Melkersson-Rosenthal syndrome is a rare granulomatous disease with a triad of facial nerve palsy, facial edema, and tongue fissures.

**Box 4.3:** Stroke in young (age <45 years).

1. **Cardiac embolus**
   - Endocarditis
   - Atrial fibrillation
   - Recent myocardial infarction
   - Dilated cardiomyopathy
   - Intracardiac thrombus
   - Cardiac tumors—atrial myxoma, cardiac rhabdomyoma, cardiac papillary fibroelastoma
   - Sick sinus syndrome
   - Valvular vegetations including nonbacterial thrombotic endocarditis
   - Nonbacterial thrombotic endocarditis—Libman-Sacks endocarditis
   - Rheumatic valvular disease
   - Prosthetic valve
   - Intracardiac tumors
   - Recent cardiac procedures—bypass graft, valvular surgery, heart transplantation, extracorporeal membrane oxygenation (ECMO)
2. **Hypercoagulable states**
   - Sickle cell disease
   - Hemoglobin SC disease
   - Polycythemia
   - Thrombocytosis
   - Thrombotic thrombocytopenic purpura
   - Paroxysmal nocturnal hemoglobinuria
   - Hyperhomocysteinemia and homocystinuria
   - Antiphospholipid antibodies
   - Lupus anticoagulant
   - Anticardiolipin antibodies Antithrombin deficiency
   - Protein C and S deficiency
   - Activated protein C resistance (including, but not limited to, Factor V Leiden mutation)
3. **Inflammatory diseases:**
   - RA
   - SLE
   - Scleroderma
   - Sjögren syndrome
   - Polymyositis
   - Polyarteritis nodosa
   - Wegener granulomatosis
4. **Infectious diseases:**
   - Neurocysticercosis
   - Varicella zoster
   - HIV
   - Bacterial (pyogenic) meningitis
   - *Chlamydia pneumoniae*
   - Hepatitis C virus and mixed cryoglobulinemia
   - Hydatid cyst embolism
5. **Cancer:**
   - Tumor emboli
6. **Hereditary disorders:**
   - Neurofibromatosis
   - Epidermal nevus syndrome
   - CADASIL
   - Sneddon syndrome
   - Williams syndrome

## Q. How do you localise peripheral facial palsy?

| Above the facial nucleus (supranuclear lesion) | • Contralateral paralysis of lower facial muscles with relative preservation of upper muscles.<br>• Lesion located either in brainstem or cortex |
|---|---|
| Pons (nuclear or fascicular lesion) | • Ventral pontine lesion (of Millard-Gubler): Ipsilateral facial monoplegia, lateral rectus palsy (VI), contralateral hemiplegia (corticospinal fibers).<br>• Pontine tegmentum lesion (of Foville): Ipsilateral facial monoplegia; contralateral hemiplegia (corticospinal fibers); paralysis of conjugate gaze to side of lesion (pontine paramedian reticular formation) |
| Cerebellopontine angle (peripheral nerve lesion) | • Ipsilateral facial monoplegia, loss of taste to anterior two-thirds of tongue, impairment of salivary and tear secretion, hyperacusis (if VIII is not affected).<br>• Additional cranial nerves may be involved: deafness, tinnitus, vertigo (VII): sensory loss over face and absence of corneal reflex (V); ipsilateral ataxia (cerebellar peduncle) |
| Facial canal between internal auditory meatus and geniculate ganglion (peripheral nerve type) | • Ipsilateral facial monoplegia, loss of taste to anterior two-thirds of tongue, impairment of salivary and tear secretion, hyperacusis<br>• Eighth nerve may be involved |
| Facial canal between geniculate ganglion and nerve to stapedius muscle | Facial monoplegia; impaired salivary secretion; loss of taste; hyperacusis |
| Facial canal between nerve to stapedius and leaving of chorda tympani | Facial monoplegia; impaired salivary secretion; loss of taste |
| After branching of chorda tympani | Facial paralysis, distribution related to site of lesion |

## Q. What is the difference between rigidity and spasticity?

**Table 4.22** depicts the difference between rigidity and spasticity.

**Table 4.22:** Difference between rigidity and spasticity.

| Rigidity | Spasticity |
|---|---|
| Resistance in all the direction | Resistance in one direction |
| In extrapyramidal involvement | In pyramidal involvement |
| Velocity independent | Velocity dependent |
| Lead pipe and Cog-wheel | Clasp-Knife |
| Affects all muscles | Affects antigravity muscles |

## Q. How do you manage of embolic stroke?

**Investigations:** Echocardiography—echocardiographic evaluation is recommended for stroke patients, primarily to investigate the conditions associated with AF.

Cardiac monitoring—for those in sinus rhythm without a history of AF, cardiac monitoring is recommended for at least the first 24 hours after the onset of ischemic stroke to identify AF or atrial flutter. However, paroxysmal AF may not be detected on short-term cardiac monitoring, such as continuous telemetry and 24- or 48-hour Holter monitors. Ambulatory cardiac monitoring for several weeks (e.g., 30 days) is suggested for all adult patients with a cryptogenic ischemic stroke or cryptogenic TIA likelihood for embolism.

### Treatment

**Reperfusion therapy:** The immediate goal of reperfusion therapy for acute ischemic stroke is to restore blood flow to the regions of brain that are ischemic but not yet infarcted. Intravenous alteplase, the mainstay of reperfusion therapy, improves functional outcome at three to six months when given within 4.5 hours of ischemic stroke onset.

Mechanical thrombectomy is indicated for patients with acute ischemic stroke caused by an intracranial large artery occlusion in the proximal anterior circulation who can be treated within 24 hours of the time last known to be well.

Anticoagulant use with an international normalized ratio >1.7 or PT >15 seconds or evidence of intracranial hemorrhage on neuroimaging are absolute contraindications to treatment with intravenous alteplase.

- **Acute thrombotic therapy:** In patients with atrial fibrillation who suffer an ischemic stroke, acute antithrombotic therapy may be warranted both to reduce disability and the risk of early recurrent stroke, which is 3–5% in the first two weeks. These benefits must be balanced against the risk of intracranial bleeding with antithrombotic therapy.
- **Long-term therapy:** Warfarin is the most studied antithrombotic therapy for prevention of recurrent stroke in patients with atrial fibrillation.
- Non-vitamin K oral anticoagulants also appear highly efficacious—dabigatran rivaroxaban apixaban.
- Due to the high risk of recurrent embolism, lifelong anticoagulation is strongly recommended for secondary prevention.
- For patients who cannot take anticoagulant medications, clopidogrel plus aspirin is recommended.
- **Low molecular weight heparin:** 5,000 U given S/C twice a day
- Dabigatran (non-valvular AF) 150 mg twice daily
- Rivaroxaban—20 mg OD

## Q. What are the difference between UMN and LMN facial palsy?

In a supranuclear, upper motor neuron or central facial palsy, there is weakness of the lower face, with relative sparing of the upper face. The upper face has both contralateral and ipsilateral supranuclear innervation, and cortical innervation of the facial nucleus may be more extensive for the lower face than the upper. The paresis is rarely complete. The lower face is weak, the nasolabial fold is shallow, and facial mobility is decreased. The upper face is not necessarily completely spared, but it is always involved to a lesser degree than the lower face.

With peripheral facial palsy, there is flaccid weakness of all the muscles of facial expression on the involved side, both upper and lower face, and the paralysis is usually complete (prosopoplegia). The affected side of the face is smooth; there are no wrinkles on the forehead; the eye is open; the inferior lid sags; the nasolabial fold is flattened; and the angle of the mouth droops.

Attempting to close the involved eye causes a reflex upturning of the eyeball (Bell's phenomenon).

### Q. What are the difference between LMN and UMN weakness?

Refer **Table 4.23**.

**Table 4.23:** Difference between LMN and UMN weakness.

| Symptom | UMN weakness | LMN weakness |
|---|---|---|
| History of stiffness/heaviness | Present | Absent |
| History of twitching | Absent | Present |
| History of wasting | Absent | Present |
| **Sign** | | |
| Atrophy | None | Severe |
| Fasciculations | None | Common |
| Tone | Spastic | Decreased |
| Distribution of weakness | Pyramidal/regional | Distal/segmental |
| Muscle stretch reflexes | Hyperactive | Hypoactive/absent |
| Babinski sign | Present | Absent |

### Q. What are the non-LMN causes of hypotonia?

- Cerebral or 'neural' shock—hemispheric stroke
- Cerebellar lesions
- Chorea

### Q. What is paratonia/gegenhalten?

Paratonia is a form of hypertonia with an involuntary variable resistance during passive movement; the nature of paratonia may vary from active assistance to active resistance; the degree of resistance depends on the speed of movement (e.g., slow → low resistance, fast → high resistance); the degree of paratonia is proportional to the amount of force applied; and the resistance to passive movement is in any direction and there is no clasp-knife phenomenon. It is a manifestation of diffuse frontal lobe disease.

### Q. What is catatonia?

There is a waxy or lead-pipe type of resistance to passive movement that may be accompanied by posturing, bizarre mannerisms, and evidence of psychosis. It may be possible to mold the extremities into any position, in which they remain indefinitely. Seen in schizophrenia.

### Q. What is hysterical rigidity?

Rigidity of psychogenic origin may be bizarre and may simulate any type of hypertonicity. Hysterical rigidity may simulate decerebration or catatonia. It may be extreme, with neck retraction and opisthotonos, the body resting with only the head and heels upon the bed (arc de cercle).

### Q. What are the conditions causing hemisensory loss?

- **Total contralateral loss of all sensations**
  - **Extensive lesion of thalamus or neighborhood:** Usually vascular
- **Contralateral loss confined to all exteroceptive sensation**
  - partial lesion of thalamus
  - Lesion laterally situated in upper brainstem
  - Associated with motor and cranial nerve involvement.
- **Contralateral loss confined to proprioceptive sensation**
  - Partial lesion of thalamus
  - Lesion medially situated in upper brainstem.
- **Contralateral loss of position sense and cortical sensation with disturbance of light touch and pain**
  - Indicates parietal lobe lesion or a lesion between thalamus and cortex.
- **Contralateral hyperalgesia and hyperesthesia**
  - Partial lesions of thalamus.
- **Loss of pain and temperature on one side of the face and opposite side of the body**
  - Lesion of the medulla affecting the descending root of trigeminal nerve and the ascending spinothalamic tract from the rest of the body. Lateral medullary syndrome (Wallenberg syndrome). This is due to thrombosis of posterior inferior cerebellar artery (PICA) or vertebral artery.
- **Bilateral loss of all forms of sensation below a definite level**
  - This occurs due to gross lesions of spinal cord. It is indicated by a zone of hyperesthesia. Actual level of involvement may be many segments higher than sensory level suggests. If pain and temperature only are affected, it denotes only anterior aspect of cord is involved (anterior spinal artery thrombosis).
- **Unilateral loss of pain and temperature below a definite level (Brown-Sequard syndrome/hemisection of cord)**
  - Ipsilateral motor and proprioceptive impairment and contralateral pain and temperature loss. There is a thin band of analgesia representing involvement of root entry zone. It is seen in cord compression, injury or demyelination.

#### Q. What is sacral sparing?

Sacral sparing refers to preservation of pin prick and temperature sensation in sacral dermatomes (S3, 4, 5) in the presence of sensory loss at a higher level. This is a dependable sign of intrinsic cord compression damaging inner most fibers of spinothalamic tracts while sparing those placed more laterally which subserve sacral sensation.

#### Q. What is saddle anesthesia?

Impairment of sensation over the lowest sacral segments when it affects all forms of sensation accompanied by loss of leg reflexes and sphincter control indicates major lesion of cauda equina. If touch is preserved, lesion is near conus in which plantar reflexes may be extensor and knee jerks may be retained.

#### Q. What is glove and stocking anesthesia?

Loss of all forms of sensation over a clearly defined area in one part of the body only (glove and stocking distribution). This is due to lesion of peripheral nerve or sensory root, e.g., diabetes mellitus, polyneuropathy, mononeuritis multiplex, polyarteritis nodosa.

#### Q. What are the conditions where loss of position and vibration sense alone?

This is due to lesion of posterior column as in tabes dorsalis, subacute combined degeneration, Friedreich's ataxia, also in carcinomatous and toxic (mercury) neuropathy. If lost below a level, suggests compression of posterior part of the cord. If arms are affected much greater than legs and asymmetrically, think of cervical spondylotic myelopathy or foramen magnum lesions.

#### Q. What conditions you get patchy areas of sensory loss.

It suggests chronic polyneuritis (recovery phase), leprosy, tabes dorsalis, mononeuritis multiplex and arachnoiditis. In parietal lobe involvement, there is contralateral hemineglect, hemi-inattention and a tendency not to use contralateral arm or hand. Dysesthesias are unusual. They are present only in focal sensory seizures. Seizures may last for a few seconds or hours and may be associated with motor features. They can occur unilaterally in lip, face, digits or foot or may spread as in Jacksonian march. If bilateral, there is involvement of rolandic area at and just above the Sylvian fissure. **Figure 4.26** depicts the area of sensory loss.

#### Q. What is importance of abnormal sweating?

Hyperhidrosis is the secretion of sweat in amounts greater than physiologically needed for thermoregulation. It is most commonly a chronic idiopathic condition; however, secondary medical conditions or medications should be excluded.

Idiopathic hyperhidrosis localized to certain areas of the body is called primary focal hyperhidrosis. Primary focal hyperhidrosis usually affects the axillae, palms, and soles. The condition may also affect other sites, such as the face, scalp, inguinal, and inframammary areas.

Following diagnostic criteria for primary focal hyperhidrosis.

Focal, visible, excessive sweating of at least six months duration without apparent cause.

Plus at least two of the following characteristics:
- Bilateral and relatively symmetric
- Impairs daily activities
- At least one episode per week
- Onset before age 25
- Family history of idiopathic hyperhidrosis
- Focal sweating stops during sleep

#### Q. What are the features of cortical lesions?

Aphasia, hemineglect, gaze preference, visual deficits, or apraxia. Aphasia usually corresponds to a left hemispheric stroke, since the left cerebral hemisphere controls language function in the majority of both right-handed and left-handed individuals. A nonfluent (Broca's) aphasia often accompanies a right hemiplegia of cortical origin, since the motor cortex is in close proximity to Broca's area.

Acute ischemic stroke syndromes according to vascular territory. **Table 4.24** depicts the acute ischemic stroke syndromes.

**Table 4.24:** Acute ischemic stroke syndromes.

| Artery involved | Syndrome |
| --- | --- |
| ACA | Motor and/or sensory deficit (leg>face, arm) grasp, sucking reflexes<br>Abulia, paratonic rigidity, gait apraxia |
| MCA | Dominant hemisphere: Aphasia, motor and sensory deficit (face, arm>leg>foot), homonymous hemianopia<br>Non-dominant: Hemineglect, anosognosia, motor and sensory deficit (face, arm>leg>foot), homonymous hemianopia |
| PCA | Homonymous hemianopia; alexia without agraphia; visual hallucinations, visual perseverations; sensory loss, choreoathetosis, spontaneous pain (thalamus); III nerve palsy, paresis of vertical eye movement, motor deficit (cerebral peduncle, midbrain) |
| Penetrating vessels (lacunar) | Pure motor hemiparesis<br>Pure sensory deficit<br>Pure sensory-motor deficit hemiparesis, homolateral ataxia<br>Dysarthria/clumsy hand |
| Vertebrobasilar | Cranial nerve palsies, crossed sensory deficits<br>Diplopia, dizziness, nausea, vomiting, dysarthria, dysphagia, hiccup<br>Limb and gait ataxia, motor deficit<br>Coma<br>Bilateral signs suggest basilar artery disease |
| Internal carotid | Progressive or stuttering onset of MCA syndrome, occasionally, ACA syndrome |

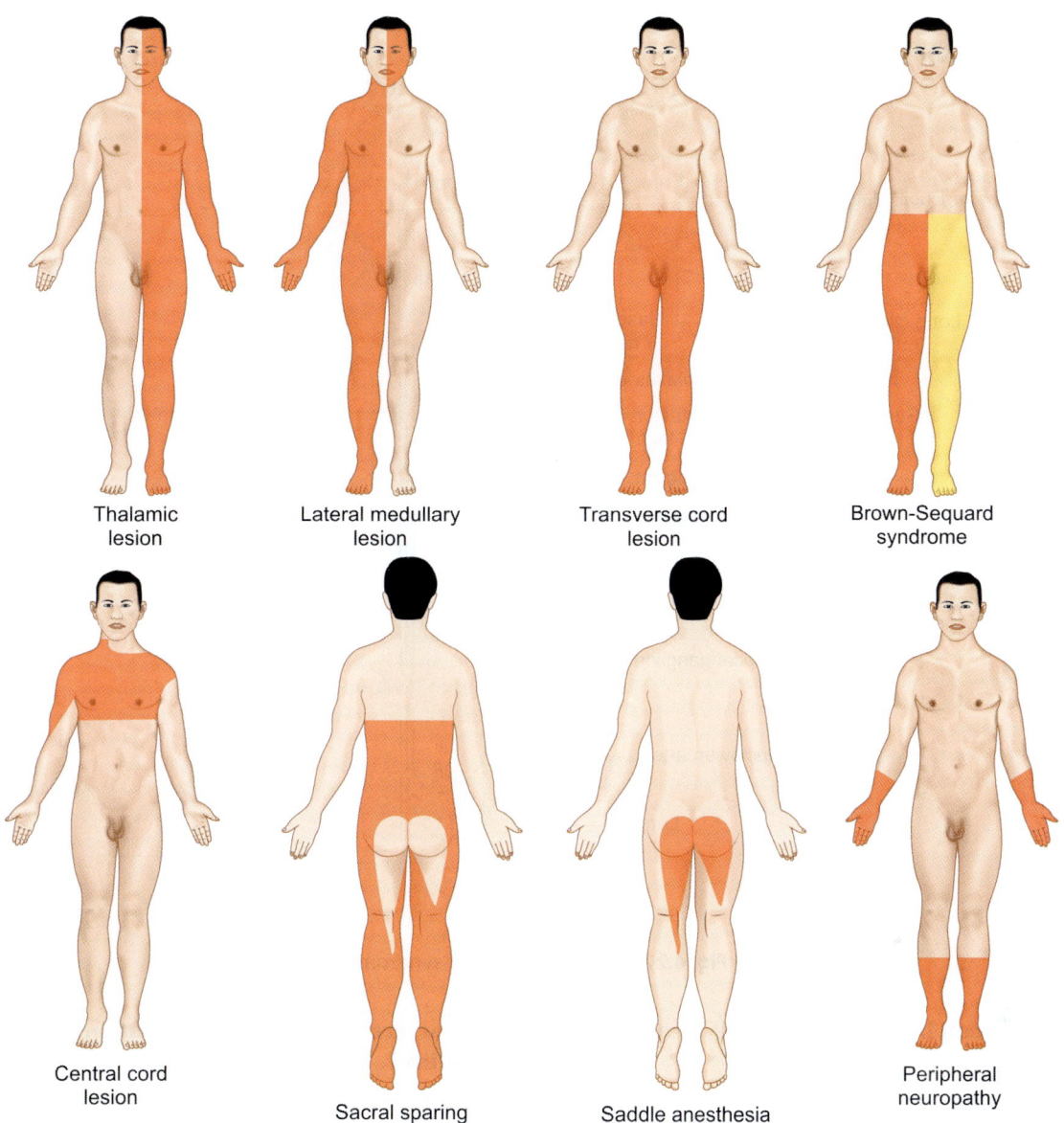

**Fig. 4.26:** Area of sensory loss.

**Q. Which stroke produces Horners syndrome—site of lesion?**

Horner syndrome is a classic neurologic syndrome whose signs include miosis, ptosis, and anhidrosis. A Horner syndrome is a common feature of cluster headache, occurring with unilateral eye or temple pain and lacrimation, generally lasting no more than an hour or two:

**First-order syndrome:** Lesions of the sympathetic tracts in the brainstem or cervicothoracic spinal cord can produce a first-order Horner syndrome. Most common cause is a lateral medullary infarction. Symptoms include vertigo, ataxia, abnormal eye movements, ipsilateral limb ataxia and dissociated sensory loss.

**Second-order syndrome:** Second-order or preganglionic Horner syndromes can occur with trauma or surgery involving the spinal cord, thoracic outlet, or lung apex. Ipsilateral axillary or arm pain often accompanies. Lumbar epidural anesthesia can also produce a Horner syndrome due to pharmacologic disruption of the preganglionic neuron as it exits the spinal cord.

**Third-order syndrome:** Third-order Horner syndromes often indicate lesions of the internal carotid artery, such as an arterial dissection, thrombosis, or cavernous sinus aneurysm. Carotid endarterectomy and carotid artery stenting can also produce a Horner syndrome **(Fig. 4.27)**.

**Q. What are the type of lesion in hypertensive stroke?**
- Ischemic—most common (Birmingham paradox)
- Lacunar stroke—due to lipohyalination
- Intracranial bleed—putamen, thalamus, pons and cerebellum

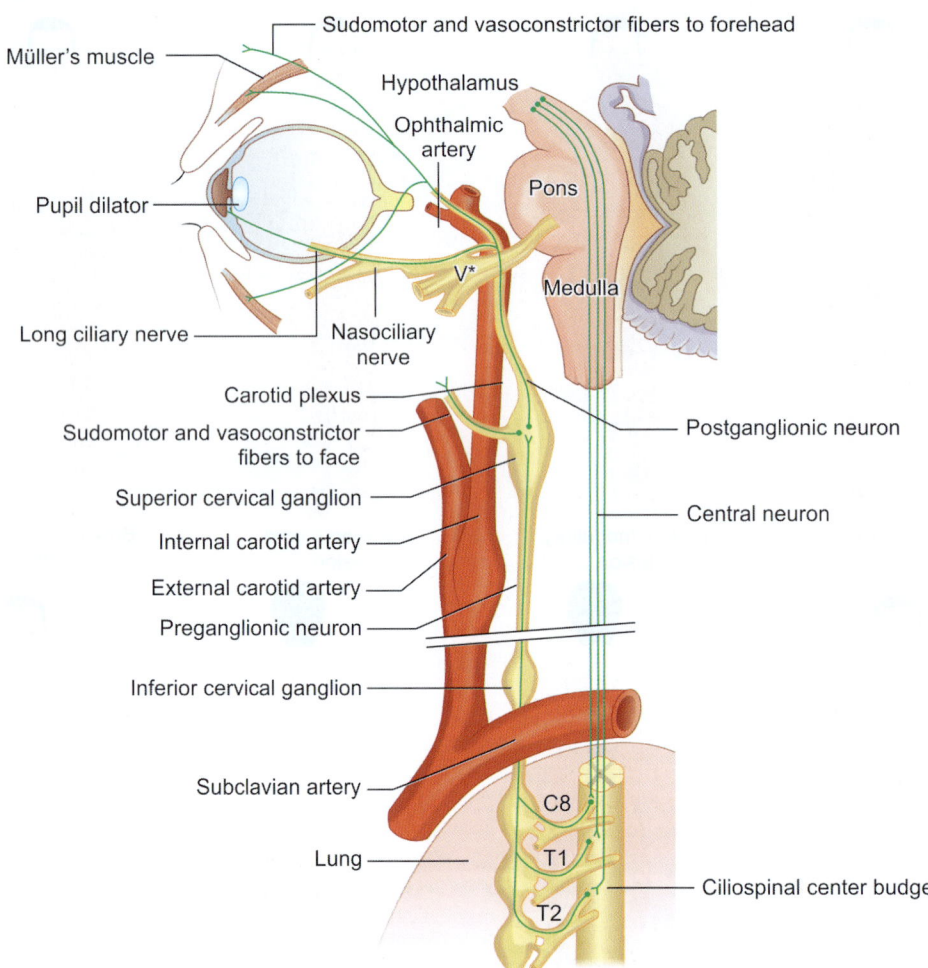

**Fig. 4.27:** Third-order Horner syndromes.

### Q. Conditions that can be picked up by BP measurement in all 4 limbs.

- Coarctation of aorta
- Vasculitis (Takayasu)
- Aortic regurgitation

### Q. When to take average of BP readings?

In severe aortic regurgitation and hyperkinetic circulatory states, diastolic pressure should be recorded both at phase IV and V.

Patients with atrial fibrillation have a significant beat-to-beat variation in their arterial pressure, which may result in underestimation of their BP. Hence, several recordings should be taken and average is noted in each limb.

### Q. What is Hill's sign?.

Popliteal cuff systolic pressure exceeds brachial cuff pressure by >20 mm Hg. It is most important indicator of severity of aortic regurgitation

- Mild AR: 20–40 mm Hg
- Moderate AR: 40–60 mm Hg
- Severe AR: >60 mm Hg

### Q. What are the conditions that producing emotional lability?

Emotional lability is a neurological condition that causes uncontrollable laughing or crying, often at inappropriate times.

- Pseudobulbar palsy
- Alzheimer's disease
- Dementia
- Multiple sclerosis
- ALS
- Traumatic brain injuries, such as coup-counter-coup

### Q. What are non-vascular causes of pseudobulbar palsy?

A pseudobulbar palsy is an upper motor neuron lesion of cranial nerves IX, X and XII.

The commonest cause is bilateral CVAs affecting internal capsule. Other causes include:

- Multiple sclerosis
- Motor neuron disease
- High brainstem tumors
- Head injury

Clinical features include:
- Gag reflex—increased or normal
- Tongue—spastic
- Palatal movement—absent
- Jaw jerk—increased
- Speech—spastic—a monotonous, slurred, high-pitched speech
- Emotions—labile
- Other—bilateral upper motor neuron limb signs

**Ataxic dysarthria:** It is an incoordination of muscles of speech, including the respiratory muscles. Speech is irregular, slurred and drunken, sometimes too loud, or too soft, the words run into each other or are spaced too far, the rhythm is jerky, sometimes explosive, staccato or scanning. There may be accompanying grimaces and gesticulations. It may be quite impossible for the patient to articulate the text phrases—intoxicated person's speech.

**Staccato speech:** Abnormal speech in which the person pauses between words, breaking the rhythm of the phrase or sentence, especially seen in multiple sclerosis.

### Q. What is the tongue position in 12th nerve lesion?

Hypoglossal nerve is a motor nerve which innervates all the extrinsic and intrinsic muscles of the tongue, except palatoglossus which is innervated by the vagus nerve.

An injured hypoglossal nerve causes wasting of tongue and it will not be able to stick out straight. At rest, if the nerve is injured a tongue may appear to have "bag of worms" (fasciculations or wasting (atrophy).

- Right hypoglossal nerve palsy—reduction in size of affected side, excessive ridging and wrinkling, and the curve of tip and median raphe towards the side of the lesion.
- Bilateral wasting and spasticity in motor neuron disease-restricted perfusion, surface indentations and reduction in size without deviation.
- Myotonia—characteristic prolonged dimpling after percussion of tongue.

### Q. Name the muscle that pushes the tongue.

Genioglossus is one of the paired extrinsic muscles of the tongue supplied by hypoglossal nerve. It is the major muscle responsible for protruding the tongue **(Fig. 4.28)**.

### Q. What is circumduction gait in hemiplegia?

Adapted swing phase of gait typical of cerebrovascular accident or any form of head injury causing motor cortex or cerebellar damage; characteristic forward drag of affected limb (moving foot through an arc away from the body, whilst toes remain in contact with the support surface), loss or marked reduction of arms wing, and leaning towards the unaffected side to create sufficient hip height on the affected side to accommodate adapted leg.

**Causes:** Stroke, anterior thigh pain, brain laceration, acute disseminated encephalomyelitis, pyramidal tract lesion, etc.

**Double hemiplegia:** Total or partial inability to move both sides of the body, but for the fact that one side is significantly more affected than the other.

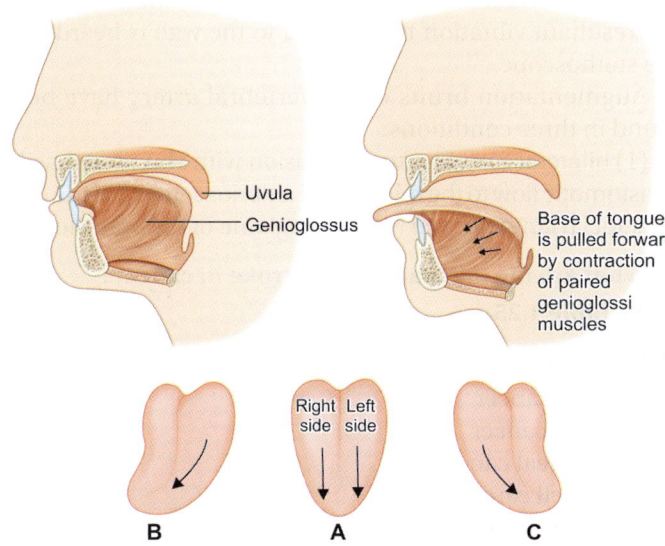

Figure XII-5 Action of the genioglossus muscle in sticking out the tongue.
A. Balanced action of both genioglossus muscles is required to stick the tongue out in the midline.
B. When the right genioglossus muscle is weak or paralyzed, the left genioglossus muscle pushes the tongue to the weak side.
C. When the left genioglossus muscle is weak or paralyzed, the right genioglossus muscle pushes the tongue to the weak side.

**Fig. 4.28:** Action of genioglossus.

### Q. What is vertebral artery bruit?

A bruit is an audible vascular sound associated with turbulent blood flow. Although usually heard with the stethoscope, such sounds may occasionally also be palpated as a thrill **(Fig. 4.29)**.

Vertebral artery bruit is moderately loud and is heard along the course of vertebral artery from the supraclavicular fossa to the mastoid region. The line of greatest intensity lies posterior to the carotid vessels, along the posterior border of the sternocleidomastoid muscle.

It is associated with an increased blood flow along one or both vertebral arteries. When flow in a vessel is augmented

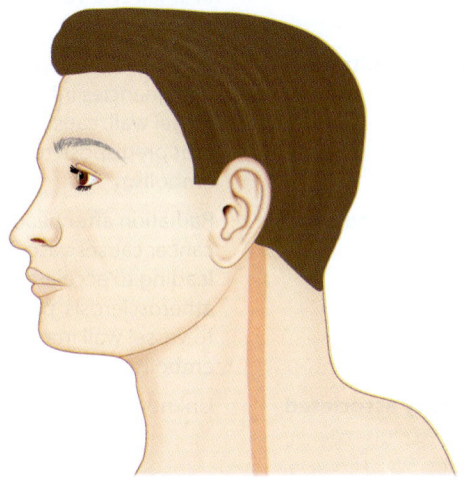

**Fig. 4.29:** Site for auscultation for vertebral artery bruit.

beyond a certain limit, turbulence arises in the stream and the resultant vibration transmitted to the wall is heard with the stethoscope.

Augmentation bruits of the vertebral artery have been found in three conditions:

(1) bilateral carotid artery occlusion with abundant basilar anastomotic flow to the middle and anterior cerebral territories; (2) subclavian steal; and (3) hemangioma of the brainstem.

**Q. What are the mechanisms of stroke in cancer?**
Refer **Table 4.25**.

**Q. Smoking as a risk factor for malignancies.**
- Bladder cancer
- Cervical cancer
- Esophageal cancer
- Renal cell carcinoma
- Laryngeal carcinoma
- Leukemia
- Carcinoma lung
- Oral cancer
- Pancreatic cancer
- Carcinoma stomach

**Q. What are the features of pseudobulbar palsy?**
A more appropriate term for this is supranuclear bulbar palsy. Pseudobulbar palsy (or spastic bulbar palsy) develops when there is disease involvement of the corticobulbar tracts that exert supranuclear control over those motor nuclei that control speech, mastication, and deglutition. The prefix pseudo distinguishes this condition from true bulbar palsy that results from pure LMN involvement in brainstem motor nuclei. Articulation, mastication, and deglutition are impaired in both pseudobulbar and bulbar palsies, but the degree of impairment in pseudobulbar palsy is generally milder. Spontaneous or unmotivated crying and laughter uniquely characterize pseudobulbar palsy. This is also termed emotional lability, hyper emotionality, labile affect, or emotional incontinence and is often a source of great embarrassment to the patient.

**Table 4.25:** Mechanism of stroke in cancer.

| Mechanism | Causal factor | Associated tumors | Stroke characteristics |
|---|---|---|---|
| Hypercoagulability | Adenocarcinomas especially that secrete mucin; tumors activate coagulation cascade; release procoagulant cytokines | Adenocarcinoma of breast, lung, prostate, etc. Also brain, kidney or hematologic malignancies | Embolic appearing infarcts, end vessels |
| Venous-to-arterial embolism | PFO, right-to-left shunt | Uncertain, likely similar to tumors of hypercoagulable state | Embolic appearing |
| Non-bacterial thrombotic endocarditis | Sterile vegetations, clumps of platelets and fibrin develop on aortic valve | Adenocarcinoma is most common | Multiple widely distributed small and large strokes |
| Direct tumor compression of vessel | Tumor growth and resultant edema compresses major intracranial vessel | Glioblastoma multiforme, metastasis to brain | Large vessel, MCA common |
| Tumor embolism | Rare—cardiac tumor causes embolization of malignant cells | Atrial or aortic valve myxoma, metastatic tumors to heart | Embolic appearing |
| Hyperviscosity | Rare—"Thickened" blood causes hyperviscous obstruction of small end vessels | Polycythemia vera, multiple myeloma, Waldenstrom's macroglobulinemia, leptomeningeal carcinomatosis | Small end-vessels strokes |
| Angioinvasive/infiltrative | Rare—hematologic malignancies infiltrate blood vessel wall, causing irregularities that predispose to arterial embolism | B-cell lymphoma | Multiple vascular territory infarcts |
| Post-radiation vasculopathy | Radiation after head and neck cancer causes vasculopathy leading to accelerated atherosclerosis, predisposing to vessel wall irregularities and embolism | Squamous cell carcinoma, other head and neck tumors | Embolic stroke from the affected carotid |
| Chemotherapy associated | Unknown | Associated with as cisplatin, methotrexate, L-asparaginase, thalidomide, lenalidomide, and bevacizumab | Varied |

## Q. What are the tools to asses nutrition?

Ask about weight loss
- Dietary history
- **Body mass index (Quetelet index):** Body weight (in kilograms), divided by the height (in meters) squared.
- Mid-upper arm circumference
- Skin fold thickness
- Waist/hip ratio
- Malnutrition universal screening tool **(Table 4.26)**.

**Table 4.26:** Malnutrition universal screening tool.

| Micronutrient | Deficiency syndromes | Principal symptoms/signs |
|---|---|---|
| Vitamin A (retinol) | | Night blindness, keratomalacia |
| Vitamin B1 (thiamine) | Wernicke's encephalopathy Korsakoff psychosis, beriberi | Nystagmus, 6th cranial nerve palsy, ataxia, acidosis, dementia, paresthesia, neuropathy and cardiac failure |
| Vitamin $B_2$, riboflavin | Ariboflavinosis | Angular stomatitis, glossitis, magenta tongue |
| Niacin, nicotinic acid | Pellagra | Dermatitis of sun exposed areas, dementia, poor appetite, difficulty sleeping, confusion, sore mouth |
| Vitamin $B_6$, pyridoxine | | Poor appetite, lassitude, oxaluria |
| Pantothenic acid | | Nausea, abdominal pain, paresthesiae, burning feet |
| Biotin | | Dermatitis, depression, lassitude, muscle pains, electrocardiogram abnormalities, blepharitis |
| Folic acid | | Macrocytic anemia, thrombocytopenia and megaloblastic bone marrow |
| Vitamin $B_{12}$ | | Subacute combined degeneration, macrocytic anemia |
| Vitamin C, ascorbic acid | Scurvy | Poor wound healing fatigue, limb pain, shortness of breath, difficulty sleeping, gingivitis, perifollicular purpura, hyperkeratosis |
| Vitamin D, ergo/cholecalciferol | Rickets/ Osteomalacia | Bone pain, proximal myopathy |
| Vitamin E, tocopherol | | Hemolysis, posterior column signs, ataxia, muscle wasting, retinitis pigmentosa, such as changes, night blindness |
| Vitamin K, phylloquinone and other menaquinones | | Bruising, purpura, nose and GI bleeds |
| **Trace elements** | | |
| Iron | | Koilonychia, smooth tongue, anemia, esophageal web |
| Zinc | Acrodermatitis enteropathica | Peristomal/perinasal/perineal erythema, thin hair, diarrhea, apathy, anorexia, growth failure, hypoglycemia |
| Copper | | Microcytic hypochromic anemia, neutropenia, scurvy like bone lesions, osteoporosis |
| Chromium | | Peripheral neuropathy, hyperglycemia |
| Selenium | | Cardiomyopathy |
| Iodine | | Goiter |

## Q. What are the features of non-dominant hemisphere lesions?

A wide variety of behavioral abnormalities may follow stroke in the hemisphere non-dominant for speech and language. The non-dominant hemisphere deficits are:
- Neglect
- Extinction
- Impersistence
- Prosopagnosia
- Topographical disorientation
- Constructional apraxia
- Dressing apraxia
- Confabulation—reduplicative paramnesia and anosognosia

## Q. What are the causes of loss of sudden onset loss of consciousness?

- Hypoglycemia hypotension stroke
- Seizures
- Arrhythmogenic right ventricular cardiomyopathy hypertrophic cardiomyopathy.
- Brugada syndrome.
- Familial polymorphic ventricular tachycardia, also called "catecholaminergic polymorphic VT.

**Q. What is hypoglycemia symptoms?**
Refer **Table 4.27**.

| Table 4.27: Symptoms of hypoglycemia. | |
|---|---|
| **Sympathetic symptoms** | **Neuroglycopenic symptoms** |
| Palpitations, tremor anxiety, sweating, increased hunger | Cognitive impairment, confusion Behavioral changes, weakness, parasthesias, lack of motor coordination, slurred speech, visual disturbances, vertigo, focal neurological deficits, seizures, coma and death |

**Q. What is hypoglycemic awareness?**
Individuals with long-standing diabetes or frequent hypoglycemia may lose their protective autonomic response and develop neuroglycopenic symptoms without warning. Most typically associated with long-standing type 1 diabetes, hypoglycemia unawareness can also complicate the management of patients with insulinoma and the diabetes that follows pancreatectomy **(Fig. 4.30)**.

Hypoglycemia unawareness (HU) is defined as the onset of neuroglycopenia before the appearance of autonomic warning symptoms or as the failure to sense a significant fall in blood glucose below normal levels.

**Q. What is locked-in syndrome?**
The locked-in syndrome (LIS) is a catastrophic condition caused most often by ischemic stroke or hemorrhage, affecting the corticospinal, corticopontine, and corticobulbar tracts in the brainstem. Because consciousness and higher cortical functions are spared, patients can sometimes communicate through eye movements.

There are two requisites for the diagnosis of locked-in syndrome:

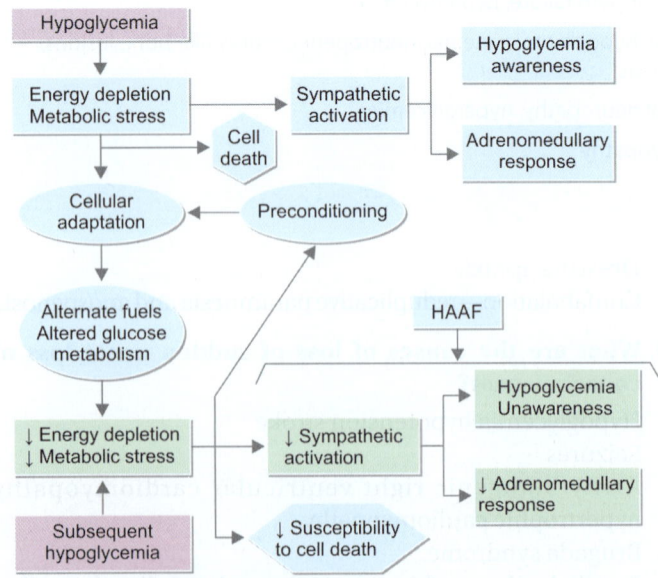

**Fig. 4.30:** Hypoglycemic unawareness.

1. Retained alertness and cognitive abilities
2. Paralysis of the limbs and oral structures such that the individual cannot signal with the limbs or speak

**Etiology:** Ischemic infarction of the ventral pons is usually due to basilar artery embolism or thrombosis pontine hemorrhage, which is most often related to hypertension but can also result from vascular malformations.

**Q. How CVA produces loss of consciousness? Role of reticular activating system.**
The reticular acting system is a complex neural network connecting the reticular formation of the brainstem to the cerebral cortex through excitatory relays in the intralaminar nuclei of the thalamus. Assessing the ascending reticular activating system (RAS) is crucial in the diagnosis and management of patients with impaired consciousness.

Strokes of the midbrain can affect the RAS and lead to hypersomnia and cognitive impairment.

**Q. What are the significance of jaw jerk reflex?**
- The jaw jerk reflex or the masseter reflex is a stretch reflex used to test the status of a patient's trigeminal nerve (cranial nerve V) and to help distinguish an upper cervical cord compression from lesions that are above the foramen magnum.
- The mandible or lower jaw is tapped at a downward angle just below the lips at the chin while the mouth is held slightly open. In response, the masseter muscles will jerk the mandible upwards. Normally, this reflex is absent or very slight. However, in individuals with upper motor neuron lesions the jaw jerk reflex can be quite pronounced.

**Q. What are the specific signs of anterior circulation and posterior circulation?**
Refer **Table 4.28**.

**Q. What is Parinauds syndrome?**
Parinaud syndrome, also known as the dorsal midbrain syndrome, is a supranuclear vertical gaze disturbance caused by compression of the tectal plate. It is characterized by a classic triad of findings:
- Upward gaze palsy, often manifesting as diplopia
- Pupillary light-near dissociation (pupils respond to near stimuli, but not light)
- Convergence-retraction nystagmus

Its importance lies in that recognition of Parinaud syndrome localizes pathology to impingement of or origin in the tectal plate, most frequently due to a posterior commissure or pineal region mass (typically solid tumors rather than pineal cysts).

**Q. What is top of basilar artery syndrome?**
Top of the basilar syndrome, also known as rostral brainstem infarction, occurs when there is thromboembolic occlusion of

| Table 4.28: Signs of anterior circulation and posterior circulation. | |
|---|---|
| **Anterior circulation stroke** | **Posterior circulation stroke** |
| **Dominant hemispheric lesion**<br>✦ Right hemiparesis—variable involvement of face and upper and lower extremity<br>✦ Right-sided sensory loss in a pattern similar to that of the motor deficit—usually involves all modalities, decreased stereognosis, and graphesthesia<br>✦ Right homonymous hemianopia<br>✦ Dysarthria<br>✦ Aphasia, fluent and nonfluent<br>✦ Alexia<br>✦ Agraphia<br>✦ Acalculia<br>✦ Apraxia<br>**Non-dominant hemispheric lesion**<br>✦ Left hemiparesis—same pattern as on right<br>✦ Left-sided sensory loss—similar pattern that of the motor deficit<br>✦ Left homonymous hemianopia—same pattern as on right<br>✦ Dysarthria<br>✦ Neglect of the left side of environment<br>✦ Anosognosia<br>✦ Asomatognosia<br>✦ Loss of prosody of speech<br>✦ Flat affect | ✦ Dizziness or vertigo<br>✦ Dysarthria<br>✦ Nausea or vomiting<br>✦ Loss or alteration of consciousness<br>✦ Limb weakness<br>✦ Ataxia nystagmus |

the top of the basilar artery. This results in bilateral thalamic ischemia due to occlusion of perforator vessels.

### Clinical presentation

Clinically, top of the basilar syndrome is characterized by:
- Visual and oculomotor deficits
- Behavioral abnormalities
- Somnolence, hallucinations and dreamlike behavior
- Motor dysfunction is often absent Radiographic features
  On CT the finding that should not be missed is that of a hyperdense basilar artery. Imaging features are discussed further in the more general article on acute basilar artery occlusion. Angiography (CT, MR, catheter) can be used to confirm the finding by demonstrating a filling defect.

### Differential diagnosis

The pattern of established infarction can be mimicked by:
- Artery of Percheron infarct
- Bilateral internal cerebral vein thrombosis (dural venous sinus thrombosis)
- Other causes of thalamic restricted diffusion

### Q. What is light near association?

Argyll Robertson pupils (AR pupils or, colloquially, "prostitute's pupils") are bilateral small pupils that reduce in size on a near object (i.e., they accommodate), but do not constrict when exposed to bright light (i.e., they do not react to light). They are a highly specific sign of neurosyphilis; however, Argyll-Robertson pupils may also be a sign of diabetic neuropathy. In general, pupils that accommodate but do not react are said to show light-near dissociation (i.e., it is the absence of a miotic reaction to light, both direct and consensual, with the preservation of a miotic reaction to near stimulus (accommodation/convergence).

### Q. What is neurosyphilis—eye signs?

Interstitial keratitis, anterior, intermediate, and posterior uveitis, chorioretinitis, retinitis, retinal vasculitis and cranial nerve and optic neuropathies.

### Q. What are the causes of pseudobulbar palsy? How is it different from bulbar palsy?

Refer **Table 4.29**.

| Table 4.29: Causes of bulbar and pseudobulbar palsy. | |
|---|---|
| **Bulbar palsy** | **Pseudobulbar palsy** |
| **Etiology:**<br>✦ Motor neuron disease<br>✦ Syringobulbia<br>✦ Guillain-Barre syndrome<br>✦ Poliomyelitis<br>✦ Subacute meningitis (carcinoma, lymphoma)<br>✦ Neurosyphilis<br>✦ Brainstem CVA<br>**Clinical features**<br>✦ Gag reflex—absent<br>✦ Tongue—wasted, fasciculations, "wasted, wrinkled, thrown into folds and increasingly motionless"<br>✦ Palatal movement—absent<br>✦ Jaw jerk—absent or normal<br>✦ Speech—nasal<br>✦ "indistinct (flaccid dysarthria), lacks modulation and has a nasal twang"<br>✦ Emotions—normal<br>✦ Other—signs of the underlying cause, e.g., limb fasciculations | **Etiology:**<br>✦ Bilateral CVA affecting internal capsule (most common)<br>✦ Multiple sclerosis<br>✦ Motor neuron disease<br>✦ High brainstem tumors<br>✦ Head injury<br>**Clinical features**<br>✦ Gag reflex—increased or normal<br>✦ Tongue—spastic "it cannot be protruded, lies on the floor of the mouth and is small and tight"<br>✦ Palatal movement—absent<br>✦ Jaw jerk—increased<br>✦ Speech—spastic: "a monotonous, slurred, highpitched, 'Donald Duck' dysarthria" that "sounds as if the patient is trying to squeeze out words from tight lips"<br>✦ Emotions—labile<br>✦ Other—bilateral upper motor neuron (long tract) limb signs |

**Q. What is artery of Percheron and mention its clinical significance??**

The artery of Percheron is where a single thalamic perforating artery arises from the proximal PCA (P1 segment) between the BA and PCOM and supplies the rostral mesencephalon and both paramedian thalami. Proximal embolism is thought to be the most common etiology of stroke in this territory with this variant.

Asymmetric thalamic involvement is seen in two-thirds of cases and midbrain infarction is present in over half. Patients with bilateral paramedian thalamic lesions may develop altered sensorium, vertical gaze palsy, and memory impairment. Conventional vascular imaging does not routinely demonstrate these tiny perforating vessels. Hypoplastic or absent P1 segments are more likely to be seen with this variant. Other vascular causes of bilateral thalamic injury include venous thrombosis, top of the basilar occlusion, and hypoxic–ischemic injury.

**Q. What are the causes of altered consciousness?**

**Symmetrical non structural:**

- **Toxins:**
  - Lead
  - Thallium
  - Mushroom
  - Cyanide
  - Methanol
  - Carbon monoxide
  - Ethylene glycol
- **Drugs:**
  - Sedatives
  - Barbiturates
  - Hypnotics
  - Bromides
  - Alcohol
  - Opiates
  - Paraldehyde
  - Salicylate
  - Psychotropics
  - Anticholinergics
  - Amphetamines
  - Lithium
  - MAO inhibitors

**Symmetrical structural:**

- **Supratentorial:**
  - Bilateral internal carotid occlusion
  - Bilateral anterior cerebral artery occlusion

**Asymmetrical structural:**

- **Supratentorial:**
  - Thrombotic thrombocytopenic purpura
  - Disseminated intravascular coagulation
  - Non-bacterial thrombotic endocarditis
  - Subacute bacterial endocarditis
  - Fat embolus
  - Unilateral hemisphere mass with herniation
- **Metabolic:**
  - Hypoxia
  - Hypercapnea
  - Hypernatremia/hyponatremia
  - Hypoglycemia
  - Hyperglycemic non-ketotic coma
  - Diabetic ketoacidosis
  - Lactic acidosis
  - Hypercalcemia
  - Hypocalcemia
  - Hypermagnesemia
  - Hyperthermia
  - Hypothermia
  - Reye's encephalopathy
  - Aminoaciduria
  - Wernicke encephalopathy
  - Porphyria
  - Hepatic encephalopathy
  - Uremia
  - Dialysis encephalopathy
  - Addisonian crisis
- **Subarachnoid hemorrhage:**
  - Thalamic hemorrhage
  - Trauma—contusion, concussion
  - Hydrocephalus
- **Subdural hemorrhage, bilateral:**
  - Intracerebral bleed
  - Pituitary apoplexy
  - Massive or bilateral supratentorial infarction
  - Multifocal leukoencephalopathy
  - Creutzfeldt-Jacob disease
  - Adrenal leukodystrophy
  - Cerebral abscess
  - Cerebral vasculitis
- **Infections:**
  - Bacterial meningitis
  - Viral encephalitis
  - Postinfectious encephalomyelitis
  - Syphilis
  - Sepsis
  - Typhoid fever
  - Malaria
  - Waterhouse-Friderichsen syndrome
- **Psychiatric:** Catatonia
- **Others:**
  - Postictal

- Diffuse ischemia (myocardial infarction, arrhythmia, congestive heart failure)
- Hypotension
- Fat embolism
- hypertensive encephalopathy
- Hypothyroidism

♦ **Infratentorial:** Basilar occlusion, midline brainstem tumor, pontine hemorrhage

♦ **Subdural empyema:**
  - Thrombophlebitis, multiple sclerosis
  - Leukoencephalopathy associated with chemotherapy, acute disseminated encephalomyelitis

**Q. What is gaze preference/deviation and where do you see it?**

Frontal eye fields are responsible for contralateral conjugate horizontal gaze. With frontal lobe lesions there occurs gaze palsy with or without gaze deviation.

Paramedian pontine reticular formation governs the ipsilateral conjugate horizontal gaze.

So a destructive frontal lobe lesion, causes gaze deviation to the same side of lesion and away from the side of hemiparesis. The deviation is generally of large amplitude and prominent. These deviations usually resolve in a few days.

In the pontine destructive lesions the gaze deviation is to the side of hemiparesis and crossed hemiplegia is seen (hemiplegia + LMN cranial nerve palsy). The deviation is usually subtle. The deviation is persistent or permanent.

Irritative lesions of the frontal lobe cause gaze deviation to opposite side of lesion whereas the irritative lesions of brainstem cause gaze deviation to the side of lesion.

**Q. What is the cause of hyponatremia in neurologic diseases? What are differences between cerebral salt wasting syndrome (CSW) and syndrome of inappropriate ADH secretion (SIADH)?**

In neurological diseases, the hyponatremia may be due to SIADH or cerebral salt wasting syndrome. SIADH is due to inappropriately high ADH levels causing volume expansion whereas in CSW high ADH levels are due to volume depletion from salt loss with negative fluid balance. Elevated levels of ANP and BNP favor the diagnosis of CSW. Decreased BUN or serum uric acid levels are usually seen in CSW. SIADH and CSW can be differentiated with the help of Fractional excretion of uric acid which remains high even after the correction of hyponatremia in CSW.

Diagnosis of CSW can be done when there is volume depletion, low CVP, polyuria, high fractional excretion of sodium, uric acid and high urine osmolality.

Management of CSW is with saline replacement and addition of fludrocortisone whereas SIADH requires fluid restriction. **Table 4.30** depicts the differences between CSW and SIADH.

**Table 4.30:** Differences between CSW and SIADH.

| | CSW | SIADH |
|---|---|---|
| Cerebral injury | Usually evident | May be present |
| Volume status | Hypovolemic/dehydrated | Euvolemic/hypervolemic |
| Central venous pressure | Decreased | Normal/increased |
| Serum sodium | Decreased | Decreased |
| Urine volume | Increased | Normal/decreased |
| Urine osmolality | Increased | Increased |
| Urinary sodium concentration | Increased | Increased |
| Fractional excretion of uric acid | High | |
| Remains high even after correction of sodium | High | |
| Brain natriuretic peptide | Normal/increased | Normal |
| Treatment | Salt and water repletion with fludrocortisone | Salt intake with free water restriction |

**Q. What is oculocephalic reflex and in which conditions it can be done?**

In comatose patient oculocephalic reflex (Doll's eye phenomenon) and caloric testing can be done.

Oculocephalic reflex can be done by sudden rotation of head by examiner laterally and also flexion and extension of the neck. In normal oculocephalic reflex (normal or positive Doll's eye phenomenon), the conjugate eye movement occurs in opposite direction related to the movement of head. This test helps in identifying subtle ocular palsies. Abnormal disconjugate movements occur with cranial nerve palsies, internuclear ophthalmoplegia or restrictive eye disease.

Supratentorial lesions and metabolic processes (except Wernicke encephalopathy) do not alter this reflex but brainstem lesions affecting the pathway and nuclei involved in ocular movements show abnormal oculocephalic reflex. Disconjugate movements indicate lesion of medial longitudinal fasciculus or CN 3 or 6 pathway such as in case of brainstem lesions **(Table 4.31)**.

**Q. What is Balint syndrome?**

This was described by Balint in 1909 when the patient acts blind yet can see the minor details of objects in central vision field. This is seen in bilateral hemisphere lesions involving parietal and frontal lobes. It can occur secondary to bilateral parieto-occipital strokes and bilateral posterior hemisphere degeneration conditions.

**Table 4.31:** Eye movements.

| Method | Response | Interpretation |
|---|---|---|
| Lateral head rotation | Eyes remain conjugate, move in direction opposite to head movement and maintain position in space | Normal |
| | No movement in either eye on rotating head to left or right | Bilateral pontine gaze palsy, bilateral labyrinthine dysfunction, drug intoxication, anesthesia |
| | Eyes move appropriately when head is rotated in one direction but do not move when head is rotated in opposite direction | Unilateral pontine gaze palsy |
| | One eye abducts, the other eye does not adduct | Third nerve palsy and internuclear ophthalmoplegia |
| Vertical head flexion and extension | Eyes remain conjugate, move in direction opposite to head movement and maintain position in space | Normal |
| | No movement in either eye | Bilateral midbrain lesions |
| | Only one eye moves | Third nerve palsy |
| | Bilateral symmetrical limitation of upgaze | Aging |

It includes triad of:
- Psychic paralysis of gaze (ocular motor apraxia)—difficulty directing eyes away from central fixation
- Optic ataxia (incoordination of extremities under visual control but normal coordination under proprioceptive control.
- Impaired visual attention.
  - Partial deficits related to Balint syndrome include isolated optic ataxia due to disruption of transmission of visual information from occipital cortex to premotor areas. (dorsal visual stream comprises of dorsal occipital and parietal areas).
  - Second partial Balint syndrome deficit is simultanagnosia (loss of ability to perceive more than one item at a time) due to left occipital lesions and have associated alexia without agraphia.

### Q. What are primitive reflexes? What is their significance?

They occur either due to cortical or subcortical damage to frontal lobes. Grasp and suck reflexes are specific indicators of extensive frontal lobe disease.

Grasp reflex is by stroking patient's palm with examiner's radial aspect of index finger and rubbing the palm along with volar aspect of fingers. If the patient grasps the examiner's hand then the reflex is positive and called forced grasping reflex.

Damage to contralateral area 6 in mesial part of hemisphere is for release of grasp reflex.

**Palmomental reflex:** It consists of ipsilateral mentalis muscle contraction when the patient's palm is stroked with blunt object. This reflex indicates damage to contralateral paracentral cortex and it can be elicited by stroking the arm or even the chest.

When tapping on upper lip, if pouting movement of lips occur in the patient, it is called positive snout reflex. Curving of lips around a round object is sucking reflex and if curving of lips around a round object brought near the side of mouth or cheek occurs, it is rooting reflex.

Snout reflex indicates impairment of corticobulbar projection and suck reflex occurs with diffuse frontal premotor disease.

Corneomandibular reflex is when the patient's jaw deviates to the side opposite of the stimulated cornea.

### Q. What is the relation between degree of carotid stenosis and character of bruit?

Carotid bruit is a sign of carotid atherosclerosis leading to stenosis. Bruit is usually present if stenosis is >50%. With modest carotid stenosis, bruit will be of short duration and heard in mid-systole. As the degree of stenosis increases the duration and intensity of bruit becomes more and is pansystolic in nature. Soft, longer duration, high frequency bruits indicate hemodynamically significant stenosis. Audible bruit is absent with stenosis of more than 85%.

### Q. What is the treatment of acute ischemic stroke?

Treatment of acute ischemic stroke includes:
- Airway, breathing and oxygenation to be taken care of and supplemental oxygen should be provided to maintain $SpO_2$ >94%.
- The blood pressure of patient should be carefully lowered so that systolic BP <185 mm Hg and diastolic BP <110 mm Hg before IV fibrinolytic therapy is initiated. If indicated it is reasonable to lower BP by 15% during first 24 hours of stroke. Once the patient is neurologically stable antihypertensives can be started.
- Hyperthermia to be treated and hyperglycemia needs to be controlled so that blood glucose levels of 140–180 mg/dL is maintained.
- If patient presents within 4.5 hours of ischemic stroke symptom onset, intravenous fibrinolytics like alteplase can be administered after weighing the benefits and risks.
- Mechanical thrombectomy can be done if eligible.
- Dual antiplatelets (aspirin+clopidogrel) can be given for initial 21 days as a secondary stroke prevention measure.
- Nutrition and DVT prophylaxis to be taken care of.

- Complications and conditions related to stroke to be treated.

**Q. What are the antihypertensives used for lowering blood pressure in ischemic stroke? Why should the blood pressure be not lowered drastically?**

**Patient otherwise eligible for acute reperfusion therapy except that BP >185/110 mm Hg**
- Labetalol 10–20 mg IV over 1–2 min, may repeat 1 time or
- Nicardipine 5 mg/hr IV, titrate up by 2.5 mg/hr every 5–15 min, maximum 15 mg/hr, when desired BP reached, adjust to maintain proper BP limits or
- Clevidipine 1–2 mg/hr IV, titrate by doubling dose every 2–5 min until desired BP reached, maximum 21 mg/hr
- Hydralazine or enalaprilat can also be given
- If BP not less than 185/110 mm Hg do not administer alteplase

**Management of BP during and after alteplase or to reduce BP ≤180/105 mm Hg**

Monitor BP every 15 min for 2 hr from start of alteplase therapy then every 30 min for 6 hr, then every hour for 16 hours.

**If systolic BP>180–230 mm Hg or diastolic BP >105–120 mm Hg**
- Labetalol 10 mg IV followed by infusion 2–8 mg/min or
- Nicardipine 5 mg/hr, titrate by 2.5 mg/hr every 5–15 min, maximum 15 mg/hr or
- Clevidipine 1–2 mg/hr IV, titrate by doubling dose every 2–5 min until desired BP reached, maximum 21 mg/hr
- If BP not controlled or diastolic BP >140 mm Hg, consider IV sodium nitroprusside

As lowering the blood pressure drastically can lead to hypoperfusion of the cerebral ischemic penumbra and further ischemia, lowering of BP to lower values and hypotension should be avoided in acute ischemic stroke.

**Q. What are the doses of antihypertensives used in hypertensive emergencies?**
- **Labetalol:** 2 mg/min up to 300 mg or 20 mg over 2 min, then 40–80 mg at 10 minute intervals up to 300 mg total.
- **Enalaprilat:** 0.625–1.25 mg over 5 min 6–8 hourly and maximum dose is 5 mg/dose.
- **Nicardipine:** Initial 5 mg/hour, titrate by 2.5 mg/hour at 5–15 minute intervals, maximum is 15 mg/hour.
- **Nitroprusside:** Initial 0.3 µg/kg/min, usual 2–4 µg/kg/min and maximum is 10 µg/kg/min for 10 min.
- **Nitroglycerin:** Initial 5 µg/min then titrate by 5 µg/min at 3–5 min intervals. If no response at 20 µg/min, increments of 10–20 µg/min may be used.
- **Esmolol:** Initial 80–500 µg/kg/min then 50–300 µg/kg/min.
- **Phentolamine:** 5–15 mg bolus
- **Hydralazine:** 10–50 mg at 30 minute intervals.

**Q. Define apraxia.**

Apraxia is impaired ability (inability) to carry out (perform) skilled, complex, and organized motor activities in the presence of normal basic motor, sensory, and cerebellar functions.

**Examples of complex motor activities:** Dressing, using cutlery, and geographical orientation.

**Table 4.32** depicts the types of apraxia.

| Table 4.32: Types of apraxia. | |
|---|---|
| **Types** | |
| Ideomotor apraxia | Most common. It is the inability to perform a specific motor command/act (e.g., cough, lighting a cigarette with a matchstick) in the absence of motor weakness, incoordination, and sensory loss or aphasia. Site of lesion is bilateral parietal lobe. Buccofacial apraxia involves apraxic deficits in movements of the face and mouth. Limb apraxia encompasses apraxic deficits in movements of the arms and legs |
| Dressing apraxia | Site of lesion is nondominant parietal lobe. It is inability to wear his/her dress |
| Constructional apraxia | It is inability to copy simple diagrams or build simple blocks. Site of lesion is nondominant parietal lobe |
| Ideational apraxia | It is a deficit in the execution of a goaldirected sequence of movements even with real object (e.g., asked to pick up a pen and write, the sequence of uncapping the pen, and placing the cap at the opposite end). This is commonly associated with confusion and dementia rather than focal lesions associated with aphasic conditions |
| **Types** | |
| Gait apraxia (Bruns ataxia) | Seen in normal pressure hydrocephalus (NPH) |
| Gaze apraxia | Part of Balint syndrome |
| Other apraxias | Speech apraxia, conceptual apraxia, and conduction apraxia |

**Q. Define agnosia.**

Agnosia is failure to recognize objects (e.g., places, clothing, persons, sounds, shapes, or smells), despite the presence of intact sensory system. **Table 4.33** shows the types of agnosia. **Site of lesion:** Contralateral parietal lobe.

**Q. What is the management of stroke?**

Refer **Figure 4.31**.

**Q. What is NIHSS score?**

A severity score that quantifies neurological impairment **(Fig. 4.32)** for specific categories within the following broad domains:
- Level of consciousness, orientation, and ability to follow commands

## Table 4.33: Types of agnosia.

| Types of agnosias | |
|---|---|
| Visual agnosia | Failure to recognize what is seen with eyes despite the presence of intact visual pathways. The individual can describe the shape, color, and size without naming it. Site of lesion is in the posterior occipital or temporal lobes |
| Prosopagnosia | A type of visual agnosia in which patient cannot identify familiar faces, sometimes the reflection/his or her own face in the mirror even including their own. Site of lesion is parietooccipital lobe |
| Simultanagnosia | It is inability to perceive more than one object at a time |
| Autotopagnosia | It is a form of agnosia, characterized by an inability to localize and orient different parts of the body |
| Pseudopolymelia | The feeling of false—the feeling of false extremities. More frequent, the patients feel the extremities. More frequent, the patients feel the third hand |
| Anosognosia | It is an inability or refusal to recognize a defect or disorder that is clinically evident |
| Auditory agnosia | It consists of the loss of ability to know objects on sounds characteristic for them (clock—on ticking) |

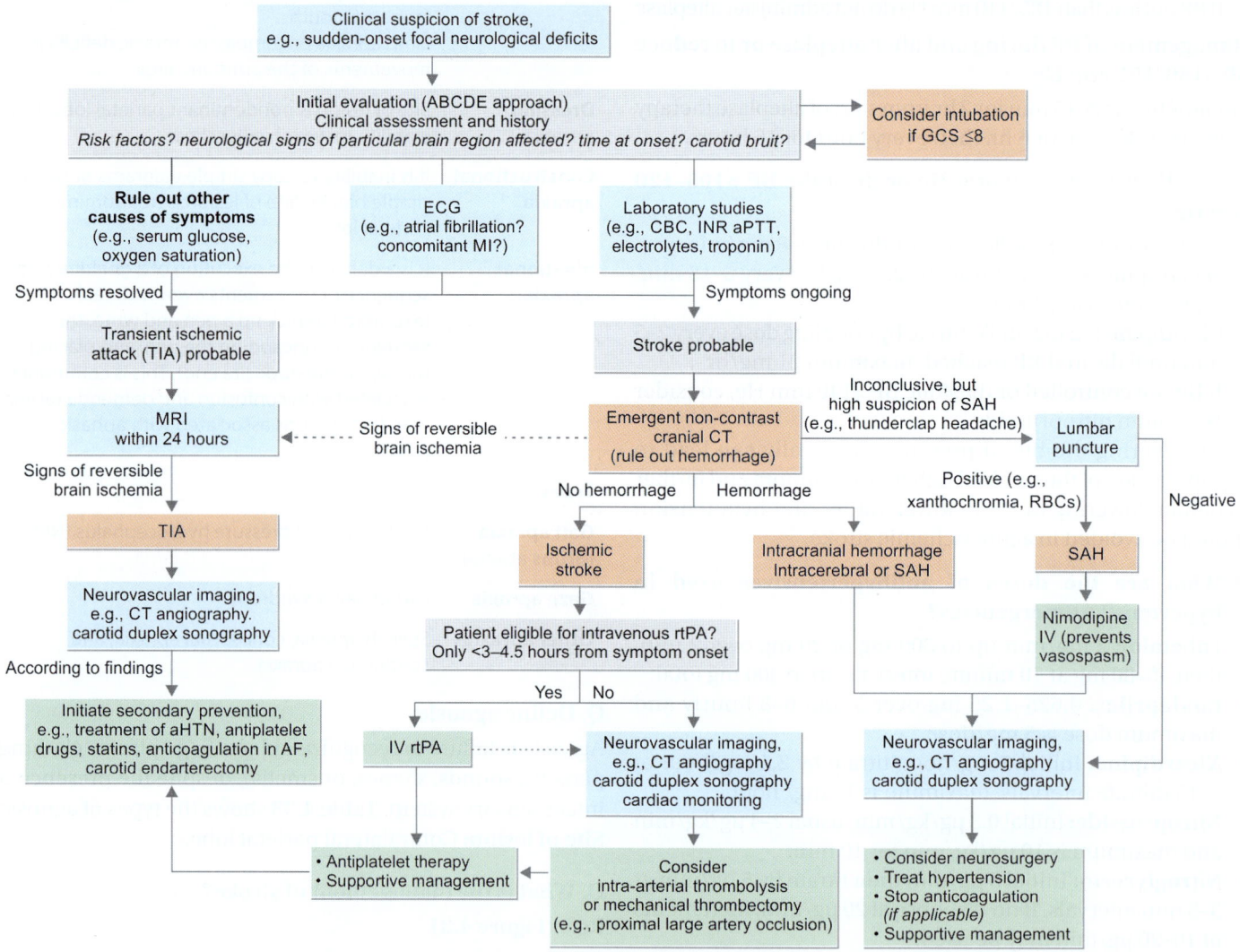

**Fig. 4.31:** Management of stroke.

- Cranial nerve palsies, e.g., visual impairment, facial droop
- Motor and sensory deficits or neglect
- Language impairment
- Coordination

**Q. What is unilateral spatial neglect?**
- Defined as a failure to report, respond, or orient to sensory stimuli presented to the side contralateral to the stroke lesion

## NATIONAL INSTITUTES OF HEALTH STROKE SCALE
### Stroke scale

| Category | Stroke scale | | | | | Score |
|---|---|---|---|---|---|---|
| **1a. Level of consciousness**<br>Alert, Drowsy, etc. | (0) Alert | (1) Drowsy | (2) Stuporous | (3) Coma | | |
| **1b. LOC questions**<br>Month, age | (0) Answer both correctly | (1) Answer one correctly | (2) Incorrect | | | |
| **1c. LOC commands**<br>Open/close eyes, make a fist and let go | (0) Obeys both correctly | (1) Obeys one correctly | (2) Incorrect | | | |
| **2. Best gaze**<br>Eyes open—patient follows examiner's fingers or face. | (0) Normal | (1) Partial gaze paisy | (2) Forced deviationect | | | |
| **3. Visual**<br>Introduce visual stimulus/threat to patient's visual field quadrants. Cover 1 eye and hold up fingers in all 4 quadrants. | (0) No visual loss | (1) Partial hernia hpsla | (2) Complete hernia hpsla | (3) Bilateral hernia hpsla | | |
| **4. Facial palsy**<br>Show teeth, raise eyebrows and squeeze eyes tightly shut. | (0) Normal | (1) Minor | (2) Partial | (3) Complete | | |
| **5a. Motor arm—left**<br>Elevate extremity to 90 degrees and score drift/movement. Count to 10 out loud and use fingers for visual cue. | (0) No drift | (1) Drift | (2) Can't resist gravity | (3) No effort against gravity | (4) No movement | |
| | NT = Amputation, joint fusion | | | | | |
| **5b. Motor arm—right**<br>Elevate extremity to 90° and score drift/movement. Count to 10 out loud and use fingers for visual cue. | (0) No drift | (1) Drift | (2) Can't resist grvity | (3) No effort against gravity | (4) No movement | |
| | NT = Amputation, joint fusion | | | | | |
| **6a. Motor leg—left**<br>Elevate extremity to 30 degrees and score drift/movement. Count to 5 out loud and use fingers for visual cue. | (0) No drift | (1) Drift | (2) Can't resist grvity | (3) No effort against gravity | (4) No movement | |
| | NT = Amputation, joint fusion | | | | | |
| **6b. Motor leg—right**<br>Elevate extremity to 30 degrees and score drift/movement. Count to 5 out loud and use fingers for visual cue. | (0) No drift | (1) Drift | (2) Can't resist grvity | (3) No effort against gravity | (4) No movement | |
| | NT = Amputation, joint fusion | | | | | |
| **7. Limb ataxia**<br>Finger to nose, heal down shin | (0) Absent | (1) Present in one limbs | (2) Present in two limbs | | | |
| **8. Sensory**<br>Pin prick to face, arms, trunk, and legs. compare sharpness side to side | (0) Normal | (1) Partial loss | (2) Severe loss | | | |
| **9. Best language**<br>Name items, describe picture, and read sentences. Do not forget glasses if they normally wear them. | (0) No aphasia | (1) Mild to moderate aphasia | (2) Severe aphasia | (3) Mute | | |
| **10. Dysarthria**<br>Evaluate speech clarity by patient reading or repeating words on list. | (0) Normal articulation | (1) Mild to moderate dysarthria | (2) Near to unintelligible or worse | | | |
| | NT = Intubated or other physical harrier | | | | | |
| **11. Extinction and inattention**<br>Use information from prior testing or double simultaneous stimuli testing to identify neglect. Face, arms, legs, and visual fields. | (0) No neglect | (1) Partial neglect | (2) Complete neglect | | | |
| NT = not testable acceptable as noted above | | | | | | |

| Score | Stroke severity |
|---|---|
| 0 | No stroke symptoms |
| 1–4 | Minor stroke |
| 5–15 | Moderate stroke |
| 16–20 | Moderate to severe stroke |
| 21–42 | Severe stroke |

TOTAL = ☐

**Fig. 4.32:** Scores are assigned for each category are combined and totals can range from 0 (no impairment) to 42 (most severe).

- More obvious forms of neglect involve colliding with environment on involved side, ignoring food on one side of plate, and attending to only one side of body
- USN is found in about 23% of stroke patients
- More common in patients with right sided lesions (42%) than left sided lesions (8%) and is more persistent with right sided strokes
- Recovery of USN common; most recovery occurs in first 6 months and later recovery is less common
- USN associated with negative prognosis for functional outcome, poorer mobility, longer LOS in rehab, and slower rates of improvement

## Case 2: Spinal Cord Diseases

### Brief History
A 47-year-old male, hailing from _____ who is working as agricultural labor came with complaints of bilateral lower limb weakness since 20 days.

### History of Presenting Illness
- Patient presented with history of sudden in onset of bilateral lower limb weakness since 20 days started left lower limb gradually progressed to right lower limb in 4 days associated with severe back pain mainly in thoracic region not radiating to lower limbs with no history of trauma.
- History of decreased sensations of both lower limbs from umbilicus region mainly touch and pain sensations of same intensity in entire both lower limbs. No history of bowel and bladder involvement disturbances. History of difficulty for sitting from supine position since 10 days.
- No history of upper limb weakness, difficulty in rolling over bed or lifting neck in supine position.
- No history of abdominal pain, behavioral disturbances, convulsion.
- No history of runny nose, loose stools, abdominal pain prior to the presentation. No history of recent vaccination.
- No history of diminished vision/double vision/drooping of eyelids/facial asymmetry/drooling of saliva/difficulty in chewing/deafness/tinnitus/vertigo/difficulty in swallowing/nasal regurgitation of food. No history of trauma/dizziness/vertigo/bowel and bladder disturbance.

### Past History
- No history of similar events in the past.
- Patient was diagnosed to have lung cancer 8 months back completed chemotherapy. He also had newly diagnosed diabetes since one week. History of insertion of tube into the left side of lung 8 months back. No history of thyroid disorders, hypertension, ischemic heart disease (IHD), tuberculosis (TB), asthma, epilepsy.

### Treatment History
- Currently patient was on radiation therapy.
- Patient was also on diabetic medication which was recently diagnosed. Patient was on steroids.
- He completed six cycles of chemotherapy 5 months back.

### Family History
- No similar complaints in family
- Married 18 years back
- Three children all are healthy.

### Personal History
- Consumes mixed diet
- No history of alcohol intake and smoking
- History of areca nut intake present
- No history of high-risk behavior
- No history of substance abuse
- History of weight loss and appetite present

### Summary
A 47-year-old male with k/c/o carcinoma of lung with sudden onset of weakness of both lower limbs with decreased sensations of both lower limbs associated with severe back pain without involvement of bowel and bladder involvement and cranial nerves involvement, I would like to consider differential diagnosis as:
- Acute myelopathy
- Acute peripheral neuropathy
- Anterior spinal artery thrombosis

### General Physical Examination
- Patient is conscious, cooperative, well-oriented to time, place and person.
- BMI could not be calculated (patient could not stand for weight measurement).

### Vitals:
- Pulse: Rate: 90/min regular, normal volume and character, vessel wall-normal. All peripheral pulses well felt and equal on both sides.
- Blood pressure: 130/80 mm Hg right arm supine position. No postural drop JVP not raised
- Afebrile at the time of examination pallor present.

### Vitals:
- Pulse: Rate: 90/min regular, normal volume and character, vessel wall-normal. All peripheral pulses well felt and equal on both sides.
- Blood pressure: 130/80 mm Hg right arm supine position. No postural drop JVP not raised
- Afebrile at the time of examination pallor present.
- Clubbing present of grade 3
- No cyanosis, icterus, pedal edema, lymphadenopathy
- No palpable peripheral nerves
- No neurocutaneous marker
- Callosities present on the lateral aspect of left foot
- Hyperpigmented popular itchy lesions present on the shoulders, thoracic region, back bedsore present in the sacral area.

### Nervous System Examination
Higher mental functions:
- Right-handed individual
- Literacy—7th standard
- Conscious and oriented
- Memory and intelligence—normal, no emotional lability
- No evidence of hallucinations or delusions
- Speech—comprehension/word output/naming/repetition/reading/writing—normal.

## Cranial Nerve Examination

| Cranial nerves | Right | Left |
|---|---|---|
| Olfactory | Normal | Normal |
| Optic nerve | | |
| Fundus | Normal | Normal |
| Visual acuity | Normal | Normal |
| Color vision | Normal | Normal |
| Field of vision | Normal | Normal |
| Oculomotor, trochlear abducens | Normal | Normal |
| Extraocular movements | Normal | Normal |
| Pupils | Normal | Normal |
| Light reflex | Normal | Normal |
| Trigeminal nerve Sensations over face | Normal | Normal |
| Motor (temporalis, masseters, pterygoids) | | |
| Reflexes: Corneal reflex Jaw jerk | Absent | Absent |
| Facial nerve: Forehead wrinkling No deviation of angle of mouth Nasolabial fold | Normal Normal Normal | Normal Normal Normal |
| Vestibulocochlear nerve: Nystagmus | Absent | Absent |
| Rinne test | Normal (air conduction >bone conduction) | Normal |
| Weber test | Not lateralized | |
| Glossopharyngeal and vagus nerve: Uvula central palatal movements, gag reflex | Normal Present | Normal Present |
| Spinal accessory nerve: Trapezius | Normal | Normal |
| Sternocleidomastoid-XII Hypoglossal nerve | Normal No fasciculation or deviation of tongue | Normal |

## Motor Examination

| Attitude Upper limb Lower limb | Adducted at shoulder, extended at elbow, wrist Extended | Same as right side Extended |
|---|---|---|
| Bulk Upper limb Arm Forearm | 24 | 24 |
| No wasting of small muscles of hand Lower limb | 23 | 23 |
| Thigh | 34 | 32 |
| Calf | 26 | 24 |
| Tone Upper limb Lower limb | Normal tone Hypotonia | Normal tone. Hypotonia |
| Power Upper limb Shoulder joint Elbow joint Wrist joint Hand grip | 5/5 5/5 5/5 Normal | 5/5 5/5 5/5 |
| Lower limb Hip joint Knee joint Ankle joint Trunk muscles Neck muscles Abdominal muscles | 1/5 1/5 1/5 Normal Normal Lower abdominal signs are weak (Beevor's sign positive) | 1/5 1/5 1/5 |
| Reflexes deep reflexes Biceps Triceps Brachioradialis Knee Ankle: | ++ ++ ++ +++ Absent | ++ ++ ++ +++ Absent |
| Superficial Corneal Abdominal Plantar | ++ Absent Extensor | ++ Absent Extensor |
| Sensory system Upper limb: Pain, temperature, touch, vibration and position sense Lower limb: Pain, temperature, touch, vibration and position sense | Normal Decreased (up to T9) | Normal Decreased (upto T9) |

### Cerebellar Signs:
No abnormal cerebellar signs.
- Signs of meningeal irritation absent
- Skull: Normal

- *Spine: Severe tenderness present in thoracic vertebrae at the level of T6, T7, T8*
- *Gait: Cannot be assessed*

**Respiratory System Examination**
- *Trachea central*
- *Bilateral chest movements equal*
- *Dull percussion: Note present in left infrascapular region and infra-axillary region*
- *Decreased breath sounds in infrascapular region and infra-axillary region*
- *No added sounds*

**Cardiovascular System Examination**
Apex beat in left 5th intercostal space 1 cm medial to midclavicular line S1, S2 heard, no murmur.

**Per Abdomen**
- *Soft, non-tender*
- *No organomegaly, no free fluid.*

**Diagnosis**
A 47-year-old man with k/c/o of carcinoma of lung presented with sudden onset of bilateral lower limb weakness associated with decreased pain, temperature, touch proprioception sensations from below the umbilicus with severe tenderness in thoracic vertebrae of T6, T7, T8 without the involvement of bowel and bladder I would like to consider the diagnosis of compressive myelopathy due to metastasis from carcinoma of lung.

**Vertical Level**
- *Motor level—T10*
- *Sensory level—T9*
- *Reflex level—T8*
- *Spinal cord level—T8*
- *Vertebral level—T6*

**Horizontal Level**
Lesion with extramedullary and extradural involvement.

## DISCUSSION

### Q. Discuss the tracts present in the spinal cord.

Refer **Figure 4.33**.

The spinal cord originates at the medulla and continues caudally to terminate at the filum terminale, a fibrous extension of the conus medullaris is that terminates at the coccyx.

The adult spinal cord is approximately 45 cm long, oval or round in shape, and enlarged in the cervical and lumbar regions, where neurons that innervate the upper and lower extremities, respectively are located. The meninges that cover the spinal cord are continuous with those of the brainstem and cerebral hemispheres.

- The adult cord consists of 31 segments, each containing an exiting ventral motor root and entering dorsal sensory root.

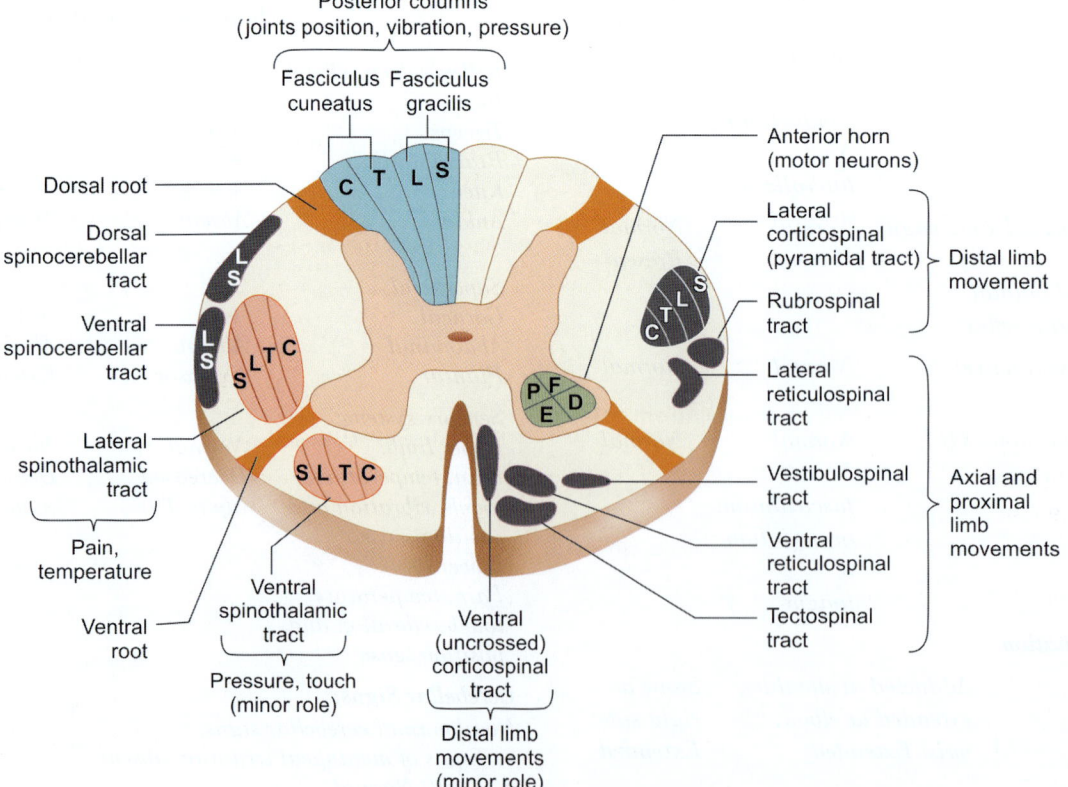

**Fig. 4.33:** Tracts of spinal cord.

- During embryologic development, growth of the cord lags behind that of the vertebral column, and in the adult spinal cord ends at approximately the first lumbar vertebral body. The lower spinal nerves take an increasingly downward course to exit via the appropriate intervertebral foramina.
- The first seven pairs of cervical spinal nerves exit above the same-numbered vertebral bodies, whereas all the subsequent nerves exit below the same-numbered vertebral bodies; this situation is due to the presence of eight cervical spinal cord segments but only seven cervical vertebrae.

### Q. How do you calculate spinal cord level from vertebral level?

The approximate relationship between spinal cord segments and the corresponding vertebral bodies are shown in **Table 4.34**.

**Table 4.34:** Relationship between spinal cord segments and the corresponding vertebral bodies.

| Spinal cord level | Corresponding vertebral body |
|---|---|
| Upper cervical | Same as cord level |
| Lower cervical | 1 level higher |
| Upper thoracic | 2 levels higher |
| Lower thoracic | 2 to 3 levels higher |
| Lumbar | T10 to T11 |
| Sacral | T12 to L1 |
| Coccygeal | L1 |

### Q. What are the classical features of spinal cord involvement?

- Presence of sensory deficit and/or motor weakness in both lower limbs and/or upper limbs.
- Bladder and bowel involvement
- Brown-Sequard type of clinical picture
- Presence of definite sensory level
- Vertebral pain.

### Q. What is the vascular supply to the spinal cord?

Refer **Figure 4.34**.

- **The anterior spinal artery:** Union of the anterior spinal branches of the vertebral artery and descends within the anterior median fissure.
- **The two posterior spinal arteries:** Originate from the vertebral arteries and descend in the posterolateral sulcus.
- By themselves not sufficient and depend on feeder arteries that join them along their course (6–10 join the ASA and 10–20 join the PSA).

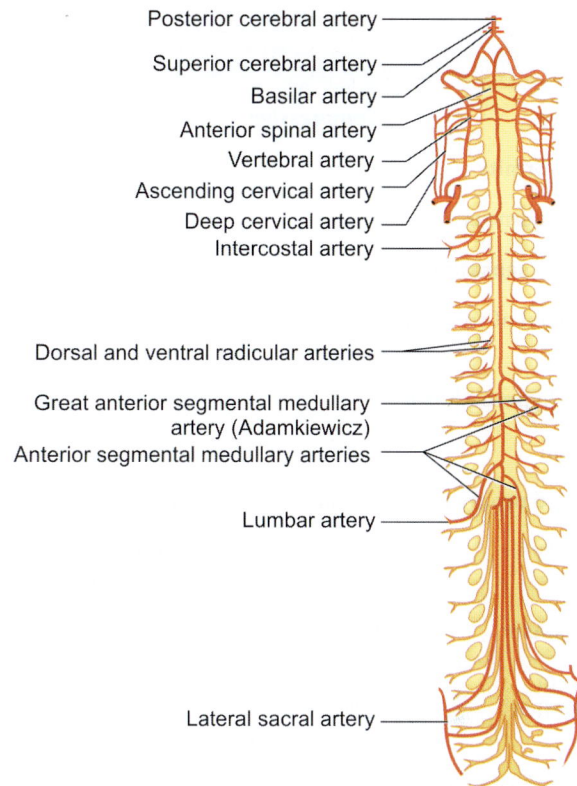

**Fig. 4.34:** Vascular supply of spinal cord.

- **Thirty-one pairs of small radicular arteries:** Supply corresponding nerve roots.
- **Some of them give a branch to spinal arteries:** The reticulospinal branches.
- **C1-4:** Vertebral artery.
- **C5-t2:** Ascending and deep cervical artery.
- **T3-T8:** Intercostal artery.
- **T9 and below:** Artery of Adamkiewicz—supplies most of the lower one-third of spinal cord; arises from a left-sided intercostal or lumbar artery (T8-L3).

### Q. What are the types of spinal cord diseases?

Refer **Figure 4.35**.

### Q. What are the differences between compressive and noncompressive myelopathy?

Refer **Table 4.35**.

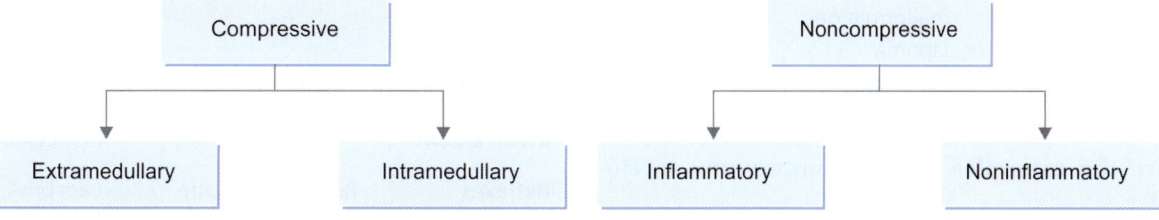

**Fig. 4.35:** Types of spinal cord diseases.

**Table 4.35:** Differentiation between compressive and noncompressive myelopathy.

| Features | Compressive | Noncompressive |
|---|---|---|
| Bony deformity | + | – |
| Bony tenderness | + | – |
| Girdle like sensation | + | – |
| Upper level of sensory loss | + | – |
| Zone of hyperesthesia | + | – |
| Root pain | + | – |
| Onset and progress | Gradual | May be acute |
| Symmetry | Asymmetrical | Majority are symmetrical |
| Flexor spasm | Common | Usually absent |
| Pattern of neurodeficit | U-shaped (Ellsberg phenomenon) | Bilaterally symmetrical |
| Bladder and bowel movement | Late | Early (acute transverse myelitis) |
| Selective tract involvement | Rare | Usually seen |

**Q. What are the examples for compressive myelopathies?**
Refer **Table 4.36**.

**Table 4.36:** Compressive myelopathies.

- Trauma
- Tumor
- Tuberculosis
- Myeloma
- Metastasis

| Extramedullary extradural | Extramedullary intradural | Intramedullary |
|---|---|---|
| • Caries spine | • Meningioma | • Ependymoma |
| • Metastasis | • Neurofibroma | • Chordoma |
| • Intervertebral disc prolapse | • Schwannoma | • Glioma |
| • Spondylosis | • Patchy arachnoiditis | • Syringomyelia |
| • Fluorosis | • Arteriovenous malformations | |
| • Trauma to vertebra | • Lipoma | |
| • Epidural abscess | • Sarcoma | |
| • Epidural hematoma | • Dermoid | |

**Q. What are the examples for noncompressive myelopathies?**
Refer **Table 4.37**.

**Table 4.37:** Noncompressive myelopathies.

*Inflammatory*
- Infectious—viral, bacterial, fungal, and parasitic
- Autoimmune—SLE, Sjogren's, sarcoidosis, Bechet syndrome, MCTD, polyarteritis nodosa, pANCA positive vasculitis
- Demyelinating—MS, NMO, ADEM, and postviral postvaccinial
- Paraneoplastic—lung carcinoma, breast, and ovary
- Encephalomyelitis

*Noninflammatory*
- Inherited—HSP, inherited metabolic disorders
- Metabolic—vitamin $B_{12}$, copper, folate and vitamin E deficiency—AIDS associated
- Toxic—cassava, lathyrism, fluorosis, SMON, nitrous oxide, TOCP, and konzo
- Vascular—anterior spinal artery thrombosis, AVM, and dural arteriovenous fistula
- Degenerative—familial spastic paraplegia
- Physical agents—electrical injury, Caisson's disease, and radiation myelopathy

(SLE: systemic lupus erythematosus; MCTD: mixed connective tissue disease; pANCA: perinuclear antineutrophil cytoplasmic antibodies; MS: multiple sclerosis; NMO: neuromyelitis optica; ADEM: acute disseminated encephalomyelitis; HSP: hereditary spastic paraplegia; AIDS: acquired immunodeficiency syndrome; SMON: subacute myelo-optic neuropathy; TOCP: triorthocresyl phosphate; AVM: arteriovenous malformation)

**Q. How do you discriminate between extramedullary and intramedullary lesions?**
Refer **Table 4.38**.

**Table 4.38:** Discriminate between extramedullary and intramedullary lesions.

| Features | Extramedullary | Intramedullary |
|---|---|---|
| Radicular pain | Common **Intradural:** Unilateral **Extradural:** Bilateral | Unusual |
| Vertebral pain | Common (extradural) | Unusual |
| Funicular pain | Rare | Common |
| Motor deficit | Ascending motor weakness, i.e., sacral → lumbar → thoracic → cervical | Descending pattern of loss, i.e., cervical → thoracic → lumbar → sacral (**Fig. 4.36**) |
| Upper motor neuron involvement | Early and prominent | • Less pronounced, late feature |
| Lower motor neuron involvement | Segmental | Marked with widespread atrophy, fasciculations seen |
| Reflexes | Brisk early feature | Less brisk, later feature |

| Features | Extramedullary | Intramedullary |
|---|---|---|
| Sensory deficit | Ascending sensory loss, i.e., sacral → lumbar → thoracic → cervical Saddle anesthesia Hemisection—contralateral loss of pain and temperature, ipsilateral loss of joint position | Descending pattern of loss, i.e., cervical → thoracic → lumbar → sacral Dissociative sensory loss Suspended sensory loss (Jacket pattern) |
| Sacral sensation | Lost (early) | Sacral sparing |
| Autonomic involvement (bladder and bowel) | Late | Early (Fig. 4.37) |
| Trophic changes | Usually not marked | Common |
| Vertebral tenderness | May be present (extradural) | No bony tenderness in vertebrae |
| Changes in cerebrospinal fluid (CSF) | Frequent (increased protein, cells) | |

(CSF: cerebrospinal fluid)

### Q. What are the differences between presentation of intradural and extradural lesion?
Refer **Table 4.39**.

**Table 4.39:** Differences between presentation of intradural and extradural lesion.

| Features | Extradural | Intradural |
|---|---|---|
| **Mode of onset** | Usually symmetrical | Asymmetrical |
| **Root pain** | Less common | More common |
| **Spinal tenderness** | Common | Uncommon |
| **Spinal deformity** | Present | Absent |

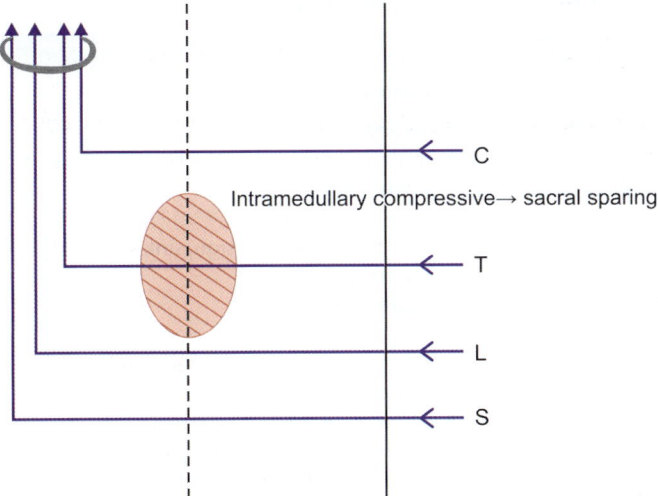

**Fig. 4.36:** Arrangement of motor fibers.

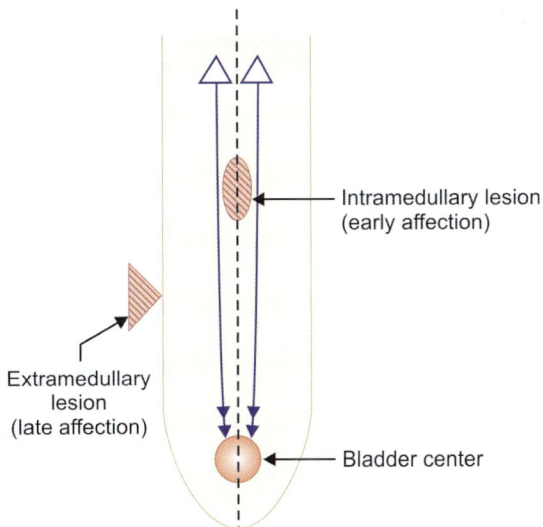

**Fig. 4.37:** Bladder involvement in spinal cord disease.

### Q. What is cervical syringomyelia?
Refer **Figure 4.38**.

### Q. What are the patterns of spinal cord diseases?
- Complete cord transection syndrome
- Brown-Sequard syndrome/hemisection of the cord
- Central cord syndrome (syringomyelia)
- Posterior column syndrome (tabes dorsalis)
- Posterolateral cord syndrome (SACD)
- Combined AHC—pyramidal tract syndrome (ALS)
- AHC syndrome
- Anterior spinal artery occlusion.

### Q. What are the features of complete cord transection?
Refer **Table 4.40**.

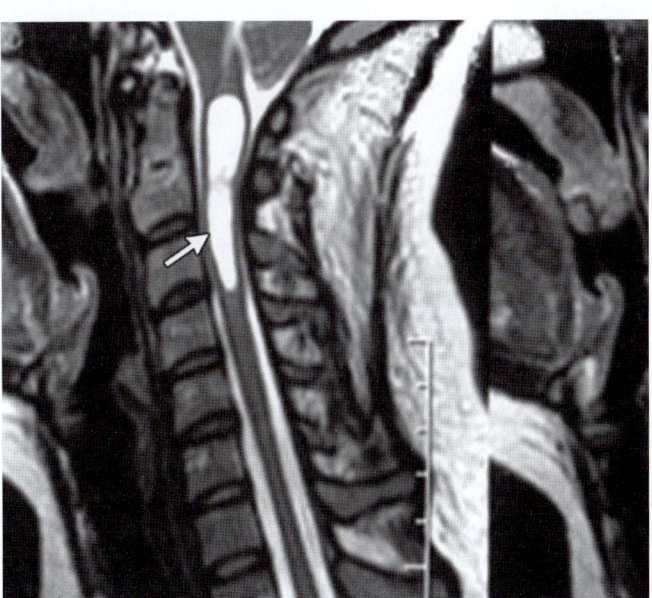

**Fig. 4.38:** MRI showing cervical syringomyelia.

### Table 4.40: Complete cord transection.

| Causes | Features |
|---|---|
| **Trauma**<br>• Metastatic carcinoma<br>• Multiple sclerosis<br>• Spinal epidural hematoma<br>• Autoimmune disorders<br>• Postvaccinial syndromes | **Sensory:**<br>• All sensations are affected<br>• Sensory level is usually 2 segments below the level of lesion<br>• Segmental paresthesia occurs at the level of lesion<br>**Motor:**<br>• Paraplegia due to corticospinal tract involvement<br>• First spinal shock followed by hypertonic hyperreflexia paraplegia<br>• Loss of abdominal and cremasteric reflexes<br>• At the level of lesion LMN signs occur<br>**Autonomic:**<br>• Urinary retention and constipation<br>• Anhidrosis, trophic skin changes, vasomotor instability below the level of lesion<br>• Sexual dysfunction can occur |

**Q. What are the features of hemisection of cord/Brown-Sequard syndrome?**

Due to damage to one lateral half of spinal cord **(Table 4.41 and Fig. 4.39)**.

### Table 4.41: Brown-Sequard syndrome.

| Causes | Features |
|---|---|
| • Caused by extramedullary lesions<br>• Usually caused by penetrating injuries (gunshot) or tumor | **Sensory:**<br>• Ipsilateral loss of proprioception due to posterior column involvement<br>• Contralateral loss of pain and temperature due to involvement of lateral spinothalamic tract 1 or 2 segments below<br>**Motor:**<br>• Ipsilateral spastic weakness due to descending corticospinal tract involvement<br>• Lower motor neuron signs at the level of lesion |

**Q. What are the features of central cord syndrome?**
Refer **Table 4.42**.

### Table 4.42: Central cord syndrome.

| Causes | Features |
|---|---|
| • Most common cause is syringomyelia<br>• Other causes are hyperextension, injuries of neck, intramedullary tumors and trauma<br>• Associated with Arnold-Chiari type 1 and 2 and Dandy-Walker malformation | **Sensory:**<br>• Pain and temperature are affected<br>• Touch and proprioception are preserved<br>• Dissociative anesthesia<br>• Shawl like distribution of sensory loss<br>**Motor:**<br>• Upper limb weakness > lower limb weakness<br>**Other features include:**<br>• Horner's syndrome<br>• Kyphoscoliosis<br>• Sacral sparing<br>• Neuropathic arthropathy of shoulder and elbow joint<br>• Early bladder involvement (exception—syringomyelia) |

**Q. What are the features of posterior column syndrome?**
Refer **Table 4.43 and Figure 4.40**.

### Table 4.43: Posterior column syndrome.

| Causes | Features |
|---|---|
| Occurs due to neurosyphilis, diabetes mellitus | **Sensory**<br>• Impaired position and vibration sense in lower limb<br>• Sensory ataxia<br>• Positive Romberg's sign, sink sign and Lhermitte's sign<br>**Abadie's sign** positive<br>• Urinary incontinence<br>• Absent knee and ankle jerk (areflexia and hypotonia)<br>• Charcot's joint<br>• Miotic and irregular pupil not reacting to light—Argyll-Robertson pupil |

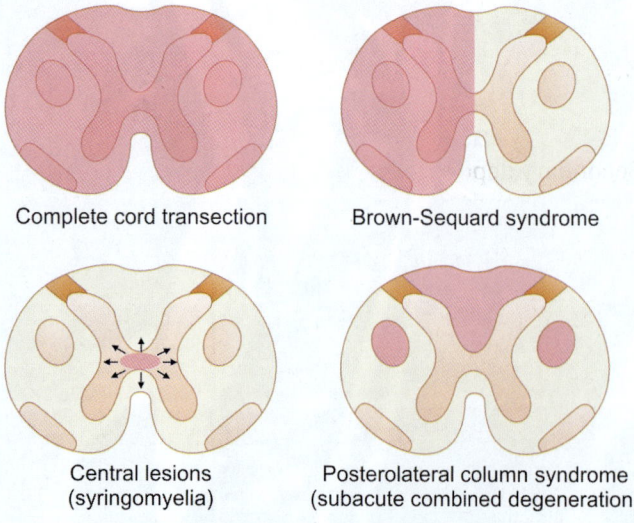

**Fig. 4.39:** Spinal cord syndromes 1.

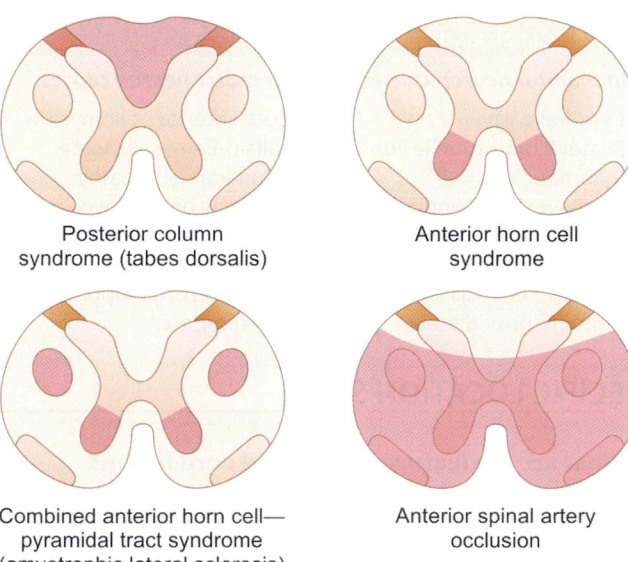

**Fig. 4.40:** Spinal cord syndromes 2.

## Q. What are the features of posterolateral column syndrome?

Refer **Table 4.44 and Figure 4.39**.

**Table 4.44:** Posterolateral column disease.

| Causes | Features |
|---|---|
| ◆ Vitamin $B_{12}$ deficiency<br>◆ AIDS<br>◆ HTLV associated myelopathy<br>◆ Cervical spondylosis | ◆ **Sensory:**<br>– Paresthesia in feet<br>– Loss of proprioception and vibration in legs<br>– Sensory ataxia<br>– Positive Romberg's sign<br>◆ **Bladder** atonia<br>◆ **Motor:**<br>– Corticospinal tract involvement—spasticity, hyperreflexia, bilateral Babinski sign<br>– AIDS-associated dementia and spastic bladder is present<br>– HTLV associated myelopathy—slowly progressive paraparesis and an increase in CSF IgG antibodies to HTLV1 |

(AIDS: acquired immunodeficiency syndrome; HTLV: human T-cell lymphotropic virus; CSF: cerebrospinal fluid; IgG: immunoglobulin G)

## Q. What are the features of anterior horn cell syndrome?

Refer **Table 4.45 and Figure 4.40**.

**Table 4.45:** Anterior horn cell syndromes.

| Causes | Features |
|---|---|
| Spinal muscular atrophy (SMA) | ◆ **Motor:**<br>– Weakness, atrophy, and fasciculations<br>– Hypotonia with depressed reflexes<br>– Muscles of trunk and extremities are affected<br>◆ **Sensory system** is not affected |

## Q. What are the features of anterior spinal artery syndrome?

Refer **Table 4.46 and Figure 4.40**.

**Table 4.46:** Anterior spinal artery syndrome.

| Causes | Features |
|---|---|
| Occurs due to syphilitic arteritis, aortic dissection, atherosclerosis of aorta, SLE, AIDS, and AV malformation | ◆ **Motor:** Flaccid and areflexic paraplegia<br>◆ **Sensory:**<br>– Loss of pain and temperature<br>– Preservation of position and vibration<br>◆ **Autonomic:**<br>– Urinary incontinence<br>– Spinal cord infarction usually occurs in T1 to T4 and L1 segment<br>◆ Abrupt onset, radicular, or girdle pain |

(SLE: systemic lupus erythematosus)

## Q. What are the features of posterior spinal artery syndrome?

Refer **Table 4.47**.

**Table 4.47:** Postspinal artery syndrome.

| Cause | Features |
|---|---|
| Rare | ◆ Loss of proprioception and vibratory sense<br>◆ Pain and temperature are preserved<br>◆ Absence of motor deficit |

## Q. What are the features of involvement of anterior horn cell and pyramidal tract?

Refer **Table 4.48**.

**Table 4.48:** Anterior horn cell and pyramidal tract.

| Causes | Features |
|---|---|
| ALS—amyotrophic lateral sclerosis | ◆ LMN signs<br>◆ UMN signs<br>◆ Sensations preserved<br>◆ Onuf's nucleus spared—hence no bladder and bowel involvement |

### Cord involvement at multiple sites

- Arachnoiditis (in tubercular, there is patchy involvement)
- Neurofibromatosis
- Multiple sclerosis
- Secondary deposits
- Cervical spondylitis.

## Q. What are causes of spastic paraplegia?

**Gradual onset**

- Cerebral causes—parasagittal meningioma, hydrocephalus, etc.
- Spinal causes:
  - Compressive or transverse lesion in the spinal cord
  - Noncompressive or longitudinal lesion or systemic disease of the spinal cord.
- Motor neuron disease (MND), e.g., amyotrophic lateral sclerosis

- Multiple sclerosis, Devic's disease
- Friedreich's ataxia
- Subacute combined degeneration (i.e., from vitamin B12 deficiency)
- Lathyrism
- Syringomyelia
- Hereditary spastic paraplegia
- Erb's spastic paraplegia
- Tropical spastic paraplegia
- Radiation myelopathy.

**Sudden onset**

- Cerebral causes—thrombosis of unpaired anterior cerebral artery, superior sagittal sinus thrombosis
- Spinal causes
- *Compressive causes*
  - Injury to the spinal cord (fracture-dislocation or collapse of the vertebra)
  - Prolapsed intervertebral disc
  - Spinal epidural abscess or hematoma.
- *Noncompressive causes:*
  - Acute transverse myelitis
  - Thrombosis of anterior spinal artery
  - Hematomyelia (from arteriovenous malformation, angiomas, or endarteritis)
  - Radiation myelopathy electrical injury.

**Q. What are the causes of flaccid paraplegia?**

- UMN lesion in shock stage, transverse myelitis, spinal injury
- *Lesion involving anterior horn cells:*
  - Acute anterior poliomyelitis
  - Progressive muscular atrophy (variety of MND).
- Diseases affecting nerve root—tabes dorsalis, radiculitis, Guillain-Barré (GB) syndrome
- *Diseases affecting peripheral nerves:*
  - Acute infective polyneuropathy (GB syndrome)
  - High cauda equina syndrome
  - Disease of peripheral nerves involving both the lower limbs
  - Lumbar plexus injury (psoas abscess or hematoma).
- *Diseases affecting myoneural junction:*
  - Myasthenia gravis, Lambert-Eaton syndrome
  - Periodic paralysis due to hypo- or hyperkalemia.
- Diseases affecting muscles—myopathy.

**Q. What are the causes of quadriplegia?**

Weakness of all the 4 limbs can occur in the lesions from cortex to C5 level of spinal cord and various LMN lesion affecting anterior horn cells, roots, peripheral nerve, neuromuscular junction (NMJ), and muscles **(Table 4.49)**.

**Table 4.49:** Causes of quadriplegia.

| Upper motor neuron causes | Lower motor neuron causes |
|---|---|
| • Cerebral palsy | • Acute anterior poliomyelitis |
| • Bilateral brainstem lesion (glioma) | • Guillain-Barré syndrome |
| • Craniovertebral anomaly | • Peripheral neuropathy |
| • High cervical cord compression | • Myopathy or polymyositis |
| • Multiple sclerosis | • Myasthenia gravis and crisis |
| • Motor neuron disease | • Periodic paralysis |
| | • Snake bite, organophosphate poisoning, etc. |

## SPECIFIC LOCATION SIGNS

**Q. What are the features of cervical cord lesion?**

In general, cervical cord disorders are best localized by the pattern of weakness that ensues, whereas sensory deficits have less localizing value.

- High cervical cord lesions (lesions above C5) are frequently life-threatening, produce quadriplegia and weakness of diaphragm, the main respiratory muscle innervated by the phrenic nerve (C3-C5).
- Extensive lesions near the junction of the cervical cord and medulla are usually fatal owing to involvement of adjacent medullary centers, which results in vasomotor and respiratory collapse.
- Compressive lesions near the foramen magnum may produce weakness of the ipsilateral shoulder and arm followed by weakness of the ipsilateral leg, then the contralateral leg, and finally the contralateral arm (cartwheel pattern or Ellsberg phenomenon).
- Lesions at C4-C5 produce quadriplegia with preserved respiratory function.
- At the midcervical (C5-C6) level, there is relative sparing of shoulder muscles and loss of biceps and brachioradialis reflexes.
- Lesions at C7 spare the biceps but produce weakness of finger and wrist extensors and loss of the triceps reflex.
- Lesions at C8 paralyze finger and wrist flexion, and the finger flexor reflex is lost.
- Horner's syndrome (miosis, ptosis, and facial hypohidrosis) may also occur ipsilateral to cervical lesions at any level.

**Q. What are the features of thoracic cord lesion?**

Lesions of the thoracic cord are best localized by identification of a sensory level on the trunk.

- Useful markers in terms of sensory dermatomes are at the nipples (T4), xiphisternum (T6), subcostal margins (T8), umbilicus (T10), and pubic symphysis (T12).
- The abdominal wall musculature, supplied by the lower thoracic nerves is observed during movements of respiration or coughing or by asking the patient to interlock the fingers behind the head in the supine position and attempt to sit up.

- Lesions at T9-T10 paralyze the lower, but spare the upper, abdominal muscles, resulting in upward movement of the umbilicus when the abdominal wall contracts (Beevor's sign) and in loss of lower, but not upper, superficial abdominal reflexes.
- With unilateral lesions, attempts to contract the abdominal wall produce movement of the umbilicus to the normal side; superficial abdominal reflexes are absent on the involved side.
- Midline back pain is a useful localizing sign in the thoracic region.

### Q. What are the features of lumbar cord lesion?

**Effect of various root lesions in lumbar region (Table 4.50)**
- Lesions at L2-L4 paralyze flexion and abduction of the thigh, weaken leg extension at the knee, and abolish the patellar reflex.
- Lesions at L5-S1 paralyze movements of the foot and ankle, flexion at the knee, and extension of the thigh, and abolish the ankle jerk (S1).
- A cutaneous reflex useful in localization of lumbar cord disease is the cremasteric reflex, which is segmentally innervated at L1-L2.

**Table 4.50:** Features of lumbar cord.

| Roots | Motor deficit (most rapidly demonstrated) |
|---|---|
| L2 | Hip flexion and thigh adduction |
| L3 | Knee extension and thigh adduction |
| L4 | Inversion of foot |
| L5 | Dorsiflexion to toes and foot |
| S1 | Plantarflexion and eversion of foot |

### Q. What are the features of sacral cord/conus medullaris?

The conus medullaris is the tapered caudal termination of the spinal cord, comprising the lower sacral and single coccygeal segments. Isolated lesions of the conus medullaris spare motor and reflex functions in the legs.

### Q. What is conus medullaris syndrome?
- Bilateral saddle anesthesia (S3-S5), prominent bladder and bowel dysfunction (urinary retention and incontinence with lax anal tone), and impotence.
- The bulbocavernosus (S2-S4) and anal (S4-S5) reflexes are absent.
- Muscle strength is largely preserved.

### Q. What is cauda equina syndrome?
- The cluster of nerves derived from the lower cord as they descend to their exits in the intervertebral foramina (L2-3 to coccygeal nerve roots).
- Cauda equina lesions are characterized by severe low back or radicular pain, asymmetric leg weakness or sensory loss, variable areflexia in the lower extremities, and relative sparing of bowel and bladder function **(Fig. 4.41)**.

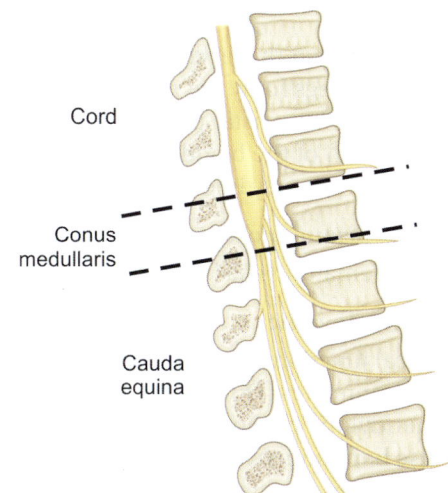

**Fig. 4.41:** Conus—cauda equina syndrome.

- Mass lesions in the lower spinal canal may produce mixed clinical picture in which elements of both cauda equina and conus medullaris syndromes coexist.

### Q. List the differences of conus medullaris versus cauda equina syndrome?

Refer **Table 4.51**.

**Table 4.51:** Conus medullaris versus cauda equina syndrome.

| | Conus medullaris syndrome (S24) | Cauda equina syndrome (L3 root and below) |
|---|---|---|
| Presentation | Sudden and bilateral | Gradual and unilateral |
| Reflexes | Knee jerk is preserved but ankle jerk is affected | Both knee and ankle jerks are affected |
| Radicular pain | Less severe | More severe |
| Low back pain | More | Less |
| Sensory symptoms and sings | Numbness is symmetrical and bilateral, sensory dissociation occurs, saddle anesthesia present | Numbness is asymmetrical, may be unilateral, no necessary dissociation |
| Motor strength | Typically symmetric hyperreflexia, distal paresis of lower limbs | Asymmetric areflexic paraplegia |
| Impotence | Frequent | Less frequent |
| Sphincter dysfunction | Overflow urinary incontinence and fecal incontinence, tend to present early in course of disease | Urinary retention tends to present late in course of disease |
| Trophic changes | Common | Less marked |

**Q. What is epiconus?**

Lesion of lumbar cord at the level of L4-S2 characterized by a flaccid paralysis of legs (only the roots are affected causing peripheral paralysis, i.e., distal paraplegia). Reflex but not conscious evacuation of the bladder is present, and rectum is preserved. Sexual potency is lost.

**Q. What are the various causes of myelopathies?**

**Congenital:** Diastematomyelia (spinal notochord syndrome)

**Traumatic spondylogenic**
- Craniocervical junction abnormalities
- Atlantoaxial anomalies (Down's syndrome)
- Cervical spondylotic myelopathy
- Cervical disc herniation with spinal cord compression
- Thoracic disc herniation with thoracic spinal stenosis
- Diffuse idiopathic skeletal hyperostosis (Forestier's disease)
- Ossification of the posterior longitudinal ligament
- Rheumatoid disease of the spine (RA)
- Cervical/thoracic spine pachymeningitis
- Thoracic cord compression by rheumatoid nodules
- Thoracic spinal cord infarction due to vasculitis
- Syringomyelia due to cervical cord compression
- Transverse myelopathy associated with antiphospholipid antibodies
- Transverse myelitis due to sulfadiazine

**Myelopathy in** systemic lupus erythematosus (SLE):
- SLE myelopathy
- Transverse myelopathy associated with antiphospholipid antibodies
- Herpes zoster myelitis
- Compression fracture (long-term corticosteroid use) with spinal cord compression
- Spinal epidural/subdural hemorrhages
- Epidural lipomatosis
- Tuberculous spondylitis
- Atlantoaxial subluxation

**Spondyloarthropathies demyelinating**
- Multiple sclerosis
- Devic's neuromyelitis optica
- Acute disseminated encephalomyelitis
- Postinfectious and postvaccinal myelopathies
- Inflammatory transverse myelitis
- Osmotic demyelination syndrome
- Leukodystrophies

**Infectious**
- Bacterial (tuberculosis, pyogenic infections)
- Viral (e.g., HIV, HTLV-1)
- Parasitic (e.g., schistosomiasis, hydatid disease)
- Other (e.g., syphilis, Lyme disease, mycoplasma)

**Granulomatous disorders**
- Sarcoidosis
- Wegener's granulomatosis

**Vascular**
- Vasculitis
- Spinal artery (anterior, posterior) occlusion
- Venous spinal cord infarction
- Vascular malformations

**Metabolic**
- B12 deficiency
- Copper deficiency
- Hyperthyroidism
- Diabetes mellitus
- Mitochondrial disorders

**Spinal tumors: Nontumoral myelopathies**
- Subacute necrotizing myelopathy of Foix and Alajouanine
- Subacute paraneoplastic necrotizing myelopathy (lung carcinoma, lymphomas)

**Drugs and toxic myelopathies**
- Neurolathyrism
- Subacute myelo-optic neuropathy
- Methotrexate, cytosine

**Systemic disorders**
- Portocaval encephalomyelopathy
- Inflammatory bowel disease
- Celiac disease

**Physical agents**
- Electrical or lightning injuries
- Radiation
- Caisson disease (decompression sickness)

**System degeneration**
- Hereditary spastic paraplegia
- Spinal muscular atrophies
- Amyotrophic lateral sclerosis (sporadic/familial)

**Inherited disorders**
- Syringomyelia
- Chiari malformations

**Q. Can cortical lesion cause paraplegia?**

Yes, thrombosis of azygos/anomalous anterior cerebral artery causes paraplegia with bladder incontinence (disinhibited bladder), paracentral meningiomas can also cause paraplegia.

**Q. What are the watershed zones of spinal cord?**

T6, 8, 10 are the least vascular zones of spinal cord prone to infarction.

**Q. How does TB affects spine?**

- Tubercular osteomyelitis involves mainly the thoracic and lumbar vertebrae (known as Pott's disease) followed by knee and hip. There is extensive necrosis and

bony destruction with compressed fractures (with kyphosis).
- The direction in which it spreads is influenced by the anatomical arrangement of the tissues, and possibly to some extent by gravity, and the abscess may reach the surface at a considerable distance from its seat of origin.
- The psoas abscess, which may originate in the dorsal vertebra, extend downwards within the sheath of the psoas muscle, and finally appear in the thigh.
- Presents as a mass in the inferior lumbar region through the lumbar triangle of Jean-Louis Petit.
- Drains via the intercostal space to produce empyema necessitans.

### Q. How the tubercle bacilli reach bone/spine?

The spinal disease is always secondary to a primary lesion and occurs due to hematogenous spread.

Tuberculous osteomyelitis and arthritis are generally believed to arise from foci of bacilli lodged in the bone during the original mycobacteremia of primary infection. The primary focus may be active or quiescent, apparent or latent, either in the lungs or in the lymph glands of the mediastinum, mesentery or cervical region, or kidney or other viscera. Alternatively, tuberculosis bacilli may travel from the lung to the spine by Batson's paravertebral venous plexus or by lymphatic drainage to the para-aortic lymph nodes. In most otherwise healthy individuals, the cellular immune response is able to contain the bacilli present in these sites, but not eradicate them **(Fig. 4.42)**.

There are four common sites of vertebral tuberculosis: Paradiscal type (most common), central type, anterior type, appendiceal type **(Fig. 4.43)**.

The intervertebral disc is not involved primarily because it is a relatively avascular structure.

### Q. What is the pathogenesis of spinal tuberculosis?

- **Inflammatory edema:** Vascular stasis, toxins
- **Extradural mass:** Tuberculous osteitis of vertebral body and abscess
- **Meningeal changes:** Dura as a rule not involved
- **Bony disorders:** Sequestra, internal gibbus
- **Infarction of spinal cord:** Endarteritis, periarteritis or thrombosis of tributary to anterior spinal artery.
- **Changes in spinal cord:** Thinning (atrophy), myelomalacia and syrinx.
- Recently, two distinct patterns of spinal TB can be identified, the classic form called spondylodiscitis (SPD) and an increasingly common atypical form characterized by spondylitis without disk involvement (SPwD). SPwD seems to be the most common pattern of spinal TB.

### Deformity

Limitation of extension to start with. Scoliosis occasionally.

As the disease advances, the involved level shows prominence of spinous process. This is knuckle deformity due

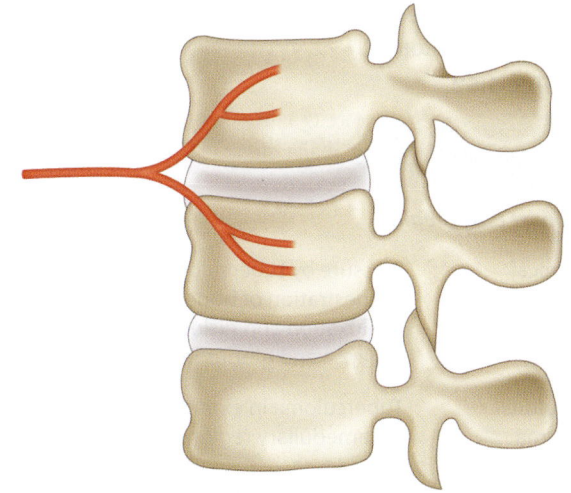

**Fig. 4.42:** Mechanism how TB involves adjacent vertebrae.

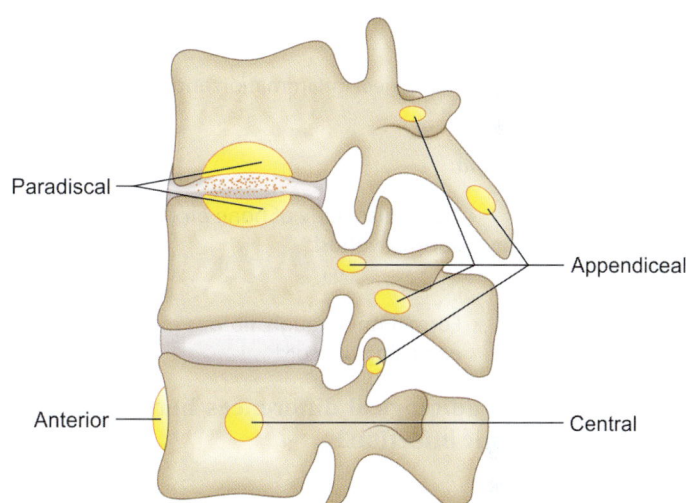

**Fig. 4.43:** Site of spinal TB.

to anterior destruction of one vertebra. Gibbus occurs when more than one vertebra is destroyed. Occasionally generalized kyphosis is seen when minimal involvement anteriorly of more than two vertebrae.

### Abscess

Children, most often present with the abscess may be paraspinal, Petit's triangle, psoas, below inguinal ligament, in the thigh or in course of femoral or sciatic nerve. If abscess bursts, a sinus may be formed.

### Vertebral lesion

- *Paradiscal*—destruction of adjacent endplates and diminution of disc space.
- *Appendiceal (posterior)*—involvement of pedicles, laminae, spinous process.
- *Central*—cystic or lytic, concertina collapse.
- Tuberculosis can cause both compressive and noncompressive myelopathy.

**Q. What are the mechanisms of paraplegia/tetraplegia in spinal tuberculosis?**

Refer **Table 4.52**.

**Table 4.52:** Mechanisms of paraplegia/tetraplegia in spinal tuberculosis

*Early onset paraplegia*

| | |
|---|---|
| Mechanical pressure | Pressure by tuberculous debris, sequestration of bone or disk, abscess, subluxation and dislocations, concertina collapse and gibbus internal |
| Tuberculous granuloma | Tuberculoma in extradural, intradural or intramedullary regions |
| Tuberculous myelitis | Uncommon, may involve spinal cord parenchyma |
| Spinal artery thrombosis | Infective thrombosis of anterior spinal artery |
| Tuberculous arachnoiditis | Meningeal inflammation and fibrosis |

*Late onset paraplegia*

| | |
|---|---|
| Transection of spinal cord by bony ridge | Transverse ridge of bone produced by severe kyphosis |
| Fibrosis of dura (pachymeningitis) | Formation of tough, fibrous membrane encircling the cord |

**Q. What are the radiological differences between spinal TB and pyogenic infection?**

Refer **Table 4.53**.

**Table 4.53:** Radiological differences between spinal TB and pyogenic infection.

| | *Tuberculosis* | *Pyogenic* |
|---|---|---|
| Commonly involved region | Thoracolumbar | Lumbar |
| Levels | Frequently multiple | Usually paradiscal |
| Disc preservation | Variable | Involved early |
| Subligamentous spread | Frequently extensive | Limited |
| Skip lesions | Frequent | Rare |
| Paraspinal soft tissue | Well defined, large | Less well defined, small |
| Enhancement of abscess wall | Thin, smooth | Thick, irregular, nodular |
| Calcification on computed tomography | May be present | Absent |

**Q. What are the differences between infectious and metastasis spine involvement?**

Refer **Table 4.54**.

**Table 4.54:** Differences between infectious and metastasis spine involvement.

| Features | Spinal TB | Pyogenic spondylitis | Metastatic spine disease | Brucella spine involvement |
|---|---|---|---|---|
| Disease location | Lumbar and dorsal | Lumbar | Dorsal | Lumbar |
| Predilection | Involvement of vertebral disc and bodies Soft tissue involvement prominent | Involvement of vertebral disc and bodies Soft tissue involvement minimal | Posterior body wall, pedicles, lamina | Involvement of vertebral disc and bodies Soft tissue involvement minimal, sacroiliitis present |
| Risk factors | Exposure to tuberculosis | Underlying diabetes, etc., predisposing to infection | Known systemic malignancy | Exposure to unpasteurized milk |
| Radiological features | Destruction of vertebral body and disc with extensive soft tissue involvement with rim enhancement | Destruction of vertebral body and disc, epidural abscess prominent contrast enhancement | Lesions have T1 hypo- and T2-hyperintense signal, heterogenous enhancement | Vertebral architecture preserved despite extensive vertebral osteomyelitis Destruction at the anterior superior corner of the vertebra, (Pedro Pons' sign) |

The differential diagnosis of the tuberculous spine includes:
- Spinal infections—pyogenic, brucella and fungal
- Neuropathic spine
- Neoplastic commonly lymphoma/metastasis
- Degenerative.

**Q. How does syphilis affect spinal cord?**

Neurosyphilis may be symptomatic or asymptomatic. Symptomatic disease manifests in several ways, including chronic meningovascular disease, tabes dorsalis, and a generalized brain parenchymal disease called general paresis.

So-called benign tertiary syphilis is characterized by the formation of Gummas in various sites.

Gummas are nodular lesions probably related to the development of delayed hypersensitivity to bacteria. They occur most commonly in bone, skin, and the mucous membranes of the upper airway and mouth, although any organ may be affected.

Skeletal involvement characteristically causes local pain, tenderness, swelling, and sometimes pathologic fractures. Involvement of skin and mucous membranes may produce nodular lesions or rarely, destructive, ulcerative lesions that mimic malignant neoplasms.

## Q. What is Beevor's sign?

Charles Edward Beevor described it as follows **(Fig. 4.44)**:

- "When a patient sits up or raises the head from a recumbent position, the umbilicus is displaced toward the head. This is the result of paralysis of the inferior portion of the rectus abdominal muscle, so that the upper fibers predominate pulling upwards the umbilicus."
- Indicates lesion at T10.
- The upper abdominal muscles supplied by T8-T10 pull the umbilicus up.

**Beevor sign can be present in the following conditions:**

- Spinal cord lesion between T10 and T12 segment
- Facioscapulohumeral muscular dystrophy (FSHD) is autosomal dominant muscle dystrophy. Beevor sign is considered as a 'sine qua non' clinical sign of this disease.
- Rarely in
  - Pompe disease: type 2 glycogen storage disease
  - GNE myopathy (autosomal recessive myopathy
  - Tubular aggregate myopathy
  - Myotonic dystrophy
  - Sporadic inclusion body myositis (IBM)
  - Amyotrophic lateral sclerosis
  - Acid maltase deficiency

## Q. Classify CVJ anomalies.

1. Skeletal and neural or a combination of both.
2. Skeletal
   - Basilar invagination and basilar impression
   - Atlantoaxial dislocation
   - Malformation of axis
   - Malformation of atlas
   - Malformation of the occipital bone
3. Neural
   - Chiari malformations
   - Syringohydromyelia
   - A combination of the above two
   - Dandy-Walker syndrome

## Q. What are the acquired anomalies of the CVJ?

- Trauma—to the bones or the supporting ligaments of the CVJ
- Inflammatory—rheumatoid arthritis, ankylosing spondylitis
- Genetic syndromes—Down syndrome, achondroplasia, osteogenesis imperfecta
- Malignancies—chondrosarcoma, multiple myeloma, metastatic deposits

## Q. What are radiological findings of CVJ?

*Lateral projection of skull X-ray*

- Palato-occipital (Chamberlain's line)
- Palato-suboccipital line (McGregor line)
- Foramen magnum line (McRae line)
- Height of the posterior cranial fossa (Klaus index)
- Wackenheim clival canal line
- Bull's angle (atlanto-palatal angle)
- Atlanto-temporomandibular index (Fischgold)

*Frontal projection of skull X-ray*

- Bimastoid line (Fischgold and Metzer)
- Bidigastric line (Fischgold and Metzer)
- Condylar angle (Schmidt and Fischer)

## Q. How do you diagnose platybasia?

- Basal angle (Welcher)
- Boogard's angle

Measurements commonly used in evaluating the craniovertebral junction (CVJ) on lateral projection or sagittal view in **Table 4.55, and Figures 4.45A and B.**

**Table 4.55:** Radiology in CVJ anomalies.

| | Figures 4.39A and B | Normal range | Remarks |
|---|---|---|---|
| Chamberlain line (palato-occipital line) | A to B | Dens apex <5 mm above this line, anterior arch of C1 typically lies below | Diagnosis of basilar invagination. (posterior rim of foramen magnum shows great anatomic variability and also it may be difficult to radiologically pinpoint opisthion) |
| McGregor line (palate-suboccipital line) | A to C | Dens apex <7 mm above this line, anterior arch of C1 typically lies below | Diagnosis of basilar invagination |

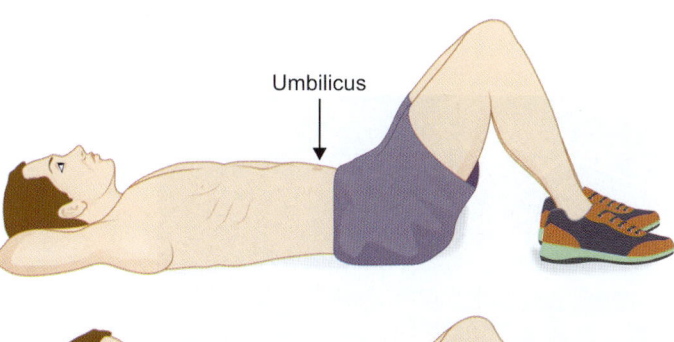
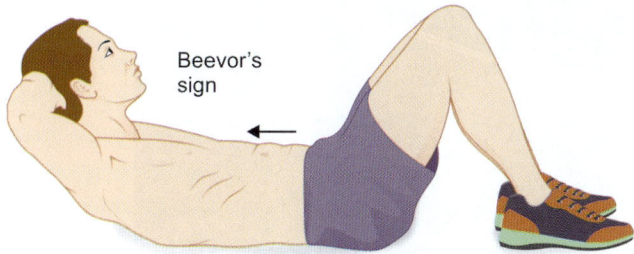

**Fig. 4.44:** Beevor's sign.

## SECTION 4: Nervous System

| | Figures 4.39A and B | Normal range | Remarks |
|---|---|---|---|
| McRae line (foramen magnum line) | B to D | Tip of dens below this line | Assess the decrease in content injury |
| Wackenheim line (craniovertebral or clivus-canal angle) | D to E | Line falls tangent to, or intersects, the posterior one-third of the odontoid | Assessment of CVJ traumatic injuries |
| Welcher basal angle | Angle D-F-G | <140 degrees | Assessment of platybasia |

### Q. What is OS odontoideum?

This term first introduced by Giacomini in 1886, refers to an independent osseous structure lying cephalad to the axis body in the location of the odontoid process.

The anterior arch of the atlas is rounded and hypertrophic but the posterior arch is hypoplastic.

As the gap between the os odontoideum and the body of axis usually extends above the level of the superior articular facet of the axis, cruciate ligament incompetence and atlantoaxial instability (AAI) are common.

### Q. What are the clinical features and association of Klippel-Feil syndrome?

- Described first by Klippel and Feil in 1912.
- Etiology is unknown.
- Due to failure of the normal segmentation of cervical somites during the third and eighth weeks of gestation.
- Classic triad of low posterior hair line, short neck and limited neck ROM found in less than 50% of cases.
- The most consistent finding is limitation of neck motion.
- Generally, flexion and extension are better preserved than side—bending and rotation.

### Associated conditions

- Scoliosis—up to 60% have >15 degrees curve.
- Genitourinary—up to 65%. Most common is absence of kidney.
- Sprengel's deformity—approximately 35%
- Cardiopulmonary—5–15%, most commonly ventricular septal defect (VSD).
- Deafness—30%, all types, MC mixed.
- Synkinesis—mirror motions have been described in up to 20% of patients under the age of 5.
- Craniocervical abnormalities (25%)—includes C1-C2 hypermobility and instability, basilar invagination (BI) and Chiari malformation, diastematomyelia and syringomyelia.
- 20% of patients may show facial asymmetry, torticollis and neck webbing (pterygium colli).
- Ptosis of the eye, Duane's eye contracture, lateral rectus palsy, facial nerve palsy and cleft palate.
- Upper extremity abnormalities, i.e., syndactyly, hypoplastic thumb, supernumerary digits and hypoplasia of the upper extremity.

### Q. What are the clinical features of basilar invagination?

Basilar invagination (BI) implies that the floor of the skull is indented by the upper cervical spine, and hence the tip of odontoid is more cephalad protruding into the foramen magnum.

There are two types of basilar invagination—primary invagination, which is developmental and more common, and secondary invagination, which is acquired.

Primary invagination can be associated with occipitoatlantal fusion, hypoplasia of the atlas, a bifid posterior arch of the atlas, odontoid anomalies.

BI is associated with high incidence of vertebral artery anomalies.

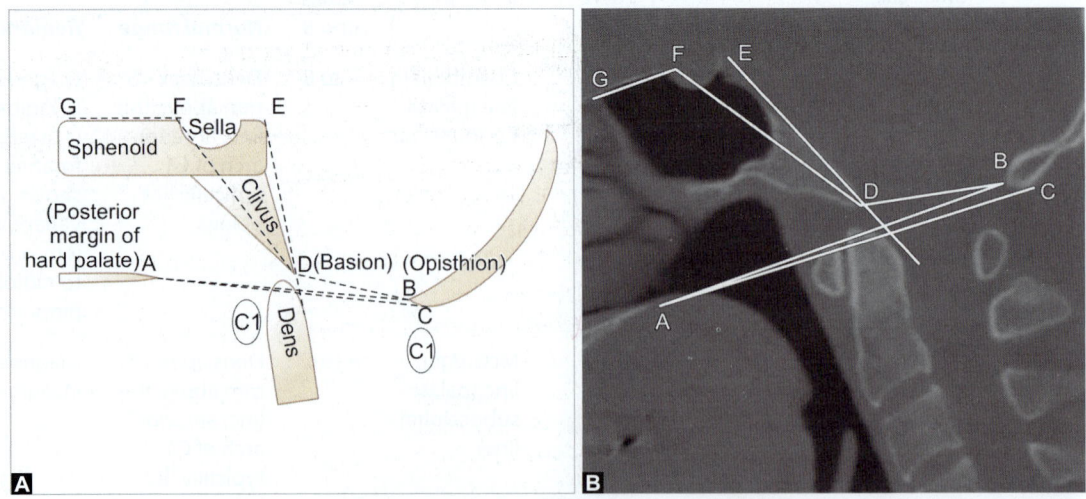

**Figs. 4.45A and B:** Radiology of CVJ anomalies.

## Signs/symptoms

- Usually occur in 2nd or 3rd decade.
- Short neck (78%), torticollis (68%)
- Signs/symptoms of associated Arnold Chiari malformation (cerebellar and vestibular disturbances) and syringomyelia (25–35%).
- Motor and sensory disturbances (85%).
- Lower cranial nerves involvement
- Headache and pain in the nape of neck (greater occipital nerve)
- Signs/symptoms of raised ICP due to posterior encroachment which causes blockage of aqueduct of Sylvius.
- Compression of cerebellum and vestibular apparatus leading to vertical or lateral nystagmus (65%) (not due to direct pressure from posterior rim of foramen magnum but rather due to a thickened band of dura).

**Q. What is basilar impression?**

Basilar impression refers to secondary or acquired forms of BI and is due to softening of the bone and is seen in conditions such as rickets, hyperparathyroidism, osteogenesis imperfecta, Paget disease, neurofibromatosis, skeletal dysplasias, and rheumatoid arthritis and infection producing bone destruction with or without ligamentous laxity.

**Q. What are the types of Arnold-Chiari malformations?**
Refer **Table 4.56**.

**Q. How do you classify atlantoaxial dislocations?**

Atlantoaxial dislocation refers to a loss of stability between the atlas and axis (C1–C2), resulting in loss of normal articulation The atlantoaxial joints can lose stable articulation from traumatic, inflammatory, idiopathic, or congenital abnormalities **(Box 4.4)**.

**Q. What are the non-traumatic causes of atlantoaxial dislocation?**

- Down syndrome due to laxity of the transverse ligament

**Box 4.4:** Classification of atlantoaxial dislocations.

| Wadia classification | Greenberg classification |
|---|---|
| ◆ Group I: AAD with occipitalization of atlas and fusion of C2 and C3.<br>◆ Group II: Odontoid incompetence due to its maldevelopment with no occipitalization of atlas.<br>◆ Group III: Odontoid dislocation but no maldevelopment of dens or occipitalization of atlas. | ◆ Reducible and irreducible<br>**Fielding and Hawkins classification**<br>◆ Anterior, posterior, lateral and rotational<br>**Wang classification system**<br>◆ Instability (type I), reducible dislocation (type II), irreducible dislocation (type III), and bony dislocations (type IV) |

- Grisel syndrome—atlantoaxial subluxation associated with inflammation of adjacent soft tissues of the neck
- Tuberculosis—compression of CMJ could be due to granulation tissue, cold abscess or bony instability and displacement
- Rheumatoid arthritis—from laxity of the ligaments and destruction of the articular cartilage
- Osteogenesis imperfecta
- Neurofibromatosis
- Morquio syndrome
- Other arthritis (psoriasis, lupus)

**Q. What are the different CNS manifestations of carcinoma of lung?**

- Neurologic—myopathic syndromes like Lambert-Eaton myasthenic syndrome (LEMS) (most common with small cell lung cancer)
- Retinal blindness
- Peripheral neuropathies
- Subacute cerebellar degeneration
- Cortical degeneration
- Polymyositis
- Paraneoplastic induced conditions like encephalomyelitis, sensory neuropathies cerebellar degenerations, limbic encephalitis, brainstem encephalitis
- Metastasis to the brain causing space occupying lesions
- Metabolic encephalopathy due to syndrome of inappropriate antidiuretic hormone secretion (SIADH)
- Pancoast tumor causing C8, T1 compression leading to ulnar palsy manifestations
- Pancoast tumor causing Horner syndrome
- Mediastinal lymphadenopathy due to carcinoma lung causing compression of recurrent laryngeal nerve palsy
- Carcinomatous leptomeningitis
- Malignancy is prothrombotic state causing cortical venous thrombosis and stroke
- Radiation induced myelopathy
- Chemotherapy induced peripheral neuropathy

**Table 4.56:** Types of Arnold-Chiari malformations.

| Malformation type | Description of congenital malformation |
|---|---|
| Type I | Elongation of the tonsils and the medial parts of the inferior lobes of the cerebellum into cone-shaped projections, which accompany the medulla oblongata into the spinal canal |
| Type II | Displacement of the parts of the inferior vermis, pons, and medulla oblongata together with elongation of the fourth ventricle (most cases are associated with spina bifida) |
| Type III | Herniation of the entire cerebellum into the cervical canal. This is associated with severe neurologic deficits |
| Type IV | Cerebellar hypoplasia |

- Metastasis to thoracic vertebrae causing compression myelopathy

**Q. What is mass reflex?**

Mass reflex is seen in paraplegia flexion which indicates severe spinal cord lesion. If the skin of the lower limbs or the lower abdominal wall is stimulated below the level of lesion there is reflex flexion of the lower trunk muscles and the lower limbs, piloerection, penile erection, evacuation of the bowel and bladder and semen, and sweating.

**Q. Infectious causes of spinal osteomyelitis?**

- Bacterial
  - Mycobacterial tuberculosis
  - Brucellosis
  - *Staphylococcus*
  - Melioidosis
- Fungal
  - *Aspergillosis*
  - *Candida* species
  - Blastomycosis
  - Histoplasmosis
  - Cryptococcosis
  - Coccidioidomycosis.

**Q. How to rule out arachnoiditis in this case?**

Because of absence of root pain and there is no patchy involvement of motor and sensory symptoms.

**Q. How to differentiate the metastatic lesion from tubercular lesion in case of vertebral involvement?**

In case of tubercular spine usually body of the vertebrae is affected, but in metastatic lesions of spine pedicles are involved because marrow is more in pedicles which is affected due to hematogenous spread of tumor cells.

**Q. What is Pierre Marie-Foix reflex?**

It is the reflex to test whether paraplegia extension is going to flexion, it is a withdrawal reflex done by applying firm passive plantar flexing of the toes and the foot. This will result in spontaneous flexion of the hip, knee, dorsiflexion of the ankle.

**Q. Conditions causing absent ankle reflex with plantar extensor?**

- Subacute combined degeneration spinal cord
- Friedreich's ataxia
- Conus medullaris
- Combined cervical spondylosis with diabetic neuropathy
- Tabes dorsalis (syphilis)
- Motor neuron disease

**Q. What are the types of bladder dysfunction in neurology?**

The term neurogenic bladder refers to bladder dysfunction caused by disease of the nervous system **(Table 4.57)**.

- **Uninhibited bladder:** Forebrain lesions—cause loss of voluntary bladder control but do not affect the spinobulbo-

**Table 4.57:** Types of bladder.

| Type | Uninhibited bladder/Detrus or hyper-reflexia | Automatic bladder/detrusor sphincteric dyssynergia | Autonomous bladder/detrusor areflexia | Sensory atonic bladder | Motor or bladder |
|---|---|---|---|---|---|
| Site of lesion | Suprapontine lesions (mostly frontal lobe) | UMN lesion of suprasacral spinal cord | LMN lesion in sacral cord | LMN lesion in peripheral nerve | LMN lesion in peripheral nerve |
| Causes | Frontal tumors, parasagittal meningioma, NPH, ACA aneurysm | Spinal cord trauma, compressive myelopathy, myelitis | Cauda equina syndrome, conus medullaris lesion, spinal shock | Diabetes, amyloidosis, tabes dorsalis | Tethered c syndrome, lumbar carcinoma stenosis, meningomyelocele |
| Bladder sensation | Preserved | Interrupted | Absent | Absent | Intact |
| Ability to initiate voiding | Present | Absent | Absent | Present | Lost |
| Type of incontinence | Urge social disinhibition | Urge | Overflow | Overflow | Overflow |
| Residual urine | Nil | Small | Large | Large | Large |
| Anal sphincter tone | Normal | Normal | Lost | Normal | Lost |
| Perianal sensation | Normal | Normal | Absent | Absent | Present |
| Anal reflex | Normal | Normal | Absent | Absent | Present |
| Treatment | Anti cholinergic medication | Self-intermittent catheterization | Continuous catheterization | Continuous catheterization | Continuous catheterization |

spinal reflex. Bladder tone remains normal. Bladder distention causes contraction in response to the stretch reflex. There is frequency, urgency, and incontinence that are not associated with dysuria. Hesitancy may precede urgency. Bladder sensation is usually normal. There is no residual urine.

- **Reflex neurogenic bladder:** This occurs with severe myelopathy or extensive brain lesions causing interruption of both the descending autonomic tracts to the bladder and the ascending sensory pathways above the sacral segments of the cord. The bladder capacity is small, and micturition is reflex and involuntary. The residual urine volume is variable.

**Automatic**

- **Autonomous bladder:** This is without external innervation. It is caused by neoplastic, traumatic, inflammatory, and other lesions of the sacral spinal cord, conus medullaris or cauda equina, S2-S4 motor or sensory roots, or the peripheral nerves, and with congenital anomalies such as spina bifida. There is destruction of the parasympathetic supply. Sensation is absent and there is no reflex or voluntary control of the bladder; contractions occur as the result of stimulation of the intrinsic neural plexuses within the bladder wall. The amount of residual urine is large, but the bladder capacity is not greatly increased.
- **Sensory paralytic bladder:** This is found with lesions that involve the posterior roots or posterior root ganglia of the sacral nerves, or the posterior columns of the spinal cord. Sensation is absent, and there is no desire to void. There may be distention, dribbling, and difficulty both in initiating micturition and in emptying the bladder. There is a large amount of residual urine.
- **Motor paralytic bladder:** This develops when the motor nerve supply to the bladder is interrupted. The bladder distends and decompensates, but sensation is normal. The residual urine and bladder capacity vary.

### Q. What are the features of anterior cerebral artery stroke?

Contralateral weakness involving primarily the lower extremity and to a lesser extent, the arm is characteristic of infarction in the territory of the hemispheric branches of the ACA. Other characteristics include abulia, akinetic mutism (with bilateral mesiofrontal damage), impaired memory or emotional disturbances, transcortical motor aphasia (with dominant hemispheric lesions), deviation of the head and eyes toward the lesion, paratonia (gegenhalten), discriminative and proprioceptive sensory loss (primarily in the lower extremity), and sphincter incontinence.

### Q. What is unpaired anterior cerebral artery?

In unpaired anterior cerebral artery syndrome, instead of right and left ACA, only a single artery is present irrigating the mesial surface of both hemispheres. When an unpaired artery or an artery with broad bihemispheric distribution is occluded, an identical syndrome to that produced by blocking both ACA can occur.

### Q. What are the differential diagnosis of spastic paraplegia?

- Hereditary spastic paraplegia
- HTLV-1 associated myelopathy (tropical spastic paraparesis)
- HTLV-2 associated myelopathy
- Neurolathyrism
- Adrenomyeloneuropathy
- Copper deficiency

### Q. What are the conditions which can present like spastic paraparesis?

- Cerebral palsy
- Hydrocephalus
- Myelopathy
- Degenerative/infiltrative/inflammatory disorders—multiple sclerosis (MS), amyotrophic lateral sclerosis (ALS), spinocerebellar ataxia (SCA), leukodystrophy
- Infections—syphilis, HIV, HTLV
- Levodopa responsive dystonia
- Metabolic or toxic damage (vitamin B12-SACD)
- Vitamin-E deficiency
- Copper deficiency
- Lathyrism
- Paraneoplastic disorder

### Q. How to elicit Hoffmann's sign?

The patient's relaxed hand is held with the wrist dorsiflexed and fingers partially flexed. With one hand, the examiner holds the partially extended middle finger between her index finger and thumb or between her index and middle fingers.

With a sharp, forcible flick of the other thumb, the examiner nips or snaps the nail of the patient's middle finger, forcing the distal finger into sharp, sudden flexion followed by sudden release. The rebound of the distal phalanx stretches the finger flexors **(Fig. 4.46)**.

If the Hoffmann sign is present, this is followed by flexion and adduction of the thumb and flexion of the index finger, and sometimes flexion of the other fingers as well. If only the thumb or only the index finger responds, the sign is "incomplete".

### Q. How to elicit Tromner's sign?

The examiner holds the patient's partially extended middle finger, letting the hand dangle, then, with the other hand, thumps or flicks the finger pad **(Fig. 4.47)**. The response is the same as that in the Hoffmann test. The two methods are equivalent, and either manner of testing may be used; both are sometimes referred to as the Hoffmann test.

### Q. What is vacuolar myelopathy?

Vacuolar myelopathy (VM) is the most common chronic myelopathy associated with HIV, incidence is less now due

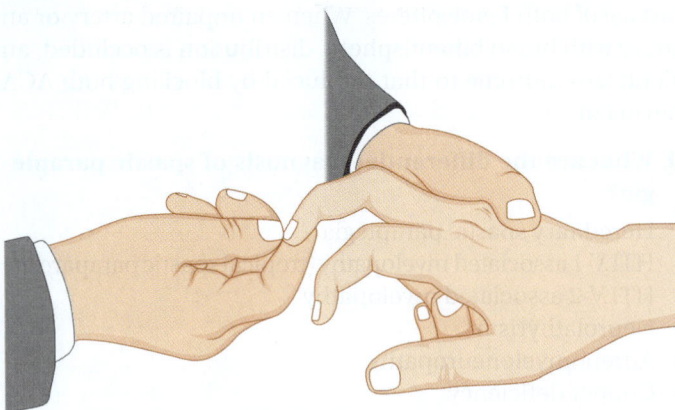

Fig. 4.46: Hoffman's sign.

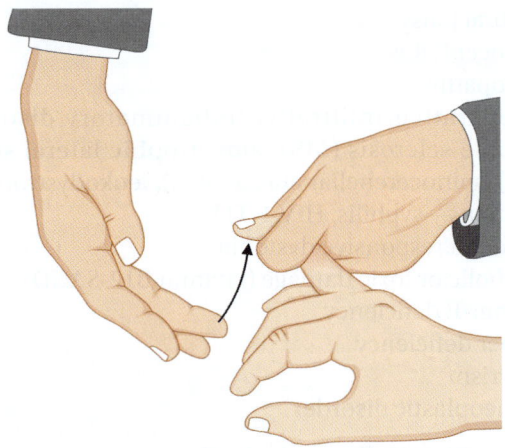

Fig. 4.47: Tromner's sign.

to newer antiretroviral therapy (HAART), VM occurs during the late stages of AIDS, when CD4+ lymphocyte counts are very low, often in conjunction with AIDS dementia complex, peripheral neuropathies, and opportunistic infections or malignancies of the central or peripheral nervous system (e.g., cytomegalovirus, progressive multifocal leukoencephalopathy, lymphoma).

Several hypotheses have been proposed to explain the development of vacuolar myelopathy (VM). One hypothesis is infiltration by HIV-infected mononuclear cells that secrete neurotoxic factors, including cytokines, possibly in conjunction with neurotoxic astrocyte factors. Transgenic mice that express HIV gene products in oligodendrocytes develop clinical and histologic features that resemble the human disease. Although direct HIV infection of astrocytes and neurons is reported in the brain and dorsal root ganglia, it is not a major feature in VM. Impaired utilization of vitamin B12 as a source of methionine in transmethylation metabolism for myelin maintenance in the spinal cord may be a contributing factor.

Vacuolar myelopathy (VM) typically presents as a posterolateral spinal cord syndrome often limited to the thoracic cord. It manifests as a slowly progressive, painless spastic paraparesis with sensory loss, imbalance, and sphincter dysfunction. Relapsing-remitting courses have been described.

Backpain is not prominent. Arm function is usually normal except for advanced cases.

VM is often associated with AIDS dementia complex and peripheral neuropathy. In such cases, patients have cognitive decline and distal limb pain and numbness.

**Physical examination**
The following may be noted:
- Slowly progressive spastic paraparesis; signs and symptoms may be asymmetric early on
- Hyperreflexia and extensor plantar responses
- Dorsal column-type sensory loss
- Ataxic gait
- Incontinence
- Erectile dysfunction may be an early sign
- Rare involvement of upper extremities
- A discrete sensory level is usually absent; if present, this strongly suggests other causes of myelopathy.

**Q. What are the differential diagnosis for vacuolar myelopathy?**
- HIV-associated transverse myelitis during seroconversion
- Herpes simplex (HSV) or zoster (VZV) virus infection
- Cytomegalovirus (CMV) infection
- Neurosyphilis
- Cervical disk syndromes
- Other HIV-associated conditions (e.g., Kaposi sarcoma, lymphoma, toxoplasmosis) in the spinal canal
- *Mycobacterium tuberculosis* infection
- Compressive myelopathy (e.g., tumor, abscess, herniated disc, arteriovenous malformation)
- Human T-cell lymphotropic virus type 1 (HTLV-1/2)—associated myelopathy/tropical spastic paraparesis (can co-exist with HIV infection)
- Spinal epidural abscess in HIV-infected parenteral drug users
- Multiple sclerosis
- Vitamin B12 deficiency
- Copper deficiency

**Q. Which spinal cord lesions present with early bladder involvement?**
Noncompressive myelopathies, among compressive myelopathies intramedullary lesions and conus medullaris lesions present with early bladder and bowel involvement.

**Q. What are the other features of intramedullary lesions?**
Burning type of pain, dissociative sensory loss (loss of pain and temperature with normal touch sensation), sacral sparing, marked lower motor neuron type of involvement with wide spread atrophy and fasciculation. Early trophic changes.

**Q. What are the causes of intramedullary lesions?**
Trauma, tumors (ependymoma, glioma, astrocytoma), metastases, syringomyelia (**Table 4.58**).

| Table 4.58: Causes of intramedullary lesions. | |
|---|---|
| **Intramedullary spinal cord tumors** | |
| **Tumors of neuroepithelial tissue** | |
| ✦ Ependymal cell tumors<br>  – Ependymoma (WHO grade II)<br>  – Subependymoma (WHO grade I)<br>✦ Astrocytic tumors<br>  – Diffuse astrocytoma (WHO grade II)<br>  – Pilocytic astrocytoma (WHO grade I)<br>  – Anaplastic astrocytoma (WHO grade III)<br>  – Glioblastoma (WHO grade IV)<br>  – Pleomorphic xanthoastrocytoma (WHO grade II) | ✦ Oligodendroglial tumors<br>  – Oligodendroglioma (WHO grade II)<br>  – Anaplastic oligodendroglioma (WHO grade III)<br>✦ Oligoastrocytic tumors<br>  – Oligoastrocytoma (WHO grade II)<br>  – Anaplastic oligoastrocytoma (WHO grade III)<br>✦ Neuronal and mixed neuronal glial tumors<br>  – Ganglioma (WHO grade I)<br>  – Paraganglioma (WHO grade I) |
| **Mesenchymal tumors**<br>Hemangioblastoma (WHO grade I) | **Other tumors (<1%)**<br>✦ Metastases<br>✦ Lymphoma |

### Q. What are the neurocutaneous syndromes?

They are also called as phakomatoses/neuro-oculocutaneous syndromes.
- They are group of inherited syndromes characterized by involvement of central nervous system, skin, retina due to a common embryological origination from ectoderm.
- Most commonly inherited as autosomal dominant pattern (except Sturge-Weber syndrome—sporadic)
- Common neurocutaneous syndromes include **(Table 4.59)**:

| Table 4.59: Neurocutaneous syndromes. | |
|---|---|
| **Neurofibromatosis I and II** | **Waardenburg syndrome 1 and 2** |
| Tuberous sclerosis | Hypomelanosis of Ito |
| Von Hippel-Lindau disease | Ataxia telangiectasia |
| Sturge-Weber syndrome | Xeroderma pigmentosum |
| Klippel-Trenaunay-Weber syndrome | Cockayne's syndrome |
| Osler-Weber-Rendu syndrome | Rothmund-Thomson syndrome |
| Wyburn-Mason syndrome | Sjogren-Larsson syndrome |
| Neurocutaneous melanosis | Werner syndrome and progeria |

**Neurofibromatosis:** Neurofibromas, café-au-lait spots, hamartoma of iris (Lisch nodules), axillary/inguinal freckling, optic nerve glioma, scoliosis.
- **Tuberous sclerosis:** Multiple benign hamartomas (brain, eyes, heart, lung, skin), cutaneous lesions—adenoma sebaceum, ash leaf macules, shagreen patches, ependymomas and subependymal giant cell astrocytomas.
- **Von Hippel-Lindau syndrome:** Retinal angiomas, cerebellar hemangioblastomas, hemangioma of spinal cord and brainstem.
- **Sturge-Weber syndrome:** Angiomas that involve the leptomeninges [leptomeningeal angiomas (LAs)] and the skin of the face, typically in the ophthalmic (V1) and maxillary (V2) distributions of the trigeminal nerve. The hallmark of SWS is a facial cutaneous venous dilation, also referred to as a nevus flammeus or port-wine stain (PWS). It is also characterized by choroidal hemangiomas, seizures and mental retardation.
- **MRI:** Tram track calcifications.

### Q. What is tethered cord syndrome?

Tethered cord syndrome (TCS) is stretch-induced dysfunction of the caudal spinal cord and conus, caused by attachment of the filum terminale to inelastic structures caudally. TCS may occur independently or in association with any of the other dysraphic lesions, whether open or closed. This syndrome is closely associated with spina bifida. When TCS occurs independently, it is usually due to anomalous regression of the human tail, part of the normal involution of the caudal cell mass.

The filum terminale is normally viscoelastic in nature, and serves to dampen movements of the spine during flexion and extension, without applying undue traction to the moving spinal cord. In TCS, the spinal cord is attached to abnormally inelastic structures caudally, such as a fibrous or fat-infiltrated filum, tumor, meningoceles or myelomeningoceles, scars, or septa [as seen in spilt spinal cord malformation (SSCM)]. This causes the caudal portion of the spinal cord to stretch between the point of tethering and the dentate ligaments that fix the cord proximally. Progressive dysfunction occurs because of repeated extension or flexion of the spine. The progressive dysfunction has also been attributed to differential growth of the vertebral column as compared to the spinal cord, but there is controversy on this point.

In the short-term, stretching of the spinal cord causes biochemical and electrophysiological changes that are still reversible if the stretch is released surgically. It is estimated that 20–50% of children with spina bifida defects repaired shortly after birth will require surgery at some point to untether the spinal cord.

T2 sagittal magnetic resonance imaging (MRI) study of a patient with tethered cord syndrome (TCS) **(Fig. 4.48)**.

### Q. What are the differences between paraplegia in flexion and extension? What are the important signs associated with it?

Paraplegia in extension and paraplegia in flexion occur only after the spinal shock has ceased **(Table 4.60)**. Paraplegia in extension indicates an increase in the extensor muscle tone owing to the overactivity of gamma efferent nerve fibers to muscle spindles as the result of the release of these neurons from the higher centers. Also, extrapyramidal descending

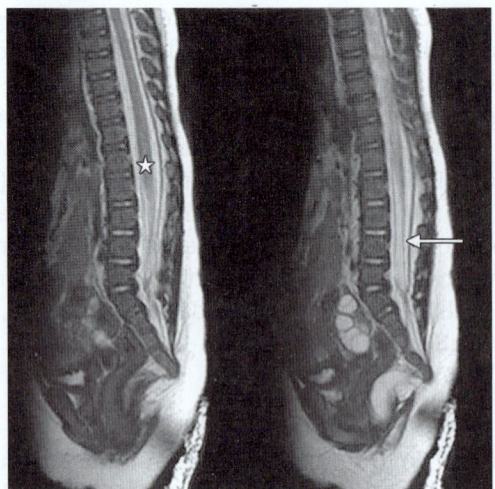

**Fig. 4.48:** T2 sagittal magnetic resonance imaging (MRI) study of a patient with tethered cord syndrome (TCS). See the thickened filum (arrow) and the low-lying conus (asterisk).

**Table 4.60:** Paraplegia in flexion and extension.

| Features | Paraplegia in extension | Paraplegia in flexion |
|---|---|---|
| Definition | Lower limb takes an extension attitude and extensor muscles are spastic | Lower limb muscles take an attitude of flexion |
| Pathology | Only pyramidal tract involved | Both pyramidal and extrapyramidal tract involved (reticulospinal tracts). Occurs in late stage of paraplegia |
| Evolution | Early | Late |
| Tone | Clasp knife spasticity in extensor group | Tone is increased in flexor groups |
| Deep tendon reflex (DTR) | Deep tendon reflexes are exaggerated Clonus may be present | DTR's are present but diminished No clonus |
| Plantar reflex | Extensor plantar response | Extensor plantar associated with flexor spasm |
| Mass reflex** | Absent | Present |

**\*\*Mass reflex:** Any stimulation (scratching of skin) below the level of lesion produces an interoceptive response resulting in flexor spasms, spontaneous emptying of bowel and bladder, profuse sweating and piloerection and seminal emission.

tracts (vestibulospinal and rubrospinal tracts) may escape injury in incomplete spinal cord injury leading to increased activity in extensor motor neurons.

Paraplegia in extension may convert to paraplegia in flexion if the damage to the spinal cord increases, leading to destruction of the above-mentioned extrapyramidal tracts. Paraplegia in flexion may be associated with mass reflex where there is spontaneous urination, defecation and sweating on scratching the skin over the medial side of the thigh.

**Flexor spams**—after recovery from spinal shock, many types of innocuous or noxious cutaneous or muscle stimuli to the lower limb can elicit a prolonged, coordinated pattern of hip flexion and ankle dorsiflexion similar to flexion withdrawal. It is due to increased hyperexcitability of spinal cord circuitry and leads to flexor spasms.

### Q. What are the different types of vertebral deformities?

The normal spine is structurally balanced for optimal flexibility and support of the body's weight. When viewed from the side, it has three gentle curves. The lumbar (lower) spine has an inward curve called *lordosis*. The thoracic (middle) spine has an outward curve called *kyphosis*. The cervical spine (spine in the neck) also has a lordosis. These curves work in harmony to keep the body's center of gravity aligned over the hips and pelvis. When viewed from behind, the normal spine is straight.

Abnormal curvature in the spine can put it out of alignment. Abnormal curvature seen from the side is called sagittal imbalance. Types of sagittal imbalance include *kyphosis, flat back syndrome,* and *chin-on-chest syndrome.* Abnormal curvature of the spine seen from the back is called *scoliosis*.

Each of these conditions can arise for a variety of reasons, including congenital deformity (deformity present at birth), age-related degeneration, disease processes like tumors or infections, other conditions, or *idiopathic* causes (causes that are not yet understood).

- **Kyphosis:** Spinal deformity in which the spine curves excessively outward, creating the appearance of a hunchback. Occasionally called *hyperkyphosis*, to differentiate it from the normal kyphosis of the thoracic spine.
- **Chin-on-chest syndrome:** Cervical and upper thoracic kyphosis that is so severe the chin drops to the chest. Also referred to as dropped head syndrome or head ptosis.
- **Lordosis:** A rare spinal deformity in which the lower back curves excessively inward. Occasionally called *hyperlordosis* to differentiate it from the normal lordosis of the lumbar spine. Hyperlordosis may occur to compensate for hyperkyphosis elsewhere.
- **Flatback syndrome:** Spinal deformity in which the lumbar spine loses its normal lordosis.

### Q. What are the features of Leriche syndrome?

- Occlusive aortic disease is usually confined to distal abdominal aorta below the renal arteries, frequently this extends to the iliac arteries. This is called Leriche syndrome.
- Claudication involving the buttocks, thighs and calves.
- Impotence—erectile dysfunction in males.
- Physical findings—absence of femoral and other distal pulses bilaterally and detection of an audible bruit over the abdomen and the common femoral arteries.
- Atrophic skin, loss of hair, and coolness of lower extremities are seen. In advanced ischemia, rubor on dependency and pallor on elevation can be seen.

### Q. What is the importance of spinal artery of Adamkiewicz?

- Spinal artery of Adamkiewicz, also called arteria radicularis magna, is the only major arterial supply feeding the anterior spinal artery along the lower thoracic, lumbar and sacral spinal cord.
- It derives from single posterior intercostal artery originating from the aorta between the levels of T9 to L5 most commonly between T9 and T12.
- This artery is the only major artery supplying this zone resulting in a watershed area that is susceptible to ischemia.
- An identifying feature specific this artery is its unique shape in the hairpin configuration.
- Damage to this artery will result in decreased perfusion of thoracoabdominal region of the anterior spinal artery because of the lack of collateral blood flow **(Fig. 4.49)**.

### Q. What is middle aortic syndrome?

- A clinicopathological study was conducted in KEM Mumbai Hospital by Sen et al, of 16 cases of inflammatory disease of the aorta in which the middle portion of the vessel—between the arch and bifurcation is involved.
- This occurs in children and young adults, predominantly females.
- Presenting complaints—hypertensive disease, lower limb claudication, abdominal angina.
- Features—weak pulse in one or other superior extremity, low placed systolic murmur over the dorsum of the abdomen.
- Histologic examination of the aorta showed a nonspecific aortitis, probably of allergic origin.
- An associated tuberculous focus was seen elsewhere in 75% of these cases suggested tubercle bacillus as a possible allergen.

### Q. What are the features stage of spinal shock?

- Sudden separation from suprasegmental levels leads to loss of all function and reflexes below level of lesion.
- Muscular flaccidity, weakness, loss of reflexes
  - Loss of autonomic function
  - Gastric atony, paralytic ileus
  - Atonic bladder—overflow incontinence
  - Atonic rectum—retention of feces
- Can usually last up to 2 weeks in humans
- Spinal shock **may be prolonged** in cases of infections (UTI, bedsore) or co existing nutritional deficiencies.
- When there is a cervical or thoracic cord injury, it is likely that absence of the bulbocavernosus reflex or negative reflex would be a result and would also signify presence of spinal shock and injury.
- The spinal shock may progress but then may resolve within 48 hours after injury.
- Return of the reflex would thankfully indicate end of spinal shock.

### Q. What are the different types of spinal pain?

- **Radicular pain** is characterized as a unilateral, lancinating, dermatomal pain often exacerbated by cough, sneeze, or Valsalva's maneuver. Radicular pain is common with extradural growths and rare with intramedullary lesions. An example of an extramedullary tumor causing radicular pain is the neurilemmoma (usually an intradural extramedullary lesion).
- **Vertebral pain** is characterized by an aching pain localized to the point of the spine involved in the compressive process and often accompanied by point tenderness. Spinal pain is common with neoplastic or inflammatory extradural lesions and infrequent with intramedullary or intradural extramedullary lesions.
- **Funicular (central) pain** is common with intramedullary lesions and very unusual with extradural lesions. It is described as deep, ill-defined painful dysesthesias, usually distant from the affected spinal cord level (and therefore of poor localizing value), probably related to dysfunction of the spinothalamic tract or posterior columns.
- With dysfunction of the posterior columns in the cervical region, neck flexion may elicit a sudden "electric-like" sensation down the back or into the arms (**Lhermitte's sign** or "barber's chair syndrome).

### Q. What are the differences between neurogenic and vascular claudication?

Refer **Table 4.61**.

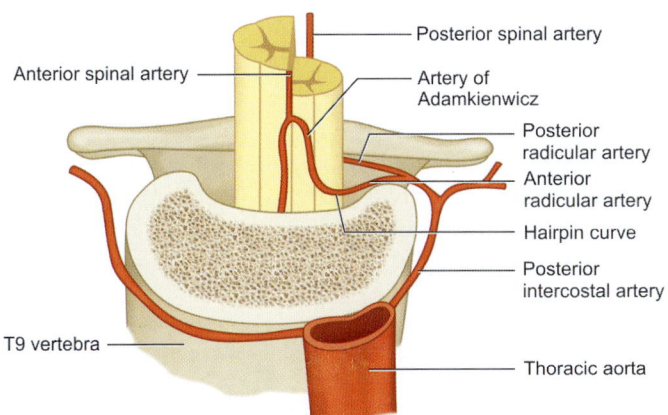

**Fig. 4.49:** Artery of Adamkienwicz.

*Note:* The artery of Adamkiewicz (AKA) originates most frequently as a branch of the left posterior intercostal artery. The AKA is most commonly found originating from a posterior intercostal artery branching from the aorta between the spinal levels of T9 and T12; however, its variability allows it to be found anywhere from the spinal levels of T9 and L5. Immediately following its point of origin, the AKA extends through the intervertebral foramen of the corresponding spinal level. It then ascends the anterior surface of the spinal cord as many as two and a half vertebrae before it undergoes its characteristic 'hairpin curve' after which it immediately anastomoses with the anterior spinal artery.

**Table 4.61:** Differences between neurogenic and vascular claudication.

| Findings | Neurogenic claudication | Vascular claudication |
|---|---|---|
| Pain type and location | Lower extremity aching, burning, paresthesias | Calf tightness and cramping |
| Radiation | Proximal to distal | Distal to proximal |
| Exacerbation | Lumbar extension including standing, and upright exercise | All lower extremity exercise |
| Walking distance | Variable | Constant |
| Relief | Lumbar flexion and rest | Cessation of lower extremity exercise |
| Back pain | Common | Rare |
| Bicycle/tredmill test | Bicycle generates minimal symptoms, treadmill generates symptoms | Bicycle and treadmill generate symptoms |
| Hill walking | Walking uphill generates minimal symptoms, walking downhill generates symptoms | Walking uphill and walking downhill generates symptoms |
| Lower extremity appearance | Normal | Vascular changes including hair loss, toenail atrophy, edema |
| Pulses lower extremity | Normal | Diminished |
| Lumbar range of motion | Diminished, painful | Normal |

## Case 3: Peripheral Neuropathy

*Brief History*
A 39-year-old male Mr. _____, hailing from _____ District, and Electronic Service Technician by profession came with chief complaints of:
- History of paranesthesia and numbness in both lower limbs and upper limbs, since 1½ months
- History of imbalance while walking since 1½ months.
- History of weakness of lower limb and upper limb since 1½ months

*History of Presenting Complaints*
Patient was apparently alright 1½ months back. Since when he noticed paresthesia and numbness in both lower limbs started simultaneously which gradually progressed to involve upper limbs over span of one week, which is present throughout the day. History of inability to appreciate firmness of ground and feeling the ground like cotton wool. No history of root pain. No history of loss of appreciation of touch, pain. No history of loss of appreciation of hot and cold sensations. No history of ulcer in the limbs. No history of band like constriction around toe or foot.
- History of imbalance while walking since 1½ months insidious in onset which is gradually progressive increased since 2 weeks requiring the support of one person.
- History of unsteadiness increases on standing and closing his eyes. No history of difficulty in reaching the object or target.
- History of weakness of lower limbs and upper limbs since 1½ months. Lower limb weakness in the form of slipping of slippers, later progressed to difficulty in gripping slippers and now progressed and history of buckling of feet.
- History of difficulty in getting up from squatting position, climbing stairs up and down.
- History of weakness of upper limbs in the form of difficulty in holding glass, buttoning and unbuttoning shirt, mixing food.
- Patient also gives history of difficulty in lifting the arm above head.
- No history of twitching of muscles. No history of recurrent fall. No history of speech disturbance. No history of involuntary movement. No history of wasting of muscles.
- No history of bladder disturbances like feeling the sensation of bladder fullness. No history of difficulty in initiation of micturition. No history of bowel disturbances. No history of catheterization. No history of erectile dysfunction.
- No history of loss of sensation of smell.
- No history of decreased vision or loss of vision.
- No history of double vision.
- No history of tingling numbness over the face. No history of difficulty in chewing.
- No history of facial asymmetry, dribbling of saliva from angle of mouth. No history of stasis of food in the mouth.
- No history of vertigo, tinnitus, deafness.
- No history of hoarseness of voice, nasal regurgitation, dysphagia.
- No history of dysarthria, no history of speech disturbances.
- No history of headache, fever, projectile vomiting, blurred vision.
- No history of convulsions.
- No history of loose stools/vaccinations.
- No history of decreased appetite, loss of weight.
- No history of palpitations, giddiness, syncope, excessive sweating.

*Past History*
- K/C/O diabetes mellitus for 5 years was not on regular medication.
- K/C/O bronchiectasis for 10 years on homeopathy medication.
- No history of similar complaints in the past. No previous history of hypertension (HTN)/ischemic heart disease (IHD). No history of any previous hospitalization. No previous history of vaccination.

*Family History*
No history of similar complaints among the family members.

*Personal History*
- Diet: Mixed, predominantly veg
- Appetite: Decreased
- Sleep: Normal
- Bladder: Regular
- Bowel: Regular
- No history of smoking/alcohol consumption

*Summary*
Middle aged male, K/C/O bronchiectasis, diabetes mellitus presented with bilateral, symmetrical, distal more than proximal, lower limb more than upper limb sensory motor involvement not associated with cranial nerve involvement. Absent bowel, bladder autonomic involvement with subacute to chronic in onset.

*Possible Diagnosis*
- Subacute to chronic demyelinating polyneuropathy.
- Peripheral neuropathy involving symmetric, distal, starting in lower limbs usually of systemic origin.

| Neurological deficit | Anatomical localization | Pathological localization | Etiology |
|---|---|---|---|
| Quadriparesis (buckling) | LMN | Demyelinating polyneuropathy | Based on investigation |
| Numbness—large fiber, posterior column sensory dysfunction | Peripheral nerve | | |

## General Examination

Middle aged male moderately built and nourished, conscious and cooperative.
- Height: 159 cm
- Weight: 57 kg
- BMI: 20 kg/m²
- No pallor, no icterus, no cyanosis, grade 1 clubbing
- No lymphadenopathy, no pedal oedema.

### Vital Signs:
- Pulse rate: 84 bpm, regular, good volume, normal character, no radioradial delay, no radiofemoral delay, no vessel wall thickening
- All peripheral pulses are equally felt
- BP: 140/80 mm Hg, right arm, supine position
- 140/70 mm Hg, right arm, sitting position 140/80 mm Hg, left arm, supine position
- RR: 20/minute
- Temperature: Afebrile
- JVP: Not elevated.
- No nerve thickening
- No neurocutaneous markers.
- No external markers of atherosclerosis.
- No signs of nutritional deficiency

### Nervous System Examination
- Right handed individual
- Literate 9th standard.

### Higher Mental Functions

Patient is conscious, oriented to time, place and person.
- Memory: Immediate, remote, recent memory is intact
- Intelligence: Normal.
- Mood/emotion: No emotional lability
- Concentration and calculation: Normal

### Speech:
- Comprehension—preserved
- Fluency normal
- Repetition is normal
- Reading normal
- Writing—unable to perform
- Naming objects: Phonation normal
  - No aphasia
  - No dysarthria
- Apraxias—absent
- Hemineglect—absent
- Hallucinations, delusions—absent

### Cranial Nerve Examination:

|  | Right | Left |
|---|---|---|
| Olfactory—I nerve: | Normal | Normal |
| Optic—II nerve | | |
| • Visual acuity | 6/6 | 6/6 |
| • Visual field | Normal | Normal |
| • Color vision | Normal | Normal |
| Fundus | Normal | Normal |

| Oculomotor, trochlear Abducens—III, IV, VI nerves: Eyelids | | |
|---|---|---|
| • Position of eyeballs at rest | Normal | Normal |
| • Extraocular movements | Normal | Normal |
| • Binocular movements | Normal | Normal |
| • Uniocular movements | Normal | Normal |
| Pupil: | | |
| • Size (in mm) | 3 mm | 3 mm |
| • Shape | Round | Round |
| Reaction | | |
| • Direct light reflex | Present | Present |
| • Consensual light reflex | Present | Present |
| • Accommodation reflex | Present | Present |
| Nystagmus | Absent | Absent |
| Trigeminal nerve—V nerve: Sensory: | | |
| • Touch | Normal | Normal |
| • Pain | Normal | Normal |
| • Temperature | Normal | Normal |
| Motor: | | |
| • Jaw deviation | Absent | Absent |
| • Hollowing above and below zygoma | Absent | Absent |
| • Clenching teeth | Normal | Normal |
| • Open mouth against resistance | Normal | Normal |
| • Side to side movement of jaw | Normal | Normal |
| Reflexes: | | |
| • Corneal | Present | Present |
| • Jaw jerk | Absent | Absent |
|  | Absent | Absent |
| Facial nerve—VII nerve: | | |
| Facial asymmetry | Absent | Absent |
| Motor: | | |
| • Frontalis | Normal | Normal |
| • Orbicularis oculi | Normal | Normal |
| • Buccinator | Normal | Normal |
| • Orbicularis oris | Normal | Normal |
| • Platysma | Normal | Normal |
| Sensory: | | |
| • Anterior 2/3rd tongue taste | Normal | Normal |
| • Lacrimation | Absent | Absent |
| • Hyperacusis | Absent | Absent |
| • Emotional fibers | Preserved | Preserved |
| Vestibulocochlear nerve—VIII nerve: | | |
| • Rinnes test | AC > BC | AC > BC |
| • Weber's test | Not lateralized | Not lateralized |

| | | |
|---|---|---|
| Glossopharygeal, vagus IX, X nerve: | | |
| Position of uvula | Central | Central |
| Movement of uvula on saying 'ah' gag reflex | No deviation present | No deviation present |
| Spinal accessory—XI Nerve: | | |
| Sternocleidomastoid | Normal | Normal |
| Trapezius | Normal | Normal |

**Motor System Examination:**

Attitude:
- Upper limb—bilaterally adducted at shoulder, extended at elbow wrist.
- Lower limb—bilaterally extended and externally rotated at hip joint and knee, plantar flexed.

Bulk:
- Inspection—bilaterally symmetrical in upper limb and lower limb. No deformities, no claw hand, no foot drop.
- Left hand small muscle wasting present.

| Measurement (cm) | Right | Left |
|---|---|---|
| Arm | 24 | 24 |
| Forearm | 21 | 21 |
| Thigh | 40 | 40 |
| Leg | 32 | 32 |

Bulk: Bilateral upper limb and lower limb hypotonia.
Power: Neck
- Flexors: Normal
- Extensors: Normal

| Upper limb | Right | Left |
|---|---|---|
| Shoulder | | |
| • Abduction | 5/5 | 5/5 |
| • Adduction | 5/5 | 5/5 |
| • Flexion | 5/5 | 5/5 |
| • Extension | 5/5 | 5/5 |
| Elbow | | |
| • Flexion | 5/5 | 5/5 |
| • Extension | 5/5 | |
| Wrist | | |
| • Flexion | 4/5 | 4/5 |
| • Extension | 3/5 | 3/5 |
| Hand grip (long flexors) | Weak | Weak |
| Thenar muscles | | |
| Opponens pollicis, abductor pollicis brevis, flexor pollicis brevis | Weak | Weak |
| Hypothenar muscles | | |
| Opponens digiti minimi, abductor digiti minimi, flexor digiti minimi brevis | Weak | Weak |
| Four lumbricals | Weak | Weak |
| Interossei | | |
| Abduction (dorsal interossei) and adduction (palmar interossei) | Weak | Weak |
| Palmaris brevis | Weak | Weak |
| Adductor pollicis | Weak | Weak |
| Trunk | | |
| Beevor's sign | Absent | Absent |
| Abdominal binding (intercostal muscle) | Normal | Normal |
| Intercostal binding (diaphragmatic movement) | Normal | Normal |
| Lower limb | | |
| Hip | | |
| • Flexion | 5/5 | 5/5 |
| • Extension | 5/5 | 5/5 |
| • Abduction | 5/5 | 5/5 |
| • Adduction | 5/5 | 5/5 |
| Knee | | |
| • Flexion | 5/5 | 5/5 |
| • Extension | 5/5 | 5/5 |
| Ankle | | |
| • Plantar flexion | 4/5 | 4/5 |
| • Dorsiflexion | 3/5 | 3/5 |

**Reflexes**

| Superficial reflexes | Right | Left |
|---|---|---|
| Corneal | Present | Present |
| Abdominal | Present | Present |
| Cremasteric | Present | Present |
| Anal reflex | Present | Present |
| Plantar | Flexor | Flexor |
| Deep tendon reflexes | Right | Left |
| Jaw jerk | Absent | Absent |
| Biceps | Absent | Absent |
| Triceps | Absent | Absent |
| Knee jerk/quadriceps/ patellar reflex | Absent | Absent |
| Ankle jerk | Absent | Absent |

| | | |
|---|---|---|
| Clonus | Absent | Absent |
| Even after reinforcement all DTR absent | | |
| Primitive reflex | | |
| Glabellar tap, palmomental (both sides), sucking, rooting, pout, snout grasp | | Absent |

No involuntary movements

Coordination: Under cerebellum

### Sensory System Examination

| Primary sensations | | |
|---|---|---|
| Touch | Present | Present |
| Pain | Present | Present |
| Temperature | Present | Present |
| Vibration | | |
| Metatarsophalangeal joints: | | |
| • Ankle | Absent | Absent |
| • Knee | Absent | Absent |
| • Iliac spines | Absent | Absent |
| Joints of fingers: | | |
| • Ulnar styloid | Absent | Absent |
| • Olecranon | Absent | Absent |
| Joint | Absent | Absent |
| Position | Impaired | Impaired |
| Sense | Absent | Absent |

| Cortical sensations | |
|---|---|
| Tactile localization (topognosis) Two point discrimination Stereognosis Graphesthesia (figure identification) Sensory extinction | Not checked as primary sensations absent |

### Cerebellum

| Upper extremity | Right | Left |
|---|---|---|
| • Limb ataxia | Present | Present |
| • Outstretched arm test finger-nose test | Could not be assessed as power is weak | Could not be assessed as power is weak |
| • Nose-finger-nose test finger-finger test | | |
| • Rapid movements | | |
| • Rapid hand tapping pronation-supination thigh slapping | | |
| • Pointing and past pointing | | |
| • Writing (macrographia) Rebound phenomenon (arm) | | |

| | | |
|---|---|---|
| Tremors (intention) | Absent | Absent |
| Lower limbs | Right | Left |
| Heel knee test | Normal | Normal |
| Pendular knee jerk | Absent | Absent |
| Finger toe test | Could not be assessed | Could not be assessed |
| Rapid alternating movements— foot tapping | Could not be assessed | Could not be assessed |
| General | | |

No titubation

No nystagmus no tremors

No hypotonia

No truncal ataxia

Tandem walking could not be assessed

Gait could not be assessed

*Romberg's test*

Could not be assessed

Gait: Could not be assessed

No signs of involvement of autonomic nervous system

Meningeal signs of irritation
- No neck stiffness
- Kernigs sign: Absent
- Brudzinskis sign—neck, leg: Absent

***Skull and spine***
- No deformities
- No tenderness
- No short neck

***Respiratory system examination***
- Trachea—central
- Bilateral chest movements equal,
- Left infraclavicular area bronchial
- Breath sounds present bilateral infra-axillary coarse crepitations heard

***CVS***
- S1, S2, heard and normal
- No murmurs

***Per Abdomen***
- Soft, non-tender
- No organomegaly,
- Bowel sounds—present

***Clinical diagnosis***

Middle aged male pt. with subacute to chronic onset of weakness of bilateral upper and lower limbs with predominantly sensory symptoms, absent bowel, bladder, autonomic nerve involvement, generalized areflexia, hypotonia on examination Most probable diagnosis is subacute to chronic demyelinating polyneuropathy.

## DISCUSSION

**Q. List the nerve fibers and their function.**

Various nerve fibers and their functions are depicted in **Figure 4.50**.

**Q. What is polyneuropathy? What are the causes?**

It is the most common variety of neuropathy. The nerve fibers are affected in a length-dependent pattern; toes and soles are affected first and hands later. A majority of these cases occur due to metabolic, toxic, or systemic disorders **(Table 4.62)**.

**Q. What is mononeuropathy? What are the causes?**

Mononeuropathy refers to single peripheral nerve involvement and usually occurs due to trauma, compression, or entrapment **(Table 4.63)**.

**Q. What is mononeuritis multiplex? What are the causes?**

**Multiple mononeuropathies/mononeuritis multiplex** refers to the involvement of multiple, separate non-contiguous peripheral nerves either simultaneously or sequentially **(Table 4.64)**.

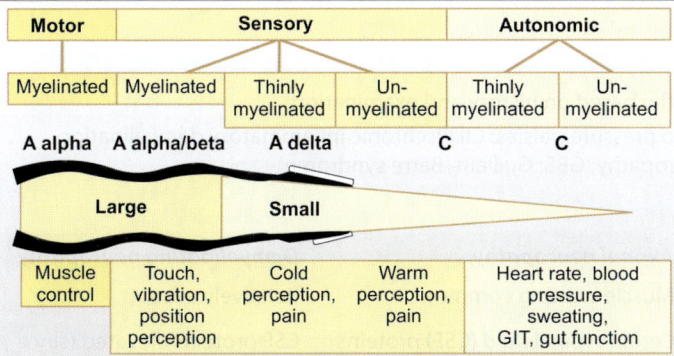

**Fig. 4.50:** Various nerve fibers and their functions. (GIT: gastrointestinal tract)

**Table 4.62:** Causes of polyneuropathy.

**Mnemonic: DANG THERAPIST**
- **D**iabetes mellitus
- **A**lcohol
- **N**utritional (B12 deficiency)
- **G**uillain-Barré syndrome
- **T**oxins (Pb, As, Zn, and Hg)
- **H**ematologic (paraproteins)
- **E**ndocrine (hypothyroid)
- **R**heumatologic (systemic lupus erythematosus, rheumatoid arthritis, and vasculitis)
- **A**myloid
- **P**orphyria
- **I**nfectious (syphilis, human immunodeficiency syndrome)
- **S**arcoid
- **T**umor (paraneoplastic)

**Table 4.63:** Causes of mononeuropathy.

**Acute:** Sustained pressure, e.g., tourniquet
**Chronic:** Entrapment
**Causes** (according to site of compression)

| | |
|---|---|
| Carpal tunnel | Median nerve |
| Cubital tunnel | Ulnar nerve |
| Spiral groove of humerus | Radial nerve |
| Inguinal ligament | Lateral cutaneous of thigh (meralgia paresthetica) |
| Neck of fibula | Common peroneal nerve |
| Flexor retinaculum | Posterior tibial nerve (tarsal tunnel) |

**Entrapment neuropathies are commonly seen in:**
- Endocrinal (diabetes mellitus, myxedema, acromegaly)
- Amyloidosis
- Hereditary neuropathy susceptible to pressure palsy
- Pregnancy
- Arthritis (rheumatoid)

**Table 4.64:** Causes of mononeuritis multiplex.

Leprosy (most common)
Diabetes mellitus
Vasculitis
Sarcoidosis
Amyloidosis
Malignancy
Neurofibromatosis
HIV infection
Idiopathic multifocal motor neuropathy

**Q. What are the features of sensory neuronopathy and motor neuronopathy?**

Refer **Table 4.65 and Figure 4.51**.
- *Neuronopathies (pure sensory or pure motor):*
  - Sensory neuronopathies (ganglionopathies)
  - Motor neuronopathies (motor neuron disease)

**Table 4.65:** Features of sensory neuronopathy and motor neuronopathy.

| Sensory neuronopathy | Motor neuronopathy |
|---|---|
| Ganglion cells predominantly affected | Disorder of anterior horn cells. Weakness, fasciculation, atrophy not truly a process of peripheral nerves |
| Both proximal and distal involvement | |
| Sensory ataxia is common | |
| No weakness | |
| *Example:* | |
| ◆ Cancer (paraneoplastic) | |
| ◆ Sjogren's syndrome | |
| ◆ Cisplatin and other analogs | |
| ◆ Vitamin B6 toxicity | |
| ◆ HIV-related sensory neuronopathy | |

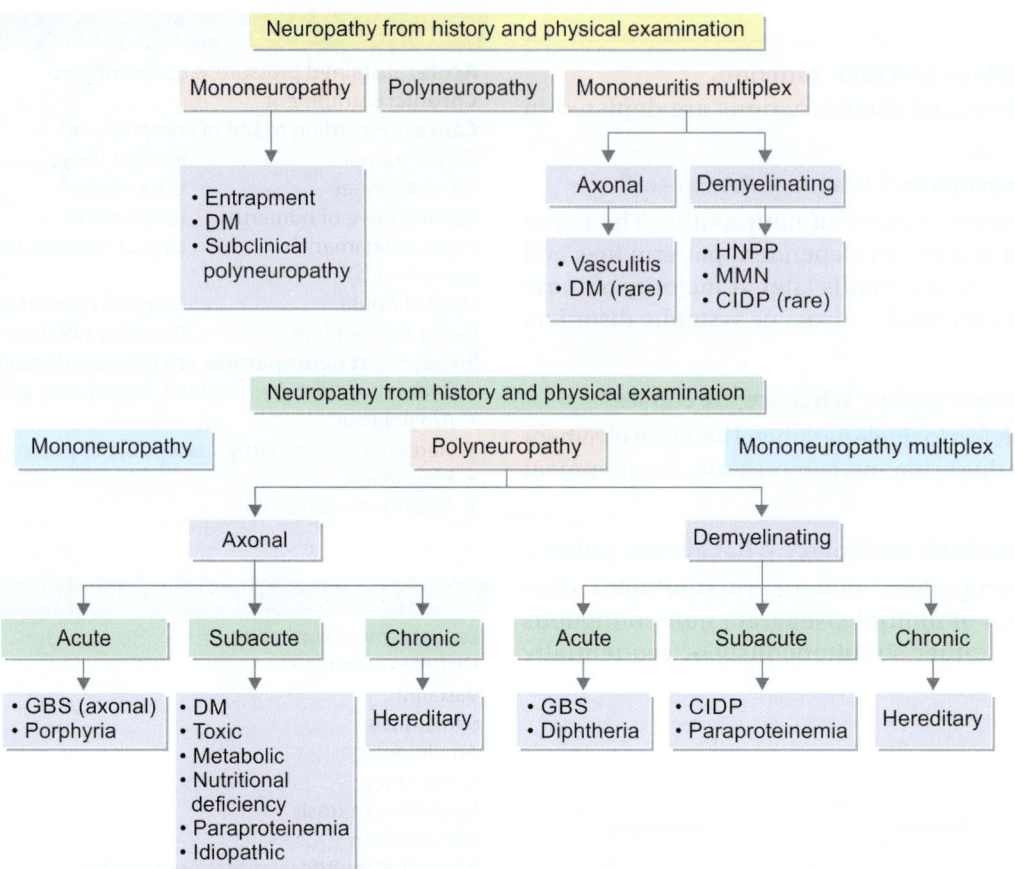

**Figs. 4.51A and B:** Classification of neuropathy based on history and examination.
(DM: diabetes mellitus; HNPP: hereditary neuropathy with liability to pressure palsies; CIDP: chronic inflammatory demyelinating polyneuropathy; MMN: multifocal motor neuropathy; GBS: Guillain–Barré syndrome)

*Peripheral neuropathies (usually sensorimotor):*
- Myelinopathies
- Axonopathies

**Q. What are the differences between axonal and demyelinating neuropathy?**
Refer **Table 4.66**.

**Table 4.66:** Differences between axonal and demyelinating neuropathy.

| Axonal neuropathy | Demyelinating neuropathy |
|---|---|
| Usually gradual and insidious onset | Usually acute or subacute |
| Large and long axons are affected early, hence initially lower extremities are affected | Diffuse process, starts in lower limbs. But not always distal |
| Stocking-glove sensory motor loss results in symmetrical distal clinical signs in legs and arms | Generalized weakness and mild sensory loss |
| Distal involvement | Proximal and distal involvement |
| Ankle jerk lost early and proximal tendon reflexes preserved | All reflexes are lost early |

| Axonal neuropathy | Demyelinating neuropathy |
|---|---|
| Muscle wasting common | Relatively absent |
| Cerebrospinal fluid (CSF) proteins normal | CSF proteins elevated (since nerve roots are involved) |
| Slow recovery | Rapid recovery |
| Residual deformity common | Residual deformity less common |
| Nerve conduction normal or slightly lowered | Nerve conduction is slowed |

**Q. What are the approach to polyneuropathy?**
Refer **Table 4.67**.

**Table 4.67:** Polyneuropathy approach.

**What is the onset and temporal evolution?**
Acute (days to 4 weeks) Subacute (4–8 weeks)
Chronic (>8 weeks)

| Acute onset | • Guillain-Barré syndrome<br>• Acute intermittent porphyria<br>• Critical illness polyneuropathy<br>• Thallium toxicity |
|---|---|

| | |
|---|---|
| Subacute onset | • Toxins or medications<br>• Nutritional deficiency<br>• Metabolic abnormality<br>• Paraneoplastic syndrome |
| Chronic | • Hereditary motor and sensory neuropathy (HMSN)<br>• CIDP<br>• CKD |
| Relapsing/ remitting course | • Guillain-Barré syndrome<br>• CIDP<br>• HIV/AIDS<br>• Porphyria |

(CIDP: chronic inflammatory demyelinating polyneuropathy; CKD: chronic kidney disease; HIV: human immunodeficiency virus; AIDS: acquired immunodeficiency syndrome)

**Q. What are the symptoms of neuropathy?**

Refer **Table 4.68**.

**Table 4.68:** Symptoms and signs of neuropathy.

**Motor symptoms**

| Negative symptoms | Positive symptoms |
|---|---|
| • Weakness<br>• Wasting<br>• Loss of dexterity | • Cramps<br>• Tremors<br>• Fasciculations<br>• Spasms |

In the early stage, weakness in peripheral neuropathy is distal; however, early proximal weakness is a feature of demyelinating neuropathy and porphyric neuropathy

**Neuropathic disorders that may have only motor symptoms at presentation**
- Motor neuron disease
- Lead intoxication
- Acute porphyria
- Guillain-Barre syndrome
- Hereditary motor neuropathy
- Chronic inflammatory demyelinating polyneuropathy
- Diphtheria
- Brachial neuritis
- Diabetic lumbosacral plexus neuropathy

**Sensory symptoms**

| Negative symptoms | Positive symptoms |
|---|---|
| Numbness, loss of sensation in hands and feet | Burning, pain, walking on cotton wool, band-like sensation on feet or trunk, stumbling, tingling, pins, and needles |
| **Large fiber neuropathy—neuropathy of signs/ataxic neuropathy**<br>There are few symptoms (numbness, ataxia) but lots of signs (loss of vibration, joint position sense, diminished reflexes, Romberg's sign positive) | **Small fiber neuropathy—neuropathy of symptoms**<br>Lots of symptoms (PAIN—burning, shock like, stabbing, prickling, shooting, lancinating, allodynia, tight band like pressure. Insensitive to heat and cold) but very few signs (loss of pain, temperature) |

Examples:
- Sjogren's syndrome
- Vitamin B12 neuropathy
- Cisplatin
- Pyridoxine neurotoxicity
- Friedreich's ataxia

Examples:
- Diabetes
- Amyloidosis
- Fabry's disease
- HIV
- Tangier's disease
- Hereditary sensory and autonomic neuropathy
- Sjogren's syndrome
- Chronic idiopathic small fiber sensory neuropathy

**Small and large fiber neuropathy—pan sensory: Global sensory loss**

Example:
- Carcinomatous sensory neuropathy
- Hereditary sensory neuropathy
- Diabetic sensory neuropathy
- Vacor intoxication
- Xanthomatous neuropathy of primary biliary cirrhosis

**Peripheral neuropathies that are often associated with pain**
- Cryptogenic sensory or sensorimotor neuropathy
- Diabetes mellitus
- Vasculitis
- Guillain–Barré syndrome
- Amyloidosis
- Toxic (arsenic and thallium)
- HIV related distal symmetrical polyneuropathy
- Fabry's disease

**Autonomic symptoms**

Enquire if the patient has fainting spells or orthostatic lightheadedness, sweating abnormalities or any bowel, bladder, or sexual dysfunction.

Examples:
*Acute:*
- Pandysautonomia
- Botulism
- Porphyria
- Guillain-Barré syndrome
- Amiodarone
- Vincristine

*Chronic:*
- Amyloid
- Diabetes
- Sjogren's
- HSN 1 and 3
- Chagas disease
- Paraneoplastic

**Q. List the patterns of neuropathy with examples.**

**Pattern 1**

***Symmetric proximal and distal weakness with sensory loss*** Inflammatory demyelinating polyneuropathy (GBS and CIDP).

## Pattern 2
***Symmetric distal weakness with sensory loss***
Metabolic disorders, hereditary toxins drugs.

## Pattern 3
***Asymmetric distal weakness with sensory loss***
- Multiple nerves—vasculitis
- Single nerves/regions—compressive mononeuropathy and radiculopathy.

## Pattern 4
***Asymmetric distal weakness without sensory loss***
- Motor neuron disease—with upper motor neuron findings
- Multifocal motor neuropathy—without upper motor neuron findings.

## Pattern 5
***Asymmetric proximal and distal weakness with sensory loss***
- Polyradiculopathy or plexopathy due to diabetes mellitus
- Meningeal carcinomatosis.

## Pattern 6
***Symmetric sensory loss without weakness***
Cryptogenic sensory polyneuropathy (CSPN), metabolic (diabetes and others) drugs, and toxins.

## Pattern 7
***Symmetric sensory loss and distal areflexia with upper motor neuron findings***
B12 deficiency, HIV, and hepatic disease.

## Pattern 8
***A symmetric proprioceptive sensory loss without weakness***
Sensory neuronopathy (ganglionopathy).

## Pattern 9
***Autonomic symptoms and signs***
Neuropathies associated with autonomic dysfunction.

## Pattern 10
***Syndrome of acute ascending motor paralysis***
- Guillain-Barré syndrome/acute idiopathic polyneuritis
- Diphtheria
- Porphyria
- Triorthocresyl phosphate (TOCP) poisoning
- Paraneoplastic
- Postvaccinial.

## Pattern 11
***Syndrome of subacute sensory motor neuropathy***
- deficiency—alcoholic beriberi, pellagra, and vitamin B12
- Toxins—arsenic, lead, Hg, and Pb
- Drugs—nitrofurantoin, INH, dapsone, disulfiram, and clioquinol
- Uremic
- DM, PAN and sarcoidosis.

**Q. What are the findings in general examination relevant to neuropathy?**

Refer **Table 4.69**.

**Table 4.69:** General examination in neuropathy.

| | |
|---|---|
| Purpura, livedo reticularis | Vasculitis |
| Skin hypopigmentation | Leprosy |
| Hyperpigmentation | Osteosclerotic myeloma—POEMS |
| Bullous lesions | Variegate porphyria |
| Purpura | Vasculitis, cryoglobulinemia |
| Ichthyosis | Refsum's disease |
| Mees' lines | Arsenic/thallium intoxication |
| Alopecia | Thallium poisoning |
| Curled hair | Giant axonal neuropathy |
| Nerve thickening | • Leprosy<br>• CMT<br>• CIDP<br>• Amyloidosis<br>• Neurofibromatosis<br>• Refsum's disease |
| | • Dejerine-Sottas disease<br>• Roussy Levy syndrome<br>• Acromegaly<br>• Idiopathic |

(POEMS: polyneuropathy, organomegaly, endocrinopathy, monoclonal gammopathy and skin changes; CMT: Charcot-Marie-Tooth; CIDP: chronic inflammatory demyelinating polyneuropathy)

**Q. What are the types of polyneuropathy?**

Refer **Figure 4.52**.

**Q. What are the cranial nerve abnormalities you may find in a case of neuropathy?**

- Anosmia—Refsum's disease and B12 deficiency
- Optic atrophy—demyelinating disease may suggest an inherited syndrome, $B_{12}$ deficiency
- Anisocoria and impaired pupillary light reflexes—parasympathetic damage and may be isolated, as in Adie's syndrome, diabetic neuropathy or acute dysautonomia as in GBS
- Impaired ocular mobility suggests botulism or Miller Fisher syndrome
- Facial weakness—GBS, CIDP, Lymes disease, and leprosy
- Trigeminal sensory loss—Sjogren neuropathy
- Lower cranial nerve palsies—Kennedy's disease.

**Q. List the drugs causing neuropathy.**

Refer **Table 4.70**.

**Q. Classify diabetic neuropathy.**

Refer **Box 4.5**.

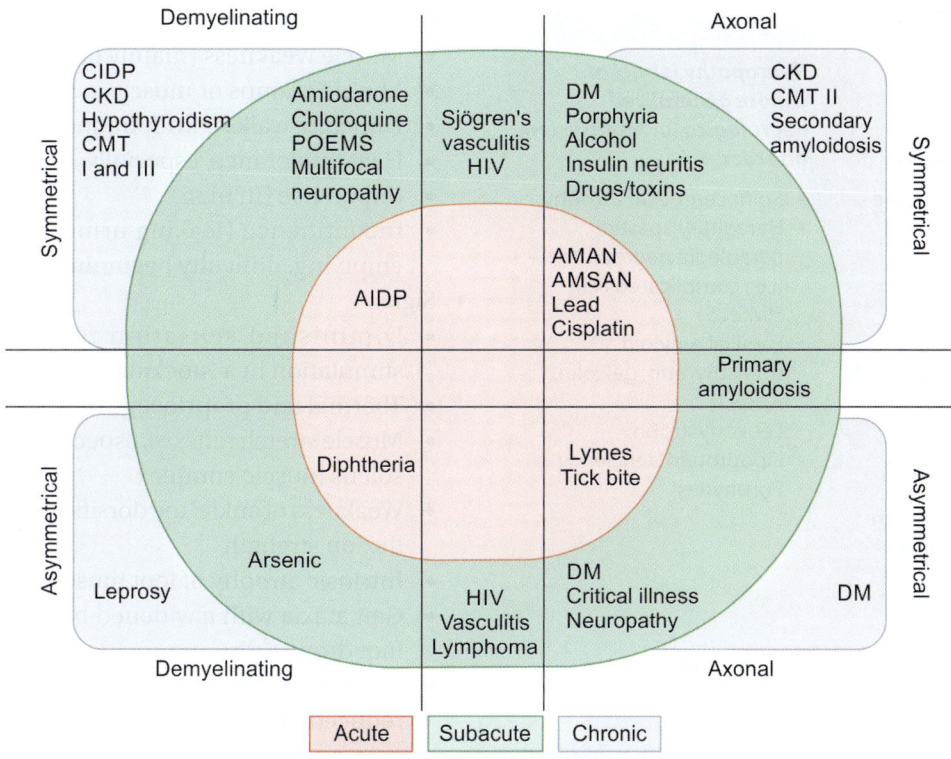

**Fig. 4.52:** Simplified diagram showing types of polyneuropathy.
(CIDP: chronic inflammatory demyelinating polyneuropathy; CKD: chronic kidney disease; CMT: Charcot-Marie-Tooth; POEMS: polyneuropathy, organomegaly, endocrinopathy, monoclonal gammopathy and skin changes; DM: diabetes mellitus; HIV: human immunodeficiency virus; AIDP: acute inflammatory demyelinating polyneuropathy; AMAN: acute motor axonal neuropathy; AMSAN: acute motor and sensory axonal neuropathy)

| Table 4.70: Medications causing neuropathies. ||
|---|---|
| ♦ **Axonal** | – Disulfiram |
| – Vincristine | – Chloroquine |
| – Paclitaxel | – Ethambutol |
| – Nitrous oxide | – Amitriptyline |
| – Colchicine | ♦ **Demyelinating** |
| – Isoniazid | – Amiodarone |
| – Hydralazine | – Chloroquine |
| – Metronidazole | – Suramin |
| – Pyridoxine | – Gold |
| – Didanosine | ♦ **Neuronopathy** |
| – Lithium | – Thalidomide |
| – Dapsone | – Cisplatin |
| – Phenytoin | – Pyridoxine toxicity |
| – Cimetidine | |

**Q. What are the causes of neuropathy in HIV?**

♦ **Seroconversion**
 • Guillain-Barre syndrome
 • Chronic inflammatory demyelinating polyneuropathy (CIDP).
♦ **Symptomatic stage:** Mononeuritis multiplex axonal type subacute or chronic
♦ **Late symptomatic stage:** Distal symmetrical sensory polyneuropathy, most common neuropathy frequently coexists with symptomatic encephalopathy and myelopathy
 • Toxic polyneuropathy (drugs)
 • Subacute asymmetrical polyneuropathy of cauda equina, caused by cytomegalovirus.

**Box 4.5:** Classification of diabetic neuropathy.

**Polyneuropathy**
♦ Symmetrical, mainly sensory and distal
♦ Asymmetrical, mainly motor and proximal (including amyotrophy)

**Mononeuropathy and mononeuritis multiplex**
♦ Cranial nerve lesions
♦ Isolated peripheral nerve lesions

**Autonomic (visceral) neuropathy**
♦ Cardiovascular
♦ Gastrointestinal
♦ Genitourinary
♦ Sudomotor
♦ Vasomotor
♦ Pupillary

**Polyradiculopathies**
♦ Diabetic amyotrophy (lumbar polyradiculopathy)
♦ Thoracic polyradiculopathy
♦ Diabetic neuropathic cachexia

**Treatment-induced neuropathy of diabetes**

| Table 4.71: Types of neuropathies. | |
| --- | --- |
| **Neuropathy is the sole or primary part of the disease** | **Neuropathy is part of a more generalized neurological or multisystem disorder** |
| • Charcot-Marie-Tooth disease—CMT1 (demyelinating) and CMT2 (axonal)<br>• HMSN-III (or *Dejerine–Sottas neuropathy*)<br>• Hereditary sensory and autonomic neuropathy (HSAN)<br>• Distal hereditary motor neuropathy (dHMN)<br>• Hereditary brachial plexus neuropathy (HBPN)<br>• Hereditary neuropathy with liability to pressure palsies (HNPP) | • Spinocerebellar atrophy<br>• Hereditary spastic paraplegia neuropathy (i.e., complicated HSP, HMSN 5)<br>• Familial amyloid (transthyretin, gelsolin, ApoA1)<br>• Leukodystrophy<br>• Lipoprotein deficiency<br>• Porphyrias |

**Q. Give examples for hereditary neuropathies.**

Refer **Table 4.71**.

**Q. What is the importance of occupation in peripheral neuropathy?**

- **Lead exposure:** Battery manufacturing and recycling, ammunition manufacturing, automotive/radiator repair, soldering, painting, plumbing and welding.
- **Arsenic exposure:** Smelters, wood preservative works, pesticides and fertilizer industries.
- **Mercury exposure:** Smelters, cement industries, sewage disposal, caustic soda factories, pig-iron industries and battery industries.
- **Coal-tar industry, screen printing, textile workers:** organic solvents like hexacarbons, perchloroethylene, hexane.

**Q. General physical examination in case of peripheral neuropathy?**

- Trophic ulcers, deformities of digits and hypopigmented anesthetic skin patch (dry, hair loss), madarosis: *Leprosy*.
- **Pallor and Burtonian line:** *Lead poisoning*.
- **Mees lines:** *Arsenic toxicity*,
- **orange tonsils:** *Tangier's disease*
- **Anisocoria and impaired pupillary light reflexes:** *dysautonomia, diabetes*.
- **Oral candidiasis, hairy leukoplakia, herpetic vesicles and papular exanthema:** HIV
- **Gynecomastia:** *Kennedy's disease*.
- **Umbilical keratomas:** *Fabry's disease*.
- **Wax-colored papules, nodules around the face, lips and ears, shoulder-pad sign, macroglossia:** *Amyloidosis*
- **High arch palate, cataract and icthyosis:** *Refsum's disease*.
- **Foot and spinal deformities**: *Charcot-Marie-Tooth disease*.

**Q. What are the clinical features of alcoholic neuropathy?**

- Symptoms:
  - Numbness and pins and needles in the arms and legs
  - Muscle weakness (mainly distal lower>>upper limb),
  - Muscle cramps or muscle aches
  - Difficulty walking with frequent falls,
  - Heat intolerance, especially after exercise
  - Impotence (in men)
  - Incontinence (leaking urine), feeling of incomplete emptying, difficulty beginning to urinate
- Signs:
  - Diminished sensation to vibration or pinprick stimulation in a 'stocking-to-glove' distribution
  - Thermal and proprioceptive sensation abnormalities
  - Muscle stretch reflexes, especially of the gastrocnemius-soleus muscle complex
  - Weakness of ankle/toe dorsiflexion and/or ankle plantar flexion strength
  - Intrinsic atrophy of foot muscles in advanced cases
  - Gait ataxia with a widened base of support or bilateral foot drop
  - Patellar and Achilles deep tendon reflexes are often reduced or absent

**Q. Which vitamin deficiency causes peripheral neuropathy?**

Cobalamin (B12), thiamine, vitamin E, pyridoxine and niacin (pellagra).

**Q. What are the clinical presentation of subacute combined degeneration?**

- **Symptoms:** Weakness of legs (symmetrical, progresses distal to proximal), arms, trunk; tingling and numbness that progressively worsens. Vision changes and change of mental state may also be present. Sensory ataxia.
- **Signs**
  - Optic atrophy, nystagmus, small reactive pupils
  - Sense of vibration, posture and passive movement affected first in lower, later in upper limbs.
  - Glove and stocking sensory loss.
  - Tenderness of calf muscles
  - Reflexes: Variable—ankle jerk lost, knee jerk may be absent. Both knee and ankle jerk may be exaggerated if lateral column lesion predominates.
  - Positive Rhomberg's sign.

**Q. How to say a palpable nerve is abnormal?**

Presence of tenderness, anesthetic skin patch, asymmetrical (when compared to opposite side).

**Q. What are the causes of autonomic neuropathy?**

Refer **Table 4.72**.

| Table 4.72: Causes of autonomic neuropathy. | |
|---|---|
| **Acquired** | **Inherited** |
| ✦ Diabetic neuropathy<br>✦ Paraneoplastic neuropathy<br>✦ Lymphoma<br>✦ Thallium, arsenic, mercury toxicity<br>✦ Thiamine deficiency<br>✦ Vincristine (Oncovin, Vincosar PFS) toxicity<br>✦ Guillain-Barré syndrome<br>✦ Alcoholic neuropathy<br>✦ Acute pandysautonomia | ✦ Familial amyloid poly neuropathy<br>✦ Hereditary sensory<br>✦ Autonomic neuropathy<br>✦ Fabry disease<br>✦ Porphyria |

**Q. Name the first muscle involved in carpal tunnel syndrome.**

**Abductor pollicis brevis**

**Note:** The opponens pollicis and abductor pollicis brevis are normally innervated by the median nerve. The flexor pollicis brevis can be innervated by the median or ulnar nerve. The adductor pollicis is typically innervated by the ulnar nerve.

**Q. Testing small muscles of hand?**

♦ **Test of interossei and lumbricals:** Test the patient's ability of flex his MCP joints and to extend the DIP joints. Remember, the palmar interossei are adductors and dorsal interossei are abductors of fingers.

♦ **Test of 1st dorsal interosseous**: Ask the patient to abduct his index finger against your resistance. The muscle can be seen and felt to contact.

**Q. How to test these small muscles?**

♦ **Abductor pollicis brevis:** The patient is asked to abduct his thumb in a plane at right angles to the palmar aspect of Index finger, against resistance of your thumb. The muscle can be felt to contract. This muscle is affected first in carpal tunnel syndrome.

♦ **Adductor pollicis:** Give the patient a book and ask him to grasp it firmly between the thumb and other fingers of both hands. In a normal subject the thumb of the affected hand will be flexed.

♦ **Opponens pollicis:** Ask the patient to touch the tip of all the fingers with his thumb. You can oppose the movement with your thumb or index finger, or you can ask the patient to swing the thumb across the palm.

**Figure 4.53** shows the tests for small muscles of hand.

**Q. What are the causes of proximal and distal muscle weakness?**

**A. Proximal muscle weakness:**
- Myopathies:
  - Polymyositis
  - Dermatomyositis
  - Muscular dystrophy
  - Hypothyroidism
  - Hypokalemic periodic paralysis
- Proximal neuropathies:
  - Diabetic amyotrophy
  - Amyloidosis
  - Porphyria
  - HIV neuropathy
  - Tangier's disease
  - GBS

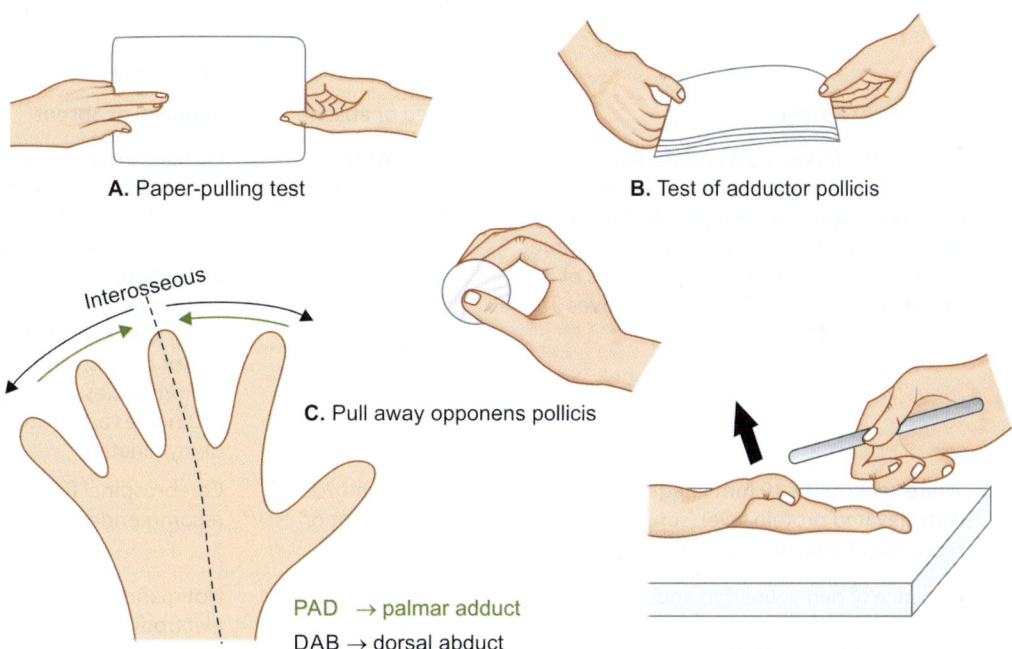

**Fig. 4.53:** Tests for small muscles of hand.

**B. Distal myopathies:**
- Myotonic dystrophy
- Welander's myopathy
- Tibial muscular dystrophy
- Markesberry-Griggs myopathy
- Laing's myopathy
- Miyoshi's myopathy
- Myofibrillar myopathies

### Q. How to elicit cremasteric reflex?

It is elicited by stroking or lightly scratching the skin on the upper, inner aspect of the thigh. The response is contraction of the cremastric muscle with elevation of the ipsilateral testicle.
Root value: L1-L2

### Q. What is lathyrism?

- Neuropathy due to prolonged consumption of *Lathyrus sativus* (khesri dhal, grass pea).
- Common in India (Madhya Pradesh)
- Characterized by gradual weakness of legs and spasticity.
- Paresthesia, numbness, formication in the legs, frequency and urgency of micturition, impotence and sphincteric spasms are present.
- **Toxin:** Neuroexcitatory amino acid BOAA (beta-N-oxalylaminoalanine).

### Q. What is the diagnostic criteria for CIDP?
Refer **Table 4.73**.

### Q. What are the causes for cutaneous vasculitis?
Refer **Box 4.6**.

### Q. What are the neurological manifestations of SLE?

The 1999 ACR Nomenclature Committee has identified 19 different NPL (neuropsychiatric lupus) conditions those are part of lupus complex of which 12 are CNS-related and 7 are PNS-related. This new set in 19 NP definitions with proper clinical judgment could be used to expand the neuropsychiatric criteria of the ACR classification criteria of SLE from just seizures and psychosis. These NPL case definitions are:

- Acute confusional state
- Acute inflammatory demyelinating polyradiculoneuropathy (AIDP) (Guillain-Barre syndrome)
- Anxiety disorder
- Aseptic meningitis
- Autonomic disorder
- Cerebrovascular disease
- Cognitive dysfunction (most common manifestation of diffuse CNS lupus)
- Demyelinating syndrome

**Table 4.73:** Diagnostic criteria of CIDP.

| Feature | ANN criteria | Saperstein criteria | INCAT criteria |
| --- | --- | --- | --- |
| Clinical involvement | Motor dysfunction, sensory dysfunction of >1 limb, or both | Major—symmetric proximal and distal weakness—minor exclusively distal weakness or sensory loss | Progressive or relapsing motor and sensory dysfunction of more than 1 limb |
| Time course (mo) | ≥2 | ≥2 | ≥2 |
| Reflexes | Reduced or absent | Reduced or absent | Reduced or absent |
| Electrodiagnostic test results | Any 3 of the following 4 criteria: Partial conduction block of ≥1 motor nerve, reduced conduction velocity of ≥2 motor nerves, prolonged distal latency of ≥2 motor nerves, or prolonged F-wave latencies of ≥2 motor nerves of the absence of F-waves | 2 of the 4 AAN Electrodiagnostic criteria | Partial conduction block of ≥2 motor nerves and abnormal conduction velocity or distal latency or F-wave latency in 1 other nerve; or, in the absence of partial conduction block, abnormal conduction velocity, distal latency, or F-wave latency in 3 motor nerves; or electrodiagnostic abnormalities indicating demyelination in 2 nerves and histologic evidence of demyelination |
| Cerebrospinal fluid | White cell count <10 mm³, negative VDRL test; elevated protein level (supportive) | Protein >45 mg/dL; white cell count of <10/mm³ (supportive) | Cerebrospinal fluid analysis recommended but not mandatory |
| Biopsy findings | Evidence of demyelination and remyelination | Predominant features of demyelination; inflammation (not required) | Not mandatory (except in cases with electrodiagnostic abnormalities in only 2 motor nerves) |

Box 4.6: Causes of cutaneous vasculitis.

* Associated chronic disorders
  - Rheumatoid arthritis
  - Sjogren syndrome.
  - Systemic lupus erythematosus
  - Hypergammaglobulinemic purpura
  - Paraneoplastic vasculitis
  - Cryoglobulinemia
  - Ulcerative colitis
  - Cystic fibrosis
  - Antineutrophil cytoplasmic or antiphospholipid antibody syndrome
* Precipitating events
  - Bacterial, viral, and mycobacterial infections
  - Therapeutic and diagnostic agents
* Idiopathic disorders
  - Henoch-Schonlein syndrome
  - Acute hemorrhagic edema of childhood
  - Urticarial vasculitis and variants
  - Erythema elevatum diutinum
    - Nodular vasculitis
    - Livedoid vasculitis
    - Genetic complement deficiencies
    - Eosinophilic vasculitis
    - Idiopathic

♦ Headache
♦ Mononeuropathy (single/multiplex)
♦ Mood disorders
♦ Movement disorder (chorea)
♦ Myasthenia gravis
♦ Myelopathy
♦ Neuropathy, cranial
♦ Plexopathy
♦ Polyneuropathy
♦ Psychosis
♦ Seizure and seizure disorder

**Q. What are the difference between compressive myelopathy versus GB syndrome?**

Refer **Table 4.74**.

**Table 4.74:** Difference between compressive myelopathy versus GB syndrome.

| Cord compression | AIDP |
| --- | --- |
| Symmetrical/asymmetrical | Symmetrical |
| Bladder involvement present | Absent |
| No cranial nerve involvement | May be present |
| Upper level of sensory deficit present | Absent |

**Q. What is cocaine-levamisole-induced cutaneous vasculitis?**

The reason for the addition of levamisole to various forms of cocaine is unclear, but is thought to potentiate nicotinic acetyl cholinergic effects in the brain when used in combination. Both cocaine and levamisole had been implicated in causing cutaneous vasculitis. Levamisole has been sporadically linked to the development of hypersensitivity reactions manifesting as leukopenia, hemolytic anemia with hepatosplenomegaly, arthralgias, and cutaneous vasculitis. Levamisole induced cutaneous vasculitis is characterized by the involvement of the external pinna, ranging in severity from purpuric papules or plaques, to hemorrhagic bullae often accompanied by musculoskeletal symptoms. Cocaine has been reported to cause rheumatologic syndromes ranging from Raynaud's phenomenon, cutaneous vasculopathy or vasculitis, digital or limb necrosis, cerebral vasculitis, Churg-Strauss syndrome, to a syndrome with sinonasal destruction termed cocaine-induced midline destructive lesions (CIMDL) that mimics limited Wegener's granulomatosis.

**Q. Name the causes of small muscle wasting of the hand.**

Small muscle of the hand is supplied by C8 and T1 segments

**Causes**

♦ Lesion in the anterior horn cells
  • Acute anerior poliomyelitis
  • Motor neuron disease (MND)
  • Syringomyelia
  • Intramedullary tumors like glioma, ependymoma
♦ Lesions in the nerve roots
  • Extramedullary lesion, e.g., patchy arachnoiditis
  • Cervical spondylosis
  • Neuralgic amyotrophy
  • Leptomeningitis (syphilitic)
  • Lesion in the spinal nerve
  • Cervical rib
  • Trauma
  • Thoracic inlet syndrome
  • Metastasis
  • Lesion in the median/ulnar nerve
  • Peripheral neuropathy
  • Carpal tunnel syndrome
  • Muscle diseases
  • Distal myopathy of Gowers
  • Myotonia dystrophica
  • Volkmann ischemic contracture
  • Peripheral vascular disease
  • Reflex wasting due to disuse atrophy—rheumatoid arthritis, postparalytic, postfracture
  • Systemic wasting—malignancy, tuberculosis, diabetes mellitus, thyrotoxicosis, AIDS

**Q. Name the myopathies causing small muscle wasting of the hand.**

♦ Distal myopathy of Gowers
♦ Myotonia dystrophica
♦ Volkmanns ischemic contracture
♦ Peripheral vascular disease

### Q. What are the signs of ulnar nerve palsy?

Ulnar nerve supplies all muscles of the hand except the thenar muscles and the two lateral lumbricals (which are supplied by median nerve).

**Muscles affected in ulnar nerve palsy are:**

- **Flexor carpi ulnaris**—flexion and adduction at the wrist are weak **flexor digitorum profundus (medial part)**—flexion of terminal pharyngeal of ring and little finger is affected.
- **Hypothenar muscles**—movements of little finger affected.
- **Interossei**—abduction and adduction of fingers are weak.
- **Ulnar claw hand (partial)**—medial two digits being most affected. Complete claw hand is seen in combined lesion of both ulnar and median nerve.

### Q. What is ulnar paradox?

A *proximal* injury to the ulnar nerve will causes less deformity compared to a *distal* injury.

An ulnar claw may follow an ulnar nerve lesion which results in the partial or complete denervation of the ulnar (medial) two lumbricals of the hand. Since the ulnar nerve also innervates the 3rd and 4th lumbricals, which flex the MCP joints (aka the knuckles), their denervation causes these joints to become extended by the now unopposed action of the long finger extensors (namely the extensor digitorum and the extensor digiti minimi). The lumbricals and interossei also extend the IP (interphalangeal) joints of the fingers by insertion into the extensor hood; their paralysis results in weakened extension. The combination of hyperextension at the MCP and flexion at the IP joints gives the hand its claw like appearance.

### Q. Name the muscle supplied by median nerve.

The following muscles are supplied by the median nerve (**Figs. 4.54A and B**):

- Pronator teres
- Flexor carpi radialis
- Palmaris longus
- Flexor digitorum superficialis
- Flexor pollicis longus
- Flexor digitorum profundus (lateral part)
- Pronator quadratus
- Thenar muscles (FPB, APB, OP)
- First and second lumbricals

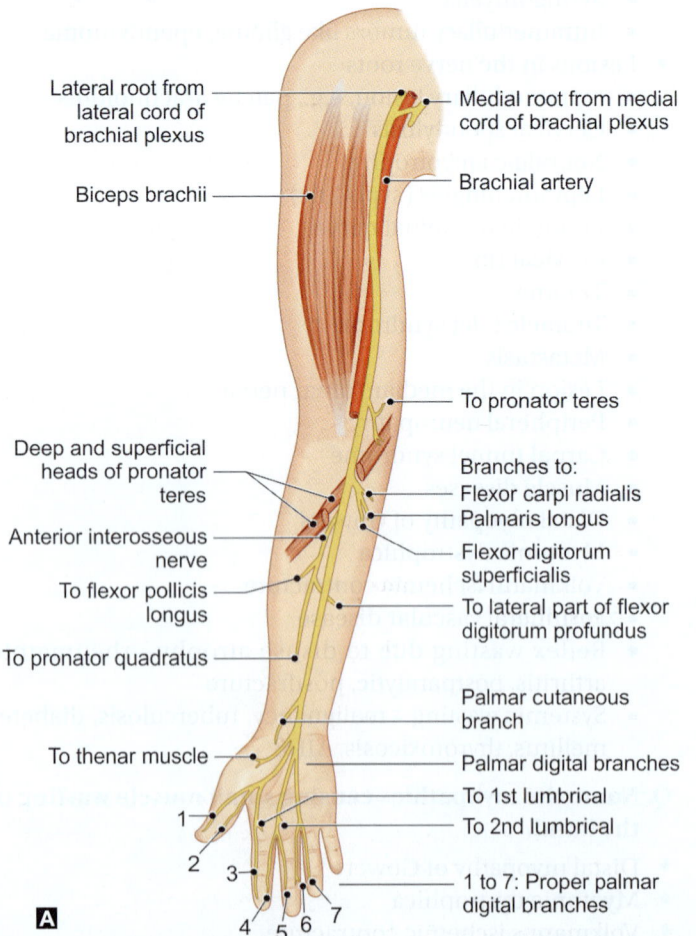
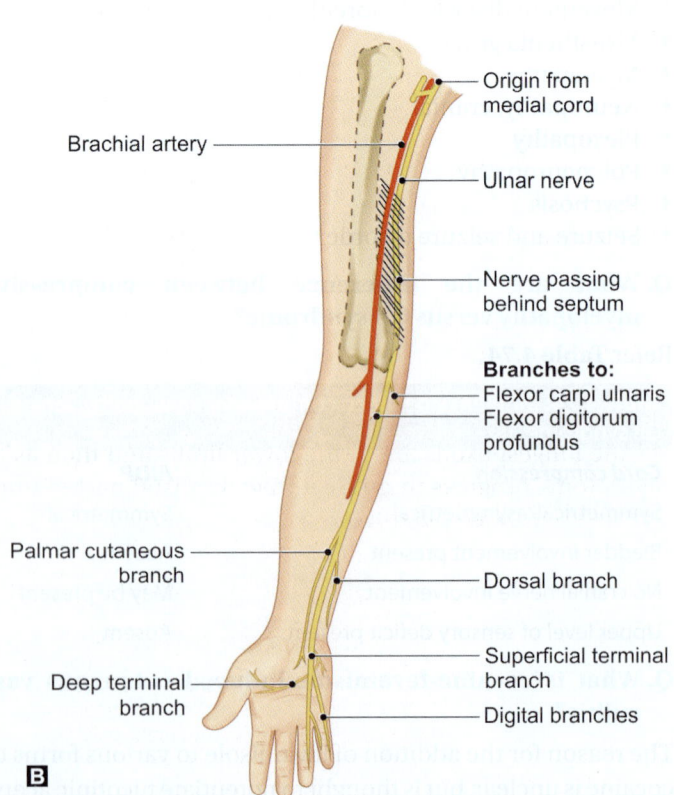

**Figs. 4.54A and B:** Ulnar nerve branches and supply.

**Q. What is Froment's sign?**

It is seen in ulnar nerve injury. It tests for adductor pollicis and first palmar interossei. The patient is asked to grasp a book between the extended thumb and the other fingers. If the ulnar nerve is injured these two muscles will be paralyzed and the patient will hold the book by flexing the thumb with the help of flexor pollicis longus. This is known as Froment's sign **(Fig. 4.55)**.

**Q. What is card test?**

A card is inserted between the two fingers which are kept extended. The patient is asked to hold the card by adducting these two fingers as tightly as possible. The clinician will try to pull the card out of his fingers. This will give an idea about the strength of the palmar interossei. This test is known as the card test **(Fig. 4.56)**.

**Q. What are the patterns of involvement in neuropathy?**
- Pattern of involvement in neuropathy. Mononeuropathy/plexopathy/mononeuropathy multiplex
- Unilateral/bilateral; symmetrical/asymmetrical, proximal/distal pure motor, pure sensory/mixed
- Upper limb predominance/lower limb predominance
  - Associated autonomic or cranial nerve involvement
  - Onset—acute/subacute/chronic; relapsing—remitting
- The common type of neuropathy is bilateral symmetrical distal sensory/sensory motor neuropathy.

**Q. Name the common systemic causes for peripheral neuropathy.**
- Deficiency disorders—vitamin $B_1$, $B_6$, $B_{12}$
- Endocrine—hypothyroidism/hyperthyroidism
- Metabolic—diabetes, CKD, amyloidosis
- Toxic—alcohol, heavy metals, organophosphorus, TOCP.
- Drugs—INH, vincristine, digoxin, lithium
- Autoimmune disorders
- Paraneoplastic—GI lymphomas, paraproteinemia

**Q. Name the course/characteristic of diabetic neuropathy.**

The common variety of peripheral neuropathy is diabetic in origin, simply because diabetes is the common medical disorder affecting a large population. Diabetic neuropathy typically B/L symmetrical and distal affecting first the feet as the longest axons are in the lower limbs and then as the symptoms progress to mid-calf region, distal part of upper limbs are affected (length dependent).

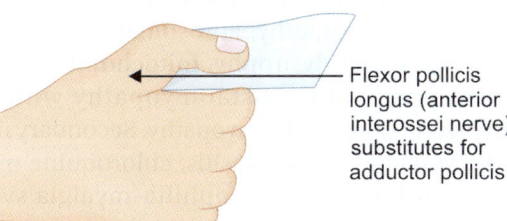

**Fig. 4.55:** Froment's sign.

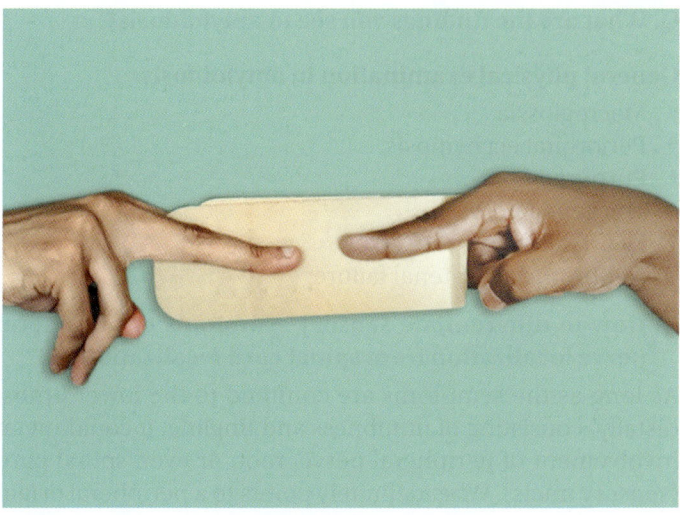

**Fig. 4.56:** Card test.

**Risk factor:** Long standing, poorly controlled DM and the presence of retinopathy and nephropathy.

**Nerve compression palsies:** Most common carpal tunnel syndrome. Ulnar nerve compression at the elbow and peroneal nerve compression at the fibula common and may occur in sequence and produce a syndrome. These nerve palsies are recoverable with appropriate decompression and pressure avoidance.

**Vascular nerve lesions:** Cranial mononeuropathies, seventh nerve palsies are relatively common but may have other. In diabetics, a third nerve palsies most common, followed by sixth nerve, and less frequently, fourth nerve palsies. Diabetic third nerve palsies are characteristically pupil-sparing.

**Q. What are the causes for acute motor paralysis with the site of lesion peripheral nerve?**
- Guillain-Barre' syndrome
- Acute axonal form of GBS
- Acute sensory neuropathy and neuronopathy syndrome
- Diphtheritic polyneuropathy
- Porphyric polyneuropathy
- Certain toxic polyneuropathies (thallium, triorthocresyl phosphate)
- Rarely, paraneoplastic
- Acute pandysautonomic neuropathy
- Tick paralysis
- Critical illness polyneuropathy.

**Q. How to assess lesion based on wearing slippers?**
- Difficulty in initiation of putting the feet into slippers is due to cerebellar lesion
- Difficulty to grip slippers is motor weakness.
- If one is aware of slippers slipping off the feet it is motor weakness; if unaware it is sensory deficit.

### Q. What are the findings you see in amyloidosis?

**General physical examination in amyloidosis:**
- Macroglossia
- Periorbital ecchymosis
- Purpuras
- Thickened nerves
- Heart failure
- Nephromegaly—renal failure

### Q. How to differentiate sensory symptoms of peripheral nerve localization from spinal cord localization?

As long as the symptoms are confined to the lower limbs, distally, consisting of numbness and tingling, it could mean involvement of peripheral nerve, root, or even spinal cord (sensory tracts). What definitely points to a peripheral origin is shock like sensation, burning pain aggravated by touching of the clothes so much so that they cannot wear socks or even cover themselves with the bed sheet. All these Point to the involvement of peripheral sensory involvement.

Characteristically the sensory symptoms ascend up to the midcalf and then jump to the fingers and hand (length dependent neuropathy), evading thighs. This pattern is diagnostic of peripheral neuropathy. A situation where tingling continues to spread upward from the feet involving the entire lower limbs and the lower abdomen suggests spinal cord localization.

### Q. What are the causes of myloneuropathies?
- HIV
- Subacute combined degeneration
- Tabes dorsalis
- Conus cauda.

### Q. What is timed vibration?

**Vibration test**

Testing should compare side to side and distal to proximal sensation. If vibration is absent distally, the stimulus is moved proximally to the metatarsophalangeal joints, then the ankle, then the knee, then the iliac spines, and so forth.

Upper extremity areas frequently tested include the distal joints of the fingers, the radial and ulnar styloids, the olecranon and the clavicles.

Gradual loss of sensation, such as from toe to ankle to knee, favors a peripheral nerve problem. Uniform loss of vibration beyond a certain point, for example, the iliac crests, favors myelopathy.

**Timed vibration**

The threshold for vibratory perception is normally somewhat higher in the lower than in the upper extremities. There is progressive loss of vibratory sensitivity with advancing age, and the sensation may be entirely absent at the great toes in the elderly. The best control is an approximately age-matched normal, such as the patient's spouse.

### Q. Which nerve is preferred for biopsy and why?

The sural nerve is most commonly biopsied because it is a pure sensory nerve and biopsy will not result in loss of motor function. In suspected vasculitis, a combination biopsy of a superficial peroneal nerve (pure sensory) and the underlying peroneus brevis muscle obtained from a single small incision increases the diagnostic yield.

### Q. What are the differential diagnosis for asymmetrical weakness and thinning of limbs?
- MND
- Mononeuritis multiplex
- Diabetic amyotrophy
- CIDP
- Nerve entrapment syndromes
- Spinal muscular atrophy
- Multiple motor neuropathy with conduction block
- Post-polio syndrome
- Kennedy's syndrome
- Critical illness neuropathy and myopathy
- Inclusion body myositis

### Q. What is the association of neurological diseases and the heart?

Neurological disease, which most frequently manifests with cardiomyopathies are the neuromuscular disorders. Most commonly associated with cardiomyopathies are muscular dystrophies, myofibrillar myopathies, congenital myopathies and metabolic myopathies.

- NMDs most frequently associated with HCM include Emery-Dreifuss muscular dystrophy, Becker muscular dystrophy, facioscapulohumeral MD, limb girdle muscular dystrophy, myotonic dystrophy, myofibrillar myopathy, rigid spine syndrome, metabolic myopathy, or Friedreich ataxia, mitochondrial myopathy, Senger's disease, glycogenosis, eosinophilia-myalgia syndrome, or arthrogryposis multiplex congenita.
- Dilated cardiomyopathy (DCM) include dystrophinopathies, limb girdle muscular dystrophies, congenital myopathies, myofibrillar myopathies, or metabolic myopathies, congenital muscular dystrophies, Barth syndrome, oculopharyngodistal myopathy, or inclusion body myopathy. Rarely DCM occurs in patients with secondary myopathies, such as polymyositis, dermatomyositis, or inclusion body myositis.
- RCM (restrictive cardiomyopathy) has been reported in myofibrillar myopathy, autosomal dominant Emery-Dreifuss muscular dystrophy, mitochondrial myopathy, multicore myopathy, distal myopathy with rimmed vacuoles, and nonspecific myopathy. Secondary myopathy with RCM include polymyositis, chloroquine myopathy, tryptophan-induced eosinophilia-myalgia syndrome, and polyneuropathy, organomegaly, endocrinopathy, M-protein, and skin changes (POEMS) syndrome,

mitochondrial disorders (CPEO, MELAS, MERRF, KSS, MM).
- Takotsubo-CMP has been reported in association with a number of hereditary and non-hereditary NMDs. These include amyotrophic lateral sclerosis, myasthenia gravis, metabolic myopathy, neurofibromatosis I, Guillain-Barre syndrome, hereditary neuropathy, mitochondrial myopathy, or rhabdomyolysis.

### Q. Which is the first muscle to get involved in ulnar nerve and median nerve injury?
- Ulnar nerve: Abductor digiti minimi
- Median nerve: Abductor pollicis brevis

### Q. What are trick movements and their importance while checking small muscles of hand?
Trick movements are when prime movers of a joint are paralyzed and other muscles take over their function.
- **Radial nerve:** In a complete nerve lesion it is possible for the patient to extend IP joint of the thumb because the short abductor and short flexor have an insertion into the extensor expansion, the patient has to bring the thumb into palmar abduction before the IP joint can extend.
- **Ulnar nerve:** Complete lesion the adductor of the thumb is paralyzed and attempts to bring the thumb to the index finger, with the forearm held with the radial aspect pointing towards the ground to eliminate gravity resulting in marked flexion of IP joint, this trick action of the long flexor is known as Froment's sign. Although the interossei are the abductors and adductors of the fingers, when the long extensors contract strongly can give the appearance of some abduction, similarly long flexors can give some adduction.
- **Median nerve:** In a complete median nerve lesion attempts, to oppose the thumb to the little finger, he cannot bring the thumb away from the hand as the short abductor and the opponens are paralyzed, he therefore flexes the IP joint of the thumb in an attempt to oppose. This movement puts the thumb in a lively splint which supports the thumb in palmar abduction, thus putting the long flexor in an advantageous position to give some opposition to the fingertips.

### Q. What are the bedside tests for autonomic dysfunction?
- **General examination:** Color of skin, especially of extremities, local or general flushing or cyanosis, feel temperature of skin in different areas (recent sympathetic lesions produce warmth and redness in affected area), sweating (complete sympathetic lesions produce absence of sweating, partial lesions produce profuse sweating), change in color, texture and quantity of hair and nails, look for presence of Horner's syndrome.
- **Cardiovascular reflexes:**
  - Postural hypotension: A fall in systolic BP below 20 mm Hg and diastolic BP below 10 mm Hg of baseline within 3 minutes in upright position is abnormal (seen in sympathetic lesions).
  - Blood pressure response to pressor stimuli: Mental arithmetic, sustained handgrip or exposure to cold causes a rise in BP. Handgrip dynamometer allows a quantifiable test, less than 10 mm Hg rise in diastolic pressure is abnormal (seen in sympathetic lesions).
  - Heart rate responses: Change of posture from lying to standing is followed by an immediate increase in heart rate and then relative bradycardia, quantified by using a continuous ECG recording (parasympathetic lesion will slow down or abolish the response).
  - The Valsalva maneuver: In the first exhalation (against a closed glottis), the BP drops and the HR increases. On releasing (by opening the glottis), the BP 'overshoots' the resting value and the HR slows. Test is performed by the patient exhaling into a mouth piece connected to a manometer or sphygmomanometer to hold the pressure at 40 mm Hg for 15 seconds, an ECG records the HR response (afferent or efferent parasympathetic lesions impair the response).
- **Skin responses:**
  - Erythema: Scratching skin will produce a line surrounded by a spreading flare and followed by a wheal with central pallor (exaggerated below the level of a transverse cord lesion, at the level of lesion even normal response may be absent)
  - Temperature: Measurement of skin temperature by accurate skin thermometers (increased temperature below recently denervated level, decreased temperature following chronic neurological lesions, increased response to warming of the part or of distal parts over denervated areas in sympathetic lesions).
  - Pilomotor response: Produced by sharp scratching or by touching the warmed body with cold metal.
  - Scrotal response: Touching the scrotum with a cold object normally results in a vermicular contraction of the dartos, without elevation of the testicles, differing it from cremasteric reflex (absent in sympathetic paralysis).
  - Sweating test: Spoon test to check adequacy of sweating. A spoon is lid over the part to be tested and the resistance encoureted in subjectively assessed (normal sweating spoon will encounter some resistance, areas of reduced sweating the resistance encountered is less and spoon moves easily).
  - Alternatively, area to be tested is thoroughly dried and liberally dusted with Quinizarin powder, the patient is then placed under a heat cradle, and given a hot drink combined with 0.5 g acetylsalicylic acid, areas of sweat are clearly outlined as the powder turns black when exposed to moisture (sympathetic lesions, segmental loss of sweating is present; below a transverse cord lesion sweating maybe absent in the early stages, but

later becomes abnormally profuse, at the level of a recent lesion the response is exaggerated).
- **Examination of bladder function:** Testing of sacral segments, bladder swelling may be palpable. The superficial anal reflex must be tested. Assessment of detrusor function can be made by asking a patient while passing urine to breathe deeply, interrupting abdominal muscle straining, if detrusor is not functioning the flow will cease. Residual urine can be assessed by a post-micturition USG.
  - Urodynamic studies
- **The rectum:** Laxity of sphincters and incontinence, the gripping of a gloved finger by internal anal sphincter will be absent even in the chronic state.
- Absence of reflex contraction on stroking of the skin near external sphincter (chronic higher spinal lesions or pontine lesions allow tonic contraction of sphincters and cause constipation).
- **Sexual function:** Cremasteric, bulbocavernosus and scrotal reflexes must be assessed.

### Q. What is intrinsic heart rate, and what is the heart rate in a transplanted heart?

The normal intrinsic heart rate is age-dependent and can be calculated using the following equation—intrinsic heart rate (beats/min) = $118.1 - (0.57 \times age)$. Normal values are ±14% for age younger than 45 years and ±18% for age older than 45 years, and approximately 5 beats/min less for women at all ages.

Autonomic blockade for evaluation of SND, and it is used to determine the intrinsic heart rate. Autonomic blockade is accomplished by administering atropine, 0.04 mg/kg, and propranolol, 0.2 mg/kg (or atenolol, 0.22 mg/kg). The resulting intrinsic heart rate represents sinus node rate without autonomic influences.

Sympathetic activity (through b1 adrenoceptors) accelerates, and parasympathetic activity (through muscarinic M2 receptors) slows, the heart. If the sympathetic and the parasympathetic drives to the heart are simultaneously and adequately blocked by a β-adrenoceptor blocker plus atropine, the heart will beat at its `intrinsic' rate. The intrinsic rate at rest is usually about 100 beats/min, as opposed to the usual rate of 80 beats/min, i.e., normally there is parasympathetic vagal 'tone', which decreases with age.

### Q. What are the diseases affecting the nerve roots of UL and LL?

Disorders of the nerve root, termed radiculopathy, lead to symptoms referable to a dermatome or myotome. Either the ventral (anterior, motor) or posterior (dorsal, sensory) root can be involved independently or after they join to form the spinal nerve. Symptoms will follow the anatomic location. Because the root must traverse the vertebral foramen, it is prone to disorders of the spine at these locations.

Radicular pain is often worsened by activities that increase intraspinal pressure, such as coughing, sneezing, straining, and other Valsalva maneuvers. The characteristics of the pain vary, but when they are exacerbated by such provocation, they are often described as sharp, shooting, electrical, and tingling. When reporting the symptoms, patients may point to or rub the distal dermatome where they are experiencing the discomfort (perceived pain). Patients also may report specific positions that increase or decrease pain; e.g., sitting will often worsen the pain of acute lumbar disc herniation, and neck extension can produce radiating pain in cervical disc herniation or other processes that narrow the foramen, for example:

- Traumatic radiculopathies
  - Nerve root avulsion
  - Disk herniation
- Diabetic polyradiculoneuropathy
- Neoplastic polyradiculoneuropathy (neoplastic meningitis)
- Polyradiculopathy associated with sarcoidosis
- Infectious radiculopathy
  - Tabes dorsalis
  - Polyradiculopathy in HIV
  - Lyme radiculoneuropathy
  - Herpes zoster
- Acquired demyelinating polyradiculoneuropathy
  - GB syndrome
  - CIDP

### Q. Define paraneoplastic syndrome. Name the features.

Paraneoplastic neurological syndromes are a heterogenous group of disorders caused by cancers not located in the central nervous system, the pathophysiology of which is different from metastasis or other complications of cancer, such as metabolic or nutritional deficits, infections, coagulopathies, and side effects of cancer treatment.

In 65% of patient with PNS, the neurological symptoms precede the tumor diagnosis.

**Affecting CNS:**
- Cerebellar degeneration
- Encephalomyelitis
- Limbic and brainstem encephalitis
- Opsoclonus-myoclonus
- Stiff-person syndrome
- Necrotizing myelopathy
- Motor neuron syndromes (ALS; subacute motor neuronopathy; upper motor neuron dysfunction)

**Affecting visual system:**
- Retinopathy
- Optic neuritis
- Uveitis

**Affecting peripheral nervous system:**
- Sensory neuronopathy
- Vasculitis of nerve and muscle
- Subacute or chronic sensorimotor peripheral neuropathy

- Sensorimotor neuropathies associated with plasma cell dyscrasias and B-cell lymphoma
- Autonomic neuropathy
- Brachial neuritis
- Acute polyradiculoneuropathy (GB syndrome)
- Peripheral nerve hyperexcitability

**Affecting NMJ and muscle:**
- Lambert-Eaton myasthenic syndrome
- Myasthenia gravis
- Dermatomyositis
- Acute necrotizing myopathy.

### Q. What are the features and examples of axonal neuropathy?

Axonal degeneration (or axonopathy), the most common pathological reaction of peripheral nerve, signifies distal axonal breakdown and is presumably caused by metabolic derangement within neurons or vascular compromise leading to ischemia. Systemic metabolic disorders, toxin exposure, vasculitis, and some inherited neuropathies are the usual causes of axonal degeneration. The myelin sheath breaks down concomitantly with the axon in a process that starts at the most distal part of the nerve fiber and progresses toward the nerve cell body, hence the term dying-back or length-dependent polyneuropathy.

- Acute:
  - Porphyria
  - Axonal GBS
  - Tick paralysis
  - Toxins
  - Critical illness neuropathy
- Subacute:
  - Systemic diseases
  - Deficiency states
  - Toxins
  - Amyloid
  - Carcinoma
- Chronic:
  - Hereditary neuropathies
  - CMT II
  - Dysproteinemias

### Q. What is the relation between diabetes and CIDP?

Chronic inflammatory demyelinating polyneuropathy (CIDP) is a heterogeneous, progressive or relapsing–remitting, immune-mediated disorder of the peripheral nervous system that has an estimated prevalence of 1–8.9 per 1,00,000.

The prevalence of CIDP in a nondiabetic population is 6 per 1,00,000 persons, while the prevalence of CIDP in a patient population with DM is 9-fold higher at 54 per 1,00,000 persons. The association of CIDP with DM remains controversial, as both diseases have increased prevalence in patients over age 50 years. It is a challenge to identify CIDP in a diabetic population due to concomitant axonal damage.

A demyelinating neuropathy that meets the electrophysiologic criteria for chronic inflammatory demyelinating polyneuropathy (CIDP) has been increasingly recognized to occur more commonly in patients with both type 1 and type 2 diabetes. Because patients with CIDP might respond to immunomodulatory therapy, it is important to distinguish this condition from other diabetic neuropathies, particularly proximal motor neuropathy. Therefore, CIDP should be suspected in neuropathic diabetic patients in the following cases:

- A predominance of motor signs involves proximal or distal lower limb muscles.
- After some years of distal sensory neuropathy, a motor neuropathy develops with progressive symptoms and signs.
- A patient is diagnosed with proximal motor neuropathy (amyotrophy).

One study showed that diabetic patients with CIDP present with a higher frequency of autonomic dysfunction and electrophysiologic evidence of associated axonal loss, which may explain a poorer response to treatment with oral prednisolone 1 mg/kg/day with/without azathioprine 1 to 2 mg/kg over 6 months.

### Q. What are the variants of CIDP?

- Pure sensory
- Pure motor
- Lewis-Sumner variant, is also described by the acronym MADSAM (multifocal acquired demyelinating sensory and motor neuropathy)
- Distal acquired symmetrical demyelinating neuropathy, or DADS variant
- Chronic immune sensory polyradiculopathy (selective involvement of sensory nerve roots)
- Chronic inflammatory lumbosacral polyradiculopathy (a regional lower extremity variant of CIDP with weakness and sensory disturbances limited to the legs, with normal motor and sensory nerve conduction studies).

### Q. What is multiple mononeuropathy?

Multiple mononeuropathy is the new terminology for mononeuritis multiplex. Multifocal motor neuropathy (MMN), with a prevalence of 1 to 2 per 1,00,000, is a treatable but incurable immune-mediated motor neuropathy that bears a superficial clinical resemblance to motor neuron disease of the lower motor neuron type.

It is a progressive, **asymmetrical**, predominantly **distal** limb weakness in the distribution of two or more peripheral nerves, developing over months to years, with a **striking predilection for the upper** extremities and particularly hands, without upper motor signs.

### Q. Name the causes of multiple mononeuropathy.

- Vasculitis (systemic, nonsystemic)

- Diabetes mellitus
- Sarcoidosis
- Hansen disease (leprosy)
- Human immunodeficiency virus-infection demyelination
- Multifocal motor neuropathy
- Multifocal acquired demyelinating sensory and motor neuropathy
- Lewis-Sumner syndrome
- Multiple compression neuropathies (hypothyroidism, diabetes)
- Hereditary neuropathy with liability to pressure palsies

### Q. Can you get MND in paraneoplastic syndrome?

There is evidence that motor neuron disease may **rarely** be a paraneoplastic phenomenon, though the possibility that the ALS and the neoplasm are chance associations is still possible. Patients may present with features that are rather typical of pure "spinal" ALS or manifest in a manner akin either to PMA or to PLS.

### Q. Demonstrate the sites for palpation of peripheral nerves for thickening.

Refer **Figure 4.57**.

### Q. Does MND involve only the anterior horn cells in spinal cord?

**Structures involved in MND:** Amyotrophic lateral sclerosis is a neurodegenerative disorder of undetermined etiology that primarily affects the motor neuron cell populations in the motor cortex, brainstem, and spinal cord.

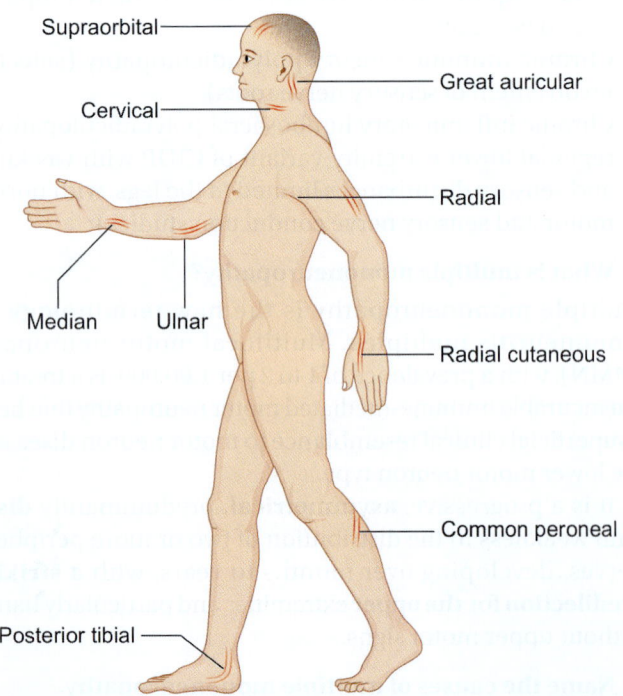

**Fig. 4.57:** Sites for palpation of peripheral nerves for thickening.

### Q. Why reflexes are preserved till late stage in MND?

Amyotrophic lateral sclerosis (ALS) characteristically involves both the upper and lower motor neurons. It produces a clinical picture of weakness and wasting due to involvement of the lower motor neurons in the anterior horn of the spinal cord, combined with weakness and hyperreflexia due to involvement of the upper motor neurons in the cerebral cortex that give rise to the corticospinal tract. There is **upper motor neuron weakness (cerebral cortex pathology) superimposed on lower motor neuron weakness (spinal cord pathology)**. ALS usually begins with focal weakness, often involving one hand or one foot.

A multi-nerve, multi-root distribution of weakness, normal or increased reflexes, and a lack of sensory loss are usually the earliest suggestions as to the nature of the problem. In ALS, the weakness early tends to be asymmetric and associated with hyperreflexia. An extremity that is both **atrophic and hyper-reflexic** is characteristic. As the condition progresses, the clinical picture evolves into one of generalized weakness.

### Q. What are the causes for painful neuropathy?
- Diabetes
- Alcohol
- Vitamin $B_1$ and $B_{12}$ deficiency
- Porphyria
- Radiculoplexopathies
- GBS
- Vasculitic neuropathy
- Toxic (arsenic, thallium, vincristine, cisplatin)
- Amyloid
- Paraneoplastic
- Sjogren's syndrome
- Uremic neuropathy
- Fabry's disease
- Hereditary sensory and autonomic neuropathy (HSAN)

### Q. What are the causes of neuropathy with cranial nerve involvement?
- GBS (7th)
- Leprosy (7th)
- Diabetes (3, 6, 7th)
- Diphtheria (3, 6, 9, 10th)
- Sarcoidosis (7th)

### Q. What are the cause for neuropathy with sensory symptoms?
- Diabetes
- Carcinoma
- Sjogren's syndrome
- AIDS
- Vitamin $B_{12}$ deficiency
- Cisplatin
- Thalidomide
- Pyridoxine intoxication

### Q. What is SMON?

Subacute myelo-optic neuropathy (**SMON**) is an iatrogenic disease of the nervous system leading to a disabling paralysis, blindness and even death. Its defining manifestation was as an epidemic in Japan during the 1960s, affecting an estimated 30,000 people. On August 3, 1978, the Tokyo District Court ruled that the cause of SMON is Clioquinol.

SMON was first observed and diagnosed in Sweden 1966, by the pediatrician and neurologist Olle Hansson.

Clioquinol was marketed as a prophylaxis to tourist diarrhea.

### Q. How do you treat vitamin $B_{12}$ deficiency?

Injection (i.e., intramuscular or deep subcutaneous) vitamin $B_{12}$, in a dose of 1000 μg (1 mg) every day for one week, followed by 1 mg every week for four weeks and then, if the underlying disorder persists (e.g., PA, surgical removal of the terminal ileum), 1 mg every month for the remainder of the patient's life. If the cause of the cobalamin (Cbl) deficiency can be eliminated (e.g., diet, drugs, reversible malabsorption syndrome) treatment can be stopped when the $B_{12}$ deficiency has been fully reversed and the cause eliminated.

### Q. In which condition vitamin $B_{12}$ is contraindicated?

- Leber's hereditary optic neuropathy
- Toxic amblyopia

### Q. What are the causes for extensor plantar with absent ankle reflex?

- Subacute combined degeneration of the spinal cord
- Motor neuron disease
- Syphilitic taboparesis
- Friedreich's ataxia
- Conus medullaris or cauda equina lesion
- Multiple sclerosis

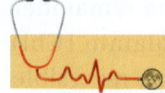

## Case 4: Guillain-Barré Syndrome

**Brief History**
A 42-year-old male business man by occupation cause with:

**Chief Complaints**
- Pain and burning sensation of bilateral hands and feet × 1 week.
- Difficulty in walking × 5 days
- Difficulty in closing eyes × 5 day
- Difficulty in speaking

**History of Presenting Illness**
In apparently normal patient present complaint started as and pain and burning sensation in bilateral hand effect region. Later patient had developed difficulty in setting up from squatting position. Walking with support and patient also has bilateral difficulty in closing eyes and history of difficulty in speaking also present. No history of fever and/no history of bowel bladder involvement

**Past History**
- Hypertension × 2 years treatment details not known.
- No history of diabetes mellitus, PTB, seizures

**Personal History**
- Mixed diet
- Sleep—normal
- Bowel and bladder—normal
- Not alcoholic and smoker

**Family History**
No significant

**General Physical Examination**
- Height 165 cm, weight 70 kg
- BML $70/(1.65)^2 = 25.6$ kg/m²
- No pallor, no icterus, no cyanosis, no clubbing, no lymphadenopathy, no edema
- BP: 160/90 mm of Hg, right arm supine position, no postural drop
- PR: 78/min regular normovolemic, no radioradial and radiofemoral delay

Respiratory rate: 20/min abdominothoracic
Temperature: 98.6°F

**Central Nervous System Examination**
Higher mental function:
- Conscious oriented to time, place, person
- Right-handed person studied up to 7th class
- Intelligence—normal
- Memory—normal

**Language**
- Labial dysarthria present
- Reading and writing naming
- Comprehension, repetition, fluency—normal.

**Cranial Nerves**
7th nerve
- Bilateral LMN facial palsy (+)
- Taste anterior 2/3 of tongue (–)
- All other cranial nerves normal.

**Motor System**
Bulk of muscles

| Bulk | Right | Left |
|---|---|---|
| Arm | 30 cm | 29.5 cm |
| Forearm | 24 cm | 23.5 cm |
| Thigh | 48 cm | 47.5 cm |
| Leg | 28 cm | 27.5 cm |

Tone: Hypotonia of all 4 limbs

**Power of Muscle**

| | | Action | Right | Left |
|---|---|---|---|---|
| Upper limb | Shoulder | Abduction | 4/5 | 4/5 |
| | | Adduction | 4/5 | 4/5 |
| | | Flexion | 4/5 | 4/5 |
| | | Extension | 4/5 | 4/5 |
| | Elbow | Flexion | 4/5 | 4/5 |
| | | Extension | 4/5 | 4/5 |
| | Wrist | Flexion | 5/5 | 4/5 |
| | | Extension | 4/5 | 4/5 |
| | Hand | | Weak | Weak |
| | Lumbricals | | Weak | Weak |
| | Interossei | | Weak | Weak |
| Hip | Flexion | 4/5 | 4/5 | |
| | Extension | 4/5 | 4/5 | |
| | Abduction | 4/5 | 4/5 | |
| | Adduction | 4/5 | 4/5 | |
| Knee | Flexion | 4/5 | 4/5 | |
| | Extension | 4/5 | 4/5 | |
| Ankle | Plantar flexion | 4/5 | 4/5 | |
| | Dorsi flexion | 4/5 | 4/5 | |
| | Eversion | | | |
| | Inversion | | | |

**Reflexes**
- All deep tendon reflexes—absent (even after reinforcement)
- Bilateral plantar—no response

Sensory system: Normal

**Cerebellar Signs**
- Could not be assessed due to weakness.
- Skull and spine: Normal
- Other system: Normal

**Diagnosis**
Acute quadriparesis with generalized areflexia and bilateral LMN facial palsy possibly acute polyneuropathy, Guillain-Barre syndrome.

## DISCUSSION

**Q. What are the probable diagnosis of peripheral neuropathy with cranial nerve palsy?**

- **Botulism:**
  - Onset of paralysis between 1 to 2 days
  - Acute descending symmetric and flaccid paralysis
  - Reflexes normal (or) decreased.
  - Pupils dilated (mydriasis), diplopia, COD of accommodation.
- **Diphtheria:**
  - Onset of paralysis between 1 to 8 weeks
  - Acute descending symmetric quadriplegia
  - Areflexia
  - Ophthalmoplegia, blurred vision, palatal paralysis.
- **Porphyria:**
  - Asymmetric motor weakness associated with abdomen pain
  - Onset precipitated by drugs like barbiturates, sulfonamides, alcohol.
  - Proximal muscle weakness with sensory symptoms but no sensory loss.
  - They may be bulbar and resp paralysis (predominantly motor neuropathy).

**Q. What is Bell's phenomenon?**

- Occurs in the case of a unilateral lower motor neuron palsy.
- It is the visible vertical rotation of globe on closing the affected eye.
- It is seen when the patient attempts to shut the eye on the affected side which causes upward movement of the eyeball and incomplete closure of the eyelid.
- This provides a test of infranuclear competence.
- Only a positive response is helpful.
- Some normal subjects do not show a Bell's phenomenon.
- In unconscious patients, a strong corneal stimulus may induce a Bell's phenomenon. If it does, it indicates midbrain-low pons intactness, i.e., cranial nerves III-VII. With structural brainstem lesions above the pons, Bell's phenomenon disappears but the jaw may deviate to the opposite side in the corneal pterygoid reflex.
- Bilateral Bell's phenomenon is found in the following conditions:
  - Myasthenia gravis
  - Sarcoidosis
  - Bilateral Bell's palsies
  - Congenital facial diplegia
  - Muscular dystrophy
  - Motor neuron disease
  - Guillain-Barré syndrome

**Q. Difference between bilateral UMN and LMN facial nerve palsy.**

Refer **Table 4.75**

**Table 4.75:** Difference between bilateral UMN and LMN facial nerve palsy.

| Bilateral UMN facial palsy | Bilateral LMN facial palsy |
| --- | --- |
| • Bell phenomenon is absent | • Bell phenomenon is present |
| • Emotional fibers—intact | • Emotional fibers—absent |
| • Jaw jerk—exaggerated | • Jaw jerk—absent |
| • Bilateral deep tendon reflex exaggerated and bilateral plantar extensor and other long tract signs—present | • Bilateral deep tendon reflex exaggerated and bilateral plantar extensor and other long tract signs—absent |

**Q. Who discovered GBS?**

Guillain-Barre syndrome (GBS) is a group of autoimmune conditions consisting of demyelinating and acute axonal degenerating forms of disease. GBS is sometimes known as Landry's ascending paralysis, French polio, acute idiopathic polyneuritis, or acute idiopathic polyradiculoneuritis. The disease is named for **Georges Guillain and Jean Alexandre Barre**, who discovered the characteristic feature of the disease—increased level of protein in cerebrospinal fluid with normal cell count—in 1916. Interestingly, however, the French physician **Jean Landry** had described the condition in 1859, a half-century earlier.

**Q. Discuss immunopathogenesis of GBS.**

- Acute respiratory infection or gastroenteritis preceding the onset of weakness is frequently an important part of the medical history.
- Six pathogens have been temporally associated with GBS in case-control studies: *Campylobacter jejuni*, cytomegalovirus, hepatitis E virus, *Mycoplasma pneumoniae*, Epstein-Barr virus and Zika virus
- Recent infection with *Campylobacter jejuni*, cytomegalovirus (CMV), Epstein-Barr virus and *Mycoplasma pneumoniae* have been serologically implicated in 32%, 13%, 10%, and 5% of patients with GBS, respectively
- *C. jejuni* infection is thought to induce an antiganglioside antibody.
- Molecular mimicry, involving similar sequences of bacterial lipo-oligosaccharides and human gangliosides, are believed to underlie autoimmune attack on axonal membranes in AMAN.
- Several gangliosides (GM1, GM1b, GD1a, and GalNAc-GD1a) on the motor axolemma were found to be likely epitopes for antibodies in AMAN.
- Preceding *M. pneumoniae* infection was linked with high titers of anti-galactosyl-ceramide antibody (anti-GalCer), and elevated anti-CMV antibody correlated with high levels of anti-GM2.
- Antibodies against GQ1b are found in patients with MFS, and this test is 85–90% sensitive
- HIV-GBS associated with HIV infection have been seen, mainly during the seroconversion period (acute retroviral syndrome or early infection). However, as the combined antiretroviral therapy (cART) are emerged, rare and

challenging cases of immune reconstitution inflammatory syndrome (IRIS)-related GBS are being reported.
- Other causes: Hodgkin's disease, SLE, paraproteinemia, sarcoidosis and may possibly occur after surgery, trauma or in postpartum period.
- Vaccines especially flu vaccine has been related to GBS.
- A relationship between administration of immuno-biologicals (e.g., tumor necrosis factor antagonists, immune checkpoint inhibitors or type I interferons) and GBS has been reported on the basis of case series information and biological plausibility.

**Q. What is the diagnostic criteria for Guillain–Barré syndrome?**

**Diagnostic criteria for Guillain–Barré syndrome** by the National Institute of Neurological Disorders and Stroke (NINDS) **is shown in Box 4.7.**

### Features required for diagnosis
- Progressive bilateral weakness of arms and legs (initially only legs may be involved)
- Absent or decreased tendon reflexes in affected limbs (at some point in clinical course)

**Box 4.7:** GB syndrome diagnostic criteria.

- Features required for diagnosis:
  - Progressive motor weakness of more than one limb
  - Areflexia or marked hyporeflexia
- Features strongly supportive of the diagnosis:
  - Progression over days to <4 weeks
  - Relative symmetry
  - Pain, often significant, at onset
  - Mild sensory symptoms or signs
  - Cranial nerve involvement
  - Autonomic dysfunction
  - Absence of fever at onset of symptoms
  - Onset of recovery 2–4 weeks after onset of plateau phase
- Laboratory features:
  - Elevated cerebrospinal fluid protein level after one week of symptoms
  - <10 leukocytes in cerebrospinal fluid
  - Slowed conduction or conduction block on electromyography

Modified with permission from Asbury, AK, Cornblath, Dr. Assessment of current diagnostic criteria for Guillian-Barre syndrom. Ann Neurol. 1990;7(suppl 1):S22.

### Features that strongly support diagnosis
- Progressive phase lasts from days to 4 weeks (usually <2 weeks)
- Relative symmetry of symptoms and signs
- Relatively mild sensory symptoms and signs (absent in pure motor variant)
- Cranial nerve involvement, especially bilateral facial palsy
- Autonomic dysfunction
- Muscular or radicular back or limb pain
- Increased protein level in cerebrospinal fluid (CSF); normal protein levels do not rule out the diagnosis
- Electrodiagnostic features of motor or sensorimotor neuropathy (normal electrophysiology in the early stages does not rule out the diagnosis).

### Features that cast doubt on diagnosis
- Increased numbers of mononuclear or polymorphonuclear cells in CSF ($>50 \times 10^6$/L)
- Marked, persistent asymmetry of weakness
- Bladder or bowel dysfunction at onset or persistent during disease course
- Severe respiratory dysfunction with limited limb weakness at onset
- Sensory signs with limited weakness at onset
- Fever at onset
- Nadir <24 hours
- Sharp sensory level indicating spinal cord injury
- Hyperreflexia or clonus
- Extensor plantar responses
- Abdominal pain
- Slow progression with limited weakness without respiratory involvement
- Continued progression for >4 weeks after start of symptoms
- Alteration of consciousness (except in Bickerstaff brainstem encephalitis)

**Q. What is the differential diagnosis of Guillain–Barré syndrome?**

Refer **Box 4.8**.

**Box 4.8:** Differential diagnosis of Guillain–Barré syndrome.

**Central nervous system**
- Inflammation or infection of the brainstem (for example, sarcoidosis, Sjögren syndrome, neuromyelitis optica or myelin oligodendrocyte glycoprotein antibody-associated disorder)
- Inflammation or infection of the spinal cord (for example, sarcoidosis, Sjögren syndrome or acute transverse myelitis)
- Malignancy (for example, leptomeningeal metastases or neurolymphomatosis)
- Compression of brainstem or spinal cord
- Brainstem stroke
- Vitamin deficiency (for example, Wernicke encephalopathy, caused by deficiency of vitamin $B_1$, or subacute combined degeneration of the spinal cord, caused by deficiency of vitamin $B_{12}$)

**Anterior horn cells**
Acute flaccid myelitis (for example, as a result of polio, enterovirus D68 or A71, West Nile virus, Japanese encephalitis virus or rabies virus)

**Nerve roots**
- Infection (for example, Lyme disease, cytomegalovirus, HIV, Epstein–Barr virus or varicella zoster virus)
- Compression
- Leptomeningeal malignancy

**Peripheral nerves**
- Chronic inflammatory demyelinating polyradiculoneuropathy (CIDP)
- Metabolic or electrolyte disorders (for example, hypoglycemia hypothyroidism, porphyria or copper deficiency)
- Vitamin deficiency (for example, deficiency of vitamins $B_1$ (also known as beriberi), $B_{12}$ or E)
- Toxins (for example, drugs, alcohol, vitamin $B_6$, lead, thallium, arsenic, organophosphate, ethylene glycol, diethylene glycol, methanol or N-hexane)
- Critical illness polyneuropathy
- Neuralgic amyotrophy
- Vasculitis
- Infection (for example, diphtheria or HIV)

**Neuromuscular junction**
- Myasthenia gravis
- Lambert–Eaton myasthenic syndrome
- Neurotoxins (for example, botulism, tetanus, tick paralysis or snakebite envenomation)
- Organophosphate intoxication

**Muscles**
- Metabolic or electrolyte disorders (for example, hypokalemia, thyrotoxic hypokalemic periodic paralysis, hypomagnesemia or hypophosphatemia)
- Inflammatory myositis
- Acute rhabdomyolysis
- Drug-induced toxic myopathy (for example, induced by colchicine, chloroquine, emetine or statins)
- Mitochondrial disease

**Other**
- Conversion or functional disorder

**Q. What are the causes of ascending and descending paralysis?**

Refer **Table 4.76**.

**Table 4.76:** Ascending and descending paralysis.

| Ascending | Descending |
|---|---|
| GB syndrome | Botulism |
| Ticll paralysis | Diphtheria |

Graphic representation of the pattern of symptoms typically observed in the different clinical variants of Guillain–Barré syndrome (GBS). Symptoms can be purely motor, purely sensory (rare) or a combination of motor and sensory. Ataxia can be present in patients with Miller-Fisher syndrome and both decreased consciousness and ataxia can be present in patients with Bickerstaff brainstem encephalitis. Symptoms can be localized to specific regions of the body, and the pattern of symptoms differs between variants of GBS. Although bilateral facial palsy with paresthesias, the pure sensory variant and Miller-Fisher syndrome are included in the GBS spectrum, they do not fulfil the diagnostic criteria for GBS.

**Q. What are the variants of GB syndrome?**

Refer **Table 4.77 and Figure 4.58**.

**Table 4.77:** Variants of GB syndrome.

| Common variants | Less common variants |
|---|---|
| • Acute motor and sensory axonal neuropathy (AMSAN)<br>• Acute motor axonal neuropathy (AMAN)<br>• Miller-Fisher variant<br>• Pure motor variants<br>• Pure sensory variants<br>• Pure dysautonomia variant<br>• Pharyngeal-cervical-brachial variant<br>• Paraparetic variant (Ropper variant) | • Acral paresthesias with diminished reflexes in either arms or legs<br>• Facial diplegia or abducens palsies with distal paresthesias<br>• Isolated postinfectious ophthalmoplegia<br>• Bilateral foot drop with upper limb paresthesias<br>• Acute ataxia without ophthalmoplegia<br>• Bickerstaff's brainstem encephalitis (BBE) |

**Q. What are features of variants of GB syndrome?**

Refer **Table 4.78**.

**Q. What are the causes for neuropathy with facial nerve involvement?**

- GBS

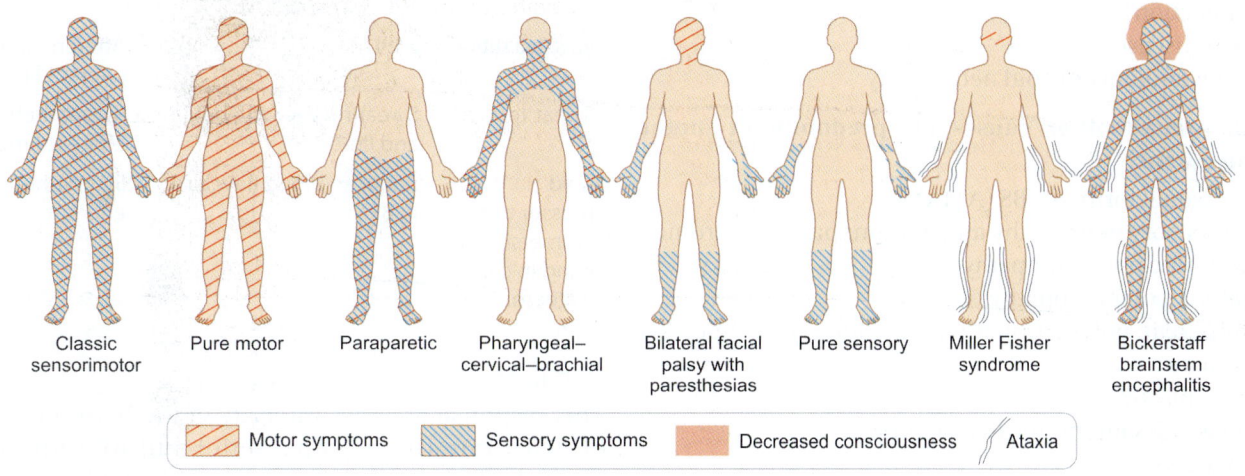

**Fig. 4.58:** Variants of Guillain-Barré syndrome.

## SECTION 4: Nervous System

**Table 4.78:** Variants of GBS.

| Variant | Frequency (% of GBS cases) | Clinical features |
|---|---|---|
| Classic sensorimotor GBS | 30–85 | Rapidly progressive symmetrical weakness and sensory signs with absent or reduced tendon reflexes, usually reaching nadir within 2 weeks |
| Pure motor | 5–70 | Motor weakness without sensory signs |
| Paraparetic | 5–10 | Paresis restricted to the legs |
| Pharyngeal–cervical–brachial | <5 | Weakness of pharyngeal, cervical, and brachial muscles without lower limb weakness |
| Bilateral facial palsy with paresthesias | <5 | Bilateral facial weakness, paresthesia and reduced reflexes |
| Pure sensory | <1 | Acute or subacute sensory neuropathy without other deficits |
| Miller Fisher syndrome | 5–25 | Ophthalmoplegia, ataxia and areflexia. Incomplete forms with isolated ataxia (acute ataxic neuropathy) or ophthalmoplegia (acute ophthalmoplegia) can occur. Overlaps with classical sensorimotor GBS in an estimated 15% of patients |
| Bickerstaff brainstem encephalitis | <5 | Ophthalmoplegia, ataxia, areflexia, pyramidal tract signs and impaired consciousness, often overlapping with sensorimotor GBS |

- Critical inflammatory poly radiculomyelopathy
- Lyme's disease
- Sarcoidosis
- HIV-infection
- Tangier disease
- Gelsolin familial amyloid neuropathy

### Q. What are all other causes for predominant motor involvement?

- Acute axonal form of GBS (AMAN)
- Acute sensory neuropathy and neuronopathy syndrome
- Diphtheritic polyneuropathy
- Porphyric polyneuropathy
- Certain toxic polyneuropathies (thallium, triorthocresyl phosphate)
- Paraneoplastic
- Acute pandysautonomic neuropathy
- Tick paralysis
- Critical illness polyneuropathy

### Q. Explain the bladder involvement in GBS.

The external urethral sphincter is involved in approximately 10–20% of cases. Retention is far more common than incontinence. Urologic studies have shown denervation of external urethral sphincter (striated muscle). Incontinence when it occurs is ascribable to overflow incontinence, since internal sphincter (smooth muscle) is not affected in AIDP and is capable of maintaining continence.

### Q. How does postural hypotension in GBS differ from postural hypotension due to other causes?

Postural hypotension in AIDP depends on loss of sympathetically mediated vascular reflexes with lowering of systemic vascular resistance. For this reason, patients with AIDP fail to demonstrate the normally encountered increase in pulse rate and diaphoresis that follow an abrupt decrease in blood pressure.

In nonneurogenic cause of orthostatic hypotension (e.g., hypovolemia), the bp drop is accompanied by a compensatory increase in heart rate of >15 beats per minute.

### Q. What are the other tests for autonomic dysfunction?

Refer **Table 4.79**.

**Table 4.79:** Tests for autonomic dysfunction.

| Test | Normal response | Main part of reflex arc tested |
|---|---|---|
| Blood pressure response to standing or vertical tilt | Fall in BP <20/10 mm Hg | Afferent and sympathetic efferent limbs |
| Heart rate response to standing | Increase 11–90 beats/min; R-R interval ratio of the HR around beat, 30:15 ratio >1.04 | Vagal afferent and efferent limbs |
| Isometric exercise | Increase in diastolic BP, 15 mm Hg | Sympathetic efferent limb |
| Heart rate variation with respiration | Maximum-minimum HR >15 beats/min; E:I ratio 1.2 | Vagal afferent and efferent limbs |
| Valsalva ratio | >1.4 | Afferent and efferent limbs |
| Sweat tests | Sweating over all body and limbs | Sympathetic efferent limb |
| Cold pressor test (immersion of hand in cold water for 3–5 min) | Reduced blood flow, rise in BP (>15 mm Hg) | Sympathetic efferent limb |

### Q. What is Valsalva response?

This response assesses integrity of the baroreflex control of heart rate (parasympathetic) and BP (adrenergic). The Valsalva response is tested in the supine position. The

**Table 4.80:** Changes during Valsalva maneuver.

| Phase | Maneuver | Blood pressure | Heart rate | Comments |
|---|---|---|---|---|
| I | Forced expiration against a partially closed glottis | Rises; aortic compression from raised intrathoracic pressure | Decreases | Mechanical |
| II early | Continued expiration | Falls; decreased venous return to the heart | Increases (reflex tachycardia) | Reduced vagal tone |
| II late | Continued expiration | Rises; reflex increase in peripheral vascular resistance | Increases at slower rate | Requires intact efferent sympathetic response |
| III | End of expiration | Falls; increased capacitance of pulmonary bed | Increases further | Mechanical |
| IV | Recovery | Rises; persistent vasoconstriction and increased cardiac output | Compensatory bradycardia | Requires intact efferent sympathetic response |

subject exhales against a closed glottis (or into a manometer maintaining a constant expiratory pressure of 40 mm Hg) for 15 s while measuring changes in heart rate and beat-to-beat BP. There are four phases of BP and heart rate response to the Valsalva maneuver **(Table 4.80)**.

### Q. What is albuminocytological dissociation?

The CSF protein content is elevated in most patients with GBS but may be normal in the first few days after onset. The CSF cell count is usually normal.

**Spinal fluid analysis:** Elevated protein without leukocytosis (usually <10 cells/mm$^3$) in ~90% at time of maximal weakness.

**Cellular CSF in GBS:** Cell count >50 cells/mm$^3$ indicates alternate diagnosis unless in setting of HIV, sarcoidosis

### Q. What are the indications of plasmapheresis?
Refer **Table 4.81**.

### Q. Discuss cranial nerve involvement in GB syndrome.

- About 50% of GBS patients have some degree of cranial nerve dysfunction during their illness.
- Facial weakness most common, especially if substantial limb weakness present.
  - Normal facial strength in the presence of marked quadriparesis very unusual in typical GBS.

**Table 4.81:** Indications of plasmapheresis.

| Substances removed by plasmapheresis | Disease |
|---|---|
| • Substances removed by plasmapheresis<br>• Autoantibodies | • Antiglomerular basement membrane disease<br>• Rapidly progressive glomerulonephritis |
| • Immune complexes<br>• Myeloma protein<br>• Cryoglobulin<br>• Complement products<br>• ADAMTS-13 (metalloproteinase)<br>• Lipoproteins<br>• Protein-bound toxins | • Hemolytic uremic syndrome<br>• TTP<br>• Renal transplant rejection<br>• Desensitization for renal transplantation<br>• Recurrent FSGS<br>• Cryoglobulinemia<br>• Systemic lupus erythematosus<br>• Guillain-Barré syndrome<br>• Myasthenic crisis |

- Facial weakness usually bilateral but may be unequal in severity; only rarely truly unilateral.
- Ophthalmoparesis see in 10–20% of patients. Abducens palsy most common; usually bilateral.
- Oropharyngeal weakness present in almost 1/4 of cases increasing the risk of aspiration.
- Rarely, patients with GBS may appear locked-in, due to paralysis of all cranial muscles, ventilatory failure, and flaccid paralysis.

### Q. What are the causes of neck muscle weakness (broken neck sign)?

- Myasthenia gravis
- Snake bite
- Gullian-Barre syndrome
- Motor neuron disease
- Myopathies
- OP poisoning—intermediate syndrome.

### Q. What you do look for in fundus in a patient with suspected GB syndrome?
Papilledema.

**Rationale:**
The elevated CSF proteins were postulated to cause a defect in the proper absorption of CSF at the arachnoid villi, giving rise to raised intracranial pressure. Edema of the spinal nerve rootlets seen in GBS has been implicated in causing decreased absorption of proteins and contribute to the raised CSF protein. Pseudotumor cerebri has also been reported with acute inflammatory demyelinating polyradiculoneuropathy.

**Association with fundus and paraplegia**
- **GB:** Papilledema
- **Transverse myelitis:** Optic neuritis
- **TB spine:** Choroid tubercles
- **Anterior spinal artery thrombosis:** Papilledema

### Q. What is the cause of pain in GB syndrome?

- Pain, especially with movement, is reported by 50–89% of patients with GBS.
- The pain is described as severe, deep, aching, or cramping (similar to sciatica) in the affected muscles or back, and is often worse at night.
- Because the pain is nociceptive and/or neuropathic, it may be difficult to control.
- Cause of the pain is possibly neuromyositis.

### Q. Discuss the investigations needed to confirm GBS.

CSF study reveals albumin cytological dissociation which sets in within a week (other causes for the same are HIV, neoplasia, spinal cord compression).

**NCV and EMG shows the following (Box 4.9 and Figs. 4.59 and 4.60):**

**Box 4.9:** NCV findings in GBS.

---
About 80% of patients have evidence of NCV slowing/conduction block at some time during disease process.
- Patchy reduction in NCV attaining values <60% of normal.
- Distal motor latency increase
- F-waves, H-wave: Absent H reflex, pronged F wave latency, absent F waves are typical
---

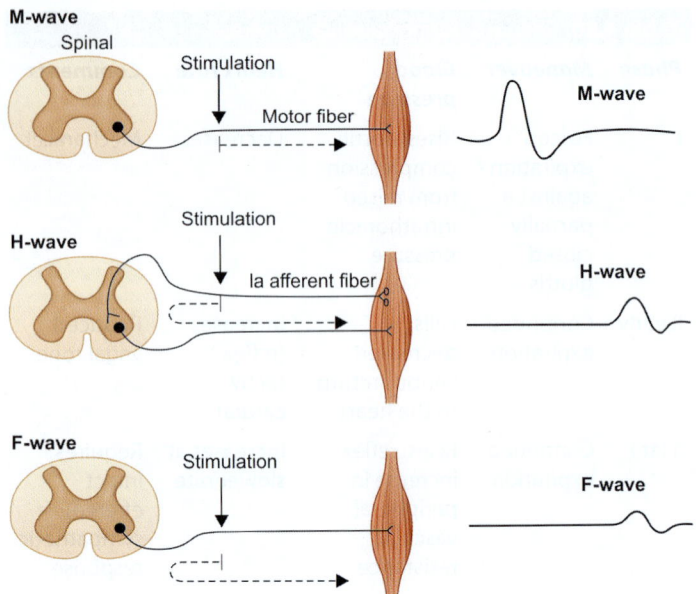

**Fig. 4.60:** Response to different waves.

- **Axonal neuropathy**: Low-amplitude potentials with relatively preserved distal latencies, conduction velocities and late potentials along with fibrillations on needle EMG, suggest an axonal neuropathy.
- **Primary demyelinating neuropathy**: On the other hand, slow conduction velocities, prolonged distal latencies and late potentials relative preserved amplitudes, and the absence of fibrillation on needle EMG imply a primary demyelinating neuropathy.

### Q. What is H-reflex?

- The H-reflex, named after Hoffmann for his original description, is an electrical counterpart of the stretch reflex which is elicited by a mechanical tap. Group 1A sensory fibers constitute the afferent arc which monosynaptically or oligosynaptically activate the alpha motor neurons that in turn generate the efferent arc of the reflex through their motor axons.
- It is elicited by selectively stimulating the Ia fibers of the posterior tibial or median nerve. Such stimulation can be accomplished by using slow (less than 1 pulse/second), long-duration (0.5–1 ms) stimuli with gradually increasing stimulation strength.
- The stimulus travels along the Ia fibers, through the dorsal root ganglion, and is transmitted across the central synapse to the anterior horn cell which fires it down along the alpha motor axon to the muscle. The result is a motor response, usually between 0.5 and 5 mV in amplitude, occurring at low stimulation strength, either before any direct motor response (M) is seen or with a small M preceding it.

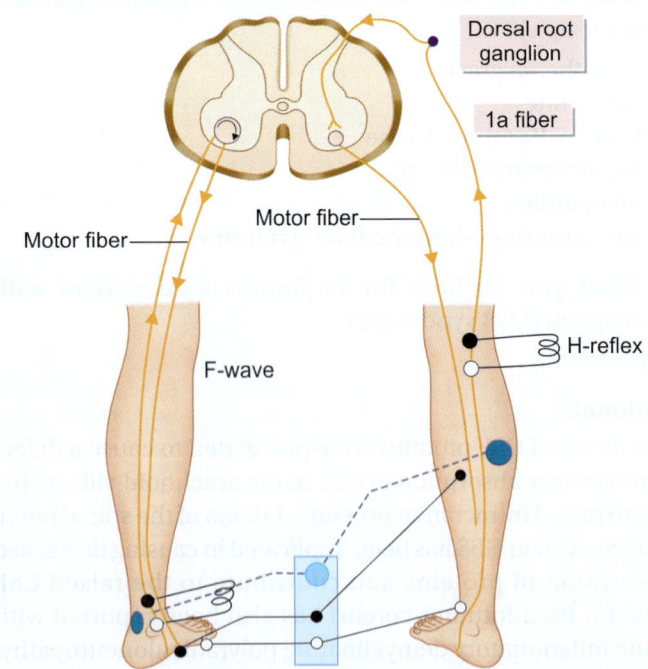

**Fig. 4.59:** Late responses include F waves, A waves, H reflex. F waves can help determine the presence of a polyneuropathy. A waves can reflect axonal damage. H reflexes provide nerve conduction measurements along the entire length of the nerve, demonstrating abnormalities in neuropathies and radiculopathies.

- The H-reflex can normally be seen in many muscles but is easily obtained in the soleus muscle (with posterior tibial nerve stimulation at the popliteal fossa), the flexor carpi radialis muscle (with median nerve stimulation at the elbow), and the quadriceps (with femoral nerve stimulation).
- Typically, it is first seen at low stimulation strength without any motor response preceding it. As the stimulation strength is increased, the direct motor response appears. With further increases in stimulation strengths, the M response becomes larger and the H-reflex decreases in amplitude. When the motor response becomes maximal, the H-reflex disappears and is replaced by a small late motor response, the F-wave.
- The H-reflex is useful in the diagnosis of S1 and C7 root lesions as well as the study of proximal nerve segments in either peripheral or proximal neuropathies.
- Clinical conditions with a depressed ankle reflex, such as polyneuropathy, sciatic neuropathy, or S1 radiculopathy, will show a diminished or absent H-reflex. Diabetic polyneuropathy is known to increase the H-reflex latency.

### Q. What is F-wave?

- The F-wave is a long latency muscle action potential seen after supramaximal stimulation to a nerve. Although elicitable in a variety of muscles, it is best obtained in the small foot and hand muscles. It is generally accepted that the F-wave is elicited when the stimulus travels antidromically along the motor fibers and reaches the anterior horn cell at a critical time to depolarize it. The response is then fired down along the axon and causes a minimal contraction of the muscle. Unlike the H-reflex, the F-wave is always preceded by a motor response and its amplitude is rather small, usually in the range of 0.2–0.5 mV.
- The F-wave is a variable response and is obtained infrequently after nerve stimulation. Commonly, several supramaximal stimuli are needed before an F-response is seen since only few stimuli reach the anterior horn cell at the appropriate time to depolarize it. With supramaximal stimulation; however, depolarization of the entire nerve helps spread the stimulus to the pool of anterior horn cells thus enhancing its chances to reach a greater number of anterior horn cells at the critical time and produce an F-wave **(Table 4.82)**.

### Q. What is the treatment of GB syndrome?

- Immunomodulatory therapy should be started if patients are unable to walk independently for 10 m
- Early treatment, each day counts,
- >2 weeks of 1st motor symptoms immunotherapy not effective

**Table 4.82:** F-wave versus H-response.

|  | F-wave | H-response |
|---|---|---|
| Response | Not a reflex, antidromic motor discharge | Monosynaptic |
| Pathway | Alpha motor neurons | IA sensory, alpha motor |
| Stimulus | Supramaximal (absent with submaximal stimulus) | Subthreshold (absent with supramaximal stimulus) |
| Persistence | Variable | Constant with low rates of stimulation |
| Latency | Variable | Constant |
| Amplitude | Usually small, 5% of M maximum | 50–100% of maximum M-wave, much larger than F-wave |
| Able to test | Almost every distal muscle | Gastrocsoleus |

- IVIg (0.4 g/kg body weight daily for 5 days OR 2 g per kg over two days, both doses are equally effective) and plasma exchange (200–250 mL plasma/kg body weight in five sessions) are equally effective treatments for GBS
- Glucocorticoid no role
- Mild cases reaching plateau-conservative treatment
- Worsening case-monitoring in ICU-VC, BP, cardiac, nutrition
- DVT prophylaxis, tracheostomy, chest physiotherapy, skin care, bed sore, joint physiotherapy daily reassurance.

### Q. What are the indications for ICU admission in GBS?

- Evolving respiratory distress with imminent respiratory insufficiency.
- Severe autonomic cardiovascular dysfunction (for example, arrhythmias or marked variation in blood pressure).
- Severe swallowing dysfunction or diminished cough reflex.
- Rapid progression of weakness
- A state of imminent respiratory insufficiency is defined as clinical signs of respiratory distress:
  - Including breathlessness at rest or during talking,
  - Inability to count to 15 in a single breath,
  - Use of accessory respiratory muscles,
  - Increased respiratory or heart rate,
  - Vital capacity <15–20 mL/kg or <1 L, or
  - Abnormal arterial blood gas or pulse oximetry measurements.

### Q. List the predictive factors of GBS.

Refer **Table 4.83**.

### Q. What is the prognosis of GBS?

- Even with treatment, about 3% of patients with GBS die.

- The median hospital stay is 7 days, and up to 25% of patients require intubation and mechanical ventilation.
- 85%—full functional recovery in months/years with minor residue.
- Worsening factors:
  - Severe proximal motor and sensory axonal
  - Advanced age
  - Rapid onset
- Relapse—5–10% classified as CIDP

**Table 4.83:** Predictive factors in GB syndrome.

**Predicts the need for mechanical ventilation**
- Bulbar symptoms
- Inability to raise the head or flex the arms
- Inadequate cough
- Maximum expiratory pressure: <40 cm $H_2O$
- Maximum inspiratory pressure: <30 cm $H_2O$
- Time from onset of symptoms to hospital admission is <7 days
- **Vital capacity:** <60% of predicated or <20 mL per kg
- Vital capacity, maximum inspiratory pressure, or maximum expiratory pressure reduced by at least 30%

**Predicts long-term disability**
- Absence of motor response
- Antecedent diarrheal illness
- Axonal involvement
- *Campylobacter jejuni* or cytomegalovirus infection
- Inability to walk at 14 days
- Older age
- Rapid progression of symptoms
- Severity of symptoms at their peak

## Case 5: Ataxia

*Brief History*
A 45-year-old male
- History of unsteadiness during walking since 5 days
- One episode of loss of consciousness 1 day back
- History of unsteadiness while walking associated with falls (3 episodes) due to instability, not associated with giddiness, vomiting, fever, weakness of the limbs, diminished vision/diplopia.
- No history of cranial nerve/sensory/bowel- bladder involvement/speech deficit/focal neurological deficit/memory deficit.
- History of one episode of loss of consciousness, 30 min, no history of aura, tonic-clonic movements, incontinence, postictal deficit/ confusion, spontaneous arousal.
- History of chronic alcohol consumption—30 years. History of GTCS 20 days back started on phenytoin. History of seizure disorder in the childhood—was on antiepileptics for few years.

*Examination*
Conscious/oriented/normal speech and memory.

*Cranial Nerves*
Nystagmus—bilateral, horizontal. No ophthalmoplegia, pupils normal, other cranial nerves normal.

*Motor System*
Normal tone, normal power in all four limbs, bilateral brisk reflexes with diminished ankle reflex. Bilateral plantar flexor.

*Sensory System*
Diminished pain, temperature, vibration in both lower limbs up to groin L > R, absent proprioception left lower limb.

*Cerebellar System*
Nystagmus +, dysdiadochokinesia, finger nose test (positive L > R), unable to perform knee heel test bilaterally, postural tremor +, ataxic gait, sways to both sides, truncal ataxia +, no rebound/pendular knee jerk. Increased swaying with eyes closed (Rhomberg test positive).

Other systems: Normal.

*Differential Diagnosis*
- Subacute combined degeneration of the spinal cord.
- Acute cerebellar ataxia—alcoholic cerebellar degeneration/ phenytoin toxicity and peripheral neuropathy.

## DISCUSSION

### Q. What are the causes of ataxia?

- **Congenital:** "Ataxic" cerebral palsy, other early insults
- **Vascular:** Ischemic stroke, hemorrhagic stroke, AV malformations
- **Infectious/transmittable:** Acute cerebellitis, post-infectious encephalomyelitis, cerebellar abscess, Whipple's disease, HIV, CJD
- **Toxic:** Alcohol, anticonvulsants, mercury, 5FU, cytosine arabinoside, lithium
- **Neoplastic/compressive:** Gliomas, ependymomas, meningiomas, basal meningeal carcinomatosis, craniovertebral junction abnormalities
- **Immune:** Multiple sclerosis, paraneoplastic syndromes, antiGAD, gluten ataxia
- **Deficiency:** Hypothyroidism, vitamin B1 and B12, vitamin E.

#### Genetic causes of ataxia
- **Autosomal recessive:** FA, AT, AVED, AOA 1, AOA 2, other inborn errors of metabolism
- **Autosomal dominant:** SCA types 1 through 28, episodic ataxias (types 1, 2, others)
- **Xlinked**
- **Mitochondrial:** NARP, MELAS, MERRF, others including POLG mutations, KearnsSayre syndrome.

#### Causes of ataxia based on tempo of disease
- Episodic—many inborn errors of metabolism; EA syndromes
- Acute (hours/days); strokes, ischemic and hemorrhagic; MS; infections; parainfectious syndromes; toxic disorders
- **Subacute (weeks/months):** Mass lesions in the posterior fossa; meningeal infiltrates; infections, such as HIV, CJD; deficiency syndromes, such as B1 and B12; hypothyroidism; immune disorders, such as paraneoplastic, gluten, and antiGAD ataxia; alcohol.
- Chronic, mass lesions, such as meningiomas; craniovertebral junction anomalies; alcoholic; idiopathic cerebellar and olivopontocerebellar atrophy; MSA. Most genetic disorders such as FA, AT; and other AR ataxias; SCAs.

### Q. What are the causes of loss of consciousness?

**Brain**
- Trauma
- Acute subdural/epidural hematoma
- Subarachnoid hemorrhage
- Bilateral strokes/hemorrhages
- Seizure
- Syncope
- Hypoperfusion

**Brainstem**
- Stroke/hemorrhage
- Herniation
- Hypoperfusion.

### Q. What are the causes of hypoglycemia?
- **Drugs**
  - Insulin or insulin secretagogue
  - Alcohol
  - Others
- **Critical illness**
  - Hepatic, renal or cardiac failure
  - Sepsis
  - Inanition
- **Hormone deficiency**
  - Cortisol
  - Glucagon and epinephrine (in insulin-deficient diabetes)
- **Nonislet cell tumor:** Seemingly well individual
- Endogenous hyperinsulinism
  - Insulinoma
  - Functional betacell disorders (nesidioblastosis)
  - Noninsulinoma pancreatogenous hypoglycemia
  - Postgastric bypass hypoglycemia
  - Insulin autoimmune hypoglycemia
  - Antibody to insulin
  - Antibody to insulin receptor
  - Insulin secretagogue
  - Other—hepatoma, leiomyoma, hemangioblastomas
- Accidental, surreptitious or malicious hypoglycemia

### Q. What is the withdrawal seizures?
**Withdrawal seizures ("Rum Fits"):** More than 90% of withdrawal seizures occur during the 7–48 hours period following the cessation of drinking, with a peak incidence between 13 and 24 hours.

During the period of seizure activity, the electro encephalogram (EEG) is usually abnormal, but it reverts to normal in a matter of days, even though the patient may go on to develop delirium tremens.

During the period of seizure activity and for days afterwards, the patient is unusually sensitive to stroboscopic stimulation; almost half the patients respond with generalized myoclonus or a convulsion.

**Treatment and prevention of withdrawal seizures**
Most patients during withdrawal do not require antiepileptic drugs, as the entire episode of seizure activity—whether a single seizure or a brief flurry of seizures—may have terminated before the patient is brought to medical attention. The parenteral administration of diazepam or sodium phenobarbital early in the withdrawal period does, however, prevent withdrawal fits in patients with a previous history of this disorder, as well as in those who might be expected to develop seizures on withdrawal of alcohol and intravenous lorazepam (2 mg in 2 mL of normal saline) was highly effective in preventing recurrent seizures after a first seizure in the same withdrawal period.

In alcoholics with a history of idiopathic or posttraumatic epilepsy, the goal of treatment should be abstinence from alcohol, because of the tendency of even short periods of drinking to precipitate seizures. Such patients need to be maintained on anticonvulsant drugs.

### Q. What are common causes of nystagmus?
Nystagmus refers to involuntary rhythmic movements of the eyes and is of two general types. In the more common jerk nystagmus, the movements alternate between a slow component and a fast corrective component, or jerk, in the opposite direction. In pendular nystagmus, the oscillations are roughly equal in rate in both directions, although on lateral gaze the pendular type may be converted to the jerk type with the fast component to the side of gaze.

Nystagmus reflects an imbalance in one or more of the systems that maintain stability of gaze. The causes may therefore be viewed as originating in: (1) structures that maintain steadiness of gaze in the primary position; (2) the system for holding eccentric gaze—the socalled neural integrator; or (3) the VOR system, which maintains foveal fixation of images as the head moves. Nystagmus can be classified as the result of a disturbance in the vestibular apparatus or its brainstem nuclei, the cerebellum, or a number of specific regions of the brainstem, such as the MLF.

Jerk nystagmus is the more common type. It may be horizontal or vertical and is elicited particularly on ocular movement in these planes, or it may be rotatory and, rarely, refractory or divergent. By custom the direction of the nystagmus is designated according to the direction of the fast component.

Drug intoxication is certainly the most frequent cause of nystagmus. Alcohol, barbiturates, other sedative hypnotic drugs, phenytoin, and other antiepileptic drugs are the common causes (mostly horizontal nystagmus).

*Nystagmus of labyrinthine origin*

This is predominantly a horizontal or vertical unidirectional jerk nystagmus, often with a slight torsional component, that is evident when the eyes are close to the central position and does not change with the direction of gaze. It is more prominent when visual fixation is eliminated (conversely, it is suppressed by fixation). The observation of suppression with visual fixation is facilitated by the use of Frenzel lenses, but most instances are evident without elaborate apparatus.

*Vestibular nystagmus of peripheral (labyrinthine) origin*

Vestibular nystagmus of peripheral (labyrinthine) origin beats in most cases away from the side of the lesion and increases as the eyes are turned in the direction of the quick phase (the Alexander law).

In contrast, nystagmus of brainstem and cerebellar origin is most apparent when the patient fixates upon and follows a moving target and the direction of nystagmus changes with the direction of gaze.

Labyrinthinevestibular nystagmus is horizontal, vertical, or oblique, and that of purely labyrinthine origin characteristically has an additional torsional component.

Nystagmus of benign positional vertigo is evoked by moving from the sitting to the supine position, with the head turned to one side. In this condition, nystagmus of vertical torsional type and vertigo develop a few seconds after changing head position and persist for another 10 to 15 s. When the patient sits up, the nystagmus changes to beat in the opposite direction.

### Q. Describe the differentiation of peripheral from central nystagmus.

Refer **Table 4.84**.

**Table 4.84:** Differentiation of peripheral from central nystagmus.

|  | Peripheral | Central |
|---|---|---|
| Visual fixation | Decrease nystagmus | Not affected or may increase |
| Form | Horizontal/rotatory bilateral (both eyes) | Any form, may change, vertical Usually unilateral |
| Vertigo | Present | Variable, unsteadiness |
| Past-pointing and falling | Towards slow phase | Towards fast phase |
| Direction of nystagmus (fast component) | Towards the opposite side of the lesion | Towards the same side of the lesion |

The nystagmus and ataxia of gait (more of a propelling, or pulsion, to one side) that accompany acute cerebellar lesions are toward the same side (the side of the lesion), while in acute vestibulopathies, nystagmus beats away from the side of the lesion and pulsion is still toward the affected side.

### Q. What is the causes of conditions with extensor plantar and absent ankle reflexes?

Causes of an absent knee and ankle reflex with extensor plantars implies a mixed upper and lower motor neuron lesion, and causes include:
- Subacute combined degeneration of the spinal cord
- Hypocupremic myelopathy
- Motor neuron disease
- Syphilitic taboparesis
- Friedreich's ataxia
- Conus medullaris or cauda equina lesion—at the conus medullaris the spinal root entry zones and the pyramidal tracts are in close proximity—they may be damaged by a small lesion, such as a neurofibroma or diabetes mellitus + cervical myelopathy.

### Q. What is the pathway of proprioceptive sensation?

The primary receptors for proprioception, or kinesthesia, are the muscle spindles. Other peripheral sense organs dealing with proprioception are located in the muscles, tendons, and joints, particularly. Pacinian corpuscles. These respond to pressure, tension, stretching or contraction of muscles fibers, joint movement, changes in the position of the body or its parts, and related stimuli **(Fig. 4.61)**.

Proprioceptors are essential for the normal coordination and grading of muscle contraction and the maintenance of equilibrium. Conscious proprioceptive impulses travel along large, myelinated fibers from the periphery to the first order neuron in the dorsal root ganglion (DRG) and then via the medial division of the posterior root.

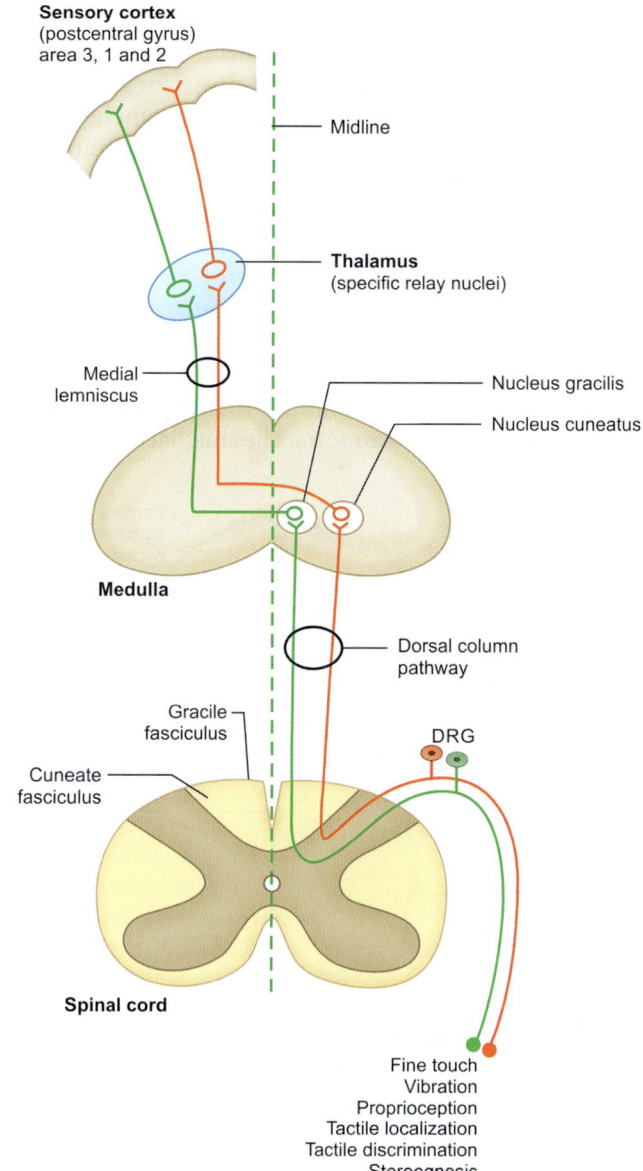

**Fig. 4.61:** The pathways for position sense and fine discriminative touch through the posterior columns and medial lemniscus.

These fibers then enter, without a synapse, the ipsilateral fasciculi gracilis and cuneatus, and ascend to the nuclei gracilis and cuneatus in the lower medulla, where a synapse occurs. Axons of the second order neuron decussate as internal arcuate fibers, and then ascend in the medial lemniscus (ML) to the thalamus. The somatotopic organization in the posterior columns and lemniscal pathways is the same as for light touch. The thalamoparietal radiations then go through the posterior limb of the internal capsule, and the fibers are distributed to the cortex.

### Q. What is the pathway of pain and temperature sensation?

The pain and thermal receptors in the skin and other tissues are free nerve endings. The pain impulses are transmitted to the spinal cord in fastconducting delta A-type fibers and slow-conducting C-type fibers. The sensations of heat and cold also travel by delta A- and C-fibers.

The axons entering the spinal cord from the posterior root ganglion proceed to the tip of the posterior gray column and divide into ascending and descending branches. These branches travel for a distance of one or two segments of the spinal cord and form the posterolateral tract of Lissauer. These fibers of the firstorder neuron terminate by synapsing with cells in the posterior gray column, including cells in the substantia gelatinosa **(Fig. 4.62)**.

The axons of the second-order neurons now cross obliquely to the opposite side in the anterior gray and white commissures within one spinal segment of the cord, ascending in the contralateral white column as the lateral spinothalamic tract. The lateral spinothalamic tract lies medial to the anterior spinocerebellar tract. In the upper cervical segments of the cord, the sacral fibers are lateral and the cervical segments are medial. The fibers carrying pain are situated slightly anterior to those conducting temperature.

As the lateral spinothalamic tract ascends through the medulla oblongata, it lies near the lateral surface and between the inferior olivary nucleus and the nucleus of the spinal tract of the trigeminal nerve. It is now accompanied by the anterior spinothalamic tract and the spinotectal tract; together they form the spinal lemniscus.

The spinal lemniscus continues to ascend through the posterior part of the pons. In the midbrain, it lies in the tegmentum lateral to the medial lemniscus. Many of the fibers of the lateral spinothalamic tract end by synapsing with the thirdorder neuron in the ventral posterolateral nucleus of the thalamus.

The axons of the third-order neurons in the ventral posterolateral nucleus of the thalamus now pass through the posterior limb of the internal capsule and the corona radiata to reach the somesthetic area in the postcentral gyrus of the cerebral cortex. The contralateral half of the body is represented as inverted, with the hand and mouth situated inferiorly and the leg situated superiorly, and with the foot and anogenital region on the medial surface of the hemisphere.

### Q. What are the functions of cerebellum and what are the clinical signs of cerebellar disorder?

The functions of cerebellum include:

- **Vestibulocerebellum:** The flocculonodular lobe receives special proprioceptive impulses from the vestibular nuclei; it is concerned essentially with equilibrium.
- **Spinocerebellum:** The anterior vermis and part of the posterior vermis—projections to these parts derive to a large extent from the proprioceptors of muscles and tendons in the limbs and are conveyed to the cerebellum in the dorsal spinocerebellar tract (from the lower limbs) and the ventral spinocerebellar tract (upper limbs). The main influence of the spinocerebellum appears to be on posture and muscle tone.
- Neocerebellum derives its afferent fibers indirectly from the cerebral cortex via the pontine nuclei and brachium pontis, hence the designation pontocerebellum; this portion of the cerebellum is concerned primarily with the coordination of skilled movements that are initiated at a cerebral cortical level.

The main function of the cerebellum was the orchestration of muscle synergies in the performance of voluntary movement—a loss or impairment of this function, i.e., asynergia or dyssynergia—resulted in irregularity or fragmentation of the normal motor sequences involved in any given act. This deficit, most apparent in the execution of rapidly alternating movements, was referred to by Babinski as dyskinesis or adiadochokinesis.

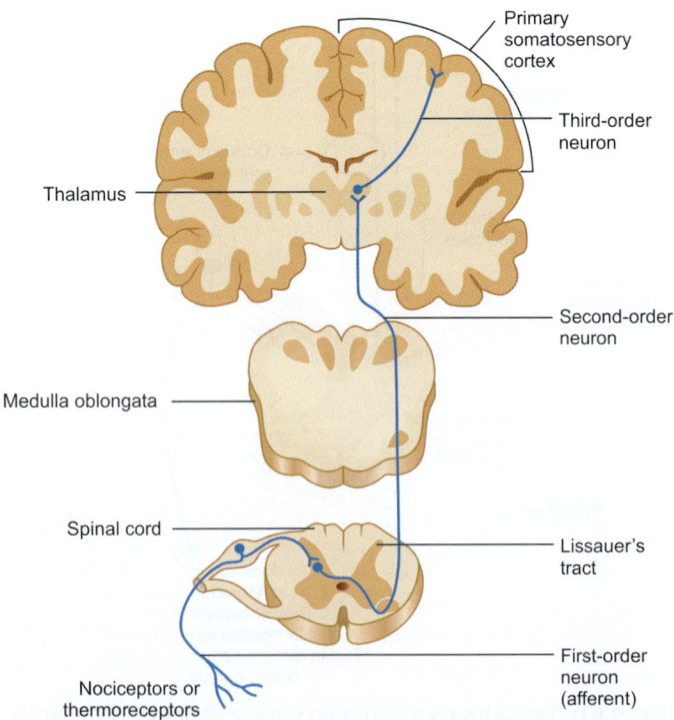

**Fig. 4.62:** Pathway of pain and temperature sensation.

Dysarthria, a common feature of cerebellar disease, is probably predicated on a similar incoordination of the muscles of articulation.

The excursion of the limb may be arrested prematurely, and the target is then reached by a series of jerky movements. Or the limb overshoots the mark (hypermetria) because of delayed activation and diminished contraction of antagonist muscles; then the error is corrected by a series of secondary movements in which the finger or toe sways around the target before coming to rest, or moves from side to side a few times on the target itself. This sidetoside movement of the finger as it approaches its mark tends to assume a rhythmic quality; it has traditionally been referred to as intention tremor, or ataxic tremor, but in reality reflects instability at the shoulder.

**Adiadochokinesis:** Defects in volitional movement are evident in acts that require alternation or rapid change in direction of movement, such as pronation-supination of the forearm or successive touching of each fingertip to the thumb.

**Wing-beating tremor/rubral tremor:** Coarse, irregular, wide-range tremor that appears whenever the patient activates limb muscles, either to sustain a posture or to effect a movement. The patient with cerebellar disease may develop a rhythmic oscillation of the fingers having much the same tempo as a parkinsonian tremor.

**Titubation:** A rhythmic tremor of the head or upper trunk (3 to 4 per second) called titubation, mainly in the anteroposterior plane.

**Speech:** Slurring dysarthria, like that following interruption of the corticobulbar tracts, or a scanning dysarthria with variable intonation, so called because words are broken up into syllables, as when a line of poetry is scanned for meter.

**Pendular nystagmus:** Unable to hold eccentric positions of gaze, resulting in a special type of nystagmus and the need to make rapid repetitive saccades to look eccentrically. Conjugate voluntary gaze can be accomplished only by a series of jerky movements.

**Ataxia:** Standing with feet together may be impossible or maintained only briefly before the patient pitches to one side or backward. Closing the eyes worsens this difficulty slightly, though the Romberg sign (which signifies impaired proprioceptive input) is absent. The pathologic changes are restricted to the anterior parts of the superior vermis. In patients with limb ataxia, the changes are found to extend laterally from the vermis, involving the anterior portions of the anterior lobes (in patients with ataxia of the legs) and the more posterior portions of the anterior lobes (in patients whose arms are affected).

**Holmes' rebound phenomenon:** Designated as an impairment of the check reflex. Thus, after strongly flexing one arm against a resistance that is suddenly released, the patient may be unable to check the flexion movement, to the point where the arm may strike the face. This is the result of a delay in contraction of the triceps muscle, which ordinarily would arrest overflexion of the arm.

**Hypotonia:** Due to depression of gamma and alpha motor neuron activity.

**Myoclonic movements:** Brief (50-100 ms), random contractions of muscles or groups of muscles—action myoclonus may be the principal residual sign of hypoxic encephalopathy, as described in the discussion of postanoxic intention, or action myoclonus.

### Q. What are the features of SACD?

Subacute combined degeneration of spinal cord: The spinal cord, brain, optic nerves, and peripheral nerves are all affected by vitamin $B_{12}$ (cobalamin) deficiency—spinal cord is usually affected first and often exclusively. The term subacute combined degeneration (SCD) is customarily reserved for the spinal cord lesion of vitamin $B_{12}$ deficiency and serves to distinguish it from other types of spinal cord diseases that happen to involve the posterior and lateral columns (loosely referred to as combined system disease).

Whether the peripheral neuropathy is a primary component of the disease or is secondary to damage of the posterior root fibers of entry in the dorsal cord has been debated, but the available pathologic evidence favors the former.

**Etiology:** Malabsorptive disorders, individuals of any age with celiac sprue; gastric or ileal resections; overgrowth of intestinal bacteria in "blind loops," anastomoses, diverticula, and other conditions resulting in intestinal stasis; and infestation with cobalaminmetabolizing fish tapeworm (*Diphyllobothrium latum*). Uncommon instances of vitamin $B_{12}$ deficiency are observed in lactovegetarians and in infants nursed by mothers deficient in vitamin $B_{12}$; vitamin $B_{12}$ deficiency may also be a result of a rare genetic defect of methylmalonyl coenzyme A (CoA) mutase.

**Clinical manifestations:** Initial symptoms include mild general weakness and paresthesias consisting of tingling, "pins and needles" feelings, or other vaguely described sensations. The paresthesias involve the hands and feet, more often the former, and tend to be constant and steadily progressive and the source of much distress. As the illness progresses, the gait becomes unsteady and stiffness and weakness of the limbs, especially of the legs, develop. If the disease remains untreated, an ataxic paraplegia evolves, with variable degrees of spasticity.

Early in the course of the illness, when only paresthesia is present, there may be no objective sign. Later, examination discloses a disorder of the posterior and lateral columns of the spinal cord, predominantly of the former.

Loss of vibration sense is by far the most consistent sign; it is more pronounced in the feet and legs than in the hands and arms, and frequently extends over the trunk. Position sense is usually impaired in parallel.

The motor signs, usually limited to the legs, include a mild symmetrical loss of strength in proximal limb muscles, spasticity, changes in tendon reflexes, clonus, and extensor plantar responses.

At first, the patellar and Achilles reflexes are diminished as frequently as they are increased; they may even be absent. With progression of the illness or with treatment, the reflexes may return to normal or become hyperactive. The gait at first is predominantly ataxic, later ataxic and spastic.

Loss of superficial sensation below a segmental level on the trunk may occur in isolated instances, A defect of cutaneous sensation may take the form of impaired tactile, pain, and thermal sensation over the limbs in a distal distribution, implicating the small fibers of the peripheral nerves or the spinothalamic tracts, but such findings are relatively uncommon.

The Lhermitte phenomenon (paresthesia down the spine or across the shoulders induced by rapid flexion of the neck) is a common finding if sought and is a sign more often allied with multiple sclerosis.

The nervous system involvement in subacute combined degeneration is roughly symmetrical and distal, and sensory disturbances precede the motor ones.

Mental signs are said to be frequent, ranging from irritability, apathy, somnolence, suspiciousness, and emotional instability to a marked confusional or depressive psychosis or intellectual deterioration.

Visual impairment because of optic neuropathy occasionally may be an early or sole manifestation of pernicious anemia; examination discloses roughly symmetrical centrocecal scotomata and optic atrophy in the most advanced cases. Some patients have symptoms of autonomic dysfunction, including urinary sphincteric symptoms and impotence.

**Neuropathologic changes:** The pathologic process takes the form of a diffuse, although uneven, degeneration of white matter of the spinal cord and occasionally of the brain. The earliest histologic event is swelling of myelin sheaths, characterized by the formation of intramyelinic vacuoles and separation of myelin lamellae. This is followed by a coalescence of small foci of tissue destruction into larger ones, imparting a vacuolated, sievelike appearance to the tissue, an appearance also observed in the myelopathy of AIDS and rarely in lupus erythematosus.

The main differential diagnostic considerations of the combined sensory and motor features are cervical spondylosis, multiple sclerosis of the cervical cord, rarities such as the female carrier state of adrenoleukodystrophy, and, most importantly, non-B$_{12}$ deficient combined system disease as a result of copper deficiency.

**Q. Describe the types of nystagmus.**
Refer **Table 4.85**.

**Table 4.85:** Types of nystagmus.

| Specific nystagmus | Probable location of structural lesion/causes |
|---|---|
| Bruns-Cushing nystagmus | Cerebellopontine angle, acoustic neuromas, meningiomas |
| Downbeat nystagmus | Cervical-medullary junction malformations, Chiari malformation, cerebellar flocculus |
| Upbeat nystagmus | Posterior fossa, caudal medulla, damage to ventral tegmental area, anterior cerebellar vermis |
| Torsional nystagmus | Brainstem |
| Seesaw nystagmus | Diencephalon, parasellar lesion, pituitary lesion, optic chiasm lesion |
| Periodic alternating nystagmus | Posterior fossa, vestibulo-ocular tract, brainstem, cerebellum |
| convergence-retraction nystagmus | Pretectum/dorsal midbrain, pinealoma |
| Pendular nystagmus | Blindness, optic neuritis, multiple sclerosis, brainstem, cerebellum |
| Dissociated Nystagmus | Medial longitudinal fasciculus (MLF) |

**Q. Define ataxia.**

- Ataxia, defined as impaired coordination of voluntary muscle movement affecting the rate, range, direction and force of movements.
- It is a physical finding, not a disease.
- Types of ataxia (**Table 4.86**):
  - Cerebellar
  - Sensory
  - Vestibular
  - Optic
  - Frontal

**Table 4.86:** Types of ataxia.

| Type of ataxia | Cerebellar | Sensory | Frontal |
|---|---|---|---|
| Stance and support | Wide based | Wide based based; looking down | Wide based |
| Velocity | Variable | Slow | Very slow |
| Stride | Irregular, lurching | Regular with path deviation | Short, shuffling |
| Romberg | +/- | Unsteady; patient falls | +/- |
| Heel-Shin | Abnormal | +/- | Normal |
| Initiation | Normal | Normal | Hesitant |
| Postural instability | + | +++ | +++++ |
| Falls | Late event | Frequent | Frequent |
| Turns | Unsteady | +/- | Multi-stepped; hesitant |

**Sensory ataxia** is due to a severe sensory neuropathy, ganglionopathy or lesions of the posterior column of the spinal cord, e.g., Sjogren's syndrome, cisplatin, chronic inflammatory demyelinating polyradiculoneuropathy (CIDP), paraneoplastic disorders, subacute combined degeneration (SACD), tabes dorsalis, Miller-Fisher syndrome, celiac disease.

- Ataxia more at night or while walking through narrow passages (coffee plantations).
- A history of falling into the sink or imbalance when splashing water on the face (Washbasin sign), passing a towel over the face or pulling a shirt over the head should also be sought.
- Pseudoathetosis—"pianoplaying" movements—when the patient has his arms outstretched and eyes closed, the affected arm will wander from its original position.
- Vibration and position sense are usually lost together.
- Positive Romberg's test is a hallmark of sensory ataxia.

**Vestibular ataxia** is due to lesion of vestibular pathways resulting in impairment and imbalance of vestibular inputs, e.g., vestibular, neuronitis, and streptomycin toxicity.

- Vertigo and associated tinnitus and hearing loss.
- Direction of the nystagmus is away from the lesion. **Optic ataxia** was first described in a man with lesions of the posterior parietal lobe on both sides of the brain, later known as **Balint syndrome**.
- Among the symptoms that characterize the syndrome are a restriction of visual attention to single objects and a paucity of spontaneous eye movements.
- Patients have difficulty in completing visually guided reaching tasks in the absence of other sensory cues. **Frontal lobe ataxia (Brun's ataxia)** is due to involvement of subcortical small vessels, Binswanger's disease, multi infarct state or normal pressure hydrocephalus (NPH).
- The gait may appear to be a combination of awkward, magnetic (stuck to the floor), cautious, slow, and shuffling. This is also known as a frontal gait disorder, referring to the frontal lobe conditions which often cause **gait apraxia.**

**Q. What is cerebellar ataxia?**
Refer **Figure 4.63**.

**Q. Discuss the functional anatomy of cerebellum.**
Refer **Table 4.87**.

**Q. What are the causes of symmetrical cerebellar ataxias?**
Refer **Table 4.88**.

**Q. What are the causes of asymmetrical cerebellar ataxias?**
Refer **Table 4.89**.

**Q. Describe the treatable causes of ataxia.**
Refer **Box 4.10**.

**Q. What is the cerebellar syndromes?**
Refer **Table 4.90**.

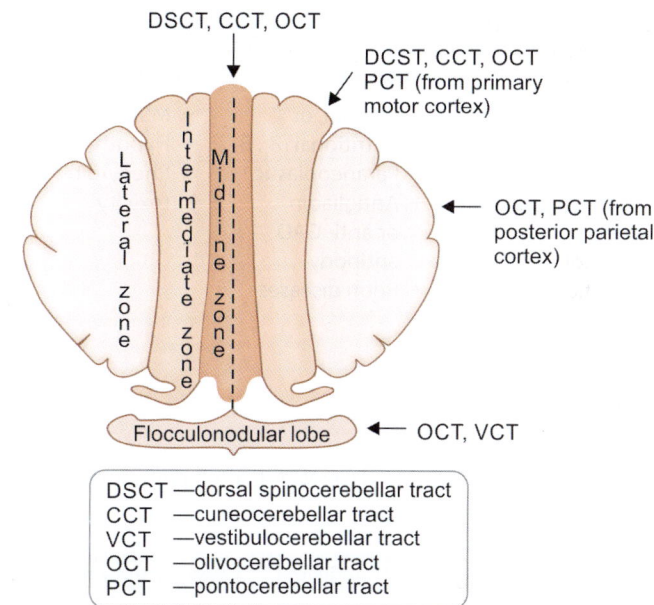

**Fig. 4.63:** Anatomical and functional areas of cerebellum.

**Table 4.87:** Areas of cerebellum.

| Zone | Corresponding anatomical site | Function | Loss of function |
|---|---|---|---|
| **Midline zone** | Anterior and posterior parts of the vermis, fastigial nucleus | Posture, locomotion, position of head relative to trunk, control of extraocular movements | Disorders of stance/gait, truncal postural disturbances, rotated postures of the head, disturbances of eye movements |
| **Intermediate zone** | Paravermal region of cerebellum and interposed nuclei (emboliform, globose) | Control of velocity, force and pattern of muscle activity | — |
| **Lateral zone** | Cerebellar hemisphere and dentate nucleus | Planning of fined and skilled movement (in connection with neurons in the Rolandic region of the cerebral cortex) | Hypotonia, dysarthria, dysmetria, dysdiadochokinesia, excessive rebound, impaired check, kinetic and static tremors, past pointing |

### Table 4.88: Causes of cerebellar ataxia.

| Acute | Subacute | Chronic |
|---|---|---|
| ✦ Drugs: Phenytoin, phenobarbitone, lithium, chemotherapeutic agents<br>✦ Alcohol<br>✦ Infectious: Acute viral cerebellitis, post-infectious<br>✦ Toxins: Toluene, glue, gasoline, methyl mercury | ✦ Alcohol, or nutritional ($B_1$, $B_{12}$)<br>✦ Paraneoplastic<br>✦ Antigliadin or anti-GAD antibody<br>✦ Prion diseases | ✦ MSA-C<br>✦ Hypothyroidism<br>✦ Phenytoin toxicity |

(GAD: glutamic acid decarboxylase; MSA-C: multiple system atrophy with cerebellar ataxia)

### Table 4.89: Asymmetrical cerebellar ataxias.

| Acute | Subacute | Chronic |
|---|---|---|
| ✦ Vascular: Cerebellar infarction or hemorrhage, subdural hematoma<br>✦ Infectious: Abscess | ✦ Neoplastic: Glioma, metastases, lymphoma<br>✦ Demyelination: MS<br>✦ HIV related: Progressive multifocal leukoencephalopathy | ✦ Congenital lesions: Arnold-Chiari malformation, Dandy-Walker syndrome |

### Box 4.10: Treatable causes of ataxia.

✦ Hypothyroidism
✦ Ataxia with vitamin E deficiency (AVED)
✦ Vitamin $B_{12}$ deficiency
✦ Wilson's disease
✦ Ataxia with antigliadin antibodies and gluten sensitive enteropathy
✦ Ataxia due to malabsorption syndromes
✦ Lyme's disease
✦ Mitochondrial encephalomyopathies, aminoacidopathies, leukodystrophies and urea cycle abnormalities
✦ Wernicke's encephalopathy

### Table 4.90: Cerebellar syndromes.

| | |
|---|---|
| **Rostral vermis syndrome** (anterior lobe)<br>*For example, alcoholics* | ✦ Wide-based stance and gait.<br>✦ Ataxia of gait; proportionally less ataxia is seen on performing heel-shin test while the patient is lying down. Normal or slightly impaired arm coordination.<br>✦ Infrequent hypotonia, nystagmus and/or dysarthria |
| **Caudal vermis syndrome** (flocculonodular, posterior lobe)<br>*For example, tumors (medulloblastoma)* | ✦ Axial disequilibrium; staggering gait. Little or no limb ataxia.<br>✦ Spontaneous nystagmus might be seen. Rotated postures of head |
| **Hemispheric syndrome** (posterior lobe, anterior variants also possible).<br>*For example, infarcts, neoplasms, abscesses.* | ✦ Incoordination of ipsilateral limb movements. More noticeable with fine motor skills<br>✦ Incoordination affects most noticeably muscles involved in speech and finger movements |
| **Pancerebellar syndrome** *For example, infectious/ parainfectious processes, hypoglycemia, paraneoplastic disorders, toxic-metabolic disorders* | ✦ Combination of all the other syndromes<br>✦ Bilateral signs of cerebellar dysfunction involving trunk, limbs, cranial musculature |

**Q. Describe signs and symptoms of localization cerebellar lesions.**

Refer **Table 4.91**.

### Table 4.91: Localization of cerebellar lesions.

| Signs and symptoms | Most probable region of involvement |
|---|---|
| Higher cognitive changes | Lateral hemispheres |
| Action tremor | Dentate and interposed nuclei OR cerebellar outflow to ventral thalamus |
| Palatal tremor | Dentate nucleus, Guillain-Mollaret triangle |
| Titubation | Any zone; especially anterior vermis and associated deep nuclei |
| Dysarthria | Posterior left hemisphere and vermis |
| Gait ataxia | Anterior vermis |
| Limb ataxia | Lateral hemispheres |
| Saccadic dysmetria | Dorsal vermis |
| Square wave jerks | Cerebellar outflow |
| Gaze evoked nystagmus | Flocculus and paraflocculus |

**Q. What is the mnemonics for cerebellar signs?**

Refer **Table 4.92**.

### Table 4.92: Cerebellar signs.

| DANISH Pen | VANISHD |
|---|---|
| **D**ysdiadochokinesia | **V**ertigo |
| **A**taxic gait | **A**taxia |
| **N**ystagmus | **N**ystagmus |
| **I**ntention tremor | **I**ntentional tremor |
| **S**canning/**S**taccato speech | **S**canning speech |
| **H**ypotonia/**H**eel-shin test | **H**ypotonia |
| **P**endular knee jerk | **D**ysdiadochokinesia |

**Q. Classify autosomal dominant cerebellar ataxia (ACDA).**

Refer **Figure 4.64**.

**Q. How do you classify SCAs?**

Refer **Figure 4.65**.

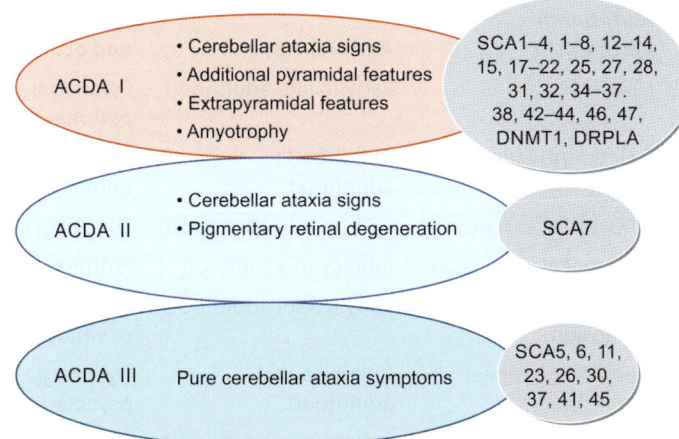

**Fig. 4.64:** Autosomal dominant cerebellar ataxia (ACDA).

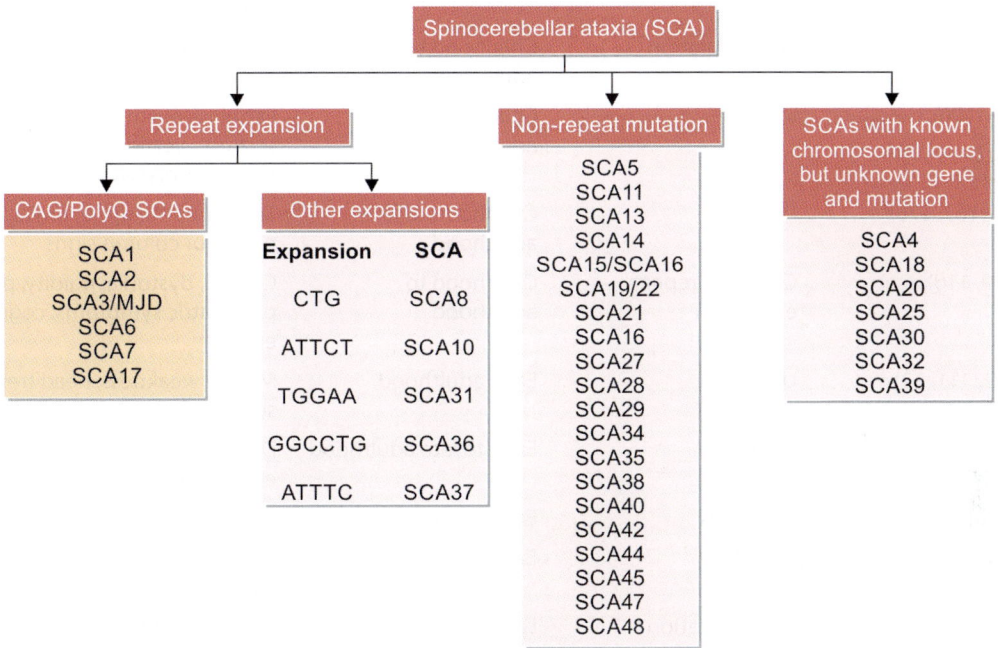

**Fig. 4.65:** Spinocerebellar ataxia.

## Q. What are the features of SCA?

Refer **Table 4.93**.

| Table 4.93: Ataxia at a glance. | | | | |
|---|---|---|---|---|
| **SCA** | **Disease gene** | **Mutational mechanism** | **Age of onset** | **Symptoms additional to ataxia, dysarthria and oculomotor symptoms** |
| SCA1 | Ataxin-1 (5, 116) | CAG repeat expansion | Early to mid-adulthood | Dysphagia, pyramidal and extrapyramidal signs, sensory deficits, cognitive decline |
| SCA2 | Ataxin-2 (73, 123, 148) | CAG repeat expansion | Early childhood to late adulthood | Dysphagia, rigidity, bradykinesia, peripheral neuropathy, executive dysfunctions, cognitive decline |
| SCA3 | Ataxin-3 (40) | CAG repeat expansion | Childhood to mid adulthood | Dysphagia, pyramidal and extrapyramidal signs, sensory deficits, peripheral neuropathy, amyotrophy and rarely Parkinsonism |

| SCA | Disease gene | Mutational mechanism | Age of onset | Symptoms additional to ataxia, dysarthria and oculomotor symptoms |
|---|---|---|---|---|
| SCA4 | 16q21.1 (43, 60) | Unknown | Early to late adulthood | Pyramidal signs, sensory neuropathy, peripheral neuropathy |
| SCA5 | SPTBN (72) | Deletion/missense | Childhood to adulthood | Facial myokymia, defects of the visual field, tremor, Writer's cramp, decreased vibration sense |
| SCA6 | CACNA1A (199) | CAG repeat expansion | Early to late adulthood | Dysphagia, tremor, somatosensory deficits |
| SCA7 | Ataxin-7 (28) | CAG repeat expansion | Infancy to adulthood | Progressive loss of vision, pyramidal signs |
| SCA8 | KLHL-1 (90) | Non-coding repeat expansion. | Early to late adulthood | Aspiration, pyramidal signs, decreased sense of vibration |
| SCA10 | Ataxin-10 (103) | Non-coding repeat expansion | Childhood to adulthood | Dysphagia, ocular dyskinesia, pyramidal signs, psychiatric symptoms, cognitive impairments |
| SCA11 | TTBK-2 (70, 189) | Frameshift | Early to late adulthood | Pyramidal signs |
| SCA12 | PPP2RB (69) | Non-coding repeat expansion. | Adulthood | Dysdiadochokinesia, head tremor, upper limb action tremor, mild Parkinsonism, pyramidal signs, psychiatric symptoms, cognitive decline |
| SCA13 | KCNC3 (63, 186) | Point mutation | Childhood to adulthood | Pyramidal signs, mental decline |
| SCA14 | PRKCG (190) | Variable | Childhood to adulthood | Facial myokymia, tremor, chorea, motor seizures, vertigo, decreased vibration sense, depression, psychosis, cognitive decline |
| SCA15/16 | ITPR-1 (167, 176) | Deletion | Childhood to late adulthood | Tremor of the upper limbs, pyramidal and posterior column signs |
| SCA17 | TBP (89, 110) | CAG/CAA repeat expansion | Childhood to adulthood | Chorea, dystonia, rigidity, pyramidal signs, psychiatric symptoms, cognitive decline and epilepsy |
| SCA18 | 7q22-32 (11, 12) | Unknown | Early adulthood | Muscle weakness, head tremor, impaired senses of vibration and proprioception |
| ScA19/22 | 11p21-q21 (23) (25, 180) | Unknown | Early to late adulthood | Dysphagia (SCA22); hyporeflexia, psychiatric, executive and cognitive dysfunctions (SCA19) |
| SCA20 | 11q12 (85) | Unknown | Early to late adulthood | Dysphonia, palatal tremor |
| SCA21 | 7p21.3-p15.1 (183) | Unknown | Early adulthood | Akinesia, tremor, rigidity, hyporeflexia, mild cognitive impairment |
| SCA23 | Prodynorphin (4) | Point mutation | Late adulthood | Reduced sense of vibration |
| SCA25 | 2p (164) | Unknown | Childhood to adulthood | Myokymia, pyramidal signs, pes cavus, and scoliosis, somatosensory deficits, autonomic dysfunctions |
| SCA26 | 19p13.3 (196) | Unknown | Early to late adulthood | — |
| SCA27 | FGF-14 (178) | Point mutation | Childhood | Tremor, cognitive deficits |
| SCA28 | AFG3L2 (19) | Missense mutation | Childhood to adulthood | Ptosis, hyperreflexia |
| SCA29 | 3p (37) | Unknown | Early childhood | Dysmetria, dysdiadochokinesia, dystonia, cognitive deficits |
| SCA30 | 4q34.3-q35.1 (166) | Unknown | Mid to late adulthood | — |
| SCA31 | TK2, BEAN (150) | Repeat insertion | Late adulthood | — |
| SCA32 | 7q32-q33 (80) | Unknown | Adulthood | Cognitive impairment, azoospermia |
| SCA34 | 16p12.3-q16.2 (51) | Unknown | Infant onset | Cutaneous plaques, decreased reflexes |
| SCA35 | TGM6 (184) | Point mutation | Mid adulthood | Ocular dysmetria, pseudobulbar palsy, tremor, hyperreflexia, torticollis, reduced position sense |

### Q. What are the features of Machado-Joseph disease?
Refer **Table 4.94**.

**Table 4.94:** Classification of Machado-Joseph disease (MJD) according to symptoms, prevalence and age of onset.

| MJD type | Age of onset | Prevalence | Symptoms |
|---|---|---|---|
| I | 5–30 years | | Limb and gait ataxia, severe dystonia, pyramidal signs, progressive external ophthalmoplegia. Fast progression of symptoms |
| II | ≈ 36 years | The most common | Ataxia, pyramidal deficits and progressive external ophthalmoplegia |
| III | ≈ 50 years | The second most common | Limb and gait ataxia, with marked pyramidal signs. The progressive external ophthalmoplegia can or cannot manifest. The third type has moderate progression and can evolve to one of the other types |
| IV | 38–47 years | In patients with the fewest CAG-repeats expansion | Slow progressive parkinsonism, responsive to the L-DOPA treatment, fasciculations and peripheral neuropathy |
| V | | | Marked spastic paraplegia with or without cerebellar ataxia. This type is usually mis-diagnosed as hereditary spastic paraplegia (HSP) |

### Q. What are the features of Friedreich's ataxia?

Friedreich's ataxia is characterized by slowly progressive ataxia with onset usually before age 25 years (mean age at onset: 10–15 years).

Friedreich's ataxia (FRDA) is typically associated with dysarthria, muscle weakness, spasticity particularly in the lower limbs, scoliosis, bladder dysfunction, absent lower limb reflexes, and loss of position and vibration sense.

Approximately two thirds of individuals with FRDA have cardiomyopathy, up to 30% have diabetes mellitus.

**Diagnostic criteria (Anita Harding)**

| Essential | • Age of onset before 25 years<br>• Progressive ataxia of gait and limbs<br>• Absent knee and ankle jerks<br>• Axonal picture on neurophysiology<br>• Dysarthria (if after five years from onset) |
|---|---|
| Additional (present in over 66%) | • Scoliosis<br>• Pyramidal weakness in lower limbs<br>• Absent reflexes in arms<br>• Large fiber sensory loss on examination<br>• Abnormal ECG |
| Others (<50%) | • Nystagmus<br>• Optic atrophy<br>• Deafness<br>• Distal amyotrophy<br>• Pes cavus<br>• Diabetes |

### Q. What is Joubert's syndrome?

Joubert's syndrome is a rare autosomal recessive disease characterized by a congenital hindbrain malformation, which can be identified on MRI as the 'molar tooth sign'. The clinical picture includes neonatal hypotonia, cerebellar ataxia, ocular motor apraxia, breathing dysregulation, and multiple organ involvement.

### Q. What is Marie's ataxia?

Marie's spastic ataxia is a variant of Friedreich's ataxia associated with features of a progressive spastic paraplegia.

It is associated with optic atrophy, nystagmus, dysarthria and dystonic choreoathetosis.

### Q. What is Gillespie syndrome?

It is a rare, congenital, neurological disorder characterized by the association of partial bilateral aniridia with non progressive cerebellar ataxia, and intellectual disability.

### Q. What is Holmes ataxia?

It is a form of autosomal recessive cerebellar ataxia and is characterized by hypogonadotropic hypogonadism, chorioretinal dystrophy and hypersegmented neutrophils.

## Case 6: Parkinson's Disease

*Brief History*
A 18-year-old male admitted with chief complaints of involuntary movements of all 4 limbs for the past 18 months which worsened in the last 3 months.

He was apparently normal 18 months back when his complaint started as difficulty in writing due to mild distal involuntary movements of the hand while he was studying in 8th standard.

It was oscillatory type of movement involving the distal part of limb, but later he noticed that it affects proximal part of limbs also. Though, it presents even at rest its frequency increases while he is trying to do some task like taking a cup of coffee. It affected all 4 limbs almost in the same time duration.

Because of the involuntary movements he was finding difficulty in gripping chappals, difficulty in walking, difficulty in getting up from squatting position.

He also has difficulty in holding coffee cup, wearing shirt, buttoning, unbuttoning.

- There is history of change in voice for the past 1 month.
- There was no history of seizures or loss of consciousness. No history suggestive of dysphagia, hearing difficulty, facial deviation, or nasal regurgitation.
- No history suggestive of neck muscle weakness or breathing difficulty.
- He gives a history of fall from bicycle and sustained injury to left knee and right hand.
- There was no history of radiating neck pain, sensory disturbances bowel and bladder disturbances fever, joint pain, or rashes.
- He discontinued his studies from 8th standard.

*Past History*
- No history of rheumatic fever or valvular heart disease.
- No history of any significant surgical or medical history in the past.
- No history of TB or bronchial asthma.

*Personal History*
He is a non-smoker, non alcoholic with normal bowel and bladder habits.

*Family History*
No history of similar illnesses in the family.

*Treatment History*
No history of any drug intake.

*On Examination*
Patient is conscious oriented, pulse rate—84/min. Regular in rhythm, all peripheral pulses felt equally.
- Blood pressure—118/70 mm Hg in right arm supine position.
- Respiratory rate—18/min.
- Weight—50 kg; height—159 cm.
- Upper segment—76 cm; lower segment—84 cm.
- There was no pallor, icterus, cyanosis, clubbing, or lymphadenopathy.
- Thyroid-normal.
- There is a golden-brown ring seen in the periphery of both the cornea.
- There were no features of liver cell failure. No evidence of rheumatic nodules.
- Bilateral prominent costochondral junction with Harrison's sulcus.

*Systemic Examination*
Central nervous system:
- Higher mental functions:
  - Right-handed individual studied up to 8th standard.
  - Conscious oriented with normal intelligence.
  - No hallucination or delusion.

*Cranial Nerves*
- Olfactory nerve normal.
- Optic nerve normal.
- Bilateral normal fundus:
  - 3, 4, 6 cranial nerve normal
  - 5, 7, 9, 10 cranial nerve normal
  - 11, 12 cranial nerve normal

*Motor System*
Bulk                     Right arm 21 cm       Left arm 21 cm
Right forearm 18 cm                   Left forearm 18 cm
Right thigh 28 cm                      Left thigh 28 cm
Right leg 22 cm                        Left leg 22 cm

*Tone*
There was cog wheel type of rigidity present on the wrist bilaterally:

| Power | | Right | Left |
| --- | --- | --- | --- |
| Shoulder | Flexor | 5/5 | 5/5 |
| | Extensor | 5/5 | 5/5 |
| | Abductor | 5/5 | 5/5 |
| | Adductor | 5/5 | 5/5 |
| Elbow | Flexor | 5/5 | 5/5 |
| | Extensor | 4/5 | 4/5 |

Wrist flexion and extension are weak. Hand-dorsal and palmar interossei weak

There was no fasciculation.

| | | Right | Left |
| --- | --- | --- | --- |
| Hip | | 5/5 | 5/5 |
| Knee | Flexor | 5/5 | 5/5 |
| | Extensor | 5/5 | 5/5 |
| Ankle | | Normal | Normal |

Both superficial and deep reflexes were normal bilateral plantar responses were flexor.

Involuntary movements: Oscillatory, rhythmic, repetitive to and fro movements of bilateral upper limb and lower limb involving more in the distal area. Aggravates on action:

Wing beating tremor also present. Sensory system normal. Cerebellar signs were negative
- No nystagmus
- No signs suggestive of meningeal irritation
- Skull and spine normal.

### Per Abdomen
On inspection, there is a white marking in the periumbilical region (branding).
- There were no dilated veins.
- On palpation there was no hepatosplenomegaly.
- No ascites.
- Normal external genitalia and hernial orifices.

### CVS
Apical beat was palpable at left 5th intercostals substance 1 cm medial to the midclavicular line.
- s1, s2 heard normal.
- No murmur.

### Respiratory System
Chest was bilateral symmetrical,
- Palpation and percussion-normal.
- On auscultation, normal bilateral vesicular breath sounds without any added sounds.

### Summary
A 18-year-old male with tremors involving all four limbs in distal more than proximal aspect which aggravates on action; and history of dysarthria with no history of rheumatic heart disease or family history of similar complaint; with cog wheel rigidity in both upper limbs (features of hyper- and hyperkinesias) and evidence of KF ring in both the eye.

Here I am considering an extrapyramidal disorder involving basal ganglia most probably Wilsons disease with neurological involvement.

### Other Differential Diagnosis
- Secondary parkinsonism (drugs, such as haloperidol, metoclopramide, phenothiazines/ post-infectious-meningitis, encephalitis/ poisoning like carbon monoxide, mercury, manganese), but no history suggestive of the same.
- Autosomal recessive parkinsonism.

## DISCUSSION

### Q. What is prodromal/premotor PD?

Even prior to the onset of nigral neurodegeneration, extranigral Lewybody pathology is believed to affect the peripheral autonomic nervous system, the caudal brainstem, as well as the olfactory bulb and may correlate to a variety of early nonmotor symptoms that have been shown to antedate the first appearance of classical motor signs. Common symptoms include hyposmia, constipation, depression, excessive daytime somnolence, and idiopathic rapid eye movement (REM) sleep behavior disorder (RBD) **(Fig. 4.66)**.

### Q. What is the idiopathic Parkinson's disease (paralysis agitans)?

It is a chronic, progressive disorder in which idiopathic parkinsonism occurs without evidence of more widespread neurologic involvement.

### Q. Describe the motor symptoms of Parkinsonism.

Always asymmetrical in onset and become bilateral within a year.
- **Tremor** is an early and presenting symptom in 70% of patients.
  - Frequency is 4–6 Hz tremor and is typically most prominent at rest and worsens with emotional stress.

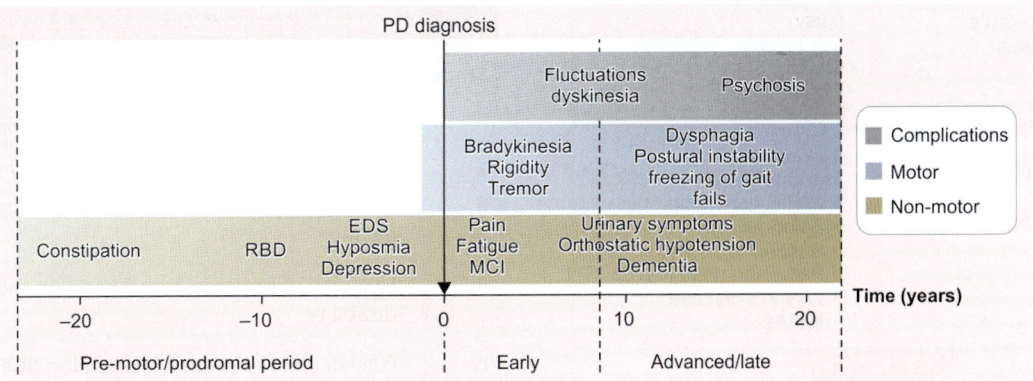

**Fig. 4.66:** Clinical symptoms and time course of Parkinson's disease progression.
(EDS: excessive daytime sleepiness; MCI: mid-cognitive impairment; RBD: rapid eye movement (REM) sleep behavior disorder)

- Typically tremor starts with the fingers and hands at rest.
- Often described as pill rolling of finger and wrist, because the patient appears to be rolling something between thumb and forefinger.
- Disappears on voluntary movement and sleep.

♦ **Rigidity:**
- Stiffness on passive limb movement is described as "lead pipe" rigidity because the increase in muscle tone is present throughout the range of movement. Unlike spasticity, it is not dependent on speed of movement.
- When tremor is superimposed on the rigidity, a ratchet like jerkiness is felt, described as "cogwheel" rigidity.

♦ **Akinesia or bradykinesia**
- Poverty/slowing of movement is the hallmark of Parkinson's disease (PD). Slowness/difficulty of initiating voluntary movement and an associated reduction in automatic movements, such as swinging of the arms when walking.
- There is fixity of facial expression (facial immobility—mask like face) with widened palpebral fissures and infrequent blinking.
- Repetitive tapping (at about 2 Hz) over the glabella (glabellar tap) produces a sustained blink response (Myerson's sign), in contrast to the response of normal subject.

♦ **Postural changes:** A stooped posture is a characteristic feature.

♦ **Gait changes:** Slow shuffling, freezing and reduced arm swing, small stride length, slow turns, festinating gait (tendency to advance rapid short steps) and catching center of gravity. Feet may be glued to floor. Postural instability and freezing may result in fall forward.

♦ **Reduced eye blink.**

**Q. Describe the nonmotor symptoms of Parkinson's disease.**

Refer **Table 4.95**.

**Q. Describe the classification of parkinsonian disorder.**

Refer **Figure 4.67**.

Atypical parkinsonisms overlap and share common features with the other parkinsonian syndromes (NBIAs, neuronal brain iron accumulation disorders; NPH, normal pressure hydrocephalus).

**Table 4.95:** Nonmotor symptoms of Parkinson's disease.

| Autonomic dysfunction | Neuropsychiatric | Sensory problems |
|---|---|---|
| ✦ Orthostatic hypotension<br>✦ Urinary incontinence<br>✦ Constipation<br>✦ Sexual problems | ✦ Anxiety<br>✦ Depression<br>✦ Apathy<br>✦ Psychosis<br>✦ Dementia | ✦ Reduced sense of smell (hyposmia)<br>✦ Pain |
| **Sleep disorders** | **Rheumatological** | **Other** |
| ✦ Restless legs<br>✦ Insomnia<br>✦ Daytime somnolence | ✦ Frozen shoulder<br>✦ Periarthritis<br>✦ Swan neck deformity | Seborrhea |

**Q. Describe the Hoehn and Yahr stage of Parkinson's disease.**

Refer **Table 4.96**.

**Table 4.96:** Hoehn and Yahr stage of Parkinson's disease.

| Stage | Disease state |
|---|---|
| I | Unilateral involvement only, minimal or no functional impairment |
| II | Bilateral or midline involvement, without impairment of balance |
| III | First sign of impaired righting reflex, mild to moderate disability |
| IV | Fully developed, severely disabling disease; patient still able to walk and stand unassisted |
| V | Confinement to bed or wheelchair unless aided |

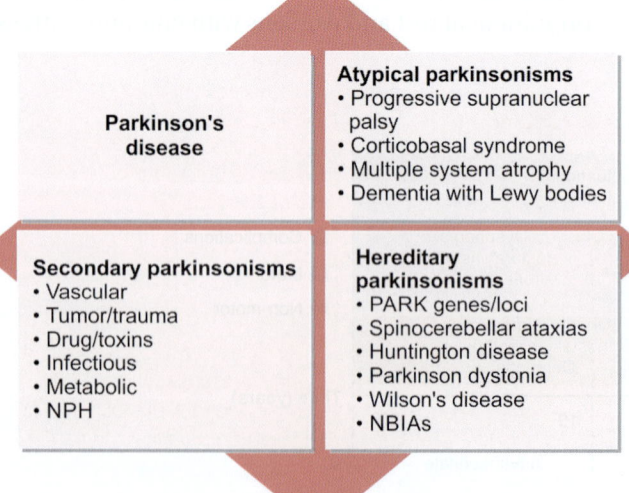

**Fig. 4.67:** Classification of parkinsonism.

## Q. What is the MDS clinical diagnostic criteria for PD?
Refer **Table 4.97**.

**Table 4.97:** MDS clinical diagnostic criteria for PD.

| Supportive | Red Flags | Exclusionary |
|---|---|---|
| • Cardinal features: **Rest tremor**, rigidity, bradykinesia (documented)<br>• Clear response to dopaminergic therapy (subjective or >30% change in UPDRS III with treatment)<br>• Marked on/off fluctuations, end-dose wearing-off<br>• Presence of levodopa-induced dyskinesias<br>• Olfactory loss<br>• Cardiac sympathetic denervation on MIBG scintigraphy | • Rapid progression of gait impairment, requiring a wheelchair within 5 years of onset<br>• Absence of progression of motor symptoms or signs over 5 years or more (absent treatment)<br>• Early bulbar dysfunction (<5 years from onset)<br>• Inspiratory respiratory dysfunction (stridor, frequent sighs)<br>• Severe autonomic failure (<5 years from onset)<br>• Recurrent (>1/year) falls from imbalance within 3 years of onset<br>• Anterocollis or limb contractures within 10 years of onset<br>• Absence of common non-motor features (sleep dysfunction, RBD, RLS/PLMS, daytime somnolence, autonomic dysfunction, hyposmia, mood disturbance)<br>• Otherwise unexplained pyramidal tract signs<br>• Bilateral symmetric parkinsonism | • Unequivocal cerebellar abnormalities (e.g., cerebellar gait, limb ataxia, oculomotor abnormalities)<br>• Downward vertical supranuclear gaze palsy or selective slowing of vertical saccades<br>• Probable behavioral variant FTD or PPA within <5 years onset<br>• Restriction of parkinsonism to lower extremities >3 years<br>• Drug-induced parkinsonism (documented prior use and link to drug, i.e., antipsychotic, etc.)<br>• Absence of response to high-dose levodopa<br>• Cortical sensory loss (evidence of graphesthesia, astereognosis) ideomotor apraxia, or primary aphasia<br>• Normal dopamine transporter imaging (presynaptic)<br>• Documentation of an alternative condition |

## Q. Describe the causes of secondary parkinsonism.
Refer **Table 4.98**.

**Table 4.98:** Causes of secondary parkinsonism.

| | |
|---|---|
| **Toxin:** Manganese, 1-methyl 4-phenyl-1,2,3,6-tetrahydropyridine (MPTP), carbon monoxide, manganese, mercury, carbon disulfide, cyanide, methanol | **Drugs:** Dopamine receptor blocking drugs, reserpine, tetrabenazine, alpha methyl dopa, lithium, flunarizine, cinnarizine |
| **Viral:** Encephalitis lethargica, Creutzfeldt-Jakob disease **Metabolic:** Wilson's disease | **Vascular:** Multi-infarct, Binswanger's disease |
| | **Trauma:** Pugilistic encephalopathy |
| **Head injury:** Punch drunk syndrome | |
| **Infectious:** Postencephalitic, human immunodeficiency virus (HIV), subacute sclerosing panencephalitis (SSPE), Prion diseases | **Others:** Parathyroid abnormalities, hypothyroidism, brain tumors, paraneoplastic, normal pressure hydrocephalus (NPH), psychogenic |

## Q. Describe the feature of Parkinson plus syndromes.
Refer **Table 4.99**.

**Table 4.99:** Parkinson plus syndromes and its features.

| Syndrome | Features |
|---|---|
| **Progressive supranuclear palsy** (PSP, Steele-Richardson-Olszewski syndrome) | Slow ocular saccades, eyelid apraxia, and restricted eye movements with particular impairment of downward gaze and reptilian stare. Frequently experience hyperextension of the neck with early gait disturbance and falls. MRI may reveal a characteristic atrophy of the midbrain with relative preservation of the pons (the 'hummingbird sign' on midsagittal images) |

| Syndrome | Features |
|---|---|
| **Multiple system atrophy (MSA)**<br>♦ Parkinsonian (MSA-P) or striatonigral degeneration<br>♦ Cerebellar (MSA-C) or olivopontocerebellar atrophy<br>♦ Autonomic (MSA-A) form or Shy-Drager syndrome | Parkinsonism in conjunction with cerebellar signs and/or early and prominent autonomic dysfunction, usually orthostatic hypotension. Cerebellar and brainstem atrophy (the pontine 'hot cross buns' sign in MSA-C) |
| **Corticobasal ganglionic degeneration**<br>(Rebeitz-Kolodny-Richardson syndrome) | Asymmetric dystonic contractions and clumsiness of one hand coupled with cortical sensory disturbances manifest as apraxia, agnosia, focal myoclonus, or alien limb phenomenon |
| **Dementia with Lewy bodies** | Early onset dementia, visual hallucinations |
| **Parkinsonism dementia complex of Guam** | Motor neuron disease plus Parkinson's |
| **Guadeloupean parkinsonism** | Levodopa-unresponsive parkinsonism, postural instability with early falls, and pseudobulbar palsy |

**Q. Discuss red flags suggesting an atypical parkinsonism.**
Refer **Table 4.100**.

**Table 4.100:** Red flags in atypical parkinsonism.

| Red flag | Suggested atypical parkinsonism |
|---|---|
| Rapid disease progression | Any atypical parkinsonism |
| Lack of a robust levodopa response | Any atypical parkinsonism |
| Bilateral symmetric parkinsonism | DLB, PSP |
| Early gait impairment, falls | Any atypical parkinsonism |
| REM sleep behavior disorder | DLB, MSA |
| Early bulbar dysfunction | PSP |
| Irregular, jerky tremor | MSA, CBD |
| Myoclonus | MSA, CBD (less common in DLB, PSP) |
| Supranuclear gaze palsy | PSP, CBD |
| Dysautonomia | DLB, MSA |
| Cerebellar signs | MSA |
| Laryngeal stridor | MSA |
| Perioral/facial levodopa-induced dyskinesias | MSA |
| Early dementia | DLB, PSP, CBD |
| Apraxia of speech or progressive nonfluent aphasia | PSP, CBD |
| Apraxia | CBD, PSP |
| Alien limb phenomenon | CBD |
| Higher cortical findings (e.g., agraphesthesia) | CBD |

**Q. Which is the best test in diagnosis of Wilson's disease?**
Liver copper after liver biopsy: >200 mg/g of Cu/dry weight of liver:
   24 hr urine Cu – Normal 25–50 mg
            >160 mg in symptomatic patients
            60–100 mg in presymptomatic patients.

**Q. What is the prognosis of Wilson's disease?**
Anticopper therapy must be lifelong in patients with Wilson's disease. With treatment liver function usually recovers after about a year although residual liver damage is usually present.
   Neurologic and psychiatric symptoms usually improves after 6–24 months of treatment.

**Q. What is D-penicillamine challenge test?**
Urine Cu of >25 ug mol/24-hours following the administration of penicillamine.
♦ Noninvasive test for Wilson's disease.
♦ At least 2 baseline measurements of 24-hours urinary Cu should be made prior to the test.
♦ 0900 h-10 mL plain sample for Cu S and ceruloplasmin. Start 24-hours urine correction for Cu.
♦ Administer 500 mg D-penicillamine.
♦ 2100 h-administer a second dose of 500 mg D-penicillamine.
♦ 0900 h-complete 24-hours urinary CU collection.

*Interpretation*
♦ Caeruloplasmin <0.2 g/L
♦ Serum Cu <12 micro mol/L
♦ Urine Cu >1.1 micro mol/24 h as an isolated test, >4 micro mol is a more useful threshold.
♦ Urine Cu post penicillamine >25 micro mol/24-hours

The diagnosis should be entertained in the absence of other liver diseases:
- Specificity 98.2%
- Sensitivity 88.2%

### Q. What is striatal toe?

A "striatal toe" has been defined as an apparent spontaneous extensor plantar response, without fanning of the toes, in the absence of any other signs suggesting dysfunction of the corticospinal tract.

It is commonly seen in dystonic syndromes, and as a feature of extrapyramidal disorders such as dopa-responsive dystonia. Striatal toe is seen in about 10% of patients with advanced Parkinson's disease.

### Q. What is Myerson's sign?

Myerson's sign or glabellar tap sign is a clinical physical examination finding in which a patient is unable to resist blinking when tapped repetitively on the glabella, the area above the nose and between the eyebrows. It is often referred to as the glabellar reflex. It is often an early symptom of Parkinson's disease, but can also be seen in early dementia as well as other progressive neurologic illness. It is named for Abraham Myerson, an American neurologist.

## Case 7: Muscle Disease

*Brief History*
A 20-year-old male admitted with c/o generalized weakness and easy fatiguability × 3 months, difficulty in getting up from squatting position × 3 months, nonpainful swelling of both calf muscles × 3 months, history of weight gain around 5 kg over past 2 months and increased sleep.
- No history suggestive of distal muscle weakness in lower limbs, upper limb involvement (proximal or distal), sensory or bladder and bowel involvement, cranial nerve involvement, diurnal variation of symptoms
- No history of similar complaints in the past
- No history of similar complaints in family
- Nonalcoholic on examination vitals: Stable

*Neurological Examination*
- Higher mental functions—normal
- Cranial nerves—normal
- Motor system:
  - Bulk—hypertrophy of both calf muscles, soft, rubbery consistency, nontender
  - Tone—normal in all 4 limbs
  - Power:
    » Both upper limbs: Deltoid and triceps muscles—4/5; other muscles—normal
    » Both lower limbs: Ilio-psoas, gluteus maximus, medius and minimus—4/5; other muscles—normal
- Reflexes
  - Superficial
    » Corneal and cremasteric—present
    » Abdominal reflex—absent
  - Deep
    » Bilateral biceps, triceps, supinator and knee—absent
    » Bilateral ankle—present (sluggish)
    » Bilateral plantar flexor
- Sensory system—normal
  - Cerebellar signs—normal
  - Skull and spine—normal
  - No signs of meningeal irritation Other system examination—normal

*Diagnosis*
Muscle disease (myopathy)

*Differential Diagnosis*
- Metabolic: Hypothyroidism (treatable cause)
- Limb girdle muscular dystrophy
- Becker's muscular dystrophy

## DISCUSSION

**Q. Discuss the features of common inflammatory myopathies.**
Refer **Table 4.101**.

**Q. Describe the dermatological manifestations in dermatomyositis.**
- **Heliotrope rash**—bluish-purple discoloration on the upper eyelids with edema
- **Gottron's sign**—erythema of the knuckles with a raised violaceous scaly eruption
- **V sign**—erythematous rash over the neck and anterior chest
- **Shawl sign**—erythematous rash over the back and shoulders
- **Mechanic's hands**—the lateral and palmar areas of the fingers may become rough and cracked, with irregular, 'dirty' horizontal lines.

At times, the muscle strength appears normal, hence the term **dermatomyositis sine myositis**.

**Q. Describe the drugs causing myopathies.**
- Lipid lowering drugs—fibric acid derivatives, HMG CoA reductase inhibitors, niacin (nicotinic acid)
- Glucocorticoids
- Zidovudine
- Drugs of abuse—alcohol, amphetamine, cocaine, heroin, phencyclidine, meperidine
- Dpenicillamine—autoimmune toxic myopathy
- Aminophilic cationic drugs—amiodarone, chloroquine, hydroxychloroquine
- Antimicrotubular drugs—colchicines

**Q. Describe statin-induced myopathy.**
Symptoms range in severity from mild muscular aches with slightly elevated CK concentrations in the serum to a rare but potentially fatal rhabdomyolytic syndrome.
- First generation—fungal metabolites (lovastatin, pravastatin, simvastatin)—infrequently implicated in muscle damage.
- Newer synthetic ones (atorvastatin, fluvastatin, cerivastatin)—more frequently toxic, especially when given with gemfibrozil (which has reportedly led to more than 50 deaths from myoglobinuric renal failure and has been removed from the market).
- Drugs in the statin class with higher lipid solubility appear to have a greater potential for toxicity as a result of their increased muscle penetration.

| Table 4.101: Features associated with inflammatory myopathies. | | | |
|---|---|---|---|
| Characteristic | Polymyositis | Dermatomyositis | Inclusion body myositis |
| Age at onset | >18 years | Adulthood and childhood | >50 years |
| Familial association | No | No | Yes, in some cases |
| Extramuscular manifestations | Yes | Yes | Yes |
| Associated conditions | | | |
| Connective tissue diseases | Yes[a] | Scleroderma and mixed connective tissue disease (overlap syndromes) | Yes, in up to 20% of cases[a] |
| Systemic autoimmune diseases[b] | Frequent | Infrequent | Infrequent |
| Malignancy | No | Yes, in up to 15% of cases | No |
| Viruses | Yes[c] | Unproven | Yes[c] |
| Drugs[d] | Yes | Yes, rarely | No |
| Parasites and bacteria[e] | Yes | No | No |

[a]Systemic lupus erythematosus, rheumatoid arthritis, Sjögren's syndrome, systemic sclerosis, mixed connective tissue disease.
[b]Crohn's disease, vasculitis, sarcoidosis, primary biliary cirrhosis, adult celiac disease, chronic graft-versus-host disease, discoid lupus, ankylosing spondylitis, Behçet's syndrome, myasthenia gravis, acne fulminans, dermatitis herpetiformis, psoriasis, Hashimoto's disease, granulomatous diseases, agammaglobulinemia, monoclonal gammopathy, hypereosinophilic syndrome, Lyme disease, Kawasaki disease, autoimmune thrombocytopenia, hypergammaglobulinemic purpura, hereditary complement deficiency, IgA deficiency.
[c]HIV (human immunodeficiency virus) and HTLV-I (human T cell lymphotropic virus type I).
[d]Drugs include penicillamine (dermatomyositis and polymyositis), zidovudine (polymyositis), and contaminated tryptophan (dermatomyositis-like illness). Other myotoxic drugs may cause myopathy but not an inflammatory myopathy (see text for details).
[e]Parasites (protozoa, cestodes, nematodes), tropical and bacterial myositis (pyomyositis).

- The mechanism of muscle damage is not well understood but it is likely that inherent enzymatic defects are present in a proportion of the severe cases. In addition, the chronic use of statin drugs reduces levels of both ubiquinone and small guanosine triphosphate (GTP) binding proteins, also plausible factors in statin-induced muscle toxicity.

**Q. Define the causes of myotonia.**

- Myotonic muscular dystrophy (type 1 and 2)
- Myotonia congenita (chloride channelopathy)
- Paramyotonia congenital (sodium channelopathy)
- Myotubular myopathy
- Myofibrillar myopathy
- Drug-induced—cholesterol lowering agents (statins, fibrates), chloroquine, cyclosporine

**Q. Describe the Gower's sign.**

Refer **Figure 4.68**.

**Q. Selection of which muscle for biopsy.**

Biopsy of a clinically involved muscle is important. Some disease processes have a patchy, rather than a diffuse, distribution. To increase the likelihood of sampling the pathologic process, **selecting a symptomatic muscle is important**. Select a muscle based on the expected distribution of the leading clinical diagnosis. For example, if the leading diagnostic consideration is polymyositis, select a proximal muscle, such as the vastus lateralis of the quadriceps, for biopsy.

Biopsy a muscle that is not too weak and atrophic. In this situation, obtaining a sample of endstage muscle is a risk. In endstage muscle, loss of myofibers is severe, and they are replaced by fibrovascular and adipose tissue without residual clues to the process that caused the muscle damage. On occasion, only the presence of a muscle spindle confirms that the specimen is a biopsy sample of skeletal muscle.

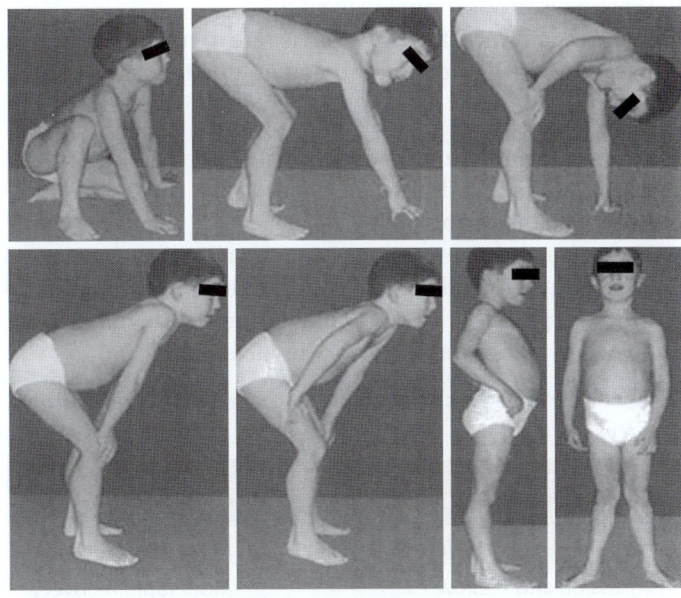

**Fig. 4.68:** The patient arises from the stooped position by using his hands to **'climb up the legs'.**

**Q. What are the possible sites of lesion?**

The patient has flaccid paralysis of bilateral lower and upper limbs. Possible sites of lesions are:

- Anterior horn cell.
- Peripheral nerves.

- Myoneural junction.
- Muscle.

Symmetrical proximal muscle weakness more than distal muscles, weakness is disproportionately greater than wasting with no sensory involvement or bowel and bladder involvement so the lesion may be in the muscle.

**Exceptions**
- Myotonic dystrophy type 1 (distal > proximal)
- Scapuloperoneal syndromes (proximal upper limbs and distal lower limbs)
- Inclusion body myositis [proximal lower limbs (quadriceps) and distal muscles of upper limb commonly wrist and finger flexors]

**Q. Why this is not neuropathy or lesions of a motor neuron?**

**Neuropathy**
- Patients with neuropathy usually present with asymmetric (mononeuropathy, radiculopathy, mononeuritis multiplex) or symmetric (polyneuropathy) weakness predominantly distal
- Tingling and numbness or loss of sensations.
- DTRs are usually absent or hypoactive.
- Wasting is proportional to weakness.
- Pain is a common feature (pain is rare in myopathy unless it is myositis of infectious etiologies, polymyositis, etc.)

**Exceptions**

Predominantly proximal muscle involvement:
- GuillainBarre syndrome
- Diabetic amyotrophy
- Hereditary motor sensory motor neuropathy type 3 (Dejerine-Sottas disease): AR disorder presents in early infancy, global areflexia, delayed motor development, enlarged nerves distal sensory involvement.

**Q. Describe the types of neuropathy based on the pathology.**
Refer **Table 4.102**.

**Table 4.102:** Types of neuropathy (axonopathy versus myelinopathy).

| Onset | Insidious | More rapid onset |
|---|---|---|
| Progression and recovery | Slow | More rapid recovery |
| Symmetry | Symmetry | Mild symmetry |
| Motor weakness | Limited to distal muscles | Proximal or diffuse weakness |
| Sensory weakness | Stocking distribution | Motor > sensory |
| Reflexes | Loss of ankle reflexes with presence other reflexes | Global loss of reflexes |
| CF | Normal CSF protein | Increased CSS protein |

**In this case with LMN type of involvement, the differential can be SMA.**

**Q. Describe the types of SMA.**
Refer **Table 4.103**.

**Table 4.103:** Types of SMA.

| Type 1 (Werdnig Hoffman) | Infancy | Autosomal recessive | Severe muscle wasting weakness associated with hypotonia |
|---|---|---|---|
| Type 2 (Werdnig-Hoffmann) | Childhood | Autosomal recessive | Slowly progressive form of SMA |
| Type 3 (Kugelberg-Welander) | Childhood and adolescence | Autosomal recessive | Proximal muscle wasting and weakness gradually progressive SMA |
| Distal form | Early adult life | Autosomal dominant | Distal weakness with wasting of small muscles |
| Bulbospinal | Adult life affects males only | X linked | Facial and bulbar weakness associated with proximal limb |

| MYOPATHY | SMA |
|---|---|
| Familial | Familial |
| Power grossly lost despite good bulk of muscle | Preservation of muscle power despite presence of gross muscle wasting |
| Proximal group of muscles | Proximal as well as distal |
| Muscle hypertrophy/pseudohypertrophy | Rare |
| Normal or sluggish DTR | Absent |
| Absent | Fasciculations |
| Markedly elevated creatine kinase, muscle dystrophy on biopsy | Mild elevation in chronic cases Evidence of muscle atrophy on biopsy |

**Q. What is myopathy?**
It means disease of the skeletal muscle (voluntary) muscle.

**Q. What is muscular dystrophy? What are the types of muscular dystrophy?**
It is a group of hereditary muscular disorder characterized by progressive degeneration of groups of muscles without the involvement of nervous system with absence or reduced dystrophin.

*The types of myopathy are:*
- **Hereditary muscular dystrophy:**
    1. Duchenne type (pseudohypertrophic) **(Fig. 4.69)**
    2. Becker muscular dystrophy
    3. Limb girdle myopathy
    4. Facioscapulohumeral dystrophy
    5. Myotonia dystrophica
    6. Myotonia congenita

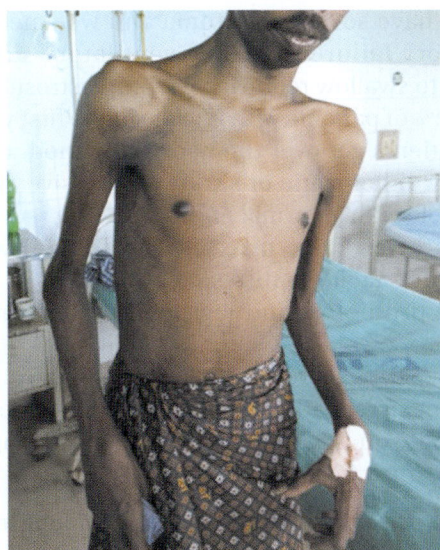

Fig. 4.69: Facioscapulohumeral dystrophy.

- **Congenital myopathy (rare):** The disease usually progresses in early life and then is static
  1. Central core
  2. Nemaline myopathy
  3. Myotubular myopathy.
- Secondary myopathy (such as endocrine disease and drugs).

### Q. What is Duchenne muscular dystrophy? What are the features?

- It is inherited as X-linked recessive disorder (30% spontaneous mutation). Duchene gene is on the short arm of X-chromosome, Xp21 and its product called dystrophin is absent (diagnosed by Western blot analysis of muscle biopsy).
- Affects only male, age of onset 3–4 years
- The child presents with difficulty in walking or getting up from sitting or lying position.
- There is history of frequent fall and delayed motor activity (e.g., walking) Gower's sign is positive (while the child gets up from lying position, he uses the hands to climb up).
- There is pseudohypertrophy in early stage involving calf and deltoid muscles. there is weakness, first involves the proximal muscles
- Gaitwaddling (ducklike)
- Other features include dilated cardiomyopathy, kyphoscoliosis and mental retardation.
- There is early respiratory involvement. Prognosis is poor, chair bound by the age of 10 years and few survive up to 20 years.
- Causes of death are dilated cardiomyopathy and respiratory failure or inanition.

### Q. What is Becker muscular dystrophy?

It is inherited as X-linked disorder, only males are affected and features are same as Duchenne type with the exception of:

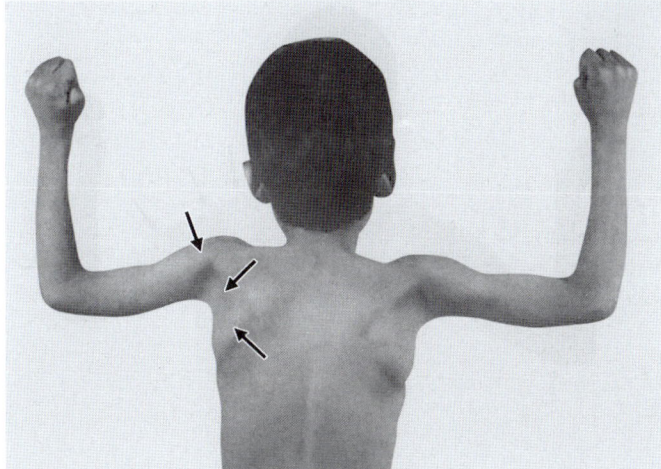

Fig. 4.70: Valley sign.

- Onset is late (5–25 years)
- Less severe, less rapid progression and less incidence of cardiomyopathy. Mental retardation and kyphoscoliosis are uncommon.
- Respiratory involvement is a late feature.
- Chair bound at about 25 years after the onset.

**Causes of pseudohypertrophy of calf muscles and signs related to muscle hypertrophy**

- Duchenne muscular dystrophy
- Becker muscular dystrophy.
- Valley sign in DMD **(Fig. 4.70)**: The patients were asked to abduct their arms to about 90° with elbows flexed to 90° and hands directed upwards. Those who could not abduct the arm to 90° were asked to do so to the maximum that they could. In this posture, on examination of pectoral girdles from behind, patients with Duchenne muscular dystrophy demonstrated a linear or oval depression (due to wasting) of the posterior axillary fold with hypertrophied or preserved muscles on its 2 borders (i.e., infraspinatus inferomedially and deltoid superolaterally), as if there were a valley between the 2 mounts. The sign was specific to Duchenne muscular dystrophy with sensitivity of about 90%.
- Poly-hill sign **(Fig. 4.71)**: Polyhill sign was elicited by asking patient to raise his arms with elbows flexed to nearly 90° and shoulders abducted to his maximum ability (around 70°). The sign shows five "hills" on either side consisted of:
  1. Enlarged infraspinatus muscle overlying the winged inferior angle of scapula
  2. Upwardly projected superior angle of scapula tenting the wasted trapezius muscle
  3. Prominence of laterally projected acromioclavicular joint
  4. Prominence of inferolateral part of the deltoid muscle due to wasting
  5. Prominent and well-preserved extensor digitorum communis/brachioradialis muscles.

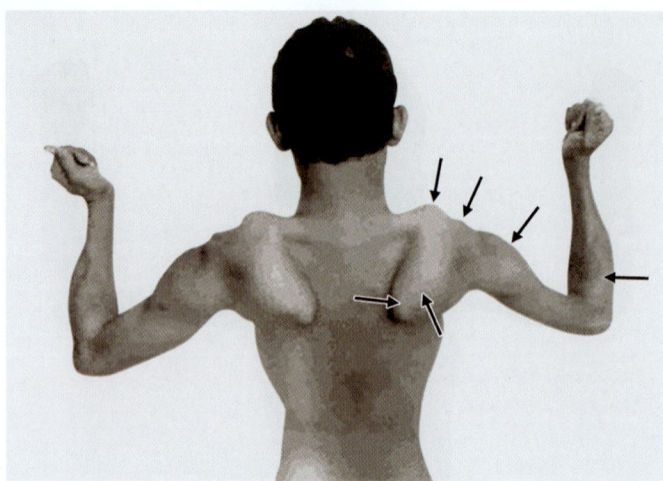

**Fig. 4.71:** Poly-hill sign.

**Q. What is the importance of birth history in myopathies?**

**Factors affecting growth are:**
- **Antenatal period:** Maternal factors—preeclampsia, diabetes, chronic renal failure can retard fetal growth and acquired infections TORCH (toxoplasmosis, rubella, Cytomegalovirus, herpes, HIV, syphilis).
- **Postnatal period:**
  - **During delivery:** Trauma while using forceps Erb's palsy and Klumpke's palsy involving brachial plexus, occasionally traumatic paraplegias are also seen. Presence of meconium aspiration or birth asphyxia can lead to cerebral palsy.
  - **Postdelivery:** Small for gestational age, low birth weight, preterm delivery, presence of jaundice, kernicterus, congenital hypothyroidism leading to infantile Hercules syndrome.

**Q. Describe the differential diagnosis for infantile hypotonia.**

The differential diagnosis of neonatal hypotonia includes:
- Perinatal asphyxia
- Metabolic disorders
- Congenital CNS abnormalities
- Spinal muscular atrophy
- Myopathies and muscular dystrophy

**Q. What is the congenital myopathies?**
- Congenital myopathies (CMs) are genetic muscle disorders characterized by structural abnormalities of myofibers and, some of them, by abnormal protein accumulation in the sarcoplasm.
- The most common CMs are core myopathies, nemaline myopathy, and centronuclear myopathy.
- CMs have a wide clinical range. At the severe end of the spectrum are conditions that are apparent even before birth because of decreased fetal movements and polyhydramnios.
- Patients have severe hypotonia and weakness at birth, respiratory failure requiring ventilatory support and inability to swallow requiring feeding gastrostomy.
- About 12% of patients with CM die in the first year of life.
- Once patients get over the neonatal period, the disease is usually either static or slowly progressive and may be compatible with a normal life span.
- Patients often have proximal and facial weakness, dysmorphic facial features, kyphoscoliosis, and other physical problems, and lag behind peers in physical prowess.
- CK is normal, as there is no myonecrosis.
- The diagnosis is made by detecting the specific structural abnormality on a muscle biopsy and increasingly also by genetic testing. CMs are genetically diverse.

**Q. Describe the congenital muscular dystrophies.**
- Congenital muscular dystrophies (CMDs) are a group of rare muscle diseases that present at birth or soon after with hypotonia, weakness, and developmental delay, similar to the congenital myopathies.
- Contractures develop early in some CMDs.
- Unlike muscular dystrophies CMDs are nonprogressive and patients are left with static, though in some cases may cause severe muscle disease.
- CK is high in some and minimally elevated or normal in others.
- The muscle biopsy shows nonspecific findings, initially myofibers atrophy and later myofibers loss with fibrosis and fat replacement. With the main finding of myofibers atrophy, it is sometimes difficult to distinguish SMA from CMD in a very young infant.
- Some CMDs are associated with severe CNS abnormalities.
- CMDs are genetic diseases; most are autosomal recessive.

**Q. What is the Lyon's hypothesis?**

This hypothesis explains why the phenotypic effect of the X chromosome is the same in the mammalian female which has two X chromosomes as it is in the male which has only one X chromosome—one of each two somatic X chromosomes in mammalian females is selected at random and inactivated early in embryonic development.

**Q. What is contracture deformity?**

A contracture develops when the normally stretchy (elastic) tissues are replaced by no stretchy (inelastic) fiberlike tissue.

This tissue makes it hard to stretch the area and prevents normal movement.

Contractures mostly occur in the skin, the tissues underneath, and the muscles, tendons, ligaments surrounding a joint. They affect motion and function in a certain body part. Often, there is also pain.

**Causes**

Contracture can be caused by any of the following:

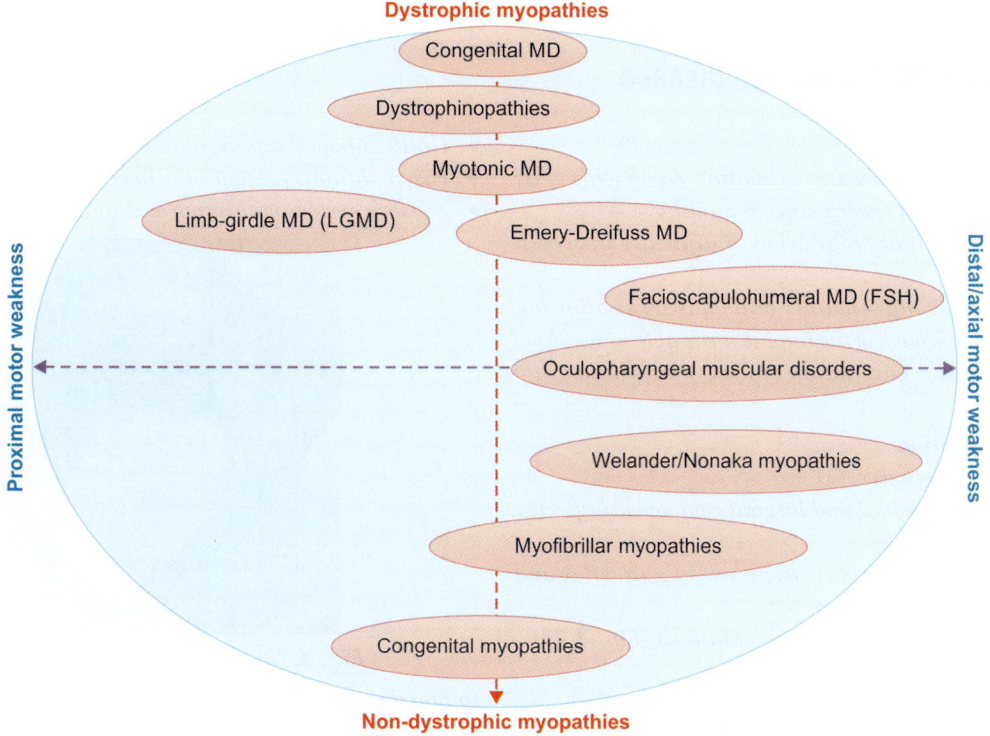

**Fig. 4.72:** Clinical spectrum of the main forms of inherited myopathies.

- Brain and nervous system disorders, such as cerebral palsy or stroke
- Duchenne and Becker muscular dystrophies
- Emery-Dreifuss muscular dystrophy
- Limb girdle muscular dystrophies (LGMD), facioscapulohumeral muscular dystrophy (FSH), myotonic muscular dystrophy type 1 and 2 (DM1 and DM2)
- Spinal muscular atrophy
- Amyotrophic lateral sclerosis
- Charcot-Marie-Tooth (CMT) or hereditary motor sensory neuropathy (HMSN)
- Reduced use (e.g., from lack of mobility)
- Scarring after traumatic injury or burns

**Q. What is the clinical spectrum of the main forms of inherited myopathies?**

Refer **Figure 4.72**.

## Case 8: Motor Neuron Disease

*Brief History*
A 62-year-old male, gardener by occupation came with chief complaints of difficulty in speech since 6 months
- Insidious onset, gradual progression of difficulty in speech since 6 months
- Difficulty in swallowing—mainly oral phase of swallowing effected (once food is back of the tongue, he is able to swallow)
- No history of nasal regurgitation of food or aspiration into lungs

*Findings on Examination*
- Pooling of oral secretions
- Dysarthria—mainly labial and lingual components affected
- Weak buccinators muscle
- Decreased palatal movements with preserved gag reflex and sensations
- Flaccid, atrophied tongue with fasciculations (Fig. 4.73)
- Other cranial nerves normal
- Absent abdominal reflexes, brisk deep tendon reflexes, no clonus, Jaw jerk present, corneomandibular reflex present, bilateral plantar reflex flexor response
- Grade 5 power and normal tone of upper and lower limbs
- Fasciculations present over lower limbs
- Sensory system within normal limits

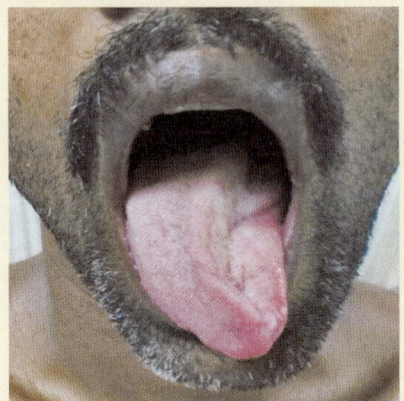

*Fig. 4.73:* Tongue wasting with atrophy.

*Impression*
Motor neuron disease—progressive bulbar palsy, ?ALS

## DISCUSSION

**Q. What are the differential diagnoses for progressive lower cranial nerve paralysis?**
Refer **Table 4.104**.

| Table 4.104: Differential diagnoses for progressive lower cranial nerve paralysis. | |
|---|---|
| Neoplasms | Myasthenia gravis |
| Brainstem glioma | Congenital myasthenic syndromes |
| Extrinsic posterior fossa tumor | Myopathies |
| Nasopharyngeal neoplasm | Intracranial infections |
| Neuromuscular transmission defect | Botulism |
| Basal meningitis: Tuberculosis, syphilis, fungal, sarcoidosis | |

**Q. How do you check for taste sensation?**
- Four primary tastes tested—bitter, sour, sweet and salty
- Cranial nerve seven—taste sensations on the anterior 2/3rd tongue
- When the tongue is retracted into the mouth, there is rapid dispersion of the test substance outside the area of interest. The tongue must therefore remain protruded throughout testing of an individual substance, and the mouth must be rinsed between tests.
- If bitter is tested, it should be last because it leaves the most aftertaste.
- Some examiners prefer to manually hold the patient's tongue with a piece of gauze to prevent retraction. Since the patient will be unable to speak with the tongue protruded, instructions must be clear in advance. The patient may raise the hand using some signaling system when taste is perceived, point to words written on paper, or make a similar nonverbal response.
- A damp applicator stick may be dipped into a packet of sugar, artificial sweetener or salt and coated with the test substance, then placed on one side of the patient's tongue and rubbed around. The patient signals whether she can identify the substance. Most patients will identify the test substance in less than 10 seconds. Taste sensation is less on the tip of the tongue, and the substance is best applied to the dorsal surface at about the junction of the anterior and middle third of the tongue.

**Q. What is corneomandibular reflex?**
**The corneomandibular reflex (von Sölder phenomenon):** Stimulation of one cornea causes contraction of the ipsilateral lateral pterygoid muscle and a twitch of the jaw to the opposite side. The jaw twitches *contralaterally* after stimulation of the cornea ipsilateral to a hemispheric lesion. A bilateral reflex may occur in coma, multiple sclerosis, or bilateral hemispheric lesions. It may indicate a UMN lesion more sensitively in amyotrophic lateral sclerosis than other UMN signs. It may also appear in parkinsonism.

**Q. What are the types of MND?**

Refer **Figure 4.74**.

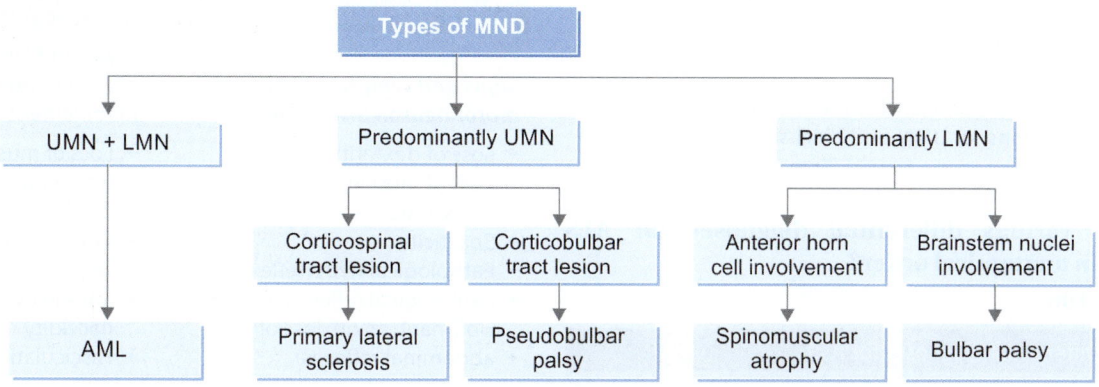

**Fig. 4.74:** Types of MND.

**Note:**

- The pathologic hallmark of motor neuron degenerative disorders is death of lower motor neurons (consisting of anterior horn cells in the spinal cord and their brainstem homologues innervating bulbar muscles) and upper, or corticospinal, motor neurons (originating in layer five of the motor cortex and descending via the pyramidal tract to synapse with lower motor neurons, either directly or indirectly via interneurons).
- Although at its onset ALS may involve selective loss of function of only upper or lower motor neurons, it ultimately causes progressive loss of both categories of motor neurons. Indeed, in the absence of clear involvement of both motor neuron types, the diagnosis of ALS is questionable.
- Bulbar palsy and spinal muscular atrophy (SMA; also called *progressive muscular atrophy*), the lower motor neurons of brainstem and spinal cord, respectively, are most severely involved.
- Pseudobulbar palsy, primary lateral sclerosis (PLS), and familial spastic paraplegia (FSP) affect only upper motor neurons innervating the brainstem and spinal cord.

**Q. What are the etiologies for MND?**

Refer **Table 4.105**.

| Table 4.105: Etiologies for MND. | |
|---|---|
| Structural lesions | • Parasagittal or foramen magnum tumors<br>• Cervical spondylosis<br>• Chiari malformation of syrinx<br>• Spinal cord arteriovenous malformation |
| Infections | • Bacterial—tetanus, lyme<br>• Viral—poliomyelitis<br>• herpes zoster retroviral —myelopathy |
| Intoxications, physical agents | • Toxins—lead, aluminum, others<br>• Drugs—strychnine, phenytoin<br>• Electric shock, X-irradiation |
| Immunologic mechanisms | • Plasma cell dyscrasias<br>• Autoimmune polyradiculopathy<br>• Motor neuropathy with conduction block<br>• Paraneoplastic<br>• Paracarcinomatous |
| Metabolic | • Hypoglycemia<br>• Hyperparathyroidism<br>• Hyperthyroidism<br>• Deficiency of folate, vitamin $B_{12}$, vitamin E<br>• Deficiency of copper, zinc<br>• Malabsorption<br>• Mitochondrial dysfunction<br>• Hyperlipidemia<br>• Hyperglycinuria |
| Hereditary disorders | • Superoxide dismutase<br>• Androgen receptor defect (Kennedy's disease)<br>• Hexosaminidase deficiency<br>• Infantile—glucosidase deficiency (Pompe's) |

**Q. What is El Escorial criteria for ALS?**

**Summary of El Escorial criteria for the diagnosis of amyotrophic lateral sclerosis (ALS) shown in Box 4.11.**

**Box 4.11:** El Escorial criteria for the diagnosis of amyotrophic lateral sclerosis (ALS).

The diagnosis of ALS requires the presence of signs of lower motor neuron (LMN) degeneration by clinical, electrophysiological, or neuropathological examination and signs of upper motor neuron (UMN) degeneration by clinical examination, and the progressive spread of these signs within a region or to other regions, together with the absence of electrophysiological or neuroimaging evidence of other disease processes that might explain these signs.

**Suspected ALS:** LMN signs only in at least two regions

**Possible ALS:**

- UMN and LMN signs in only one region, or UMN signs only in at least two regions, or LMN signs rostral to UMN signs

- **Special cases:** Monomelic ALS, progressive bulbar palsy without spinal UMN and/or LMN signs, primary lateral sclerosis without spinal LMN signs

**Probable ALS:** UMN signs in at least two regions, with some UMN signs above LMN signs

**Definite ALS:** UMN signs and LMN signs in bulbar region and at least two spinal regions, or UMN and LMN signs in three spinal regions

**Q. What are various differential diagnoses for ALS classified in anatomical order?**
Refer **Table 4.106**.

**Table 4.106:** Differential diagnoses for ALS.

| Anatomic site | Possible disorder |
|---|---|
| Muscle | • Idiopathic inflammatory myopathy<br>• Distal myopathy<br>• Nemaline myopathy<br>• Isolated neck extensor myopathy<br>• Metabolic myopathy<br>• Oculopharyngeal dystrophy |
| Neuromuscular junction | Myasthenia gravis<br>Lambert-Eaton myasthenic syndrome |
| Roots, plexus, nerve | • Radiculopathy<br>• Diabetic polyradiculoneuropathy<br>• Infectious polyradiculopathy<br>• Plexopathies<br>• Mononeuropathies<br>• Motor neuropathies |
| Anterior horn cells | • Spinal muscular atrophy<br>• Bulbospinal muscular atrophy<br>• Monomelic amyotrophy<br>• Paraneoplastic motor neuropathy<br>• Progressive post-polio muscular atrophy<br>• Hexosaminidase deficiency |
| Spinal cord | • Spondylotic myelopathy<br>• Syringomyelia<br>• Multiple sclerosis<br>• Adrenomyeloneuropathy<br>• Vitamin $B_{12}$ deficiency<br>• Familial spastic paraparesis<br>• HTLV-1 myelopathy |
| Central nervous system | • Parkinson's disease<br>• Creutzfeldt-Jakob disease<br>• Multisystem atrophy<br>• Huntington's disease<br>• Brain stem stroke<br>• Brain stem glioma<br>• Foramen magnum tumors |
| Systemic disorders | • Hyperthyroidism<br>• Hyperparathyroidism |

**Q. How do you differentiate UMN and LMN manifestations?**
Refer **Table 4.107**.

**Table 4.107:** LMN versus UMN.

| Signs and symptoms of upper motor neuron involvement | Signs and Symptoms of lower motor neuron involvement |
|---|---|
| • Loss of dexterity<br>• Loss of muscle strength (mild weakness)<br>• Spasticity<br>• Pathological hyperreflexia<br>• Pathological reflexes (Babinski, Hoffmann's sign, loss of abdominal reflexes) | • Loss of muscle strength (moderate to severe weakness)<br>• Muscle atrophy<br>• Hyporeflexia<br>• Muscle hypotonicity or flaccidity<br>• Fasciculations |
| • Increased reflexes in an atrophic limb ("probable" UMN sign)<br>• Pseudobulbar (spastic bulbar) palsy (emotional lability, brisk jaw jerk, hyperactive gag, forced yawning, snout reflex, suck reflex, slow tongue movements, spastic dysarthria) | • Muscle cramps |

**Q. What is opercular syndrome and pseudobulbar palsy?**

- In addition to dysarthria (and aphasia when on the dominant hemisphere), acute lesions of the frontoparietal operculum cause difficulty in swallowing liquids (dysphagia), which tend to come back through the nose.
- When the lesions involving the operculum or corticobulbar pathways are bilateral, dysphagia tends to last longer and may be permanent. In those cases, saliva accumulates in the mouth, aspiration of food may cause repeated bouts of pneumonia, and the patient may be aphonic.
- This array of symptoms resembles the clinical picture produced by the involvement of the bulbar muscles themselves or by the involvement of the neuromuscular junction, peripheral nerve, or medullary neurons. Therefore, it has been termed pseudobulbar palsy because, unlike actual bulbar palsy, the bulbar muscles themselves are not affected and lack atrophy.
- The **Anterior Opercular Syndrome (Foix-Chavany-Marie syndrome)** or the syndrome of Facio-pharyngo-glosso-masticatory diplegia with automatic voluntary movement dissociation) is due to bilateral anterior peri-Sylvian lesions involving the primary motor cortex and parietal opercula. Patients with this syndrome lose voluntary control of facial, pharyngeal, lingual, masticatory, and sometimes ocular muscles. Reflexive and automatic functions of these muscles are preserved. These patients may blink, laugh, or yawn spontaneously, but they cannot close their eyes or open their mouths on command. They do not have emotional lability (uninhibited laughter and crying). The gag reflex is decreased, and swallowing is severely impaired.

**Q. What are fasciculation?**

The fasciculations can be defined as visible fast, fine, spontaneous and intermittent contractions of muscle fibers (motor unit) resulting in verminous movements below the dermis. They do not move the joint **(Table 4.108)**.

**Table 4.108:** Causes of fasciculations.

| | |
|---|---|
| Fasciculations in healthy subjects | Coffee; exhaustive physical activity/fatigue; stress; cramp syndrome and benign fasciculations |
| Fasciculations associated with movement disorders | Machado-Joseph disease, SCA 3; spinocerebellar degeneration—type 36; Parkinsonism's (multiple system atrophy, ALS-plus syndromes) |
| Motor neuron diseases | Amyotrophic lateral sclerosis; progressive spinal muscular atrophies; benign monomelic amyotrophy; post-polio syndrome; Kennedy disease, Morvan syndrome |
| Systemic diseases | Hyperthyroidism; syndrome of inappropriate secretion of thyrotropin; hypophosphatemia, calcium disorders secondary to hyperparathyroidism, hypomagnesemia. |
| Drugs and/or intoxications by heavy metals pollutants | Organophosphorus poison, atropine, neostigmine; corticosteroids; succinylcholine; elemental mercury intoxication; theophylline, lithium, nortriptyline; flunarizine; isoniazid |

**Q. What are causes of polyradiculopathy?**
- Disc herniation
- Spondylosis
- GBS
- Lyme disease
- DM
- Arachnoiditis
- Tumors
- CMV in HIV patients

**Q. How to evaluate motor neuron disease?**
- MRI head/cervical spine to rule out cervical spondylosis, syringobulbia, CVJ anomalies
- Anti-GM1 antibodies for multifocal motor neuropathy
- CBC, ESR, peripheral smear
- Thyroid disorders to be ruled out
- Vitamin $B_{12}$ and folate deficiency to be ruled out
- EMG—fasciculation and fibrillation
- NCV—sensory action potential normal Motor velocity normal but decreased amplitude

**Q. What are the secondary causes of MND?**
- Toxins (lead, aluminum)
- Electric shock
- Autoimmune
- Hypoglycemia
- Hyperthyroidism
- Vitamin $B_{12}$ and folate deficiency
- Hexosaminidase deficiency
- Superoxide dismutase deficiency

**Q. When do you say fasciculations are significant?**

If fasciculations are present in a wasted weak muscle, then it is significant.

**Q. How do you precipitate fasciculations?**

Fasciculations are spontaneous, but can be seen by tapping the muscle, applying cold to the muscle or by hyperventillation.

**Q. Distinguish "benign" from "malignant" fasciculations.**

Benign fasciculations are not associated with muscle weakness, wasting, or any abnormality of reflexes. In general, benign fasciculation potentials tend to fire faster and affect the same site repetitively (e.g., eyelid twitching), as opposed to fasciculation potentials in pathologic conditions, such as motor neuron disease, which tend to be more random.

## MOVEMENT DISORDERS

**Q. What is the movement disorders?**

Movement disorders also cause motor weakness not by producing weakness but by producing hyperkinesias **(Fig. 4.75)**.

Movement disorders are classified into **(Fig. 4.76)**:
- Hyperkinetic disorder
- Hypokinetic disorder
  Categorization of movement disorders.

**Site of lesion**
- **Parkinsonism:** Contralateral substantia nigra
- **Unilateral hemiballismus:** Contralateral subthalamic nucleus
- **Chronic chorea:** Caudate nucleus/putamen
- **Athetosis, dystonia:** Contralateral putamen or thalamus
- **Myoclonus:** Cerebellar cortex/thalamus
- **Rhythmic palatal/facial myoclonus:** Central tegmental tract, inferior olivary nucleus, olivodentate fibers.

**Q. Define chorea.**

Chorea is an involuntary movement characterized by involuntary, irregular purposeless random non rhythmic hyperkinesias
- Movements are actually random and aimless:
  - Rather than disrupting a voluntary task, it appears as if fragments of movements intrude; in some cases, there is loss of motor tone, known as "motor impersistence", which appears due to lapses in the ability to perform desired action.
- When asked to hold the hands outstretched, there may be constant random movements of individual fingers (piano playing movements).
- If the patient holds the examiner's finger in her fist, there are constant twitches of individual fingers (milkmaid grip):
  - "Jack in the box" tongue/harlequin's tongue: Patient is unable to maintain tongue in protruded state and the tongue moves in and out.
- Blink rate is increased.

# SECTION 4: Nervous System

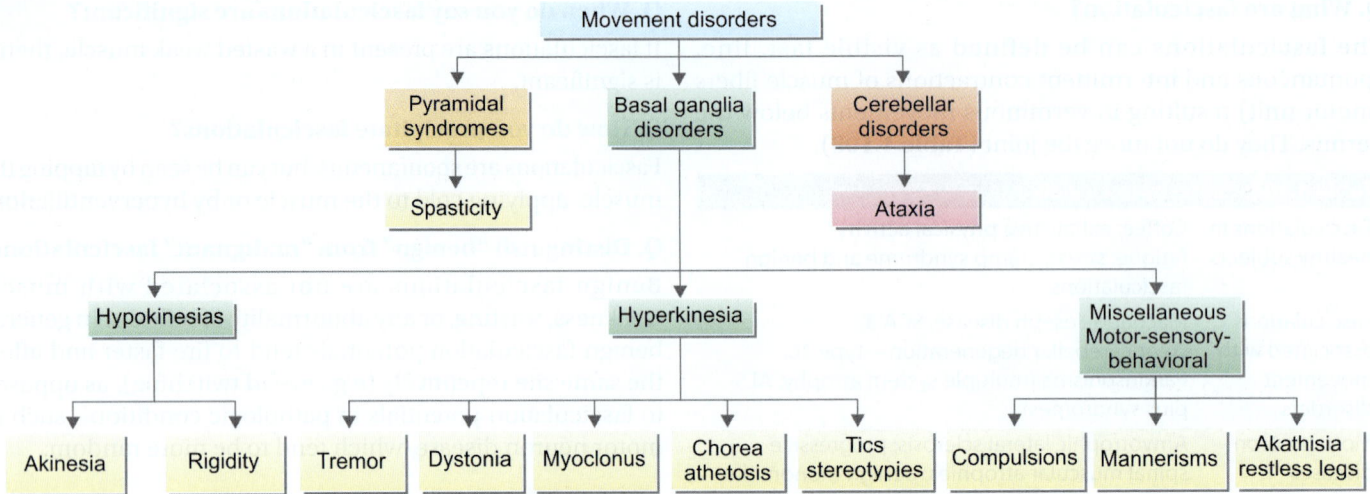

**Fig. 4.75:** Movement disorders.

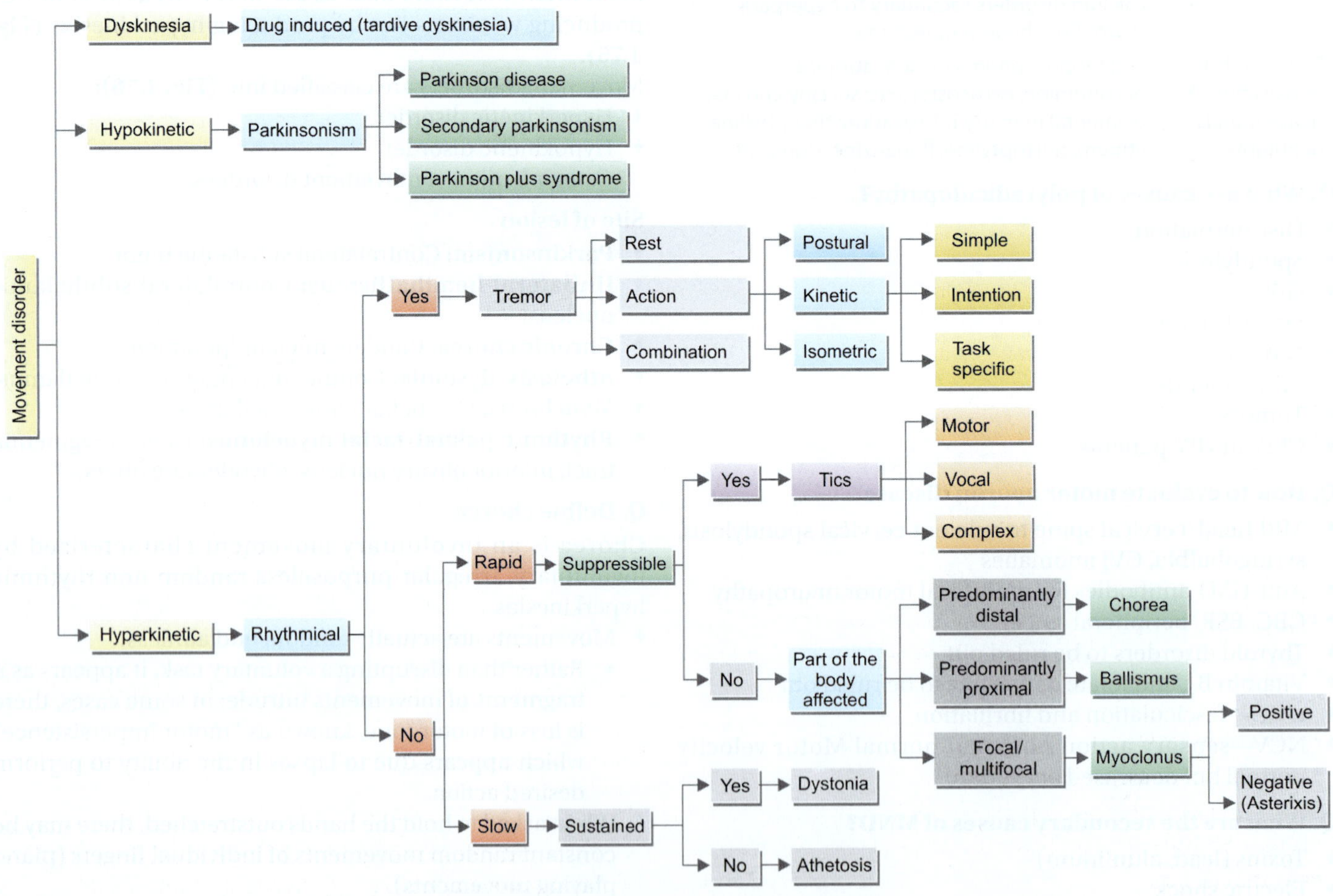

**Fig. 4.76:** Approach to movement disorders.

## Q. Name the disease characterized by chorea.

**Inherited disorders**
- Wilson's disease
- Huntington's chorea
- Benign hereditary chorea
- Neuroacanthocytosis
- Dermatorubropallidoluysian atrophy

**Rheumatic chorea**
- Sydenham's chorea
- Chorea gravidarum

**Drug-induced chorea**
- Narcoleptics (phenothiazines, haloperidol)
- OCP
- Excess dosages of L dopa and dopamine agonists

**Systemic disorder**
- SLE
- Antiphospholipid antibodies
- Thyrotoxicosis
- Polycythemia vera
- Hyperosmolar nonketotic hyperglycemia
- Toxoplasmosis in AIDS
- Paraneoplastic syndromes

**Hemi chorea**—stroke, tumors, vascular malformation

## Q. Define tremor.

A tremor is a series of involuntary rhythmic purposeless oscillatory movements. The excursion may be small or large and may involve one or more part of the body.

## Q. Define classification of tremor.

**Rest tremor**

Tremor present during relaxation and attenuate when the part is used, e.g., Parkinson's disease and other Parkinson's syndrome.

**Action tremor**
- Tremor which appears while performing some activity.
- Action tremor again divided into—postural and kinetic tremors.

**Postural tremor**

Action tremor which becomes evident when the limb are maintained in antigravity position (arms outstretched), e.g., enhanced physiological tremor, tremor of thyrotoxicosis, essential tremor.

**Kinetic tremor**

Tremors which appear when making a voluntary movement and may occur at the beginning during or at the end of the movement, e.g., intention tremor.

## Q. What is athetosis?

- Involuntary, irregular, coarse, somewhat rhythmic, and writhing or squirming in character (twisting).
- Hyperkinesias are slower, more sustained, and larger in amplitude than those in chorea.
- May involve the extremities, face, neck, and trunk.
- In the extremities, they affect mainly the distal portions, the fingers, hands, and toes:
  - Affected limbs are in constant motion (athetosis means "without fixed position")
  - Choreoathetosis refers to movements that lie between chorea and athetosis in rate and rhythmicity and may represent a transitional form.

**Causes**
- Cerebral palsy
- Congenital due to perinatal injury to the basal ganglia.

## Q. What is the hemiballismus?

Dramatic neurologic syndrome of wild, flinging (forceful), incessant (uninterrupted or continuous) movements that occur on one side of the body.

Due to infarction or hemorrhage in the region of the contralateral subthalamic nucleus.

- More rapid and forceful
- Involve the proximal portions of the extremities.
- When fully developed, there are continuous, violent, swinging, flinging, rolling, throwing, flailing (thrashing) movements of the involved extremities.
- They are usually unilateral and involve one entire half of the body.
- Rarely, they are bilateral (biballismus or paraballismus) or involve a single extremity (monoballismus).

## Q. What is the myoclonus?

Single or repetitive, abrupt, brief, rapid, lightninglike, jerky, arrhythmic, asynergic, involuntary contractions, involving portions of muscles, entire muscles, or groups of muscles.

- Seen principally in the muscles of the extremities and trunk, but the involvement is often multifocal, diffuse, or widespread.
- May involve the facial muscles, jaws, tongue, pharynx, and larynx.
- Myoclonus may appear symmetrically on both sides. Such synchrony may be an attribute unique to myoclonus.

Myoclonus has been classified in numerous ways including the following:
- Positive versus negative;
- Epileptic versus nonepileptic;
- Stimulus sensitive (reflex) versus spontaneous;
- Rhythmic versus arrhythmic;
- Anatomically (peripheral, spinal, segmental, brainstem, or cortical)
- By etiology (physiologic, essential, epileptic, and symptomatic)

- Encephalitis
- Juvenile myoclonic epilepsy (JME, Janz syndrome)
- Drug overdose
- Hypnic jerks (appear during the process of falling asleep)
- Hiccup
- Creutzfeldt–Jakob disease
- Subacute sclerosing panencephalitis (SSPE)
- Anoxic encephalopathy (Lance-Adams syndrome)

### Q. Describe the tic.

A "tic" is an involuntary movement or vocalization that is usually sudden onset, brief, repetitive, stereotyped but nonrhythmical in character, can be suppressed.

### Types

Motor tics are associated with movements. Categorized as simple or complex.

Simple motor tics involve only a few muscles usually restricted to a specific body part.

- **Examples of simple motor tics include:** Eye blinking, shoulder shrugging, facial grimacing, neck stretching, mouth movements, jaw clenching, and spitting.
  - Vocal/phonic tics are associated with sound
  - Simple vocal tics consist of sounds that do not form words, such as, throat clearing, grunting, coughing, and sniffing.
  - Common complex vocal tics include repeating words or phrases out of context.
- **Coprolalia:** Use of socially unacceptable words, frequently obscene.
- **Palilalia:** Repeating one's own sounds or words.
- **Echolalia:** Repeating the lastheard sound, word, or phrase.
  - Gilles de la Tourette syndrome—associated with chronic motor and phonic tics.

### Q. What is the dystonia?

- Refers to a syndrome of involuntary sustained or spasmodic muscle contractions involving cocontraction of the agonist and the antagonist.
- The movements are usually slow and sustained, and they often occur in a repetitive and patterned manner.
- They can be unpredictable and fluctuate.

### Partial or focal generalized

- Spasmodic torticollis
- Blepharospasm
- Oromandibular dystonia
- Writer's cramp
- Hemiplegic dystonia after stroke
- Dystonia musculorum deformans (idiopathic torsion dystonia)
- Dopamine responsive dystonia: In childhood and generally involves the legs only.
- Drug-induced dystonia (metoclopramide, phenothiazine, haloperidol, chlorpromazine)
- Symptomatic dystonia (after encephalitis, Wilson's disease)

### Blepharospasm and oromandibular dystonia

Involuntary prolonged tight eye closure (blepharospasm) is associated with dystonia of mouth, tongue or jaw muscles (jaw clenching and tongue protrusion).

Writer's Cramp = Mogigraphia = Scrivener's Palsy

Symptoms usually appear when a person is trying to do a task that requires fine motor movements such as writing or playing a musical instrument.

### Q. What is the myokymia?

Myokymia, a form of involuntary muscular movement, usually can be visualized on the skin as vermicular or continuous rippling movements.

### Q. What is the akathisia?

Akathisia is a movement disorder characterized by a feeling of inner restlessness and a compelling need to be in constant motion, as well as by actions such as:

- Rocking while standing or sitting.
- Lifting the feet as if marching on the spot.
- Crossing and uncrossing the legs while sitting.

### Q. Describe restless legs syndrome/Ekbom's syndrome.

- Spontaneous, continuous leg movements associated with paresthesia.
- These sensations occur only at the rest and relieved by movement.
- **Causes:** Familial, lumbar root disease, polyneuropathy, renal failure, and iron deficiency.

### Q. What is the synkinesis/mirror movements?

Mirror movements are characterized by involuntary movements on one side of the body mirroring voluntary movements of the other side.

### Q. Which disease is an important cause of myoclonus in children in India which characteristically occurring in children and adolescent with past history of infectious disease?

**SSPE following measles:**

It causes progressive mental decline with poor scholastic performance, myoclonus, dystonia, mutism, spasticity and finally death in 2–5 years.

### Q. Which is the vascular cause of tremor associated with hemiplegia?

**Benedict's syndrome:** It is a midbrain syndrome involving third nerve nuclei, red nucleus, cerebrospinal tract, and brachium conjunctivum.

It is characterized by oculomotor palsy with contra lateral cerebellar ataxia tremors and corticospinal signs.

# SECTION 5

# Others

## Section Outline

- Approach to Anemia
- Approach to Jaundice
- Approach to Lymphadenopathy
- Approach to Edema
- Comprehensive Geriatric Assessment
- Approach to Arthritis

## Case 1: Approach to Anemia

### Brief History
A 35-year-old woman is seen for easy fatigue for many months. Lately, she has developed a taste for eating ice. She complains of menorrhagia since last 6 months. Her last childbirth was 1 year ago.

Family and past history are negative. She does not smoke or drink.

### Examination
Physical examination is positive for pale conjunctiva, spooning of nails, and a II/VI systolic murmur at left lower sternal border.

### Laboratory Investigations
- Complete blood count (CBC)—Hg 7.1 g/dL, Hct 23%, WBC 5,400/mm$^3$ (differential is normal), platelets, 450,000/mm$^3$
- Mean corpuscular volume (MCV) is 74 fl (normal 85–95 fl); red cell distribution width (RDW) is 19.1% (normal 13–15).
- Stools are negative for occult blood.

### Diagnosis
Iron deficiency anemia.

## DISCUSSION

### Q. What is the etiology of anemia?
Etiology of anemia depends on whether the anemia is hypoproliferative (i.e., corrected reticulocyte count <2%) or hyperproliferative (i.e., corrected reticulocyte count >2%).

### Q. What are the causes of microcytic hypochromic anemia?
- Iron deficiency anemia
- Anemia of chronic disease (AOCD)
- Sideroblastic anemia (may be associated with an elevated MCV as well, resulting in a dimorphic cell population)
- Thalassemia
- Lead poisoning.

The peripheral blood smear picture of microcytic hypochromic anemia is shown in **Figure 5.1**.

### Q. What are the causes of normocytic normochromic anemia?
- Anemia of chronic disease (AOCD)
- Renal failure
- Aplastic anemia
- Pure red cell aplasia
- Myelofibrosis or myelophthisic processes
- Multiple myeloma.

Macrocytic anemia can be caused by either a hypoproliferative disorder, hemolysis, or both. Thus,

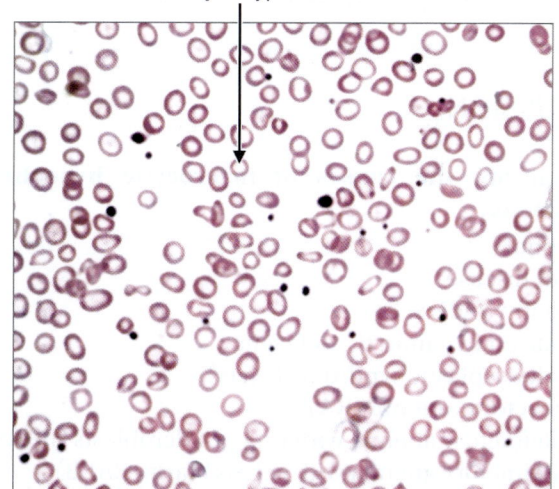

**Fig. 5.1:** Peripheral blood smear showing microcytic hypochromic.

it is important to calculate the corrected reticulocyte count when evaluating a patient with macrocytic anemia. In hypoproliferative macrocytic anemia, the corrected reticulocyte count is <2%, and the MCV is >100 fl. But, if the reticulocyte count is >2%, hemolytic anemia should be considered.

## Case 2: Approach to Anemia

*Brief History*
A 46-year-old male who consumes a strict vegetarian diet presented to hospital with history of easy fatiguability, exertional breathlessness associated with occasional left-sided chest pain. His symptoms were progressively increasing over the previous month. He had no history of any co-morbidities or addictions (alcohol/ smoking).

*Examination*
*General examination*
There was pallor. No jaundice/cyanosis/clubbing/pedal edema/ lymphadenopathy. There was evidence of glossitis. Knuckle pigmentation seen. He had no other features of nutritional deficiency.

*Vitals*
BP: 136/66, PR: 108/minute, RR: 20/minute. Venous hum could be heard over the neck.
*Systemic Examination*
- R/S: No abnormality detected.
- CVS: Apex beat was hyperdynamic. There was a midsystolic murmur over the left parasternal region near the pulmonary area. Murmur was not associated with thrill and was not radiating.
- P/A: No abnormality detected except for an old laparotomy scar.
- CNS: Romberg test was positive.

*Diagnosis*
Anemia with neuropathy possibly vitamin $B_{12}$ deficiency.

## DISCUSSION

**Q. What are the causes of macrocytic hypochromic anemias?**
- Alcohol
- Liver disease
- Hypothyroidism
- Folate and vitamin $B_{12}$ deficiency
- Myelodysplastic syndrome (MDS)
- **Refractory anemia (RA)**
  - Refractory anemia with ringed sideroblasts (RARS)
  - Refractory anemia with excess blasts (RAEB)
  - Refractory anemia with excess blasts in transformation
  - Chronic myelomonocytic leukemia (CMML)
  - Drug-induced
  - Diuretics
  - Chemotherapeutic agents
  - Hypoglycemic agents
  - Antiretroviral agents
  - Antimicrobials
  - Anticonvulsants

The peripheral blood smear picture of macrocytic hypochromic anemia is shown in **Figure 5.2**.

**Q. Classify anemia on basis red cell volume and plasma volume.**
The classification of anemia is shown in **Figure 5.3**.

**Q. What is hemolytic anemia? Classify with examples.**
Hemolytic anemia (HA) is divided into extravascular and intravascular causes.

**Extravascular hemolysis**
Red cells are prematurely removed from the circulation by the liver and spleen. This accounts for a majority of cases of HA.

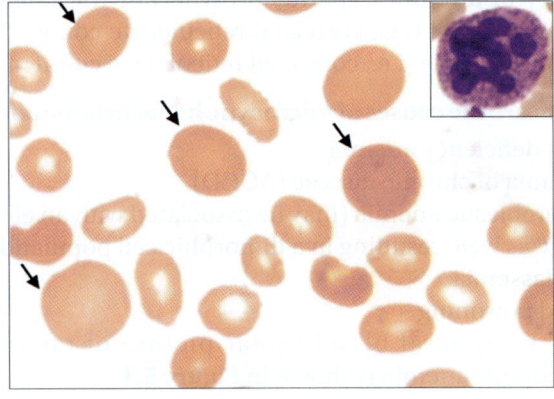

**Fig. 5.2:** Peripheral blood smear showing macro-ovalocytes.

*Hemoglobinopathies (sickle cell, thalassemias)*
- Enzymopathies (G6PD deficiency, pyruvate kinase deficiency)
- Membrane defects (hereditary spherocytosis, hereditary elliptocytosis)
- Drug-induced

**Intravascular hemolysis**
Red cells lyse within the circulation, and is less common.
- PNH
- AIHA
- Transfusion reactions
- MAHA
- DIC
- Infections
- Snake bites/venom.

**Q. What are the various sites of examination of anemia?**
- Conjunctiva **(Fig. 5.4)**
- Tongue
- Oral mucosa

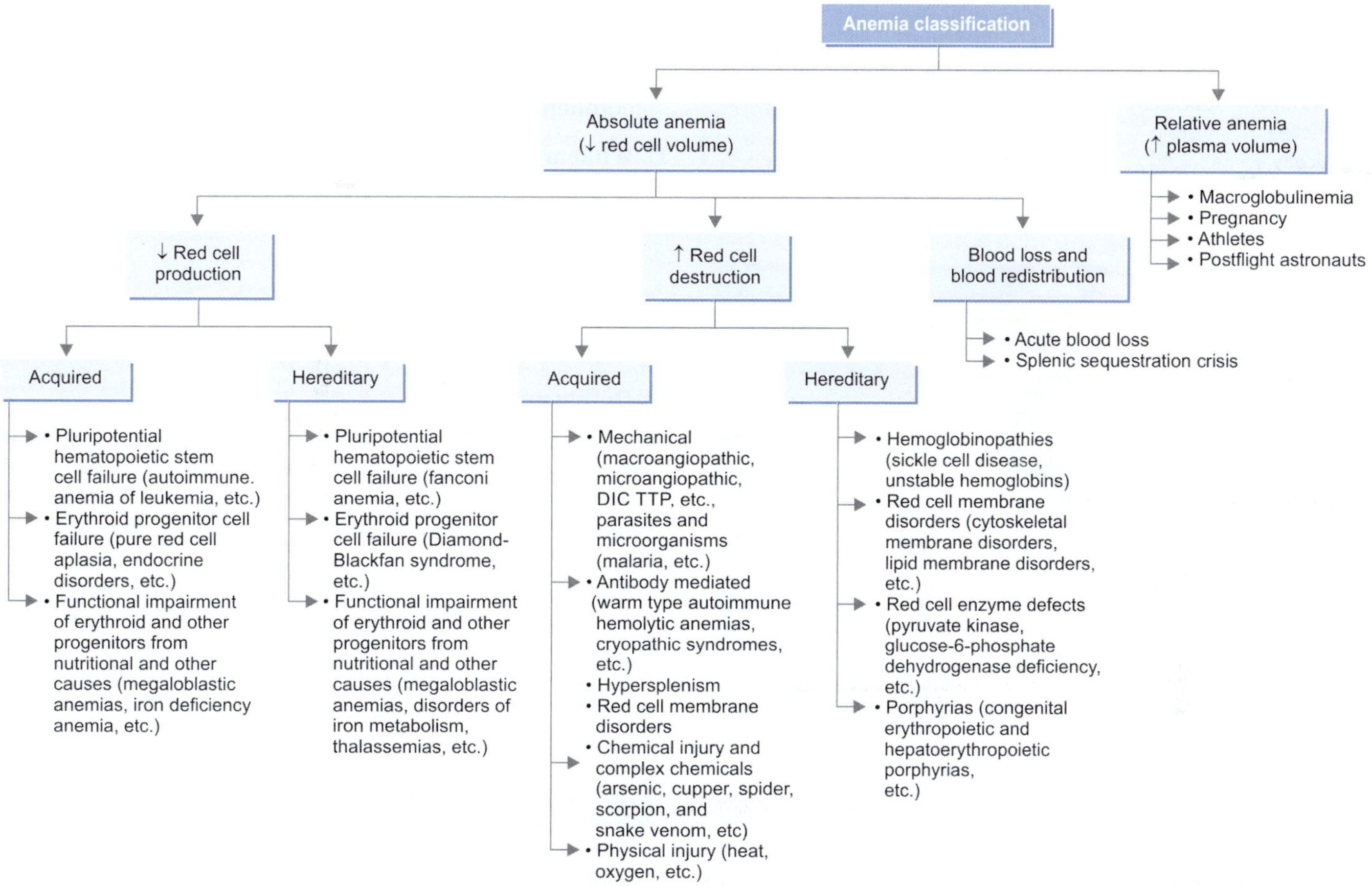

```
                            Anemia classification
                                     │
                ┌────────────────────┴────────────────────┐
       Absolute anemia                              Relative anemia
       (↓ red cell volume)                          (↑ plasma volume)
                │                                          │
                │                                          ├→ Macroglobulinemia
                │                                          ├→ Pregnancy
                │                                          ├→ Athletes
                │                                          └→ Postflight astronauts
    ┌───────────┼───────────┬──────────────┐
  ↓ Red cell   ↑ Red cell   Blood loss and
  production   destruction  blood redistribution
                                   │
                                   ├→ Acute blood loss
                                   └→ Splenic sequestration crisis
```

**Fig. 5.3:** Classification of anemia. Hypoproliferative anemias are further divided by the mean corpuscular volume into microcytic anemia (MCV <80 fl), normocytic anemia (MCV 80–100 fl), and macrocytic anemia (MCV >100 fl).

Under ↓ Red cell production:

*Acquired*
- Pluripotential hematopoietic stem cell failure (autoimmune anemia of leukemia, etc.)
- Erythroid progenitor cell failure (pure red cell aplasia, endocrine disorders, etc.)
- Functional impairment of erythroid and other progenitors from nutritional and other causes (megaloblastic anemias, iron deficiency anemia, etc.)

*Hereditary*
- Pluripotential hematopoietic stem cell failure (fanconi anemia, etc.)
- Erythroid progenitor cell failure (Diamond-Blackfan syndrome, etc.)
- Functional impairment of erythroid and other progenitors from nutritional and other causes (megaloblastic anemias, disorders of iron metabolism, thalassemias, etc.)

Under ↑ Red cell destruction:

*Acquired*
- Mechanical (macroangiopathic, microangiopathic, DIC TTP, etc., parasites and microorganisms (malaria, etc.)
- Antibody mediated (warm type autoimmune hemolytic anemias, cryopathic syndromes, etc.)
- Hypersplenism
- Red cell membrane disorders
- Chemical injury and complex chemicals (arsenic, cupper, spider, scorpion, and snake venom, etc)
- Physical injury (heat, oxygen, etc.)

*Hereditary*
- Hemoglobinopathies (sickle cell disease, unstable hemoglobins)
- Red cell membrane disorders (cytoskeletal membrane disorders, lipid membrane disorders, etc.)
- Red cell enzyme defects (pyruvate kinase, glucose-6-phosphate dehydrogenase deficiency, etc.)
- Porphyrias (congenital erythropoietic and hepatoerythropoietic porphyrias, etc.)

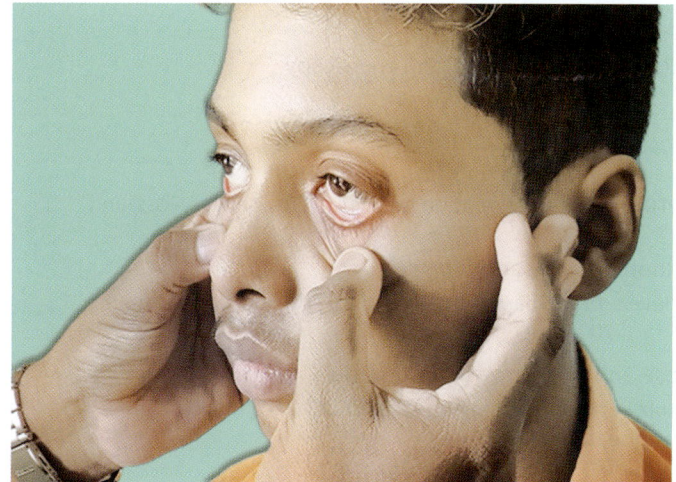

**Fig. 5.4:** Method of demonstration of pallor over conjunctiva.

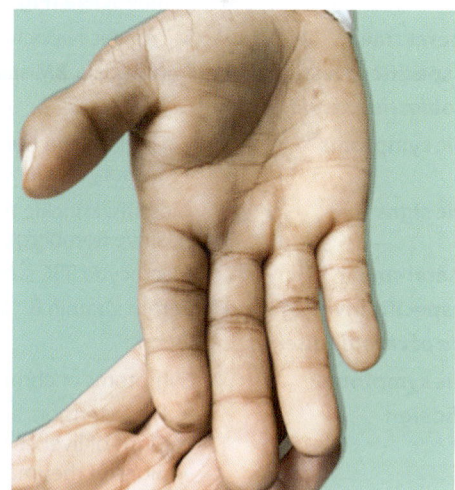

**Fig. 5.5:** Demonstration of pallor in hands.

- Palmar crease **(Fig. 5.5)**
- Nail bed (Hb <8 g/dL).

**Q. What are the grades of anemia/pallor?**
Refer **Table 5.1**.

**Q. How do you demonstrate cervical venous hum?**
Refer **Figure 5.6**.
- Auscultate the root of the neck on the right side with bell of stethoscope, with patient in standing or sitting position.
- A continuous murmur will be heard.

| Table 5.1: Grading of anemia/pallor. | | |
| --- | --- | --- |
| **Mild** | **Moderate** | **Severe** |
| Cannot be detected clinically | Clinically visible | Clinically visible plus one of the following features:<br>✦ Palmar crease disappearance<br>✦ Cervical venous hum (suggestive of chronic compensation) |

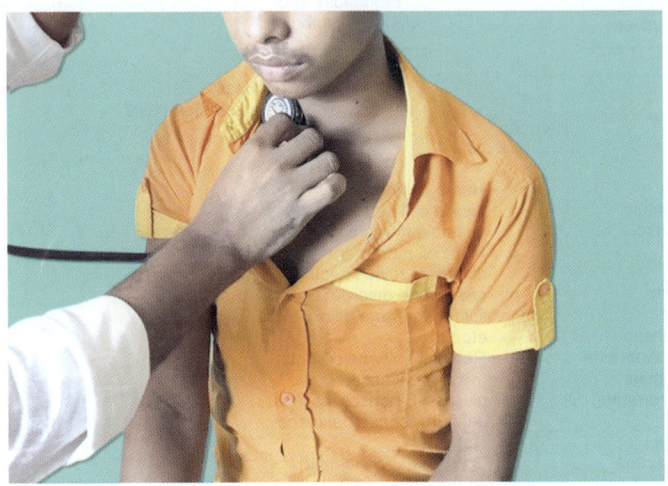

**Fig. 5.6:** Demonstration of cervical venous hum.

♦ The cervical venous hum was first described by Pontain and hence called **Pontain's murmur**.
♦ The presence of a cervical venous hum indicates chronic compensated severe anemia.

**Q. What are the conditions that cause pallor but anemia is absent?**
♦ Hypopituitarism
♦ Hypothyroidism
♦ Hypogonadism
♦ Shock
♦ Left heart failure.

**Q. Define anemia.**
Anemia is defined as decrease in circulating red blood cell (RBC) mass. It is characterized by decrease of hemoglobin concentration (Hb)/RBC count/hematocrit [packed cell volume (PCV)] below normal for the patient's age, sex, and altitude of residence.

Normal adult hemoglobin level is in the range of 13–17 g/dL in males and 12–15 g/dL in females.

**Q. What are the various clues for the etiology of different anemias?**
Refer **Table 5.2**.

| Table 5.2: Clues for etiology of anemia. | |
| --- | --- |
| *Iron deficiency anemia* | |
| Specific symptoms | Pica, dysphagia, restless leg syndrome, and melena |
| Specific signs | ✦ Bald tongue (**Fig. 5.7**)<br>✦ Koilonychia (**Fig. 5.8**)<br>✦ Blue sclera (**Fig. 5.9**) |
| Peripheral smear | Microcytic hypochromic red cells |
| Other specific investigation | Iron studies, BM staining for iron, stool/urine for occult blood, and endoscopy |
| *Megaloblastic anemia* | |
| Specific symptoms | ✦ Tingling and numbness<br>✦ Sensory ataxia |
| Specific signs | Glossitis, knuckle pigmentation (**Fig. 5.10**), absent deep tendon reflexes (DTRs), sensory loss, and positive Romberg's test |
| Peripheral smear | Macrocytic RBC's, hypersegmented neutrophils, and pancytopenia |
| Other specific investigation | Serum vitamin $B_{12}$ levels, red cell folate levels, bone marrow examination, and Schilling's test |
| *Anemia of chronic disease* | |
| Specific symptoms | Symptoms of chronic kidney, liver disease, and connective tissue disorders |
| Specific sign | ✦ Hypertension, arteriovenous (AV) fistula— chronic kidney disease (CKD)<br>✦ Signs of liver cell failure—chronic liver disease (CLD)<br>✦ Signs of rheumatoid arthritis, systemic lupus erythematosus (SLE), etc. |
| Peripheral smear | Normocytic normochromic anemia ± pancytopenia |
| Other specific investigation | Renal function test, liver function tests, autoantibodies, and raised serum ferritin |
| *Hemolytic anemia* | |
| Specific symptoms | History of associated jaundice, developmental delay, family history positivity, recurrent blood transfusions, and gallstones |
| Specific signs | ✦ Triad of anemia + jaundice + splenomegaly<br>✦ Hemolytic (Chipmunk) facies (**Fig. 5.11**)<br>✦ Hyperpigmentation) (**Fig. 5.12**), short stature, and leg ulcers |

| Peripheral smear | <ul><li>Microcytic hypochromic (thalassemia)</li><li>Microspherocytes (hereditary spherocytosis)</li><li>Sickle cells</li><li>Reticulocytosis</li></ul> |
|---|---|
| Other specific investigation | Hemoglobin electrophoresis, Coombs test, sickling test, and osmotic fragility |

*Aplastic anemia*

| Specific symptoms | <ul><li>Recurrent infections</li><li>Bleeding manifestations</li></ul> |
|---|---|
| Specific signs | <ul><li>Signs of pancytopenia</li><li>No organomegaly</li></ul> |
| Peripheral smear | Pancytopenia |
| Other specific investigation | <ul><li>Bone marrow examination</li><li>Cytogenetics</li></ul> |

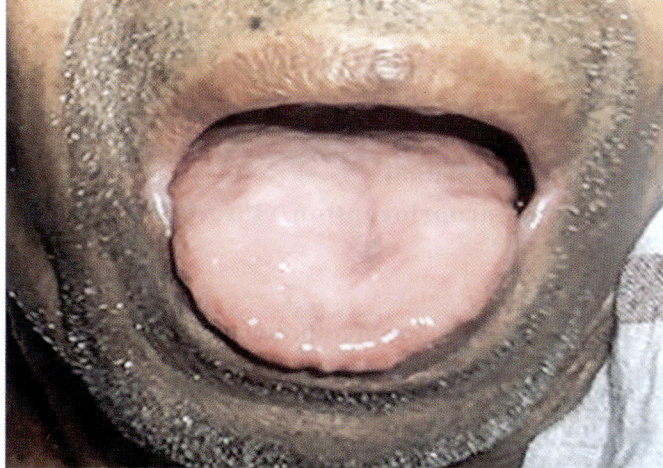

**Fig. 5.7:** Bald tongue.

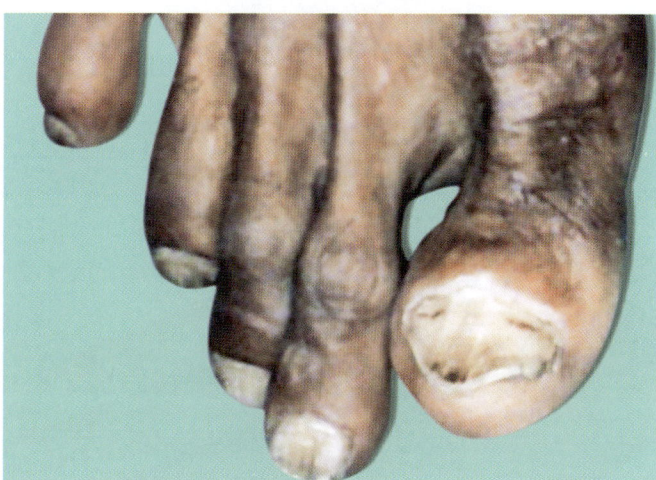

**Fig. 5.8:** Koilonychia.

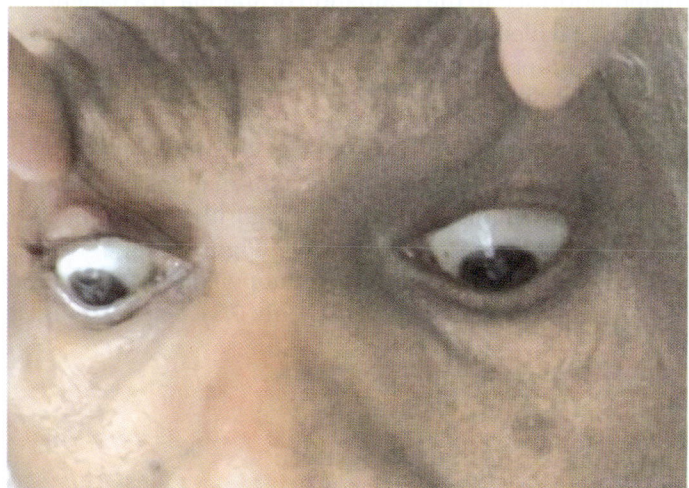

**Fig. 5.9:** Blue sclera.

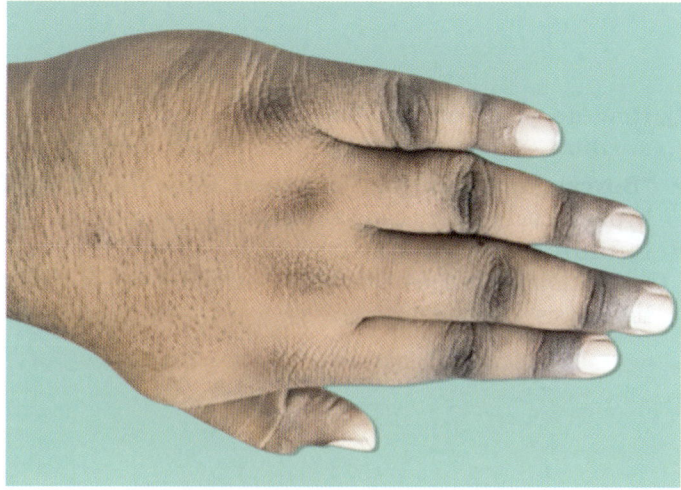

**Fig. 5.10:** Knuckle pigmentation.

# SECTION 5: Others

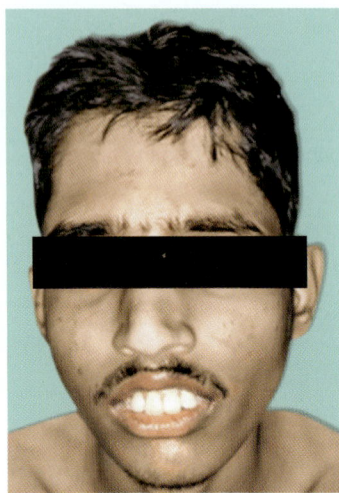

**Fig. 5.11:** Chipmunk facies.

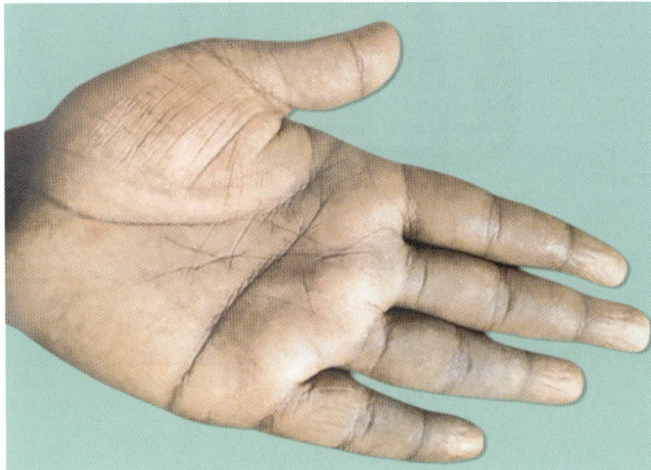

**Fig. 5.12:** Hyperpigmentation of palm.

**Q. How do you perform the systemic examination in anemia?**

- **"Boxcars" or "sausaging" of retinal veins:** Suggestive of hyperviscosity which can be seen in myelofibrosis
- **Jaundice**-elevated bilirubin is seen in several hemoglobinopathies, liver diseases and other forms of hemolysis

- **Lymphadenopathy:** Suggestive of lymphoma or leukemia
- **Glossitis (inflammation of the tongue) and cheilitis (swollen patches on the corners of the mouth):** Iron/folate deficiency, alcoholism, pernicious anemia.

### Abdominal examination
- **Splenomegaly:** Hemolysis, lymphoma, leukemia, myelofibrosis.
- **Hepatomegaly:** Alcohol, myelofibrosis.
- **Scar from gastrectomy:** Decreased absorptive surface with the loss of the terminal ileum leads to vitamin $B_{12}$ deficiency.
- **Scar from cholecystectomy:** Cholesterol and pigmented gallstones are commonly seen in sickle cell anemia are hereditary spherocytosis.

### Cardiovascular examination
- Tachycardia
- Systolic flow murmur
- Severe anemia may lead to high output heart failure

### Neurologic examination
- **Decreased proprioception/vibration:** Vitamin $B_{12}$ deficiency.

### Skin
- **Pallor of the mucous membranes/nail bed or palmar creases:** Suggests hemoglobin <9 mg/dL.
- **Petechiae:** Thrombocytopenia, vasculitis
- Dermatitis herpetiformis (in iron deficiency due to malabsorption—celiac disease)
- **Koilonychia (spooning of the nails):** Iron deficiency

### Rectal and pelvic examination
These examinations are usually overlooked and underperformed in the evaluation of anemia. If a patient has heavy rectal bleeding, one must evaluate for the presence of hemorrhoids or hard masses that suggest neoplasm as causes of bleeding.

**Q. What are the laboratory investigations in anemia?**

Different laboratory investigations for diagnosis of anemia are shown in **Figure 5.13** and the algorithmic approach to different type of anemias is shown in **Figure 5.14**.

For the diagnosis of specific hematopoietic disorders, there are some other laboratory tests **(Table 5.3)**.

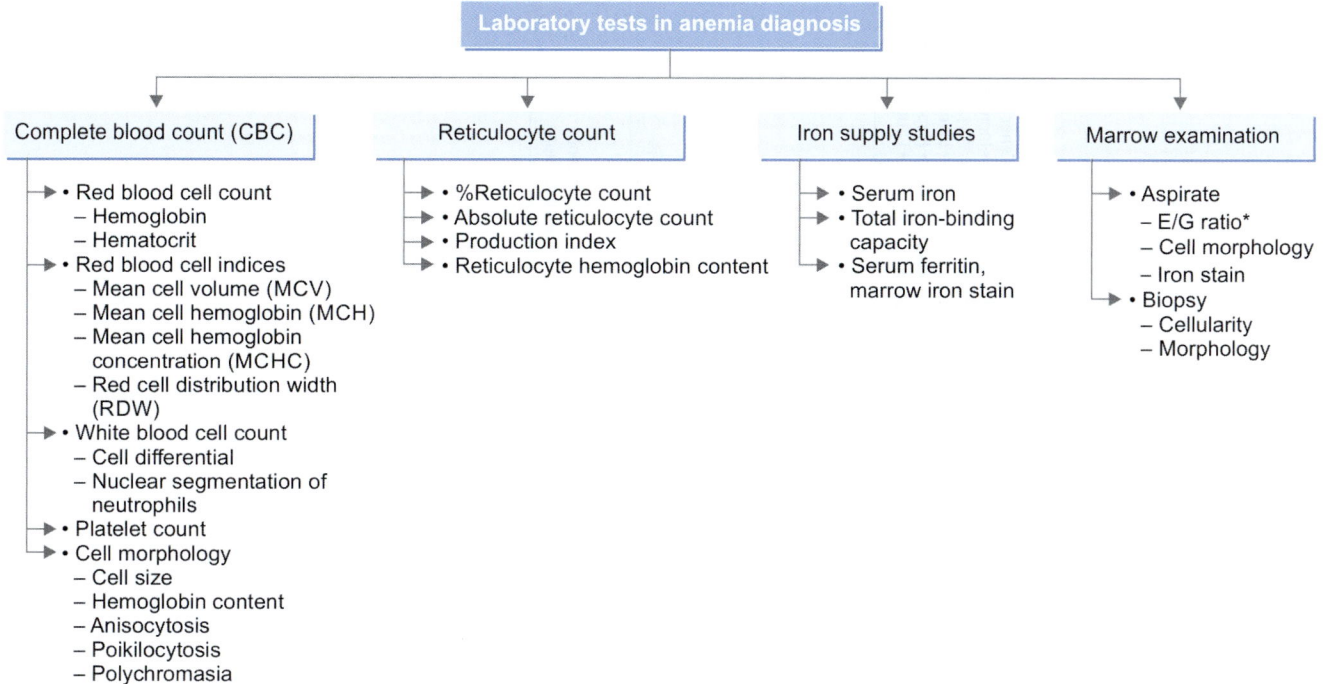

**Fig. 5.13:** Laboratory tests in anemia.
*E/G ratio, ratio of erythroid to granulocytic precursors.

| Table 5.3: Investigations required in certain subtypes of anemia. | | |
|---|---|---|
| *Hypoproliferative anemias* | *Maturation disorders* | *Hemolytic anemias* |
| ✦ **\*Cytometric assay of CD59/CD55 levels (paroxysmal nocturnal hemoglobinuria)**<br>✦ **Chromosomal analysis (leukemias)**<br>✦ **Marrow aspirate/biopsy special stains**<br>  – **Trichrome stain, silver stain for reticulin (myelofibrosis)** | ✦ Serum vitamin $B_{12}$ level (vitamin $B_{12}$ deficiency)<br>✦ Serum RBC folate level (folic acid deficiency)<br>✦ Hb electrophoresis (abnormal hemoglobins)<br>✦ Hb $A_2$ level-HPLC (β-thalassemia)<br>✦ Hb F level-HPLC (β-thalassemia) RBC protoporphyrin level (iron deficiency) Brilliant cresyl blue stain | ✦ Hb electrophoresis and HPLC (hemoglobinopathies)<br>✦ Coombs test (autoimmune hemolytic anemia)<br>✦ Cold agglutinin titer (autoimmune hemolytic anemia)<br>✦ Haptoglobin level (hemolysis)<br>✦ G6PD screen (G6PD deficiency |

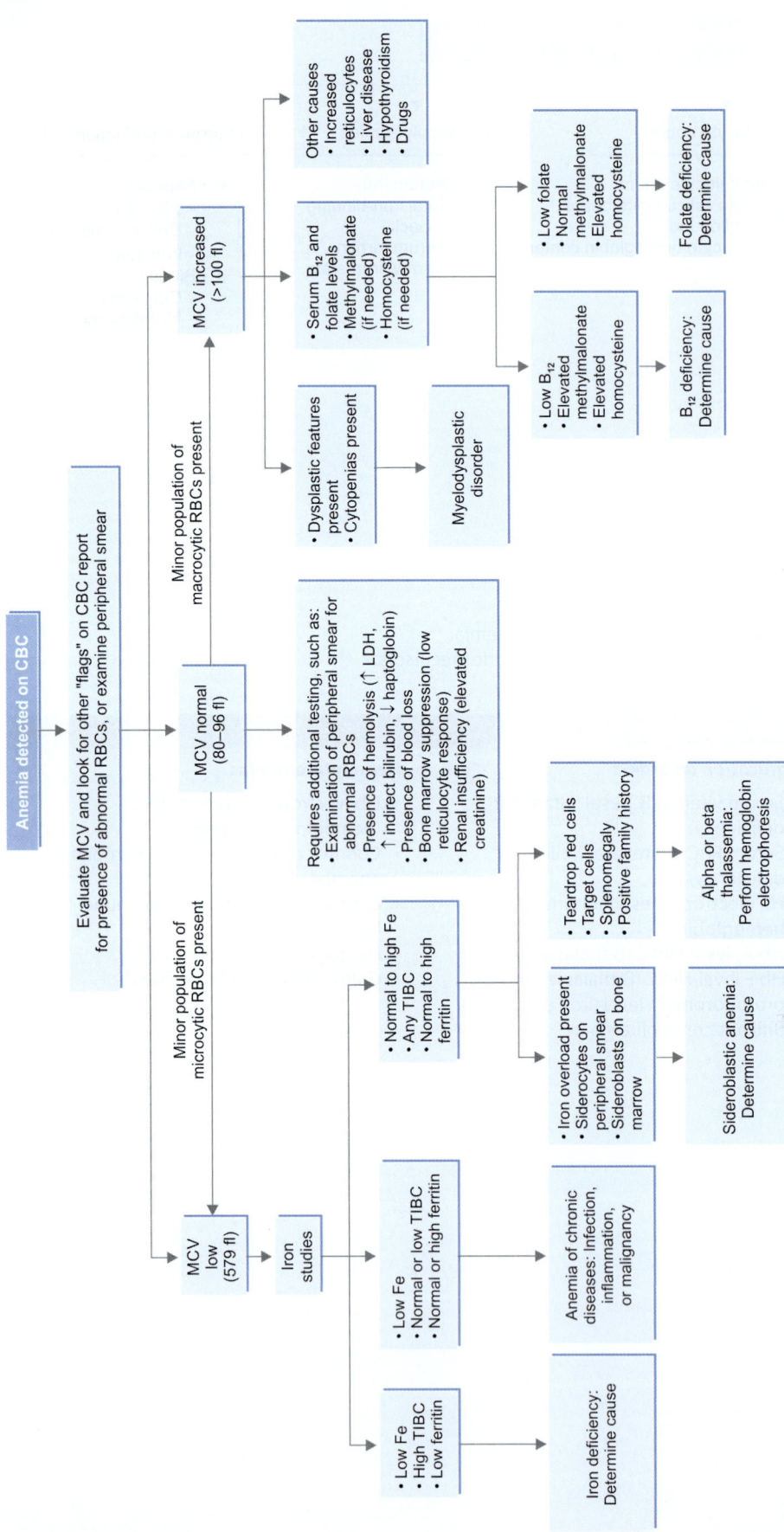

**Fig. 5.14:** Algorithm for diagnosis of anemia based on complete blood count.

[CBC: complete blood count; MCV: mean corpuscular volume; RBCs: red blood cells; Fe: iron; TIBC: total iron-binding capacity (trasferrin); LDH: lactate dehydrogenase]

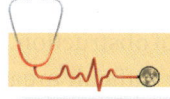

## Case 3: Approach to Jaundice

**Brief History**
Elderly male poorly built and nourished

**Examination**
- Weight—43 kg, height—172 cm, BMI—14.8 kg/m²
- Vitals stable
- Emaciated with small muscle wasting of hands and foot
- Pallor+, deep icterus (orange yellow), no cyanosis, no clubbing or pedal edema
- No signs of liver cell failure
- Scratch marks + (suggestive of pruritus)
- Left supraclavicular lymph nodes +

**P/A Examination**
- Scaphoid abdomen
- Hepatomegaly + 2 cm below the left coastal margin
- Liver span of 12 cm
- Gallbladder palpable 4 cm below the left costal margin
- No spleen
- Bowel sounds +

**Diagnosis**
A case of obstructive jaundice probably an intra-abdominal malignancy.

## DISCUSSION

### Q. How to differentiate between jaundice and carotenemia?

In hypercarotenemia (also known as carotenemia), the skin has a yellow-orange color, but the eyes do not, in jaundice, both the eyes and skin have a yellowish color.

### Q. How do you see icterus?

Icterus is seen in bright natural daylight by retracting the upper eyelids upwards and asking the patient to look downwards.

### Q. What is the cause for unilateral icterus?
- Hemiplegia
- In the presence of unilateral edema.
- Yellowish discoloration in one eye when the other eye is artificial.

### Q. What are the causes of blue sclera?
- Pseudoxanthoma elasticum
- Osteogenesis imperfecta
- Ehlers-Danlos syndrome
- Marfan's syndrome
- Alkaptonuria
- Hypophosphatasia
- Diamond-Blackfan anemia
- Juvenile Paget's disease
- Normal in newborns
- Van der Hoeve's syndrome

### Q. Name bile salts and bile pigments.

**Bile salts:** Sodium taurocholate, sodium glycocholate
**Bile pigments:** Bilirubin, biliverdin.

### Q. Why does pruritus develop in obstructive jaundice?

It is proposed that cholestasis leads to release of pruritogens from the liver; this stimulates neural itch fibers in the skin, which transmit the stimulus to the spinal cord and subsequently the brain. Pruritogens accumulating in the plasma of patients with cholestasis may also enter the brain and alter neurotransmission **(Fig. 5.15)**.

**Pruritogens**
- Lysophosphatidic acid
- Bile salts and bile acids
- Opioids
- Progesterone metabolite.

### Q. Enumerate the cholestatic conditions that manifest as jaundice.

Conditions producing cholestasis are shown in **Box 5.1**.

**Box 5.1:** Conditions producing cholestasis.

**Intrahepatic**
- Viral hepatitis
  - Fibrosing cholestatic hepatitis—hepatitis B and C
  - Hepatitis A, Epstein-Barr virus, cytomegalovirus
- Alcoholic hepatitis
- Drug toxicity
  - Pure cholestasis—anabolic and contraceptive steroids
  - Cholestatic hepatitis—chlorpromazine, erythromycin estolate
  - Chronic cholestasis—chlorpromazine and prochlorperazine
- Primary biliary cirrhosis
- Primary sclerosing cholangitis
- Vanishing bile duct syndrome
  - Chronic rejection of liver transplants
  - Sarcoidosis
  - Drugs
- Inherited
  - Progressive familial intrahepatic cholestasis
  - Benign recurrent cholestasis
- Cholestasis of pregnancy
- Total parenteral nutrition
- Nonhepatobiliary sepsis
- Benign postoperative cholestasis

- Paraneoplastic syndrome
- Veno-occlusive disease
- Graft-versus-host disease
- Infiltrative disease
  - TB
  - Lymphoma
  - Amyloidosis
- Infections
  - Malaria
  - Leptospirosis

**Extrahepatic**
- Malignant
  - Cholangiocarcinoma
  - Pancreatic cancer
  - Gallbladder cancer
  - Ampullary cancer
  - Malignant involvement of the porta hepatis lymph nodes
- Benign
  - Choledocholithiasis
  - Postoperative biliary structures
  - Primary sclerosing cholangitis
  - Chronic pancreatitis
  - AIDS cholangiopathy
  - Mirizzi syndrome
  - Parasitic disease (ascariasis)

**Q. What are the different imaging modalities for the diagnosis of jaundice?**

The ultrasound is inexpensive, does not expose the patient to ionizing radiation, and can detect dilation of the intra and extrahepatic biliary tree with a high degree of sensitivity and specificity. The absence of biliary dilatation suggests intrahepatic cholestasis, while the presence of biliary dilatation indicates extrahepatic cholestasis. False-negative results occur in patients with partial obstruction of the common bile duct or in patients with cirrhosis or primary sclerosing cholangitis (PSC) where scarring prevents the intrahepatic ducts from dilating.

Although ultrasonography may indicate extrahepatic cholestasis, it rarely identifies the site or cause of obstruction. The distal common bile duct is a particularly difficult area to visualize by ultrasound because of overlying bowel gas. Appropriate next tests include CT, magnetic resonance cholangiopancreatography (MRCP), and endoscopic retrograde cholangiopancreatography (ERCP). CT scanning and MRCP are better than ultrasonography for assessing the head of the pancreas and for identifying choledocholithiasis in the distal common bile duct, particularly when the ducts are not dilated. ERCP is the "gold standard" for identifying choledocholithiasis.

**Q. What is primary biliary cirrhosis?**

It is an autoimmune disease predominantly of middle aged women in which there is a progressive destruction of interlobular bile ducts. The diagnosis is made by the presence of the antimitochondrial antibody that is found in 95% of patients.

**Q. What is primary sclerosing cholangitis?**

It is characterized by the destruction and fibrosis of larger bile ducts. The disease may involve only the intrahepatic ducts and present as intrahepatic cholestasis. However, in 95% of patients with PSC, both intra- and extrahepatic ducts are involved. The diagnosis of PSC is made by imaging the biliary tree. The pathognomonic findings are multiple strictures of bile ducts with dilatations proximal to the strictures. Approximately 75% of patients with PSC have inflammatory bowel disease.

**Q. Evaluation of a patient with jaundice.**
Refer **Figure 5.16**.

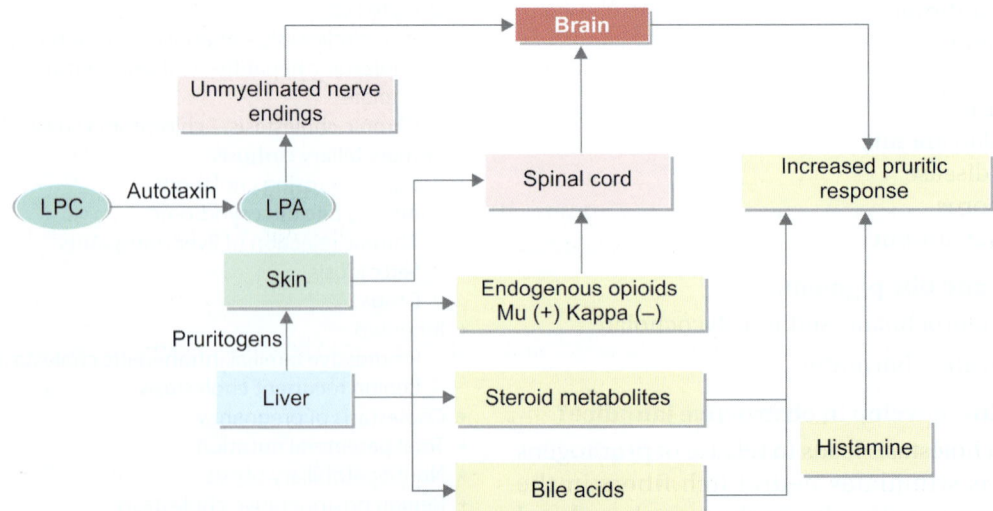

**Fig. 5.15:** Pruritus in cholestasis.

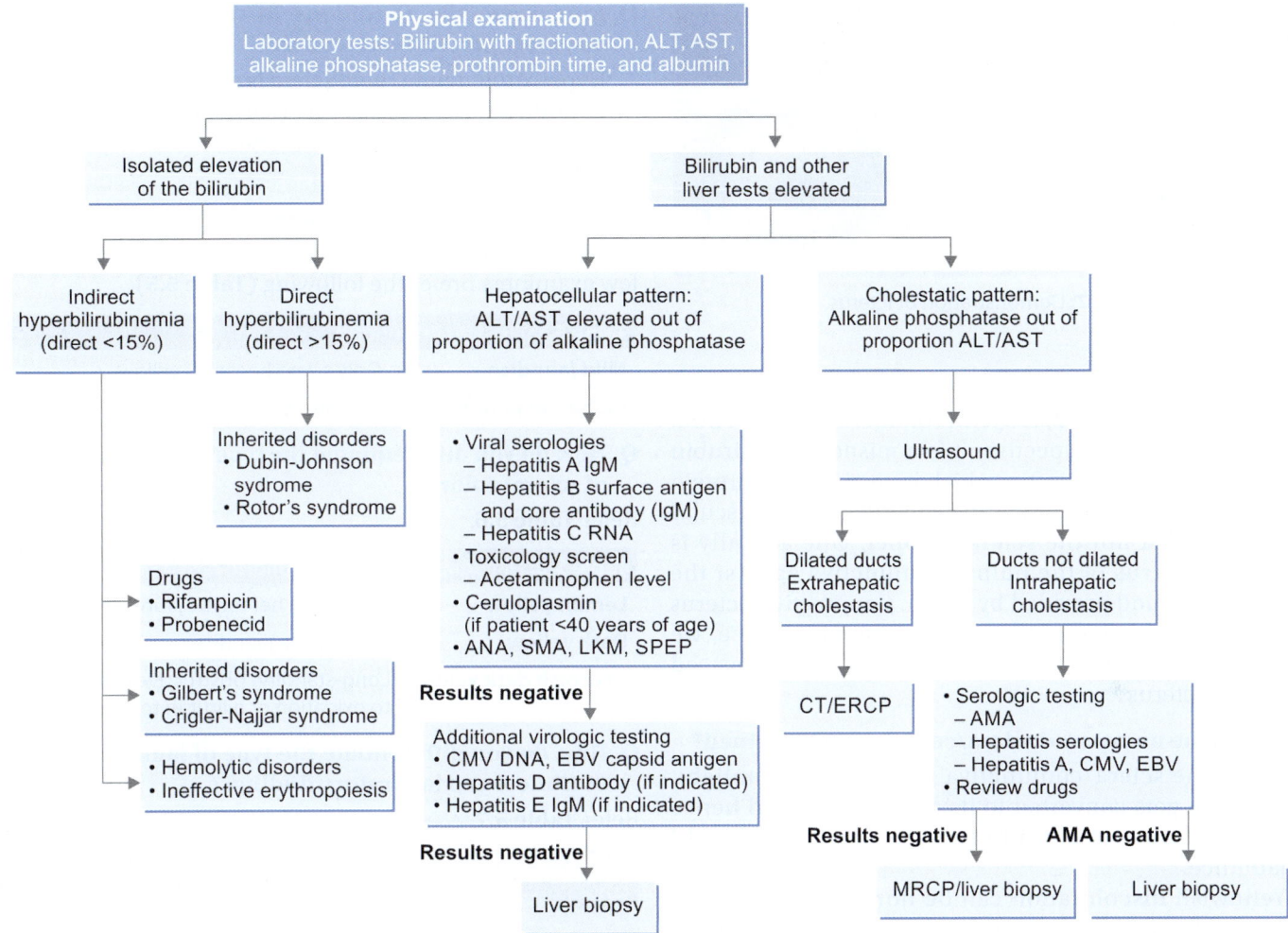

**Fig. 5.16:** Algorithm for deranged liver function tests.

### Q. What is Virchow's node?

In 1849, Rudolf Ludwig Karl Virchow, noted the involvement of remote lymph nodes in intra-abdominal cancers. 40 years later, Troisier, reporting several cases of intra-abdominal malignancy where supraclavicular lymph nodes were the only external indication of cancer, coined the term Virchow's node to describe this finding. In current usage, Virchow's node refers to a left supraclavicular lymph node that is the harbinger of an abdominal malignancy. It should be remembered that inflammatory and infectious abdominal processes can also lead an enlarged left supraclavicular lymph nodes.

The thoracic duct drainage has been implicated for the involvement of left supraclavicular lymph nodes. The thoracic duct drains the left jugular, left subclavian, and left mediastinal lymph nodes superiorly. Inferiorly, the thoracic duct drains the intercostal lymphatics, and via the cisterna chyli, the lower intercostal, gastric, superior mesenteric, inferior mesenteric, lumbar, and internal and external iliac lymphatics.

The left supraclavicular lymph nodes drain into the thoracic duct via short lymphatic channels draining into the left jugular lymphatics. Reflux into the left supraclavicular lymph nodes from the thoracic duct is relatively easy, occurs in half of patients with unobstructed lymphatic drainage, and is the proposed etiology of Virchow's node.

The right-sided lymphatic drainage, on the other hand, is not from the abdomen, being predominantly from the right subclavian, right mediastinal, and right jugular vessels.

### Q. Define icterus.

Yellowish discoloration of skin, mucous membranes, sclera, and blood vessels secondary to increased bilirubin (bile pigments have affinity for elastin tissue).

### Q. What are the sites to look for jaundice/icterus?

- Sclera **(Fig. 5.17)**
- Sublingual mucosa
- Oral cavity
- Palms and soles
- Skin.

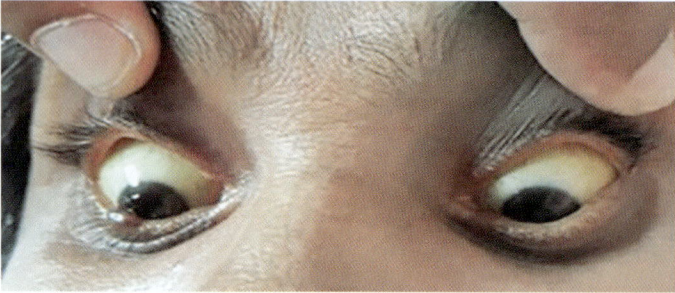

Fig. 5.17: Demonstration of icterus.

### Q. What is scleral icterus?

Scleral icterus **(Fig. 5.18)** is a term commonly used but from a histopathologic perspective, it is a misnomer. Bilirubin has a high affinity for elastin, which is an abundant protein in the conjunctivae as well as the superficial, fibrovascular episclerae, but not the sclerae proper. One actually is observing icterus of the bulbar conjunctiva against the white background provided by sclera. Conjunctival icterus is often the first sign of hyperbilirubinemia. Hence, we recommended the use of term "conjunctival icterus" instead of "scleral icterus".

### Q. Why is the unexposed sclera/conjunctiva examined?

- When the sclera/conjunctiva is exposed to sunlight, bilirubin gets converted to its soluble form and hence exposed part of conjunctiva may not reveal mild jaundice.
- Yellowish discoloration can be normally seen in the exposed parts of sclera/conjunctiva which is called as muddy sclera/conjunctiva.

### Q. How do you diagnose clinical types of jaundice on basis serum bilirubin level?

Refer **Table 5.4**.

| Table 5.4: Serum bilirubin levels and jaundice. | |
|---|---|
| 0.3–1.2 mg/dL | Normal |
| 1.2–2.5 mg/dL | Latent jaundice (generally not appreciated on clinical examination) |
| >2.5 mg/dL | Clinically appreciated |

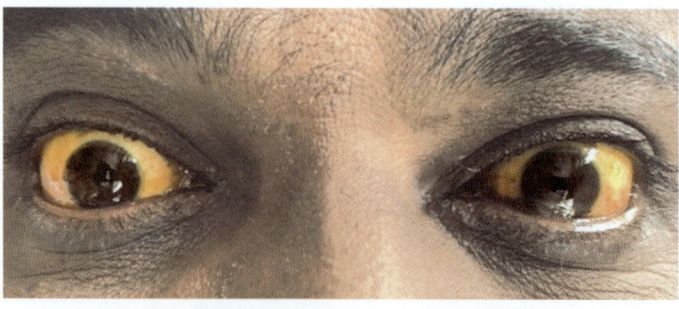

Fig. 5.18: Dark yellow icterus.

### Q. Enumerate the conditions in which there is yellow discoloration without jaundice.

- Hypercarotenemia (here sclera is not affected)
- Hypothyroidism (due to decreased metabolism of carotene)
- Excessive exposure to phenols/nitric acid
- Quinacrine intake.

### Q. What is the grading of jaundice?

**Grading:** No standard grading system is available; however, few examiners prefer the following **(Table 5.5)**:

| Table 5.5: Grading of jaundice. | |
|---|---|
| Mild jaundice | Only sclera becomes yellow |
| Moderate jaundice | Skin also becomes yellow |

### Q. How do you differentiated the type of jaundice on basis of scleral color?

Refer **Table 5.6**.

| Table 5.6: Differentiating type of jaundice based on scleral color. | |
|---|---|
| Lemon yellow | Most likely hemolytic jaundice |
| Dark yellow | Obstructive jaundice |
| Greenish dark yellow | Long-standing obstructive jaundice due to oxidation of bilirubin to biliverdin |

### Q. How do you differentiate the type of jaundice on basis of clinical and laboratory findings?

Refer **Table 5.7**.

| Table 5.7: Differentiating jaundice based on clinical and laboratory findings. | | | |
|---|---|---|---|
| | *Prehepatic (hemolytic)* | *Hepatic* | *Posthepatic (obstructive/ surgical)* |
| **History** | | | |
| Urine | Normal | Yellow | Yellow |
| Stools | Normal | Normal | Pale clay like |
| Pruritus | – | ± | ++ |
| **Examination** | | | |
| Bradycardia | – | – | + |
| Pallor | Present | Absent | Absent |
| Jaundice | Mild | Moderate | Severe |
| Splenomegaly | Present | Variable | Absent |
| Palpable gallbladder | ± | – | ++ |
| Features of liver cell failure | Absent | + (early feature) | ± (late feature) |
| **Laboratory data** | | | |
| Serum bilirubin | UCB | UCB↑ + CB | CB |
| Serum enzymes | LDH | AST↑ ALT | ALP |

|  | *Prehepatic (hemolytic)* | *Hepatic* | *Posthepatic (obstructive/ surgical)* |
|---|---|---|---|
| Urine bilirubin | – | + | + |
| Urine urobilinogen | + | + | – |
| Examples | • Thalassemia Sickle cell anemia<br>• Spherocytosis<br>• Malaria<br>• Immune hemolytic anemias | • Hepatitis (viral/ alcoholic/ drug-induced)<br>• Infiltrative disorders<br>• Ischemic hepatitis | • CBD stones<br>• Helminths in the CBD<br>• Carcinoma—head of pancreas<br>• Primary biliary cirrhosis<br>• Primary sclerosing cholangitis |

(AST: aspartate aminotransferase; ALP: alkaline phosphatase; CB; conjugated bilirubin; CBD: common bile duct; LDH: lactate dehydrogenase; UCB: unconjugated bilirubin)

**Q. Enumerate the conditions in which jaundice and anemia coexist.**
- Vitamin $B_{12}$ deficiency
- Hereditary spherocytosis
- Thalassemia major
- Sickle cell anemia

**Q. What are the causes of pulsatile liver?**
- Tricuspid regurgitation
- Aortic regurgitation
- Hemangioma of liver/arteriovenous fistula in liver

**Q. What are the causes of tender liver?**
- Acute viral hepatitis
- Congestive cardiac failure
- Pyogenic or amoebic liver abscess
- Acute Budd-Chiari syndrome
- Carcinoma of liver
- Hepatic infarct
- Cholangiohepatitis

**Q. What are the features seen on clinical examination of hemolytic jaundice?**

Refer **Figure 5.19**.
- Anemia
- Icterus
- Rashes
- Ulcers
- Cholecystectomy scar

**Q. What are the complications of hemolytic anemia?**
- Pigmented gallstones
- Chronic leg ulcers
- Severe anemia may cause heart failure.

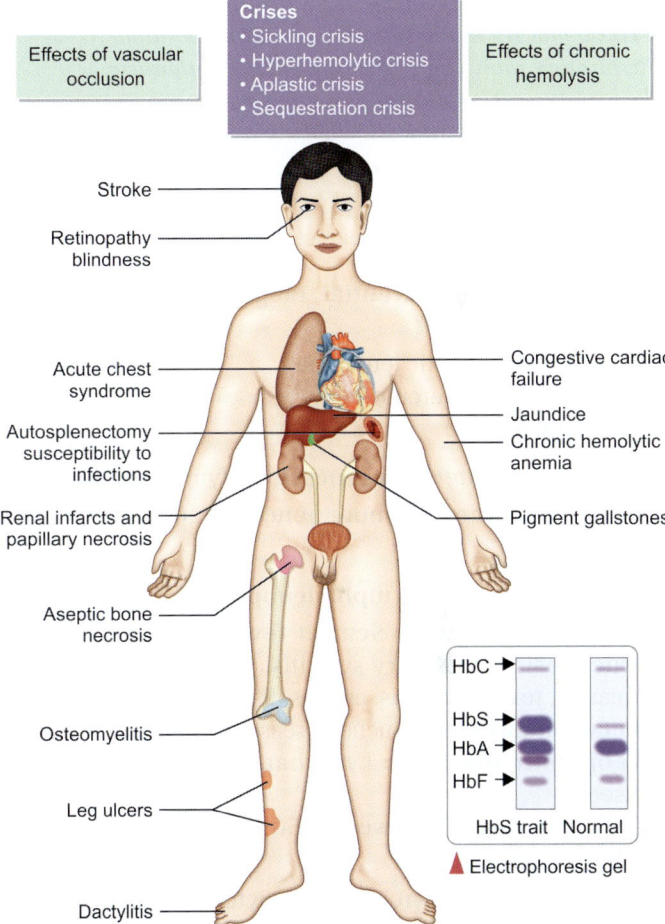

**Fig. 5.19:** Physical manifestation of hemolytic anemia.

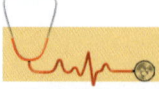

## Case 4: Approach to Lymphadenopathy

*Brief History*
A 50-year-old male, moderately built and nourished.

*Examination*
Height: 169 cm
Weight: 52 kg
BMI: 18.18
Pulse: 89/mt, regular, normal volume and character, all peripheral pulses well felt, no radiofemoral delay.
BP: 110/60 mm Hg in the right arm in supine position and 110/60 mm Hg in the right arm in sitting position.
Respiratory rate: 18/mt, regular, abdominothoracic.
Temperature: 97.4°F at right axilla.
No pallor, icterus, cyanosis, clubbing and edema.

*Generalized lymphadenopathy:* Bilateral cervical (posterior cervical, freely mobile, non- tender), right supraclavicular, bilateral axillary (4 × 4 cm, matted, L>R, non-tender), bilateral epitrochlear, bilateral inguinal (both horizontal and vertical) PER.

*Abdominal Examination:*
Hepatomegaly + palpable 5 cm below right costal margin, firm, surface smooth moves with respiration.
Splenomegaly + palpable 9 cm below left costal margin, consistency firm, notch felt.
Liver span 18 cm, bowel sounds +, no bruit.
Diagnosis: Generalized lymphadenopathy.

## DISCUSSION

**Q. What are the differential diagnosis of generalized lymphadenopathy?**
- Chronic lymphocytic leukemia
- Disseminated tuberculosis
- Retroviral disease

**Q. What are the criteria for generalized lymphadenopathy?**
Involvement of three or more noncontiguous lymph node areas.

**Causes of generalized lymphadenopathy**
- **Infectious disease:** Scarlet fever, rheumatic fever, brucellosis, secondary syphilis, rubella, tuberculosis, measles, toxoplasmosis, chagas disease, kala-azar, AIDS
- **Metabolic diseases:** Gaucher disease, Niemann-Pick disease
- **Neoplastic diseases:** Lymphatic leukemia, Hodgkin disease
- **Collagen vascular disease:** Still disease, rheumatoid arthritis, SLE

**Other causes:** Hyperthyroidism, phenytoin uses, amyloidosis, sarcoidosis.

**Q. What are the criteria for significant lymphadenopathy?**
- Any lymph node of size >2.25 cm
- Tender hard, firm, fixed, or any lesion in draining lymph node

**Q. Name the causes of hepatosplenomegaly with generalized lymphadenopathy.**
- Lymphoma
- Chronic lymphocytic leukemia
- Disseminated tuberculosis
- Systemic lupus erythematosus (SLE)
- Sarcoid
- Felty's syndrome.

**Q. What is primary complex?**
It is usually a unit comprising of the focus of primary tuberculosis and infected draining lymph nodes in any organ.

**Q. What is Ghon's focus and Ghon's complex?**
**Ghon's focus:** Focus of primary in lung is usually subpleural in middle (upper region of lower lobe or lower portion of middle lobe when on right side).
**Ghon's complex:** Ghon's focus and tracheobronchial lymph nodes.

**Q. What is the fate of a primary complex?**
- Resolve
- Progressive primary disease
- Tuberculosis pneumonia
- Cavity/calcification/scar
- Miliary tuberculosis

**Q. What is the mechanism of hepatic involvement in tuberculosis?**
- Congenital tuberculosis
- Primary hepatic tuberculosis
- Disseminated tuberculosis
- Tuberculoma
- Tuberculosis of biliary tract
- Hepatic failure
- Granulomatous tuberculosis.
Hepatic granuloma most common causes is tuberculosis, sarcoidosis.

**Q. What is the mechanism of splenic involvement in tuberculosis?**
- Disseminated tuberculosis
- Associated with hematological malignancy
- Isolated splenic tuberculosis.
Splenic involvement most commonly encountered in HIV positive individual.

Isolated splenic tuberculosis is rare, clinical case may present as splenic abscess.

### Q. List the clinical differences in lymphadenopathy.
Refer **Table 5.8**.

**Table 5.8:** Lymphadenopathy.

|  | Metastasis in | Lymphoma | Tuberculosis | Syphilis |
|---|---|---|---|---|
| Size | Small to large | Large, symmetrical | Small matted nodes | Large |
| Consistency | Hard | Firm to rubbery | Firm | Shotty |
| Tenderness | Tenderness +/− | Nontender | Nontender | Nontender |

### Significant lymphadenopathy (based on size, fixity and consistency (Table 5.9)

**Table 5.9:** Significant lymphadenopathy characteristics.

| Size >2 cm in | Inguinal region |
|---|---|
| Size >1 cm in | Extrainguinal region |
| Any size | Supraclavicular<br>Epitrochlear<br>Popliteal<br>Any lymph node with a lesion in the draining area |
| Based on fixity | Fixed to each other (matting)<br>Fixed to underlying tissues<br>Fixed to skin |
| Based on consistency | Hard/firm lymph nodes |

### Q. What are the causes of generalized lymphadenopathy?
Refer **Box 5.2**.

**Box 5.2:** Diseases associated with lymphadenopathy.

**Infectious diseases**
- Viral—infectious mononucleosis syndromes (Epstein-Barr virus, cytomegalovirus), infectious hepatitis, herpes simplex, herpesvirus-6, varicella-zoster virus, rubella, measles, adenovirus, HIV, epidemic keratoconjunctivitis, vaccinia, herpesvirus-8
- Bacterial—streptococci, staphylococci, cat-scratch disease, brucellosis, tularemia, plague, chancroid, melioidosis, glanders, tuberculosis, atypical mycobacterial infection, primary and secondary syphilis, diphtheria, leprosy
- Fungal—histoplasmosis, coccidioidomycosis, paracoccidioidomycosis
- Chlamydial—lymphogranuloma venereum, trachoma
- Parasitic—toxoplasmosis, leishmaniasis, trypanosomiasis, filariasis
- Rickettsial—scrub typhus, rickettsial pox, Q fever

**Immunologic diseases**
- Rheumatoid arthritis
- Juvenile rheumatoid arthritis
- Mixed connective tissue disease
- Systemic lupus erythematosus
- Dermatomyositis
- Serum sickness
- Sjögren's syndrome
- Drug hypersensitivity—diphenylhydantoin, hydralazine, allopurinol, primidone, gold, carbamazepine, etc.
- Angioimmunoblastic lymphadenopathy
- Primary biliary cirrhosis
- Graft-versus-host disease
- Silicone-associated
- Autoimmune lymphoproliferative syndrome

**Malignant diseases**
- Hematologic—Hodgkin's disease, non-Hodgkin's lymphomas, acute or chronic lymphocytic leukemia, hairy cell leukemia, malignant histiocytosis, amyloidosis
- Metastatic—from numerous primary sites

**Lipid storage diseases**
Gaucher's, Niemann-Pick, Fabry, Tangier

**Endocrine diseases**
Hyperthyroidism

**Other disorders**
- Castleman's disease (giant lymph node hyperplasia)
- Sarcoidosis
- Dermatopathic lymphadenitis
- Lymphomatoid granulomatosis
- Histiocytic necrotizing lymphadenitis (Kikuchi's disease)
- Sinus histiocytosis with massive lymphadenopathy (Rosai-Dorfman disease)
- Mucocutaneous lymph node syndrome (Kawasaki's disease)
- Histiocytosis X
- Familial Mediterranean Fever
- Severe hypertriglyceridemia
- Vascular transformation of sinuses
- Inflammatory pseudotumor of lymph node
- Congestive heart failure

### Q. Enumerate the medications that can cause lymphadenopathy.
Refer **Box 5.3**.

**Box 5.3:** Medications that can cause lymphadenopathy.

- Allopurinol, atenolol
- Captopril, carbamazepine
- Gold, hydralazine, penicillins
- Phenytoin, primidone, pyrimethamine
- Quinidine, trimethoprim/sulfamethoxazole sulindac

### Q. What are the causes of epitrochlear lymph node enlargement?

Lymph nodes in the arm are typically found in the epitrochlear and deltopectoral regions. The causes are cat scratch disease, leprosy, leishmaniasis and tuberculosis are a few reported benign causes of isolated epitrochlear lymph node enlargement; malignant causes include lymphoma and malignant melanoma.

**Systemic causes of epitrochlear lymphadenopathy**
- Secondary syphilis
- Non-Hodgkin's lymphoma (NHL)

- Human immunodeficiency virus
- Disseminated tuberculosis
- Sporotrichosis
- Cat-scratch disease.

### Q. What is Troisier's sign?

Virchow's node (or signal node) is a lymph node in the left supraclavicular fossa (the area above the left clavicle). It takes its supply from lymph vessels in the abdominal cavity. The finding of an enlarged, hard node (also referred to as Troisier's sign) has long been regarded as strongly indicative of the presence of cancer in the abdomen, specifically gastric cancer, that has spread through the lymph vessels. It is sometimes called the signal node or sentinel node for the same reason.

### Q. What are the areas drained by cervical, axillary and inguinal lymph nodes?

Refer **Figures 5.20 and 5.21**.

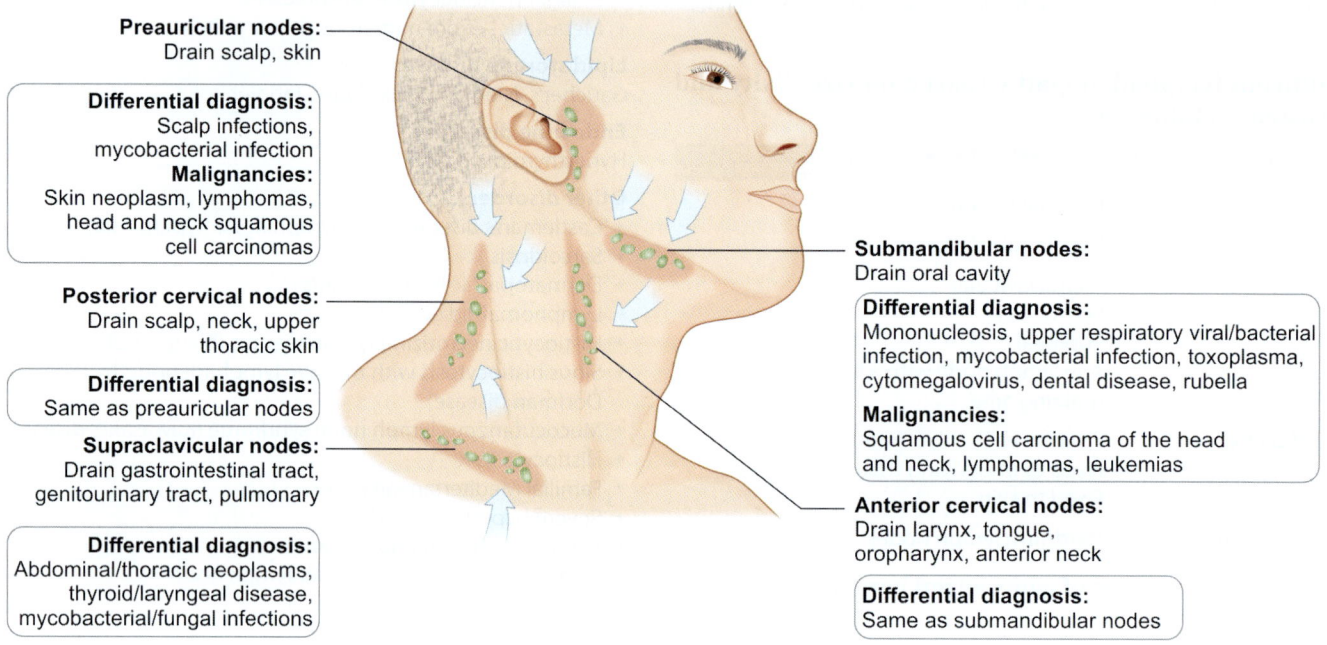

**Fig. 5.20:** Cervical lymph node with drainage.

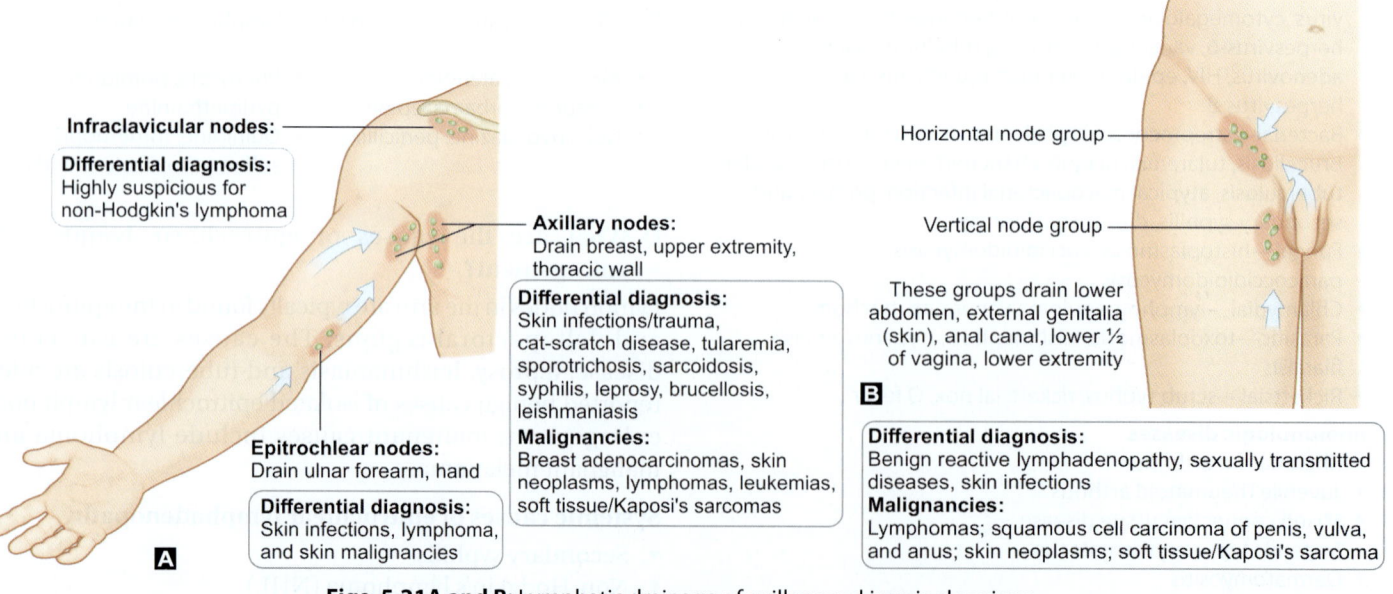

**Figs. 5.21A and B:** Lymphatic drainage of axillary and inguinal regions.

## Q. What are the causes of clubbing?
Refer **Box 5.4**.

**Box 5.4:** Causes of clubbing.

**Not associated with overt disease**
- Hereditary clubbing
- Sporadic clubbing
- Pachydermoperiostosis

**Thoracic neoplasms**
- Lung cancer especially fibrous tumors (accounts for most clubbing)
- Benign and malignant pleural tumors
- Other thoracic neoplasms, including esophageal cancer, and lymphoma

**Heart and vascular disease**
- Cyanotic congenital heart disease
- Subacute bacterial endocarditis
- Infected aortic graft
- Aortic surgery
- Takayasu's arteritis
- Behýet's disease

**Pulmonary AV shunting**
- Cyanotic congenital heart disease
- Acquired heart disease
- Pulmonary AV fistula
- Hereditary hemorrhagic telangiectasias

**Interstitial lung disease**
- Asbestosis
- Idiopathic pulmonary fibrosis
- Collagen vascular disease
- Langerhans histiocytosis
- Lipoid pneumonia

**Chronic infections**
- Bronchiectasis
- Bronchiectasis from sarcoidosis or tuberculosis
- Lung abscess
- Empyema
- Cystic fibrosis

**Gastrointestinal and liver disease**
- Inflammatory bowel disease
  - Crohn's disease
  - Ulcerative colitis
  - Polyposis coli
- Amebic colitis
  - Bacillary dysentery
- Liver disease
  - Hepatoma
  - Hepatopulmonary syndrome
- Biliary cirrhosis
- Esophageal stricture

**Hemoglobinopathy**
- Hemoglobinopathies
- Congenital methemoglobinemia

**Other**
- Thyroid acropathy
- Secondary hyperparathyroidism
- HIV related
  - Lymphoid interstitial pneumonia
  - Other infections
- Prostaglandin infusion
- Fabry's disease
- Toxic exposure to arsenic, mercury or beryllium

**Unilateral clubbing**
- Vascular disorders
  - Subclavian artery aneurysm
  - Brachial AV fistula
- Subluxation of the shoulder
- Median nerve injury
- Local trauma
- Hemiplegia

## Q. What are the named lymph nodes and their characteristic features?
Different named lymph nodes with their features are shown in **Table 5.10**.

**Table 5.10:** Named lymph nodes.

| Lymph node | Features |
|---|---|
| Virchow node | Left supraclavicular node |
| Scalene node | - Sentinel node of bronchogenic carcinoma<br>- Relax neck<br>- Palpate (deep) between the two heads of<br>- SCM |
| Winterbottom sign | - Posterior triangle lymph node enlargement<br>- Seen in early phase of African trypanosomiasis |
| Causes of posterior triangle lymph node enlargement | - Scalp infection<br>- Measles<br>- Rubella<br>- Infectious mononucleosis<br>- Trypanosomiasis |
| Node of Woods | - Jugulodigastric lymph node enlargement seen in TB when spread via tonsils |
| Delphian node | - Pretracheal node |
| External Waldeyer ring | - Commonly seen to be enlarged in non-Hodgkin's lymphoma |
| Berry's node | - Jugulo-omohyoid lymph nodes seen in thyroid malignancy |

## Case 5: Approach to Edema

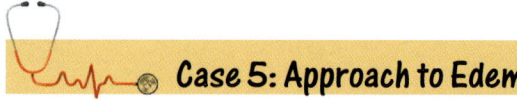

*Brief History*
A postmenopausal woman known case of diabetes, hypertension on irregular presents with history of bilateral leg swelling, shortness of breath, generalized weakness.

*Examination*
- HR 110, irregularly irregular
- BP 100/70
- RR: 26 breaths per minute
- JVP raised
- Bilateral pitting pedal edema+. No pallor, icterus, cyanosis, clubbing

*Systemic Examination*
- Cardiovascular system
  - Apical impulse is felt in left 6th ICS, 1 cm lateral to midclavicular line, hyperdynamic in nature.
  - Soft S1 is heard
  - S2 heard
  - S3 gallop
  - No murmurs
- Respiratory system: Bilateral basal crepitations heard

*Diagnosis*
Congestive cardiac failure with atrial fibrillation (edema is secondary to right heart failure)

## DISCUSSION

### Q. Define edema.

Edema is defined as the abnormal fluid accumulation in the interstitial space that exceeds the capacity of physiological lymphatic drainage.

Pedal edema is a common presentation of various systemic and nonsystemic diseases among Indian population which is always an enigma. A proper understanding of the pathophysiological basis of pedal edema and a systematic approach towards a patient can help a physician to narrow down to the right cause.

### Q. What is the mechanism of development of edema?

Interstitial fluid space is dependent on the hydrostatic and oncotic pressure gradient across the capillaries and also the lymphatic drainage. So they are dependent on four main factors, namely:
- Capillary permeability
- Capillary hydrostatic pressure
- Capillary oncotic pressure
- Lymphatic drainage

Any derangement of one or more of these four factors which are involved in the regulation of interstitial fluid results in pedal edema.

### Q. What are the causes of edema?

Generally, causes of pedal edema can be identified on the basis of their pathophysiological mechanism **(Box 5.5 and Fig. 5.22)**.

**Box 5.5:** Pathophysiology of edema.

**Increased hydrostatic pressure**
- **Volume expansion:** Kidney failure, pregnancy, medication side effect (e.g., prednisone, NSAIDs), acute salt load, heart failure
- **Venous obstruction/insufficiency:** Heart failure, pulmonary hypertension, cirrhosis, deep vein thrombosis, chronic venous stasis
- **Arteriolar vasodilation:** Dihydropyridine $Ca^{2+}$ channel blockers.

**Decreased oncotic pressure (hypoalbuminemia)**
Malnutrition, cirrhosis, nephrotic syndrome.

**Increased capillary permeability**
Sepsis, cellulitis.

**Lymphatic obstruction (lymphedema)**
- **Malignancy:** Lymph node dissection, infiltration of lymphatics, extrinsic compression of lymphatics
- **Filariasis** (e.g., *Wuchereria bancrofti, Brugia malayi*)

**Miscellaneous causes**
- **Lymphatic obstruction**—poor drainage of the interstitial fluid also results in pedal edema. It may be due to:
- **Primary:** Congenital lymphedema which is seen at birth or before 2 years, lymphedema precox, which is common in females, before 35 years of age and lymphedema tarda which is seen after 35 years of age.
- **Secondary:** Obstruction of lymphatic drainage due to tumor, trauma, radiation and infections like filariasis.
- **Lipedema:** Deposition of fluid in adipose tissue.
- **Idiopathic edema:** In females of menstruating age idiopathic or cyclical edema is seen throughout the menstruating period. It has to be differentiated from premenstrual edema which often occurs few days prior to menstruation.

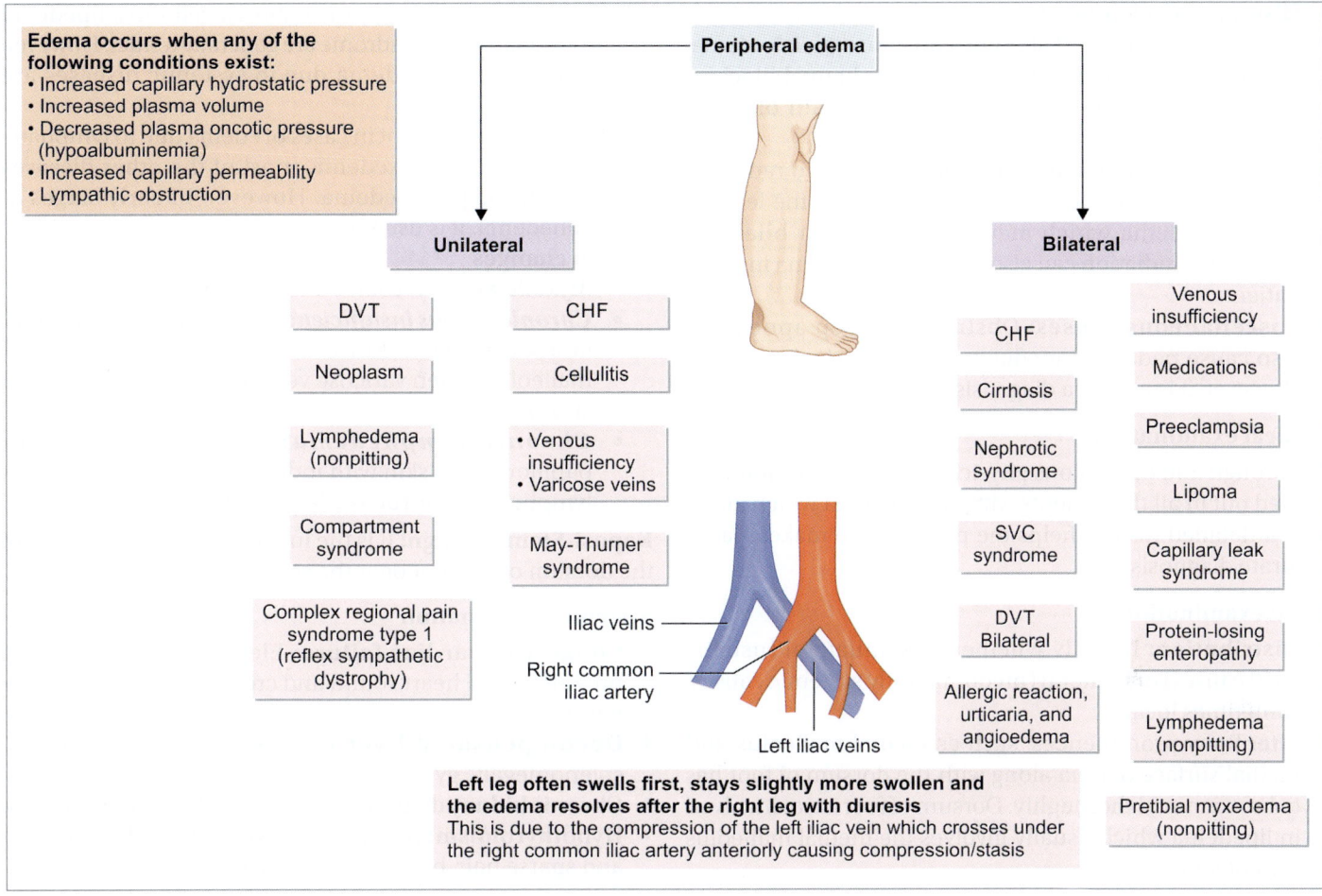

**Fig. 5.22:** Causes of peripheral edema.

**Q. What are the drugs that can cause the leg swelling?**
Refer **Box 5.6**.

**Box 5.6:** Drugs causing leg swelling.

| Anti-hypertensive drugs | Chemotherapy |
|---|---|
| • Calcium channel blockers | • Docetaxel |
| • Beta blockers | • Gemcitabine |
| • Clonidine | • Pemetrexed |
| • Hydralazine | • Lenalidomide/thalidomide |
| • Minoxidil | • Targeted immunotherapy |
| • Methyldopa | **Other** |
| **Hormones** | • Nonsteroidal anti-inflammatory drugs |
| • Corticosteroids | • Pioglitazone, rosiglitazone |
| • Estrogen | • Monoamine oxidase inhibitors |
| • Progesterone | • Pramipexole |
| **Gabapentinoids** | |
| • Pregabalin | |
| • Gabapentin | |

**Q. How will you evaluate a case of pedal edema?**

**History**

A detailed history is the most important component in the evaluation of pedal edema as it often gives a clear perspective which can pinpoint the underlying cause.

- **Site and distribution:** Whether the pedal edema is unilateral or bilateral. Unilateral edema results mainly due to local causes, such as deep vein thrombosis (DVT), cellulitis, compartment syndrome and filarial lymphatic obstruction. Bilateral pedal edema is mainly due to systemic causes like congestive cardiac failure, anemia, chronic kidney disease and chronic liver disease.
- **Duration of illness:** Short duration of the illness indicates an acute cause like cellulitis, DVT, compartment syndrome, etc., which usually occurs in 72 hours.
- **Association with pain:** Conditions like deep vein thrombosis and cellulitis are generally painful whereas edema due to heart failure, hypoproteinemia and lymphedema are painless. A dull aching type of pain is seen in chronic venous insufficiency.
- **Variability of edema:** Venous edema due to congestive cardiac failure and venous insufficiency is aggravated by standing and improves with overnight limb elevation during sleep. Idiopathic edema which is seen in females increases throughout the day during upright posture.
- **History of systemic illness:** Symptoms of systemic diseases like exertional dyspnea, orthopnea, paroxysmal nocturnal dyspnea and chest pain point to cardiac failure.

- **History of drug intake:** Drugs, such as calcium channel blockers, NSAIDs and steroids can cause pedal edema. Around 50% of patients taking calcium channel blockers and 5% of patients taking NSAIDs complain of pedal edema.
- **History of trauma and radiation:** Trauma and radiation can cause cellulitis and compartment syndrome leading to pedal edema which may be unilateral or bilateral. Long-term radiation can also cause lymphedema in some patients.
- **Miscellaneous causes:** Obstructive sleep apnea can also cause pedal edema due to right ventricular failure. However, it is always a diagnosis of exclusion.

## Clinical examination

A thorough and meticulous physical examination should be carried out in all the patients with pedal edema which along with a detailed history helps the physician to make a fairly accurate diagnosis.

## Local examination

- **Distribution:** Identify whether it is unilateral (usually local causes) or bilateral (predominantly systemic causes, sometimes local).
- **Site:** Bony prominences, such as medial malleolus and medial surface of tibia along with the dorsum of foot has to be examined thoroughly. Dorsum of foot is not involved in lipedema which usually involves the medial malleolus area of foot.
- **Tenderness:** Deep vein thrombosis, cellulitis, lipedema and compartment syndrome are generally tender. However, lymphedema and edema due to systemic diseases are painless.
- **Pitting edema:** Except in cases of edema due to lymphatic obstruction and myxedema, most of the other diseases cause pitting pedal edema. However, in early stages of lymphedema, it is usually pitting.
- **Skin changes**
  - *Myxedema:* Dry, coarse and thick skin is noted
  - *Chronic venous insufficiency:* Hemosiderin deposition causes brawny skin commonly over the medial malleolus. Often varicose veins are seen on the medial side of the leg.
  - *Chronic lymphedema:* Hyperkeratotic and papillomatous skin with induration which is known as lymphostatic verrucosis (elephantiasis).

**Kaposi-Stemmer sign:** It is the inability to pinch the skin on the dorsum of the foot near the second toe.

## Systemic examination

- **Congestive cardiac failure:** Elevated jugular venous pressure, third heart sound and crepitations over the lung bases.
- **Decompensated liver disease:** Jaundice, ascites, splenomegaly, gynecomastia and spider naevi.
- **Chronic kidney disease:** Anemia, dry skin, uremic breath.
- **Hypothyroidism:** Bradycardia, skin changes like dry skin and sparse hair, hoarseness of voice.

SECTION 5: Others 357

# Comprehensive Geriatric Assessment

## HISTORY TAKING

Name:
Hospital number:
Age:
Sex:
Date of examination: Address/contact:
Name/relationship of contact person: Contact address/number:

| Problem list | Duration |
|---|---|
| | |
| | |

## Past Medical History

| Medical condition | Duration |
|---|---|
| | |
| | |
| | |
| Vision impaired | |
| Hearing impaired | |
| Cancer | |
| OA | |
| Thyroid | |

## Family History

| Hypertension | |
|---|---|
| Diabetes | |
| Heart disease | |
| Dementia | |
| Cancer | |

## Social Assessment

| Married: | Yes | No |
|---|---|---|
| Spouse living: | Yes | No |
| Living with: | | |
| No. of children | | |
| How often do you see them? | | |
| Who assists you? | | |

| Is it sufficient? | Yes | No |
|---|---|---|
| Native language | | |
| Type of house | Independent | Apartment |
| Stairs | Present | Absent |

### Personal History

| Do you exercise daily? | Yes | No |
|---|---|---|
| If yes, minutes/day? | | |
| What type? | | |
| Weight loss/gain (3 kg) | Yes | No |
| Smoker | Yes | No |
| | Duration | |
| Alcohol | Yes | No |
| | Duration | |

| Level of independence (tick one of them) | Independent |
|---|---|
| | Dependent |
| | Needs assistance |

| Caregiver fatigue | Yes | No |
|---|---|---|

| 10-minute comprehensive screening | | | |
|---|---|---|---|
| Memory | 3 objects named | Yes | No |
| Depression | Are you often sad/depressed? | Yes | No |
| Falls | Fallen more than twice in last 1 year | Yes | No |
| | Able to walk around chair? | Yes | No |
| Urinary incontinence | Lost urine/got wet in past 1 year? | Yes | No |
| Memory recall | One object | Two objects | Three objects | None |
| Imagine this is a clock and add numbers to make it look like a clock. Draw the clock hand to show ten minutes past eleven | | | |

| Vision | Difficulty in reading | Right eye | Left eye |
|---|---|---|---|
| Hearing | | Right ear | Left ear |
| 6, 1, 9 test—stand behind the patient and say 6, 1 and 9 in normal tone and in whisper | Normally | Yes/No | Yes/No |
| | Softly | Yes/No | Yes/No |
| Constipation | | Yes | No |
| Insomnia | | Yes | No |

## Physical Functional Capacity

Are you able to_____?

| Run/walk fast to catch a bus | Yes | No |
|---|---|---|
| Do heavy work at home | Yes | No |
| Go shopping for groceries/clothes | Yes | No |
| Get to places out of walking distance? (drive/take a bus) | Yes | No |
| Bath using shower/bucket | Yes | No |
| Put on clothes/footwear | Yes | No |

## Basic Activities of Daily Living

| Bath | Yes | No | Transfer | Yes | No |
|---|---|---|---|---|---|
| Dress | Yes | No | Toilet | Yes | No |
| Toilet | Yes | No | Feeding | Yes | No |

| Montreal cognitive assessment score | |
|---|---|
| Geriatric depression score | |

## PHYSICAL EXAMINATION

| Height (m) | |
|---|---|
| Weight (kg) | |
| Body mass index (BMI) (W/H²) | |
| Pulse | |
| Blood pressure (BP) (sitting/supine) | |
| BP (standing 1 minute/3 minutes) | |
| Anemia | Yes/No |
| Skin | Normal/abnormal |
| Teeth | Normal/abnormal |
| Any other GPE abnormality | |

## SYSTEMIC EXAMINATION

| | Normal/abnormal | Describe | |
|---|---|---|---|
| Joints | | | |
| Cervical spine | | | |
| Thoracic spine | | | |
| Lumbar spine | | | |
| RS | | | |
| CVS | | | |
| P/A | | | |
| Neurological examination | | R | L |
| Muscle strength | Upper limb | | |
| | Shoulder | | |
| | Elbow | | |
| | Wrist | | |
| | Small muscles of hand | | |
| | Lower limb | | |
| | Hip | | |
| | Knee | | |
| | Ankle | | |
| Tone (describe) | Rigidity/hypotonia/spasticity | | |
| Balance | Normal/abnormal | Sensory Cerebellar Vestibular | |
| Gait | | | |
| Timed up and go test (seconds) | | | |

## CURRENT TREATMENT DETAILS

Write down name of drug, dose and dosing frequency of all the medications the patient is currently consuming, including over the counter-medications and those from alternative systems of medicine.

**Polypharmacy:** Yes/No

**Investigations:**

| *Investigations* | *Date* | *Values* |
|---|---|---|
| Complete blood picture | | |
| Creatinine | | |
| Electrolytes, blood sugar | | |
| PSA (for males) | | |
| Urine routine | | |
| Ultrasonography (USG) abdomen and pelvis | | |

## DIAGNOSIS FORMAT

### Comprehensive Geriatric Assessment Report

| Acute illness | |
|---|---|
| Comorbidity | |
| Geriatric giants | |
| Other age-related problems | |
| Social problems | |
| Economic problems | |
| Prescription modification | |

**Examples**

| Acute illness | Delirium secondary to hyponatremia<br>Postoperative fracture neck of femur |
|---|---|
| Comorbidity | Diabetes, hypertension, dyslipidemia |
| Geriatric giants | Delirium Incontinence |
| Other age-related problems | Cataract, knee osteoarthritis |
| Social problems | Stress incontinence Living alone<br>Feels lonely<br>Has nobody for emergency help |
| Economic problems | Present, not earning |
| Prescription modification | Avoid diuretics and beta-blockers |

## DISCUSSION

Comprehensive geriatric assessment (CGA) is a multidimensional, multidisciplinary diagnostic, and therapeutic process conducted to determine the medical, mental, and functional problems of older people with frailty so that a coordinated and integrated plan for treatment and followup can be developed.

Factors which make assessment/treatment of elderly different are as follows:
- Individuals become more dissimilar as they grow
- Abrupt decline in any system is always due to disease and not due to normal aging
- Multiple pathology
- Missing symptoms (e.g., angina in an elderly patient with osteoarthritis—may not manifest)
- Masking symptoms (e.g., history of fall and fracture neck of femur in an elderly female—masked a coexistent hemiparesis due to an internal capsule infarct).

When an older person is identified as being at risk of frailty, whether in an acute hospital, day hospital, community or residential care, they should be considered for a CGA. CGA should be initiated as soon as possible after admission to hospital by a skilled, senior member of the multidisciplinary team, and used to identify reversible medical problems, target rehabilitation goals, and plan all the components of discharge and postdischarge support needs.

**Q. What are the criteria for selection of patient for such assessment?**

**Strongly consider doing a CGA if three or more of the red flags are present**
- \>75 years
- Needs help with activities of daily living/instrumental activities for daily living (ADLs/IADLs) by caregiver
- Lives alone
- Falls
- Delirium/confusion
- Incontinence
- \>2 admissions to acute care hospital/year
- "Failure to thrive"

**Q. What are basic activities of daily living?**

Basic activities of daily livings (BADLs) are fundamental activities such as personal cares which are basic to independent living. Loss of basic ADLs places a heavy burden on the caregivers and is a marker of complete dependence.

For assessing autonomy in daily activities:
- Toileting, self-hygiene, bathing, grooming, dressing, feeding, and ambulation (stairs too).
- For each of the questions, enquire whether the person can perform it independently, whether he/she needs assistance or he/she is completely caregiver-dependent.

**Q. What are instrumental activities of daily living?**

Instrumental activities of daily living (IADLs) are complex tasks which enable an older adult to live independently and safely. They are not necessary for fundamental existence in the way that basic ADLs are necessary, but are an indicator of functional independence. Assessment of IADLs is useful during baseline and followup assessments among older adults. Loss of IADLs may be the first indication of deterioration in an older adult.
- Complex tasks and roles you do at home
- Shopping, meal planning and preparation, housekeeping, laundry, transit, financial management, using a telephone, medication management, and driving.

**Q. What are geriatric giants?**

The term geriatric giant was coined by Sir Bernard Isaacs. He identified a set of medical problems or syndromes which were common in older adults and which crossed several organ systems and were difficult to manage. These geriatric giant are chronic disabilities which impact multiple domains, such as physical, psychological, and social domains. Although geriatric giants are commonly to be an unavoidable part of old age, they can often be improved if they are identified and managed **(Fig. 5.23)**.

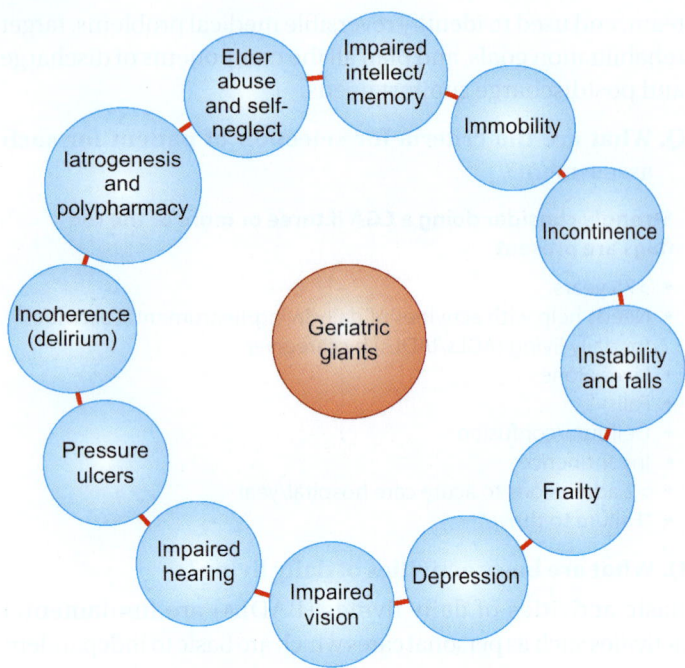

**Fig. 5.23:** Modern geriatric giants.

### Q. What is frailty?

Frailty is defined as the loss of an individual's ability to withstand minor stresses because of decreased functional reserve of several organ systems.

Two main criteria used in diagnosing frailty are Linda Fried/Johns Hopkins frailty criteria and the Rockwood frailty index.

### Five key elements form the core of the frailty cycle

*Frailty is defined as the presence of three or more of following conditions:*

- Unexplained weight loss (>5% over a year)
- Poor endurance and energy (self-reported)
- Poor strength (in lowest 20th percentile)
- Slow walking speed (poor "Get up and Go" test)
- Low physical activity (lowest 20th percentile)

### Q. What are other geriatric problems?

**Failure to thrive**
It is a syndrome of weight loss, decreased appetite, poor nutrition and inactivity, often accompanied by dehydration, depressive symptoms, impaired immune function and low cholesterol

**Sarcopenia**
- Age-related loss of muscle mass
- Increases the risk for falls, fractures, dependency, use of hospital services, institutionalization, poor quality of life, and mortality

**Anorexia of aging**
- The multifactorial decrease in appetite and/or food intake that occurs in late life
- Specific geriatric syndrome that can lead to malnutrition if not appropriately diagnosed and treated

- **Multimorbidity:** The coexistence of ≥2 chronic conditions, where one is not necessarily more central than the others
- **Polypharmacy:** Administration of more medications than clinically indicated, representing unnecessary drug use, i.e., ≥5 drugs during a 3-month period

## Case 6: Approach to Arthritis

*Brief History*
A 24-year-old girl presented to the hospital with complaints of progressive breathlessness, chest pain and pedal edema over the past 1 month.
Additional complaints included alopecia, oral ulcers, and bilateral knee joint pain. Examination: On examination she had BP 170/90 mm Hg, malar rash, and anasarca.

*Laboratory Investigations*
Basic investigation revealed Hb 9 g/dL, platelet count 1,12,000, creatinine. 2.6 mg/dL, urine showed 3 + RBC and proteinuria.

*Diagnosis*
Multisystem involvement—connective tissue disorder possibly SLE.

## Case 7: Approach to Arthritis

*Brief History*
A 52-year-old lady presented with complaints of pain in her joints.

*Examination:*
- On examination, she had pallor, BMI 19, BP 130/80 mm Hg
- She had thickening, swelling and reduced range of motion in her bilateral first, second and third metacarpophalangeal joint. She was wincing with pain when the physician tried to palpate the above mentioned joints.
- The fingers in her hands also appeared to be deformed and were stiff.
- Her left middle finger showed hyperflexion of the distal interphalangeal (DIP) joint with hyperextension of the proximal interphalangeal (PIP) joint.
- Her right hand appeared to be deviated laterally. Her left ring finger showed flexion of the proximal interphalangeal (PIP) joint with hyperextension of the distal interphalangeal (DIP) joint.
- She also had swelling in both her elbows and wrists and also complained of thickening and swelling in the ball of her big toe on both feet.

*Diagnosis*
Inflammatory polyarthritis—possibly rheumatoid arthritis.

## DISCUSSION

**Q. What are the various conditions affecting musculoskeletal system?**
- **Arthralgia (subjective):** Only pain around the joint
- **Arthritis (objective):** Pain + other signs of inflammation (redness/swelling/increased temperature/loss of function)
- **Synovitis:** Inflammation of synovial membrane
- **Tenosynovitis:** Inflammation of the tendon sheath
- **Enthesitis:** Inflammation of site of attachment of ligament, tendon or capsule to the periosteum or bone
- **Myositis:** Inflammation of muscle

**Q. What are the presenting features of arthritis?**
Refer **Table 5.11**.

**Table 5.11:** Arthritis—presentation.

| | |
|---|---|
| Duration | • Acute (presenting within hours to days)<br>• Chronic (persisting for weeks or longer) |
| Number of joints involved | • Monoarticular (only 1 joint)<br>• Oligoarticular/pauciarticular (2–4 joints)<br>Polyarticular (5 joints or more) |
| If more than one joint is involved | Symmetric (or) asymmetric additive (or) migratory |
| Type | Inflammatory or noninflammatory (see below) |
| Deformities | Present (or) absent. Deformities are usually seen in:<br>• Rheumatoid arthritis<br>• Psoriatic arthritis<br>• Osteoarthritis<br>• Reiter's disease<br>• Chronic gout |
| Precipitating factors, such as | • Sexually transmitted disease (STD) infection<br>• Trauma alcohol diarrhea |
| Associated features | Constitutional symptoms:<br>• Fever, fatigue and weight loss<br>• Extra-articular manifestations and systemic manifestations<br>• Comorbid conditions |

**Note:** Treatment history should be taken in detail.

**Q. What are the differences between inflammatory and noninflammatory arthritis?**
Refer **Table 5.12**.

**Table 5.12:** Inflammatory versus noninflammatory disease.

| Features | Inflammatory (rheumatoid arthritis) | Noninflammatory (osteoarthritis) |
|---|---|---|
| Age of onset | Usually 20–40 years but may begin at any age | Most commonly over 50 years of age |
| Speed of onset | Rapid over weeks to months | Slow; over years |
| Systemic symptoms | • Fatigue, low-grade fever, anorexia<br>• Extra-articular manifestations: Rheumatoid nodules, Sjogren's syndrome, Felty syndrome | No systemic symptoms |
| Joint affection | Symmetrical | Asymmetrical |
| Joint symptoms | Painful, swollen, stiff joints, and muscle aches | Joints painful without swelling |
| Joints involved | Primarily affects small joints [metacarpophalangeal (MCP) and proximal interphalangeal (PIP)] with sparing of DIP | • Affects large weight-bearing joints (hip, knee or the spine)<br>• Affects proximal interphalangeal (PIP) and distal interphalangeal (DIP) joints |
| Stiffness | Morning stiffness for >1 hour. Stiffness occurs after periods of rest/inactivity (the so-called "gel phenomenon") | Morning stiffness for <30 minutes. Stiffness is generally mild and occurs after periods of activity |
| Relation of movement with pain | Movement or mild to moderate activity decreases pain | Movement increases the pain (worsens with activity) and improves with rest |
| Examination of joint | Swollen, red, warm, tender, and painful | Swollen, cool, and hard on palpation. When severely inflamed (as in acute gout or septic arthritis), can have erythema of the overlying skin |
| Radiological findings | Bony erosions, soft-tissue swelling, angular deformities, periarticular osteopenia | Loss of joint space and damage to articular cartilage, osteophytes |
| Rheumatoid factor (RF) and antinuclear antibody (ANA) | Positive | Negative |
| Erythrocyte sedimentation rate (ESR) and C-reactive protein | Both are often raised | Usually normal but transient elevation of ESR may occur due to synovitis |
| White blood cell (WBC) count in the synovial fluid | WBC count is >2,000/ mm$^3$ in septic arthritis and not in rheumatoid arthritis | WBC count is <2,000/mm$^3$ |

**Q. Enumerate the causes of arthritis.**

Refer **Table 5.13**.

**Table 5.13:** Causes of arthritis.

| | |
|---|---|
| **Acute monoarthritis** | |
| Inflammatory | Crystal disease (e.g., gout), infectious disease, spondyloarthropathy, rheumatoid arthritis |
| Mechanical | Trauma, avascular necrosis |
| **Acute polyarthritis** | |
| Infectious | Bacterial, human immunodeficiency virus (HIV) |
| Noninfectious | Rheumatoid arthritis, spondyloarthropathy, other connective tissue diseases, crystal (gout), sarcoidosis, malignancy, leukemia, sickle cell anemia |
| **Chronic monoarthritis** | |
| Inflammatory | Crystal disease, infectious disease (e.g., tuberculosis, fungal), spondyloarthropathy, rheumatoid arthritis |
| Noninflammatory | Osteoarthritis, avascular necrosis, neuropathic arthropathy, villonodular synovitis |

| | Chronic polyarthritis |
|---|---|
| Inflammatory | Rheumatoid arthritis, spondyloarthropathy, other connective tissue diseases |
| Mechanical | Osteoarthritis |
| Crystal | Gout |
| Metabolic | Infiltrative, metabolic, hypothyroidism |

**Q. How do you approach to a patient with musculoskeletal complaint?**

Refer **Table 5.14**.

**Table 5.14:** Musculoskeletal complaint.

| | Distribution | | | | |
|---|---|---|---|---|---|
| | **Polyarthritis (≥4 joints)** | | **Monoarthritis/oligoarthritis (1–3 joints)** | | **Non-articular** |
| | *Acute* | *Chronic* | *Acute* | *Chronic* | |
| **Noninflammatory** | • Hemoglobinopathies<br>• Amyloid arthropathies | • Osteoarthritis | • Meniscal tear<br>• Osteoarthritis flare<br>• Reflex sympathetic dystrophy | • Osteoarthritis<br>• Osteonecrosis<br>• Neuropathic arthritis<br>• Hemochromatosis<br>• Pigmented villonodular synovitis | • Trauma<br>• Fracture<br>• Fibromyalgia<br>• Reflex sympathetic dystrophy |
| **Inflammatory** | • Viral arthritis<br>• Serum sickness<br>• Drug-induced arthritis<br>• Early onset CTD<br>• Rheumatic fever<br>• Palindromic rheumatism<br>• RS3PE | • Rheumatoid arthritis<br>• Undifferentiated polyarthritis<br>• Inflammatory osteoarthritis<br>• MCTD<br>• Lupus, scleroderma<br>• Polyarticular JIA<br>• Adult Still's disease | • Infectious arthritis<br>• Gout<br>• Pseudogout<br>• Reactive arthritis<br>• Chlamydial arthritis | • Psoriatic arthritis<br>• Spondyloarthropathies<br>• Pauciarticular JIA<br>• Indolent infectious arthritis | • Bursitis<br>• Tendinitis<br>• Polymyalgia rheumatica |

**Q. What are the findings of examination of skin, hands, and eyes?**

Table 5.15 shows the skin changes in rheumatology.

**Table 5.15:** Skin changes in rheumatology.

| | |
|---|---|
| Erythema | • Septic arthritis<br>• Crystal arthropathy |
| Palpable purpura | Vasculitis **(Fig. 5.24)** |
| Ulcers over skin | Vasculitis **(Fig. 5.25)** |
| Rash | • Systemic lupus erythematosus (SLE) (malar or discoid rash) **(Fig. 5.26)**<br>• Vasculitis<br>• Drugs<br>• Stills disease |
| Violaceous scaly lesions | Psoriasis |
| Keratoderma blennorrhagica Circinate balanitis | Reiter's disease |
| Mucosal ulcers | Behcet's disease SLE **(Fig. 5.27)** |
| Dryness of skin | Sjogren's disease |
| Thickened hard skin | • Systemic sclerosis<br>• Scleroderma **(Figs. 5.28A to C)** |
| Pyoderma gangrenosum | Inflammatory bowel disease |
| Palmar erythema | Rheumatoid arthritis |
| Photosensitivity | Development of rash on exposure to sunlight of less than 30 minutes (SLE) |
| Digital gangrene | Raynaud's and medium vessel vasculitis |
| Alopecia | • SLE<br>• Scleroderma |
| Heliotrope rash and Gottron's papules | Dermatomyositis |
| Salt and pepper appearance | Scleroderma (most prominently on the upper back and chest) |

| | |
|---|---|
| **Livedo reticularis (Fig. 5.29)** | SLE<br>Antiphospholipid antibody (APLA) syndrome<br>Sneddon's syndrome, polyarteritis nodosa |
| **Raynaud's** | Systemic sclerosis, vasculitis<br>Mixed connective tissue disorder |
| **Sclerodactyly** | Progressive systemic sclerosis |

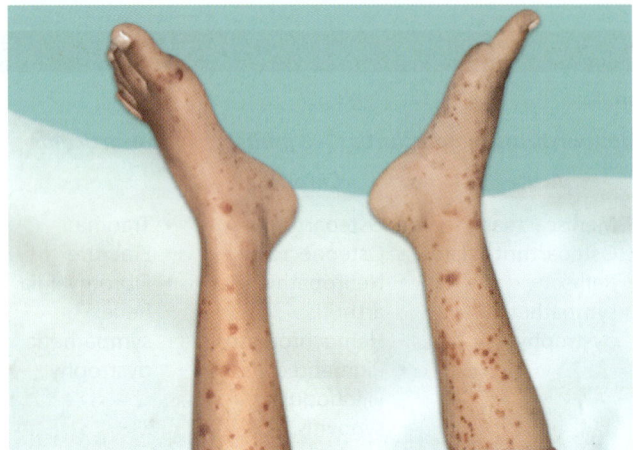

**Fig. 5.24:** Palpable purpura over lower legs in Henoch–Schönlein purpura.

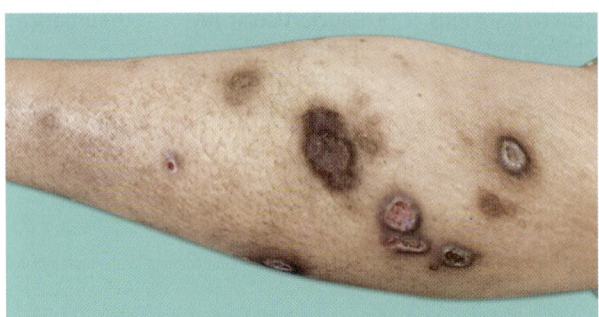

**Fig. 5.25:** Ulcers on the leg in medium vessel vasculitis.

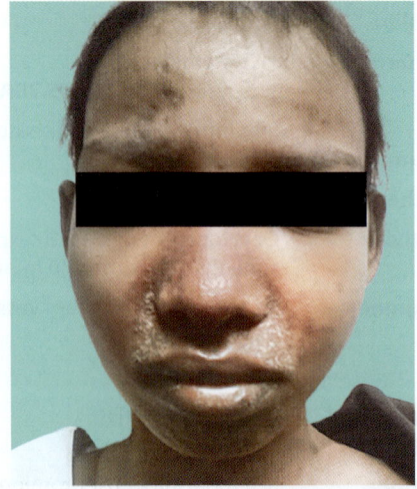

**Fig. 5.26:** Systemic lupus erythematosus with malar rash and alopecia.

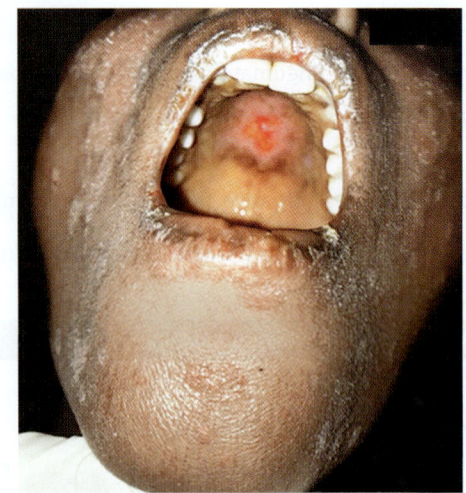

**Fig. 5.27:** Mucosal ulcers in SLE.

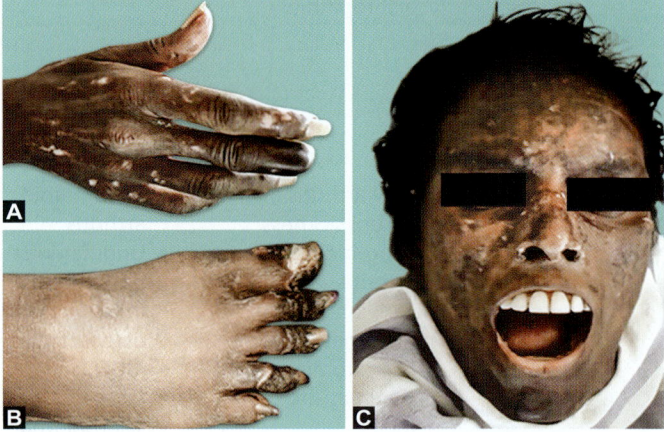

**Figs. 5.28A to C:** Systemic sclerosis: (A and B) Shiny and thickened skin of hands and feet; (C) Mask-like face with decreased oral aperture.

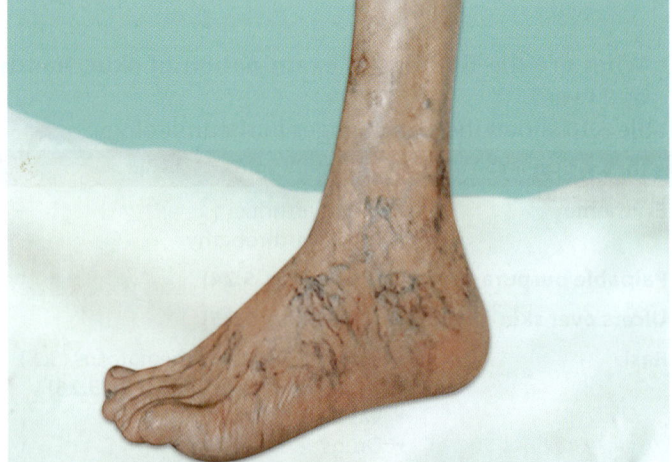

**Fig. 5.29:** Livedo reticularis.

Livedo reticularis—mottled reticulated vascular pattern that appears as a lacelike purplish discoloration of the skin. It is due to swelling of the venules caused by obstruction of capillaries.

**Q. What are the differential diagnosis of subcutaneous nodules?**
- Rheumatoid arthritis
- Rheumatic fever
- Gout
- Erythema nodosum
- Sarcoidosis
- SLE
- Hyperlipidemia.

**Q. What is erythema nodosum?**

It is a type of panniculitis characterized by painful reddish nodules in the subcutaneous tissue most commonly seen on the shin **(Fig. 5.30)**.

Common causes include:
- Tuberculosis
- Leprosy
- Sulfonamides and other drugs
- Streptococcal infection
- Sarcoidosis
- Inflammatory bowel disease.

## Nail Changes (Table 5.16)

**Table 5.16:** Nail changes.

| Clubbing | • Fibrosing alveolitis<br>• Hypertrophic<br>• Osteoarthropathy |
|---|---|
| Pitting and onycholysis | Psoriasis |
| Splinter hemorrhages | Vasculitis |

## Nail Changes in Psoriasis (Fig. 5.31)

Involvement is common and may be observed up to 50% of patients with psoriasis. These include:
- "Thimble pitting" of the nail plate
- Distal separation of the nail plate from the nail bed (onycholysis)

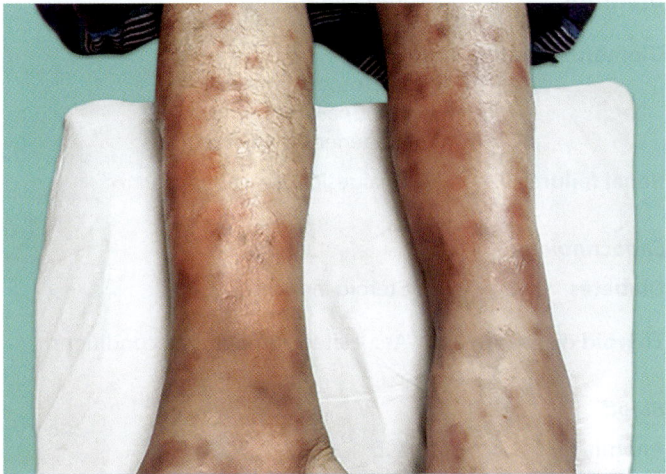

**Fig. 5.30:** Erythema nodosum.

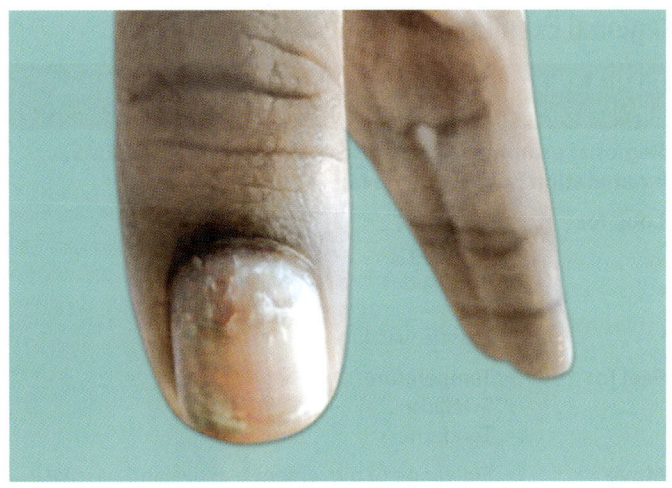

**Fig. 5.31:** Nail changes in psoriasis.

- Yellow brown discoloration underneath the nail plate ("oil drop" sign)
- Subungual hyperkeratosis
- Thickening of the nail (onychodystrophy)

**For diagnosis of nail involvement:** >6 nails should be involved with each nail should have >20 pits.

## Eye Changes (Table 5.17)

**Table 5.17:** Eye changes.

| *Dryness of eyes* | *Sjogren's syndrome* |
|---|---|
| **Episcleritis/scleritis** | Rheumatoid arthritis |
| **Iritis/iridocyclitis** | Ankylosing spondylitis |
| **Conjunctivitis** | Reiter's disease |
| **Tenosynovitis of superior oblique** | Rheumatoid arthritis (Brown's syndrome) |
| **Scleromalacia perforans** | Rheumatoid arthritis |

**Q. What are the various examinations to be done for musculoskeletal system?**

### GALS screening (Table 5.18)

**Table 5.18:** Gait, arms, legs, spine (GALS) screening.

| Gait | • Observe the gait |
|---|---|
| Arms | • Examine the range of movement of joints<br>• Joint deformities<br>• Synovial thickening |
| Legs | • Examine the range of movement of joints<br>• Joint deformities<br>• Synovial thickening<br>• Special tests |
| Spine | • Look for spine deformity<br>• Special test |

## Regional Examination (Table 5.19)

**Table 5.19:** Regional examination of musculoskeletal system (REMS) examination (look, feel, move).

| Regional examination of musculoskeletal system (REMS) examination (look, feel, move) | |
|---|---|
| Look for | <ul><li>Swellings</li><li>Redness</li><li>Rashes</li><li>Scars</li><li>Muscle wasting</li></ul> |
| Feel for | <ul><li>Temperature</li><li>Swelling</li><li>Tenderness</li></ul> |
| Move | <ul><li>Full range of movement—active and passive (Table 5.20)</li><li>Restriction—mild/moderate/severe</li></ul> |
| Function | <ul><li>Functional assessment of joint</li></ul> |
| All the joints have to be examined in the above headings. | |

## Range of Movement of Joints (Table 5.20)

**Table 5.20:** Range of movement of joints.

| | Flexion | Extension | Abduction | Adduction | Rotation |
|---|---|---|---|---|---|
| Wrist | 70° | 70° | 30° | 30° | |
| MCP | 45° | 90° | | | |
| PIP | 120° | | | | |
| DIP | 90° | 10° | | | |
| Elbow | 160° | 5° | | | |
| Shoulder | 160° | 60° | 175° | 50° | 70° |
| Hip | 110° | 30° | 30° | 30° | 45° |
| Knee | 130° | | | | |
| Ankle | 40° (dorsiflexion) | 50° (plantar flexion) | | | |

## Others

- **Subtalar joint:** Has 5° of inversion and eversion.
- **Midtarsal joint:** Has 30° of inversion and eversion.

**Q. What are the examination findings of other systems in rheumatological disorders?**

Refer **Table 5.21**.

**Table 5.21:** Other systems in rheumatological disorders.

| *Cardiovascular system* | |
|---|---|
| Pericarditis | RA, SLE |
| Endocarditis | SLE |
| Aortitis and aortic regurgitation | RA<br>Psoriasis<br>Ankylosing spondylitis Reiter's |
| Conduction defects | SLE |
| *Nervous system* | |
| Myelopathy | RA—atlantoaxial dislocation<br>Vasculitis |
| Neuropathy (entrapment/mononeuritis multiplex) | RA, SLE<br>Vasculitis (especially PAN) |
| Stroke | RA, SLE, APLA<br>Vasculitis |
| Myopathy | Polymyositis dermatomyositis |
| *Respiratory system* | |
| Upper respiratory tract | Wegener's granulomatosis |
| Pleural effusion | RA, SLE |
| Fibrosis | RA, SLE, systemic sclerosis |
| Lung nodules | RA (Caplan's syndrome) |
| Alveolar hemorrhage | Microscopic polyangiitis<br>Goodpasture's syndrome<br>Wegener's granulomatosis |
| Asthma | Churg–Strauss syndrome |
| Decreased chest expansion | Ankylosing spondylosis |
| *Gastrointestinal system* | |
| Oral ulcers | SLE<br>Behcet's disease |
| IBD | Seronegative spondyloarthropathies |
| Hepatosplenomegaly | SLE, RA<br>Stills disease |
| GI bleeding | Henoch–Schönlein purpura,<br>Other vasculitis<br>Analgesic use |
| *Genitourinary system* | |
| Urethritis | Reactive arthritis |
| Glomerulonephritis | SLE<br>Microscopic polyangiitis<br>Goodpasture's syndrome<br>Wegener's granulomatosis |
| Renal failure | Analgesics use, vasculitis |
| *Endocrinology* | |
| Diabetes | Steroid induced |
| Thyroid disease | Associated autoimmune conditions |
| *Blood* | |
| Anemia<br>Thrombocytopenia<br>Pancytopenia | SLE<br>RA (Felty's syndrome) |

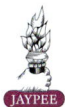 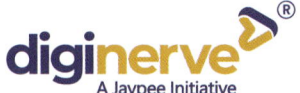

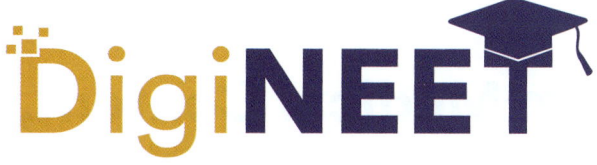

Simplify your undergraduate studies and NEET PG preparation with this comprehensive program covering all 19 subjects. Crafted by India's top faculty, it includes video lectures, printed notes, OSCEs, a QBank, test series, and the innovative Dr. Wise AI Chatbot.

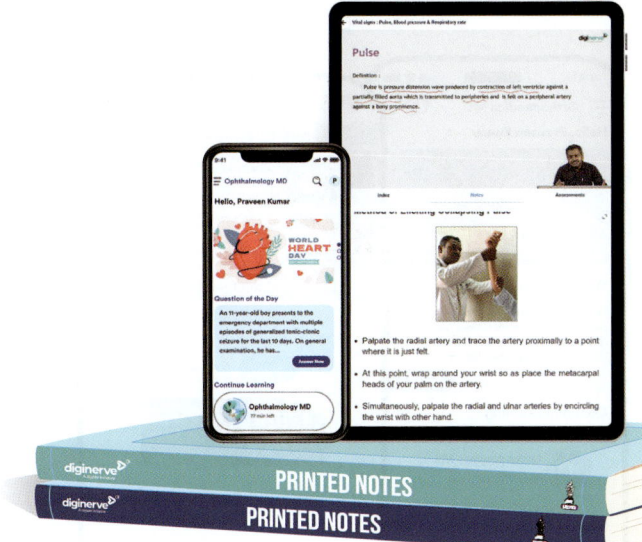

## Course Features

**1400+ hrs Video Lectures**

**1500+ Topics in Notes**

**15000+ Questions in QBank**

**1800+ GEMS**

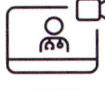
**450+ OSCEs**

**Test Series**

**Dr. Wise AI Chatbot**

**Drug Chart**

### Regular Webinars by Esteemed Faculty

## Access Anytime, Anywhere

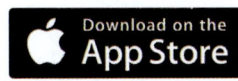 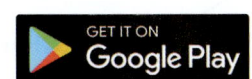 

Scan to Download

+91-8800-418-418

marketing@diginerve.com

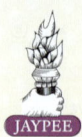 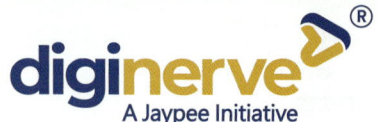

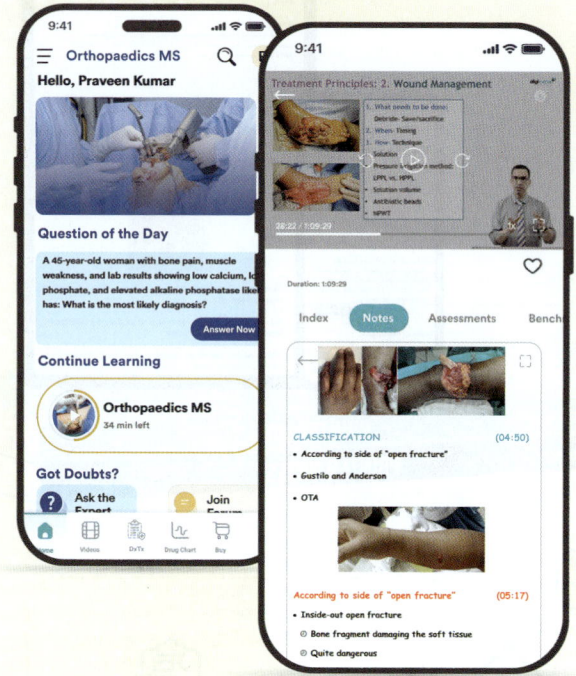

# Premium Medical Content, Anytime, Anywhere

**Trusted by 150K+ Users**

**20+** Courses | **3600+** Hrs of Video Content | **790+** Mentors

## A host of features for UnderGrads, PostGrads and Professionals

Available on 

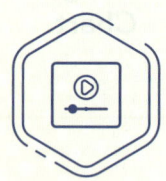 Video Lectures

 Notes

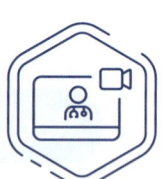 OSCEs

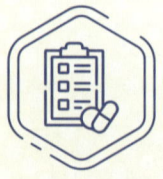 Drug Chart

 Question Bank

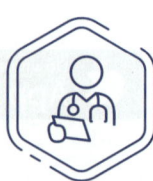 Dr. Wise AI Chatbot

+91-8800-418-418    marketing@diginerve.com

# Index

Page numbers followed by *b* refer to box, *f* refer to figure, and *t* refer to table.

## A

Abdomen, systemic examination 143
Abdominal angina 79
Abdominal distension 139
Abdominal examination 342, 350
Abdominal wall veins 149, 171
Abdominojugular reflux 171
Abductor pollicis brevis 285
Abscess 263
Absent vocal resonance 19
Acid beta glucosidase 150, 151
Acid-fast bacterium 182
Acid phosphatase 173
Acinar emphysema, distal 11
Acquired heart disease 56
Acquired immunodeficiency syndrome 24
Acute ischemic stroke syndromes 238*t*
Acute kidney injury 163
Acute liver failure 150*t*, 157
 types of 150*t*
Acute motor paralysis, causes for 289
Acute rheumatic fever 61, 130
 management of 61
Adamkiewicz artery 273*f*
Adductor pollicis 285
Adenoma 149
Adenosine deaminase 182
Adiadochokinesis 309
Adrenal tuberculosis 29
Adventitious sounds 6, 41
Agnosia 249
 types of 250, 250*t*
Airway complications 46
Akinesia 318
Akinetic mutism 228
Alcohol on nervous system, effects of 233
Alcoholic cirrhosis, pathogenesis of 159*f*
Alcoholic neuropathy, clinical features of 284
Alexia
 with agraphia 217
 without agraphia 217
Alkaptonuria 345
Alopecia 364*f*
Alveolar hemorrhage 366
Amphoric bronchial breathing 32
Amylase 24

Amyloidosis 290
 physical examination in 290
Amyotrophic lateral sclerosis
 diagnosis of 329*b*
 differential diagnoses for 330*t*
Anemia 78, 337, 338, 340, 342
 cardiovascular changes in 78
 classification of 339*f*
 diagnosis of 344*f*
 etiology of 340*t*
 grades of 339, 340*t*
 laboratory tests in 343*f*
 pale tongue in 186*f*
 subtypes of 343*t*
 thrombocytopenia pancytopenia 366
Angina
 pectoris 79
 types of 79
Angiosarcoma 149
Ankle 198
 reflex 268
Ankylosing spondylitis 99
Annulus, damage to 77
Anterior cerebral artery 215
 stroke 269
Anterior choroidal artery 215
 occlusion 228
Anterior horn cell 259, 259*t*, 294, 298
 syndrome 259, 259*t*
Anterior opercular syndrome 330
Anterior spinal artery syndrome 259, 259*t*
Anterolateral scar indications 75
Antibiotic 62
 prophylactic 179
Anton's syndrome 205*f*, 208
Aorta coarctation of 126, 230
Aortic dilation, ascending 95
Aortic dissection 95
Aortic ejection 101
 click 91
Aortic regurgitation 95, 97, 101, 104, 104*t*, 107
 acute 104, 104*t*
 causes of 99
 chronic 104, 104*t*
 complications of 99
 etiology of acute 104
 pathophysiology of 99*f*
 severe 102*t*, 105
 signs of acute 104
Aortic sclerosis, degenerative 95

Aortic stenosis 82, 82*t*, 87, 92, 93, 93*t*, 94, 94*f*, 94*t*, 95, 105, 127
 absent murmur in 92
 causes of 89
 classification of 89*b*
 etiology of 89*b*
 severity of 92*t*
 subvalvular 95
 supravalvular 89, 95
 symptoms of 89
 valvular 95
Aortic valve 105
 implantation, transcatheter 93
 involvement 99
 replacement, indications of 103
Aortic wall involvement 99
Aortopathy 131, 132
Aortosclerosis, degenerative 95, 95*t*
Apex beat, characteristics of 66*t*
Aphasia 214, 214*t*, 217, 218*f*
 approach for 218*f*
 global 217
 types of 217, 217*t*, 249*t*
Apical impulse 101
Apraxia 148, 249
Arcuate fasciculus 216
Arcus 159, 159*t*
 senilis 232, 232*f*, 232*t*
Areflexia, distal 282
Arnold-Chiari malformations, types of 267, 267*t*
Arterial spiders 144*t*
Arterial vasodilation hypothesis, peripheral 177
Arthralgia 361
Arthritis 361, 361*t*
 approach to 361
 causes of 362, 362*t*
 inflammatory 361
 noninflammatory 361
Ascending motor paralysis, syndrome of acute 282
Ascites 149, 150, 176, 183, 183*t*
 causes of 182, 182*b*, 182*t*
 classification of infected 178*t*
 clinical signs of 176, 177*f*
 different forms of 183*t*
 formation, theories of 178*f*
 grading of 176, 176*t*
 hypothesis of 176
 infectious 183
 malignant 183

management protocol of 184*f*
 protein 183
 uncomplicated 183
Ascitic fluid 181, 183
Ascitic tap 183*f*
Ashrafian sign 98
Aspirin 61
Asterixis
 bilateral 160
 causes of 160*t*
 unilateral 160
Asthma 13, 13*t*
 molecular phenotypes of 13
 targeted therapy of 14
Asymmetric distal weakness 282
 with sensory loss 282
 without sensory loss 282
Ataxia 305, 309, 310, 313, 314
 based on tempo of disease, causes of 305
 causes of 305
 endocrine cause of 224
 genetic causes of 305
 treatable causes of 311, 312*b*
 types of 310, 310*t*
Ataxic dysarthria 241
Ataxic speech 219
Atherosclerosis 228
Athetosis 331
Atlantoaxial dislocation 267
 classification of 267*b*
 non-traumatic causes of 267
Atrial fibrillation 58, 84, 93
 anticoagulants in 73*f*
 causes of 234
 diagnosis of 72*f*
 management of 72, 72*f*
 new-onset 106
Atrial septal defect 108, 111, 127
 anatomy of 112, 113*f*
 complications of 114
 coronary sinus 111
 murmurs 114*t*
 sinus venosus 111
 treatment of 115
 types of 111
Atrial septum, development of 112, 113*f*
Atrophic glossitis 187, 188*f*
Auscultation 55,, 78, 141
Austin flint murmur 68, 102, 102*t*, 103, 133
 pathogenesis of 102*f*
Autoimmune hepatitis 147, 149
 clinical features of 147, 147*t*

Automatic bladder 268
Autonomic dysfunction
    bedside tests for 291
    tests for 300, 300t
Autonomic nervous system, signs
    of 199
Autonomic neuropathy 283
    causes of 285, 285t
Autonomic signs 282
Autonomic symptoms 281, 282
Autonomous bladder 268, 269
Autosomal dominant cerebellar
    ataxia 312, 313f
Autosomal recessive 305
Avellis' syndrome 207
Axillary regions, lymphatic
    drainage of 352f
Axillary scar indications 75
Axonal neuropathy 280, 280t, 293
Axonopathy 324t
Azygous vein, opening of 154f,
    155f

# B

Bacterascites 178
Bacteria 22
Bacterial meningitis 204
Balint syndrome 208
Barrel chest 32
Basilar artery
    ischemia, clinical features of
        212, 212t
    syndrome 207
Basilar invagination, clinical
    features of 266
Basophilia 172f
Batwing opacities 70
Becker's sign 98
Beevor's sign 265, 265f
Behçet's disease 188
Bell's palsy, causes of 235
Benedict's syndrome 206, 334
Benzathine penicillin 62
Beri-beri 233
Berry aneurysms 126
Beta-blockers 93
Bicuspid aortic valve 89, 95
Bile
    pigments 345
    salts 345
Biliary cirrhosis
    primary 149
        signs of 147, 147t
        symptoms of 147, 147t
Biopsy, muscle for 323
Bisferiens pulse 101
Bite marks with hematomas 188
Bitot's spot 159f
Bladder
    dysfunction in neurology,
        types of 268
    types of 268t

Bland cholestasis 149
Blepharospasm 334
Blood
    pressure 21, 54, 78, 81b
        diastolic 249
        management of 249
        systolic 249
    smear, peripheral 172f, 337f,
        338f
Blue sclera 341f
    causes of 345
BODE index 10, 11b
Body mass index 4, 54, 140, 195,
    243
Body myositis, inclusion 323
Botulism 297
Boxcars 342
Bozzolo's sign 98
Bradykinesia 318
Brain 305
    blood supply to 214
Brainstem 306
    syndromes 206, 206t
Broca's area 216
Broken neck sign 301
Bronchial asthma 13
Bronchial breath sound 29
    characteristics of 32
Bronchial breathing 32
    types of 19, 19t
Bronchiectasis 41-43
    bilateral 43f
    causes of 42, 42b
    complications of 44, 44t
    morphological types of 42f
    proximal 42
    severity scoring of 44
    signs of 43t
    symptoms of 43
    theories of 42
Bronchitis
    chronic 9, 12, 12t, 13
    types of 9
Bronchogenic carcinoma 18, 30
Bronchophony 20, 34
Brown-Sequard syndrome 237,
    258, 258t
Brucella spine involvement 264
Brudzinski's sign 199
Budd-Chiari syndrome 156f
    causes of 156
    chronic 154
    diagnosis of 156
Bulbar palsy 222, 222t, 245
    causes of 245t

# C

Cabot-Locke murmur 133
Calcific aortic valvular disease 89
Cancer 235
Capillary permeability, increased
    354

Capillary pulsations, mechanism
    of 98
Carbon dioxide narcosis 11
Card test 289f
Cardiac anomalies 112
Cardiac catheterization,
    indications for 70, 115
Cardiac conditions 98
Cardiac defects 126, 127
Cardiac embolus 235
Cardiac enlargement, left
    ventricular type of 230
Cardiac failure, causes of 76
Cardiac lesions 88
Cardiac murmurs 136, 136f
Cardiac origin 225
Cardiac resynchronization therapy
    84
Cardiac-limb syndrome 126
Cardiomyopathy, dilated 131, 132
Cardiovascular diseases 134
Cardiovascular examination 57,
    342
Cardiovascular reflexes 291
Cardiovascular system 6, 15, 51,
    133, 200, 202, 366
    clinical diagnosis of 50, 133
    examination 74, 97, 254
Carey Coombs murmur 133
Carotenemia 345
Carotid artery, internal 205, 215
Carpal tunnel syndrome 285
Carpentier classification 85, 86f
Catamenial pneumothorax 39
Cauda equina syndrome 261,
    261f, 261t
Caudate lobe 169
    location and boundaries 169f
Cavernous bronchial breathing 32
Central cord syndrome 258, 258t
Central nervous system 15, 203,
    298
    affecting 292
    examination 296
    tuberculosis, pathogenesis of
        219
Central nystagmus 307, 307t
Central venous catheter
    extravascular migration 25
Centriacinar emphysema 11
Cerebellar ataxia
    asymmetrical 312t
    causes of 312t
    etiologies of 224, 225t
Cerebellar disorder, clinical signs
    of 308
Cerebellar drift 199
Cerebellar dysfunction 223
Cerebellar lesions, localization
    of 312t
Cerebellar signs 199, 253, 296,
    312t
Cerebellar syndromes 312t
Cerebellar system 305

Cerebellum 278, 311f
    areas of 311t
    functional anatomy of 311
    functions of 308
Cerebral artery
    acute bilateral posterior 205f
    acute right anterior 205f
    occlusion
        mainstem middle 228
        syndromes of posterior
            213t
        posterior 215
Cerebral embolism, causes of 224,
    225b
Cerebral salt wasting syndrome
    247
Cerebrovascular system 215f
Cervical cord lesion 260
Cervical lymph node with
    drainage 352f
Cervical syringomyelia 257f
Cervical venous hum 339, 340f
Charge syndrome 127
Cheilitis 342
Chest
    flat 32
    wall complications 46
    X-ray 68, 110
Chin-on-chest syndrome 272
Chipmunk facies 342f
Cholangiocarcinoma 149
Cholecystectomy, scar from 342
Cholestasis
    conditions producing 345b
    pruritus in 346f
Cholestatic hepatitis 149
Chondroectodermal dysplasia
    127
Chordae tendineae, damage to
    77
Chordal lesions 80
Chorea 61, 331, 333
    chronic 331
    drug-induced 333
Choroid tubercles 29
Chromosome 151
Chronic disease, anemia of 340
Chronic inflammatory
    demyelinating
    polyneuropathy, diagnostic
    criteria of 286t
Chronic kidney disease 283
Chronic liver disease 144, 160
Chronic liver failure 150t
Chronic obstructive pulmonary
    disease 8-10, 10b, 10f, 11,
    13, 13t
    complications of 10
    risk factor for 9, 10b
Chyliform 23
    effusion 23
Chylothorax 23, 23t
    management of 24
Chylous 23

Chylous ascites, mechanisms of formation of 181
Chylous effusion 23
Circle of Willis 126
Cirrhosis 143, 149, 158, 164f
   causes of 158b
      anemia in 160
      complications of 160, 161f
   etiology of 163
   liver disease 142
   morphological classification of 147f
   signs pointing etiology of 163t
   type of 145, 158t
   with enlarged liver, causes of 150
Claude's syndrome 206
Clicking pneumothorax 39
Climb up legs 323f
Clubbing
   causes of 353, 353b
   unilateral 353
Coanda effect 95f
Coarctation of aorta
   clinical signs of 230
   murmur in 126
Coarse crepitations 32
Cocaine use 228
Cole-cecil murmur 133
Collagen vascular disease 350
Collapse 33, 33t, 47
Collapsing pulse 100, 100f
   examination of 100f
Common neurological symptoms 194
Communicating artery, posterior 215
Compensatory emphysema 48
Complete blood count 344
Complete cord transection 257, 258f
Congenital heart disease 56, 108, 123, 124, 127
   acyanotic 60
   classification of 123f
   complex 131, 132
   stigmata of 126, 126t
Congenital malformation, description of 267
Conjunctivitis 365
Connective tissue diseases 80
Consciousness
   altered state of 193
   causes of loss of 305
   loss of 244
Constrictive pericarditis 180, 180t, 181
   peripheral signs of 180
Constructional apraxia 152
Contarini's syndrome 28
Contralateral hyperalgesia 237
Conus medullaris 261, 261t
   syndrome 261

Coprolalia 334
Cord
   compression 287
   hemisection of 237, 258
Cornelia de Lange's syndrome 127
Corneomandibular reflex 328
Coronary artery bypass graft 84
Cor-pulmonale 9
Corrigan's pulse 98, 100
Cortical lesions 238
Cortical sensation 199, 278
Cough 3
Courvoisier's law 157
Cracked pot resonance 20
Crackling rales 32
Cranial nerve 196, 197, 212, 296, 305, 316
   abnormalities 282
   dysfunction 193, 201, 253, 276
   involvement 294
   palsy 297
Craniovertebral junction
   anomalies 265, 265t
   radiology of 266f
Crepitations, types of 32
Cricosternal distance, causes of abnormal 13
Cruveilhier-Baumgarten venous hum 133
Cryptococcal meningitis, clinical features of 220
Cushing reflex 219
Cuspal lesions 79
Cutaneous vasculitis, causes of 286, 287b
Cyanosis
   causes for 114
   respiratory causes of 32
Cystic bronchiectasis 44f
Cystic fibrosis 45, 46
   genetic defect in 46

D

D'Espine sign 16
   false-positive 17
Dahl's sign 10
Daily living
   basic activities of 358, 359
   instrumental activities of 359
Danish pen 312
De Musset's sign 98
Deafness 60
Decompensation, causes of acute 160
Deep palpation 171
Deep tendon reflexes 198
Deficiency syndromes 243
Dejerine syndrome 207
Dennison sign 98

Dermatomyositis 322, 323
   sine myositis 322
Detrusor
   areflexia 268
   sphincteric dyssynergia 268
Dextrocardia with situs inversus 43f
Diabetes mellitus 280, 283
Diabetic neuropathy 282
   characteristic of 289
   classification of 283b
Diagnostic paracentesis, indications for 183
Diamond-Blackfan anemia 345
Diarrhea 60
Diastolic knock, cause of 77
DiGeorge syndrome 127
Digit symbol test 152, 153f
Diphtheria 297
Distal phalangeal distance 15
Dobutamine stress echo 93
Docks murmur 133
Dorsal midbrain syndrome 212f
Down syndrome 126
Drug, anti-arrhythmic 84
Drummond sign 98
Duke criteria, modified 130t
Dupuytren's contracture 145, 145f
Duroziez's sign 98
Dynamic auscultation 132f
Dysarthria 214, 214t, 313, 314
   types of 218, 219t
Dyspnea 3, 53, 60, 106
Dystonia 331

E

Ear 29
Ecchymoses 150
Echolalia 334
Edema 354
   causes of 354
   pathophysiology of 354b
Effusion
   causes of 22, 24
   types of 22, 23
Egophony 20, 21, 34
Ehlers-Danlos syndrome 99, 127, 345
Eisenmenger syndrome 125, 125t, 126
   signs of 124
Ekbom's syndrome 334
Elicit Hoffmann's sign 269
Elicit Tromner's sign 269
Ellis-Van Creveld syndrome 127
Embolic stroke 204, 204t, 226f, 236
Emotional fibers checking 197
Emotional lability, producing 240
Emphysema 9, 11, 12, 12t, 13, 48, 49
   irregular 12
   types of 11, 12f

Empyema 15, 23, 25t, 26
   clinical course of 16
Enalaprilat 249
Encephalitis 219
Encysted effusion, differential diagnosis of 24
Encysted pleural effusion 48
Endocardial cushion defect 127
Endocrinology 366
Endoscopy 150
Enthesitis 361
Eosinophilic effusion 24
Episcleritis 365
Epitrochlear lymph node enlargement, causes of 351
Epitrochlear lymphadenopathy, systemic causes of 351
Erythema nodosum 29, 365f
Erythrocytes 22
Esmolol 249
Esophageal varices 161f
Ewart's sign 77f
Exacerbation, causes of 11
Excessive daytime sleepiness 317
Extensive tinea corporis 29
Exteroceptive sensation 237
Extradural lesion 257
Extrahepatic portal hypertension 150
   causes of 150
Extramedullary lesions 256
Extravascular hemolysis 338
Exudative effusion 22
   transudative from 22t
Eye 29
   blink, reduced 318
   changes 365, 365t
   dryness of 365
   movements 248t
   xanthelasmas around 157f

F

Facial hair, diminished 160f
Facial myoclonus 331
Facial nerve 197
Facial palsy 219
   peripheral 236
Facioscapulohumeral dystrophy 325f
Fasciculations 189
   benign 331
   causes of 331t
   malignant 331
Fatty liver 158
   disease 165f
Fever 3
Fibrin purulent stage 16
Fibrosis 29, 33, 33t, 47, 49, 366
   causes of 33
   long-standing 30
Fibrothorax 16

Fine crepitations 32
Finger
　clubbing of 15f
　normal 15f
First-order syndrome 239
Fissures, atrophy of 188
Flaccid 219
　paraplegia, causes of 260
　tongue with fasciculations 189
Flatback syndrome 272
Flexors, long 198
Fluid
　removal 184
　thrill 176
　wave 176
Focal cerebellar signs 225
Focal disorders 148f
Foix-Chavany-Marie syndrome 330
Foot, small muscles of 198
Foville's syndrome 207
Friedreich's ataxia 315
Froment's sign 289f
Fulminant hepatitis 149
Fundoscopy 230
Fundus and paraplegia, association with 301
F-wave 303, 303t

## G

Gait 199
　abnormalities 194
　arms, legs, spine screening 365t
　changes 318
Gastrectomy, scar from 342
Gastrointestinal causes 144
Gastrointestinal disease 353
Gastrointestinal system 6, 55, 98, 137, 200, 366
Gastrointestinal tract 279f
　systemic examination 176
Genioglossus, action of 241f
Genitourinary system 366
Georges Guillain syndrome 297
Gerhardt's sign 98
Geriatric assessment, comprehensive 357, 359
Geriatric giants 359
Gerstmann syndrome 208
Ghent criteria, revised 129t
Giant cell arteritis 204
Gibbus 29
Gibson's murmur 133
Glass slide method 145f
Glomerulonephritis 366
Glossitis 342
Glossoptosis 189
Glucose 24
Gorlin's tongue sign 189
Gottron's sign 322, 323

Graham-Steel murmur 133
Granulocytic precursors, erythroid to 343
Granulomas 30
Granulomatous hepatitis 149
Granulomatous meningeal inflammation 219
Gross tremor, absence of 148f
Guillain-Barré syndrome 280, 287, 287t, 296, 298b, 299, 299f, 301
　differential diagnosis of 298b
　predictive factors in 304t
　variants of 299t, 300t
Gynecomastia 146f
　causes of 146

## H

Hackett's grading of splenomegaly 173f
*Haemophilus influenzae* 10
Hairy leukoplakia 186f, 187
Hand
　asterixis in 162f
　grip 198
　pallor in 339f
　testing small muscles of 285, 285f
Headaches 194
Head-to-toe signs 140
Healthy tongue, characteristics of 186
Hearing loss 29
Heart
　border 5
　disease 353
　　cyanotic 123
　　high-risk 131t
　failure 75, 84
　　clinical features of 75t
　　congestive 78
　　etiologies of 76t
　　left 75, 75t, 76, 76f
　　right-sided 75, 76, 76f
　　symptoms 62
　rate, reflex decrease in 219
　sounds 127
　　abnormalities 81, 81t
Heaving apical impulse 230
Heberden's angina 79
Heliotrope rash 322
Hematology 150
Hemi chorea 333
Hemiballismus, unilateral 331
Hemiplegia 203, 220
　localization of 206f
　uncrossed 232
Hemisensory loss 237
Hemodynamic consequence 64, 65

Hemoglobinopathy 338, 353
Hemolytic anemia 340, 343
　complications of 349
　physical manifestation of 349f
Hemolytic jaundice 349
Hemorrhagic effusion 23, 23t
Hemorrhagic stroke 204, 204t, 226f, 229
Hemothorax 23, 23t
　management of 24
Henoch-Schönlein purpura 364f
Hepatic encephalopathy 148, 152
　clinical grades of 148t
　evidence of 152
　grading of 152t
　types of 163, 164f
Hepatic portal hypertension 156, 156t
Hepatic ultrasound 150
Hepatic veins, anatomy of 156f
Hepatitis, chronic 149
Hepatocellular carcinoma 149
Hepatocellular disease, stigmata of 171
Hepatocellular injury, acute 149
Hepatojugular reflux 148
Hepatomegaly 168, 342
　causes of 168, 169f
　painless 168, 169, 169t
　types of 169, 170f
Hepatorenal syndrome 163, 163b
　diagnosis of 163
　diagnostic criteria for 163b
　types of 163, 163t
Hepatosplenomegaly 366
　ascites, causes of 163
　causes of 350
Hereditary muscular dystrophy 324
Hereditary neuropathy 284
Herniation
　clinical features of 223
　sites of 228t
　syndromes 228
　types of 228
Herpes simplex encephalitis 221
Heyde's syndrome 89
Hill's sign 98
Hip 198
Hoffman's sign 270f
Holmes' rebound phenomenon 309
Holosystolic murmur 79
Holt-Oram syndrome 126
Hoover's sign 10
Horner syndrome 239
　left 31f
　third-order 240f
Horseshoe dullness 176, 177f
Hot potato voice 219
Human immunodeficiency virus 203, 204, 283

Hydralazine 249
Hydropneumothorax
　causes of 39, 40
　differentiate 17
　X-ray 40f
Hydrostatic pressure, increased 354
Hyperactive malarial splenomegaly 175b
Hypercarbia, signs of 21
Hypercoagulability 242
Hypercoagulable disorders 203
Hyperesthesia 237
Hyperkinetic dysarthria 219
Hyper-reflexia 268
Hypertension, secondary 229t
Hypertensive emergencies 249
Hypertensive retinopathy 230
　malignant 230f
　stages of 229
Hypertensive stroke 239
Hypertrophic obstructive cardiomyopathy 83, 83t, 93, 93t, 101f, 127
　murmur of 94f
Hyperviscosity 242
Hypoalbuminemia 354
Hypoglossal nerve 197
Hypoglycemia
　causes of 306
　symptoms of 244t
Hypophosphatasia 345
Hypoproliferative anemias 339f, 343
Hypotension, causes of 17
Hypotonia, causes of 237

## I

Icterus 347
　dark yellow 348f
　demonstration of 348f
　with splenomegaly, causes of 174
Illness, history of 143
Indwelling pleural catheter 25, 27
Infantile hypotonia, differential diagnosis for 326
Infections, chronic 353
Infectious disease 235, 350
Infective endocarditis 130, 130t
　prophylaxis of 130t
　regimen for 131t
　signs of 129, 129f
Inferior vena cava obstruction 155f
　cardinal features of 152
Inflammatory demyelinating polyneuropathy
　acute 283
　chronic 280, 283
Inflammatory disease 235, 362t
Inflammatory myopathy 322, 323t
Inguinal lymph nodes 352

Inguinal regions, lymphatic drainage of 352*f*
Inherited disorders 30, 262, 333
Intellectual function, impairment of 152
Intercostal tube drainage, indications of 26
Internal capsule
　anatomy of 221
　blood supply of 214, 215*f*
　fibers in 227*f*
　hemorrhage in 205*f*
Internuclear ophthalmoplegia 208
Interphalangeal distance 15
Interstitial lung disease 353
　causes of 30
　classification of 47, 47*f*
Interventricular septum 90
Intracerebral hemorrhage, non-hypertensive causes of 228
Intracranial pressure, raised 194
Intracranial tuberculomas 219
Intradural lesion 257
Intrahepatic portal hypertension 150
Intramedullary lesions 256, 270
　causes of 270, 271*t*
Intramedullary spinal cord tumors 271
Intravascular hemolysis 338
Involuntary movements 194
Ipsilateral cerebellar signs 225
Ipsilateral features 206-208
Iridocyclitis 365
Iritis 365
Iron deficiency
　anemia 173
　stages of 172
Ischemic stroke 204, 249
Isolation aphasia 217

## J

Jackson's syndrome 207
Jaundice 150, 160, 345-348, 348*t*
　approach to 345
　causes of 160
　cholestatic 157
　diagnosis of 346
　grading of 348*t*
　types of 348, 348*t*
Jaw jerk 198
　reflex 244
Jean Alexandre Barre syndrome 297
Joints, range of movement of 366, 366*t*
Jones criteria, modified 130*t*
Jug handle appearance 115*f*
Jugular venous
　pressure 54
　　causes of raised 76
　pulse 54

Julian sign 98
Juvenile Paget's disease 345

## K

Kawasaki disease 204
Kayser-Fleischer ring 159, 159*t*, 232, 232*f*, 232*t*
Kerley line 70
Kernig's sign 199
Key-Hodgkin murmur 133
Kidney, left 174, 174*t*
Kinetic tremor 333
Klippel-Feil syndrome 266
Knee 198
Knuckle pigmentation 341*f*
Koilonychia 341*f*, 342
Kronig's isthmus 30
Kyphosis 29, 272

## L

Labetalol 249
Labyrinthine origin, nystagmus of 306
Lacrimation hyperacusis 197
Lactate dehydrogenase 18, 22, 25, 344
Lacunar infarcts 232
Lacunar stroke
　signs of 213*t*
　symptoms of 213*t*
Lacunar strokes 213
Landolfi's sign 98
Language 296
　and brain 216*f*
　domains of 217
Lateral medullary syndrome 207, 208*f*, 224
Lateral midbrain syndrome 211*f*
Lateral pontine syndrome 209*f*
Left atrial
　enlargement 83
　pressure, consequences of raised 63
Left ventricle 90
　dilated 121
Left ventricular
　ejection fraction 84
　end diastolic pressure, increased 66
　hypertrophy 90, 127
　　causes of 88
Leg
　flapping tremors in 162*f*
　swelling 355
　　drugs causing 355*b*
LEOPARD syndrome 126
Leriche syndrome 272
Lesion 218*f*, 323
　causative 20, 20*t*
　dominance of 84*t*
　extradural 257*t*

　extramedullary 256*t*
　intradural 257*t*
　intramedullary 256*t*
　location of 213*t*
　peripheral nerve, site of 289
　site of 205-208, 217, 331
　type of 239
Leukemias, diagnosis of 173
Leukocyte 22
　alkaline phosphatase 173
Leukonychia 145, 145*f*
Levine and Freeman's grading 75
Light house sign 98
Light's criteria 18
Limb
　asymmetrical weakness and thinning of 290
　ataxia 199
　stiffness of 194
Lincoln sign 98
Line tracing test 152, 153*f*
Livedo reticularis 364*f*
Liver
　anomalous lobe of 169*f*
　causes of false-positive measurement of 169
　cell failure 140
　cirrhosis, factors affecting 158*t*
　conditions 168*t*
　description of 168
　disease 170, 170*t*, 353
　failure, clinical features of acute 157
　function tests, deranged 347*f*
　injury, causes of drug-induced 149
　margins of 169*t*
　span 168, 168*t*
　surfaces of 169*t*
Localization cerebellar lesions
　signs of 312
　symptoms of 312
Loculated effusion 48
　chest X-ray of 17*f*
Loculated pleural effusion, causes of 16
Logue's sign 98
Lordosis 272
Low molecular weight heparin 236
Lower cranial nerve paralysis, progressive 328
Lower limbs 162, 199
Lower lobe pulmonary fibrosis 33
Lower motor neuron 206, 330*t*
　causes 260
　facial nerve palsy, bilateral 297, 297*t*
　facial palsy 236
　involvement
　　signs of 330
　　symptoms of 330
　weakness 237, 237*t*

Lower respiratory tract examination 4, 41
Lumbar cord lesion 261, 261*t*
Lung
　abscess 44, 45*f*
　　causes of 44, 45*b*
　　clinical features of 45
　　complications of 45, 46*b*
　cancer, paraneoplastic syndromes of 30
　carcinoma of 34, 267
　collapse of right 32*f*
　disease 19
　　suppurative 41
　fibrosis, drugs causing 30
　lymphatic drainage of 16
　nodules 366
　radiological zones of 29
　resonance, normal 20
Lupus vulgaris 29
Lymph imbalance theory 178
Lymph node 29, 353, 353*t*
　right supraclavicular 34
Lymphadenopathy 342, 351*b*, 351*t*
　approach to 350
　causes of generalized 350, 351
　characteristics 351*t*
　clinical differences in 351
　differential diagnosis of generalized 350
　generalized 350
Lymphatic obstruction 354
Lymphedema 354
Lymphocytic effusion 24
Lymphoma 351

## M

M2 stroke 206*t*
Machado-Joseph disease 315
　classification of 315*t*
　type 315
Macrocytic anemia 339*f*
Macrocytic hypochromic anemias, causes of 338
Macroglossia 189
Macronodular cirrhosis 158
Macro-ovalocytes 338*f*
Macrovesicular hepatitis 149
Malar rash 364*f*
Malnutrition universal screening tool 243*t*
Marfan's syndrome 88, 99, 126, 345
Mass lesion 48
Massive pleural effusion, left-sided 16*f*
Maturation disorders 343
Mayne's sign 98
Mean corpuscular volume 344
Mechanic's hands 322

Medial medullary syndrome 207, 209f
Medial midbrain syndrome 211f
Medial pontine syndrome 210f
Mediastinal complications 46
Medulla 207
Meningeal irritation, signs of 199
Meningitis, history suggesting 194
Menstrual and obstetric history 4
Mental function, higher 193, 196, 276
Metabolic causes 34
Metabolic diseases 350
Metastasis 351
    spine 264t
Metastatic spine disease 264
Microcytic hypochromic anemia, causes of 337
Microglossia 189
Micronodular cirrhosis 158
Microvesicular hepatitis 149
Middle cerebral artery 215
    lesions 205t
    occlusion 228
    stroke 205
    syndromes 225
Mill wheel murmur 133
Millard-Gubler syndrome 207
Minervini's sign 98
Mitral regurgitation 74, 81b, 82, 82t, 83, 83t, 84, 84t, 85, 85t, 94, 106, 116, 119t
    acute 81b, 84t
    causes of 79
        acute 83
    chronic 80, 81b, 84, 84t
    complications of 82
    etiology of 82
    predominant 84
    primary 77
    secondary 77
    severity of 82, 82t, 105
    signs of acute 84
    symptomatic secondary 84f
Mitral re-stenosis, chances of 85
Mitral stenosis 57, 63, 64, 66-68, 84t, 105, 106
    causes of 58, 64
        angina in 63
    classification of 64t
    complications of 67
    indicators of severity in 70
    management of 71f
    murmur 67, 67f, 102, 102t, 103
    pathogenesis of 62, 62f
    predominant 84
    salient features of 64b
    severity of 63t, 63t, 67, 70, 106
    symptoms of 65
    treatment of 71
    with fibrillation 67
    X-rays of 69f
Mitral valve 63t, 84, 105
    anatomy 70t
    apparatus 80f
        components of 79
    normal 64
    prolapse 85, 85f, 85t
    regurgitation 85
    repair 84
        transcatheter 84
    replacement 72
        indicators of 83
Mixed cirrhosis 158
Modern geriatric giants 360f
Monoarthritis 363
    acute 362
    chronic 362
Mononeuritis multiplex 283
    causes of 279t
Mononeuropathy 283
    causes of 279t
Mononucleosis 149
*Moraxella catarrhalis* 10
Morton and Mahon sign 98
Motor fibers, arrangement of 257f
Motor neuron disease 328, 331
    causes of 331
    etiologies for 329, 329t
    types of 329, 329f
Motor neuronopathy 279, 279t
Motor paralytic bladder 269
Motor response 228
Motor symptoms 281
Motor system 197, 202, 296, 305, 316
    examination 277
Movement
    disorders 331, 332f
    rapid alternating 199
Mucopurulent relapses 10
Mucosal ulcers 364f
Mucous membranes, pallor of 342
Muller's sign 98
Multidisciplinary team 84
Multifocal motor neuropathy 280
Multiple lentigines syndrome 126
Multiple mononeuritis multiplex 279
Multiple mononeuropathy
    causes of 293
    multiplex 279
Multiple sclerosis 221, 233
Multiple ulcers 189, 189f
Multisystem disorder 284
Multivalvular disease 105
Multivalvular heart diseases 104
    causes of 105
Murmur 78, 81t, 121, 133, 133t
    components of 67
    diastolic 75
    differential diagnosis of continuous 121
    mid-diastolic 68

    early
        diastolic 102
        systolic 118
    ejection systolic 102
    grading of 75
    loud 114
    mid-diastolic 67t
    systolic 75
Muscle 198, 299
    disease 322
    power of 296
    weakness, causes of proximal and distal 285
Muscular dystrophies, congenital 326
Musculoskeletal complaint 363, 363t
Musculoskeletal system 361, 365
    regional examination of 366t
Mutational mechanism 313, 314
Myasthenic dysarthria 219
Myelinopathy 324t
Myelofibrosis 172f
Myeloid leukemia, chronic 174f
Myelopathy 366
    causes of 262
    compressive 255, 256, 256t, 287, 287t
    drugs and toxic 262
    noncompressive 256t
Myeloperoxidase 173
Myloneuropathy, causes of 290
Myoclonus 331
Myopathy 324, 366
    congenital 325
    drugs causing 322
    inherited 327f
    statin-induced 322
    types of 284t, 324, 324t
Myositis 361
Myotonia, causes of 323

# N

Nail
    bed 342
    changes 365, 365f, 365t
    spooning of 342
    white 146f
Neck 198
    muscle weakness, causes of 301
Needle liver biopsy 150
Nelson's syndrome 187
Neoplastic
    cells 24
    diseases 350
Nerve
    fibers 279, 279f
    median 291
    peripheral 294, 299
    roots 298
        diseases affecting 292

Nervous system 6, 55, 98, 191, 366
    examination 196, 201, 252, 276
Neurocutaneous markers 223
Neurocutaneous syndromes 271, 271t
Neurofibromatosis 271
Neurogenic claudication 273, 274, 274t
Neuroglycopenic symptoms 244
Neurologic examination 322, 342
Neurological changes 149
Neurological disorder 284
Neuromuscular function, impairment of 152
Neuromuscular junction 299
Neuronopathies 279
Neuropathic disorders 281
Neuropathologic changes 310
Neuropathy 281, 284, 289, 324
    causes 283, 294
        for painful 294
    classification of 280f
    demyelinating 280, 280t
    drugs causing 282
    entrapment 279
    general examination in 282t
    medications causing 283t
    of diabetes, treatment-induced 283
    peripheral 275, 284
    signs of 281t
    symptoms of 281, 281t
    with facial nerve, causes for 299
    with sensory symptoms, cause for 294
Neutrophilic effusion 24
Nevus Araneus 144t
Niacin deficiency, causes of 17
Nicardipine 249
Nitroglycerin 249
Nitroprusside 249
Nodular transformation 149
Nonalcoholic fatty liver disease 165f
Non-bacterial thrombotic endocarditis 242
Noncardiac causes 59, 60
Noncardiac origin 225
Noncompressive myelopathies 255, 256, 256t
Non-dominant hemisphere lesions 243
Noninflammatory disease 362, 362t
Non-neurogenic causes 34
Nontumoral myelopathies 262
Noonan's syndrome 126
Normal apical impulse 57
Normal cardiac chamber pressures 109
Normocytic anemia 339f

Normocytic normochromic anemia, causes of 337
Nothnagel syndrome 206
N-terminal pro-brain natriuretic peptide 25
Number connection test 153f
Nutrition 243
Nystagmus
    common causes of 306
    specific 310
    types of 310, 310t

## O

Obliterative pulmonary hypertension 63
Obliterative vasculitis 219
Obstructive pulmonary disease, classification of acute chronic 11, 11b
Oculomotor symptoms 313, 314
Oligoarthritis 363
Oncotic pressure, decreased 354
Onycholysis 365
Open pneumothorax 38
Open spontaneous pneumothorax 38
Opponens pollicis 285
Optic nerve 230
    proximal part of 230
Optic tract lesion 231f
Oral candidiasis 186f
Oral hyperpigmentation, causes of 179
Organic dusts 30
Oromandibular dystonia 334
Orthopnea 59, 59t
    causes of 58
Osteoarthritis 362
Osteogenesis imperfecta 345
Overflow hypothesis 177

## P

Pain
    abdominal 139
    and temperature, loss of 237
    chest 3, 53, 60
    funicular 273
    pathway of 308f
    radicular 273
    unilateral loss of 237
    vertebral 273
Palatal paralysis 219
Palfrey's sign 98
Palilalia 334
Pallor
    grades of 339, 340t
    over conjunctiva 339f
    with splenomegaly, causes of 174
Palm, hyperpigmentation of 342f
Palmar click 98

Palmar creases 342
Palpable purpura 364f
Palpation 5, 8, 15, 78, 140, 170
    breast bud 146f
Palpitation 53, 54
Panacinar emphysema 11
Panlobular emphysema 11
Pansystolic murmur 79
    causes of 75
Papillae, atrophy of 188
Papillary lesions 80
Papillary muscle 80
    damage to 77
    dysfunction, signs of 84
Paracentesis, diagnostic 180f, 182f
Paradoxical split, basis of 91
Paralysis
    ascending 299t
    causes of 299
    descending 299t
    causes of 299
Paraneoplastic syndrome 292, 294
Paraplegia 262, 271, 272t
    mechanisms of 264, 264t
Parapneumonic pleural effusion 24, 25t
Parasternal heave, causes of left 109
Parasternal pulsations, causes of 77
Parenchymal complications 46
Parietal drift 199
Parinaud syndrome 207
Parkinson plus syndromes 319, 319t
Parkinson's disease 316, 318, 318t
    nonmotor symptoms of 318, 318t
    progression 317f
Parkinsonian disorder, classification of 318
Parkinsonism 331
    atypical 320, 320t
    causes of secondary 319, 319t
    classification of 318f
    motor symptoms of 317
Paroxysmal nocturnal dyspnea 59, 59t
Patent ductus arteriosus 121, 122t, 127
    clinical severity grading of 121t
    complications of 122
    signs of 121
    symptoms of 121
    type of 121
Patent foramen ovale 114
Pedal edema 53, 139, 355
    causes of 8
    mechanism of 9f
Pelvic examination 342
Pemberton's sign 31

Pendular nystagmus 309
Penny sign 98
Percheron stroke, artery of 207
Percussion 54, 78, 141
    note, types of 20, 20t
Percutaneous coronary intervention 84
Pericardial cavity 21
Pericarditis 61
Periodic acid-Schiff 173
Peripheral edema, causes of 355f
Peripheral nerves, sites for palpation of 294f
Peripheral nervous system, affecting 292
Peripheral neuropathy
    diagnosis of 297
    systemic causes for 289
Peripheral origin, vestibular nystagmus of 306
Peritonitis 180
    classification of 178
Periumbilical veins 171
Persistent palpitations 60
Petechiae 150, 342
Peutz-Jeghers syndrome 187
Phentolamine 249
Phlyctenular conjunctivitis 29
Physical agents 262
Physical functional capacity 358
Pierre-Marie-Foix syndrome 207
Pin head method 145f
Pitting 365
Plantar extensor 268
Plasma volume 338
Plasmapheresis
    indications of 301, 301t
    substances removed by 301
Platybasia 265
Platynychia, causes of 173
Pleura, lymphatic drainage of 16, 19, 20f
Pleural cavity 21
Pleural complications 46
Pleural effusion 15, 17, 24, 28, 28t, 49, 366
    causes of 22t
    malignant 26
    causes of predominant
        left sided 18
        right sided 18
    classification of 22t
    diagnostic algorithm of 19, 19f
    lymphadenopathy in 18
    malignant 17, 27
        treatment of 27, 27f
    with trachea, causes of 17
Pleural fibrosis 16
Pleural fluid 18, 21, 24, 25
    analysis 23
    biochemical investigations in 24
    eosinophilia 19
    causes of 19

formation of 21
increased production of 21
microscopic appearance of 24
normal 21
parameters, interpretation of 23t
production, causes of increased 21
Pleural transudate, treatment of 25f
Pleurodesis 24
Pneumothorax 36, 37, 48, 49
    classification of 37f
    closed 38
    complications of 39
    etiologies of 37
    physical signs of 37
    right-sided 39f
    spontaneous 37
    traumatic 37
    types of spontaneous 38, 38f
Polyarteritis nodosa 204
Polyarthritis 363
    acute 362
    chronic 363
Polycythemia, secondary 11
Poly-Hill sign 326f
Polymicrobial bacterascites 179
Polymyositis 323
Polyneuropathy 283
    approach to 280, 280t
    causes of 279t
    types of 282, 283f
Polyradiculopathy 283
    causes of 331
Polyuria 60
Pons 207
Pontains murmur 133
Porphyria 297
Portal ascites 183
Portal hypertension 150, 155, 155f, 157, 163, 183
    chronic 157
    classification of 155f, 165f
    hepatic causes of 171
    increases 171
Portal vein
    anatomy of 151
    thrombosis 149, 155f
Portal-systemic encephalopathy, chronic 148f
Portosystemic anastomosis 163, 164f
Portosystemic shunts, sites of 151
Posterior cerebral artery syndrome, clinical features of 213
Posterior circulation, signs of 245t
Posterior column syndrome 258, 258t
Posterior spinal artery syndrome 259
Posterolateral column
    disease 259t
    syndrome 259

Posthepatic causes 171
Post-obstructive bronchiectasis 44
Post-radiation vasculopathy 242
Post-spinal artery syndrome 259t
Post-triscupid shunts 124
Post-tussive suction 44, 45
Postural hypotension 300
    causes of 34
Postural tremor 333
Pott's disease 29
Precordium 133
Predominant motor involvement, causes for 300
Prehepatic causes 171
Prehepatic portal hypertension 156, 156t
Preserved presystolic accentuation, mechanism of 67
Preserved ratio impaired spirometry 13
Presystolic accentuation 67
Primitive reflexes 198, 248
Prinzmetal angina 79
Prophylaxis 130, 131
    of infective endocarditis, indications for 130
Proprioceptive sensation 237
Protein 22
Pruritogens 345
Pseudobronchiectasis 44
Pseudobulbar palsy 222, 222t, 242, 245
    causes of 245, 245t
    non-vascular causes of 240
Pseudochylothorax 23, 23t
Pseudochylous effusion 23
Pseudohypertrophy, causes of 325
Pseudoxanthoma elasticum 345
Psoriasis 365, 365f
Ptosis, causes for 222
Puddle sign 176, 177f
Pulmonary area, cause of diastolic murmur in 75
Pulmonary arteriovenous shunting 353
Pulmonary artery 127
    hypertension 9
    signs of 106
Pulmonary blood flow 123, 124
Pulmonary field changes 83
Pulmonary function tests 10b
Pulmonary hypertension 106, 121, 131, 132
    chronic 63
    passive 63
    reactive 63
    types of 63
Pulmonary regurgitation 104, 104t
Pulmonary stenosis 94, 94t, 127
Pulmonary valve 105

Pulmonary venous hypertension 68f
    signs of 70
    pressure 70
Pulsatile liver, causes of 169, 349
Pulse 21, 78, 81b
    abnormal 35
    irregularly irregular 75
    causes for 58
    pressure 79
Pulsus
    alternans 35, 35f
    paradoxus 21, 35
Pupils 228
Purpura 150
Pursed lip breathing 10
Pyogenic infection 264, 264t
Pyogenic spondylitis 264
Pyopneumothorax, causes of 39b
Pyramidal drift 199
Pyramidal tract 259, 259t

## Q

Quadriplegia, causes of 260, 260t
Quetelet index 243
Quincke's sign 98

## R

Radial nerve 291
Rapid eye movement 317
Raymond syndrome 207
Rectal examination 342
Recurrent fall, causes of 224, 225b
Recurrent pleural effusion, causes of 18
Recurrent pneumothorax, causes for 39
Red blood cells 344
Red cell volume 338
Re-expansion pulmonary edema 28
Reflex 198, 202, 277, 296
    arc tested, main part of 300
    neurogenic bladder 269
    superficial 198
    tachycardia 79
Reiter's syndrome 188
Renal failure 366
Renin-angiotensin-aldosterone 9
Reperfusion therapy 236
Respiration, accessory muscles of 34
Respiratory diseases 9f
    differential diagnosis of 47
Respiratory movements 5
Respiratory pattern 228
Respiratory rate 54
Respiratory system 1, 35, 37, 43, 49, 87, 199, 202, 317, 366
    examination 45, 254, 278

Respiratory tree, normal components of 12f
Restless legs syndrome 334
Restrictive cardiomyopathy 180, 180t, 181
Restrictive ventricular septal defect 117
Reticular activating system, role of 244
Retinal veins, sausaging of 342
Retinopathy, mild hypertensive 229f
Rheumatic aortic regurgitation 104, 104t
    stenosis 89
Rheumatic arthritis 61
Rheumatic chorea 169, 333
Rheumatic fever 62
    signs of 130
Rheumatic heart disease 85, 85t
    prophylaxis for 62, 62t
Rheumatoid arthritis 99, 362
Rheumatological disorders 366, 366t
Rheumatology 363t
Rhomboid glossitis, median 188, 188f
Riboflavin deficiency 187
Right lateral medullary syndrome 205f
Right ventricle 90
Risenmenger's heart disease 123
Roger's murmur 133
Romberg's test 199, 278
Rosenbach's sign 98
Roth's criteria 18b
Rubella syndrome 126
Rubral tremor 309
Rytand's murmur 133

## S

Sacral cord 261
Sailer's sign 98
Scalene lymph nodes, palpate for 16
Scar
    in apex beat 75
    types of 74
Scimitar syndrome 111
Scleritis 365
Scleromalacia perforans 365
Scoliosis 33, 34
    causes of 33
    types of 33
Scrofuloderma 29
Second-order syndrome 239
Seizures 195
Sensation, primary 199
Sensory
    atonic bladder 268
    axonal neuropathy 283
    dysfunction 194

loss 282
    area of 239f
motor neuropathy, syndrome of subacute 282
neuronopathy 279, 279t
paralytic bladder 269
symptoms 281
system 199, 305
    examination 278
Sentinel bleeds 220
Septum, development of 118f
Serum
    bilirubin level 348, 348t
    biochemistry 150
    immunology 150
Serum-ascites albumin gradient 182, 182t
Shawl sign 322
Shelly's sign 98
Sherman sign 98
Shifting dullness 176, 177f
Shone's complex 110
Shone's syndrome 110f
Shoulder 198
SIADH 247, 247t
Sickle cell 338
Significant lymphadenopathy 351
Sinus arrhythmia 64, 64f
Sinusoidal obstructive syndrome 149
Sjogren's syndrome 365
Skin 29, 342
    changes 363t
    hands, and eyes, examination of 363
    responses 291
Skinfold thickness 17
Skull 199, 278
Sleep behavior disorder 317
Small airways disease 9
Small muscle wasting of hand, causes of 287
Smear, peripheral 340
Smoking 242
Soft murmur, causes of 82
Soft neurological signs 199
Spastic paraparesis 269
    causes of 259
    differential diagnosis of 269
Spastic tongue without fasciculations 189
Speech 223, 276, 309
    areas 216
        types of 216t
    defects 214
        types of 214t
    genesis of 216f
Spider nevi 144, 144t, 145f
    demonstration of 145f
Spider telangiectasia 144t
Spiderangiomas 144t
Spinal accessory 197

Spinal cord 254, 294
  disease 252, 257, 257f
    types of 255, 255f
  involvement, classical features
    of 255
  level 255
  segments 255t
  syndromes 258f, 259f
  syphilis affect 264
  tracts of 254f
  vascular supply of 255f
  watershed zones of 262
Spinal deformity 272
Spinal osteomyelitis, infectious
    causes of 268
Spinal pain, types of 273
Spinal shock, stage of 273
Spinal tuberculosis 29, 264, 264t
  site of 263f
  tetraplegia in 264, 264t
Spinal tumors 262
Spine 199, 278
Spinocerebellar ataxia 313f
Spleen 171, 173, 174, 174t
  characteristics of normal 174t
  normal 174
Splenomegaly 171, 342
  causes of 173, 174t
  with ascites, causes of 163
  with lymphadenopathy, cause
    of 175
Splinter hemorrhages 365
Spondyloarthropathies
    demyelinating 262
Spontaneous bacterial empyema 25
Spontaneous pneumothorax,
    causes of secondary 37b
Stable angina 79
Staccato speech 219, 241
Steatohepatitis 149
Steatotic liver disease sub-
    classification 166
Steven Johnson syndrome 188
Stills murmur 133
Stomach carcinoma 158
Stony dullness 20
Straight back syndrome 29
Stroke 201, 202, 235b, 333
  anterior circulation 245
  chameleons 231
  characteristics 242
  classification of 203f
  drugs causing 232
  in cancer, mechanism of 242, 242t
  in young, causes for 204, 204t, 235
  localization of 205t
  malignancy produce 232
  management of 250f
  mimickers 231
  neuroimaging in 205f
  risk factor for 203, 203t
  types of 202

Structural heart diseases 72
Structural lesion, probable
    location of 310
Subarachnoid hemorrhage 204, 220
Subcutaneous nodules,
    differential diagnosis of 365
Subsequent neurological
    pathology 219
Subvalvular aortic
  sclerosis 96
  stenosis 89
Subvalvular thickening 70
Succussion splash, conditions
    causing 21
Sudden loss of vision, causes of 221
Superior vena cava
  obstruction of 154f, 155f
  syndrome 31
Surgery, indications for 110
Surgical aortic valve replacement 93
Suzman's sign 230
Sweating 60
Symmetric proprioceptive sensory
    loss without weakness 282
Symmetric sensory loss 282
    without weakness 282
Sympathetic symptoms 244
Syncope 53
Synovitis 361
Syphilis 189, 351
  tertiary 62
Syphilitic aortic regurgitation 104, 104t
Systemic disorder 262, 333
Systemic lupus erythematosus 364f
Systemic sclerosis 364f

## T

Takayasu's arteritis 99, 204
  clinical features of 223
Tamponade 180, 180t, 181
Taste sensation 328
Temperature sensation 308f
Tender hepatomegaly 169
  causes of 168, 169t
Tender liver, causes of 349
Tender spleen, causes of 175
Tenosynovitis 361, 365
Tension pneumothorax 38, 38t
Tetralogy of Fallot 125, 125f, 125t, 127
  associations of 124
  complications of 125
  components of 124
  signs of 124
  surgical
    management of 125
    shunts in 125

Thalamus, extensive lesion of 237
Thalassemias 338
Therapeutic paracentesis,
    indications for 184
Therapeutic thoracocentesis 16
Thinker's sign 10
Third-order syndrome 239
Thoracic cord lesion 260
Thoracic neoplasms 353
Thrombosis, risk factors for 224, 226t
Thrombotic stroke 204, 204t, 226f
Thrombotic therapy, acute 236
Thyroid disease 366
Tic, types 334
Titubation 309
Toluidine blue 173
Tone 197, 316
Tongue 189
  alligator 189
  angry looking 189
  bald 187, 188f, 341f
  beefy red 186, 186f
  black-colored 187f
  blue-colored 187, 187f
  bluish red color 187
  changes in movements of 189
  characteristics of 186
  chewing 189
  cobblestone 189
  crocodile 189
  deviation of 189
  dry 188
    red 188, 189f
  examination of 186
  fissured 188, 188f
  geographic 187, 188f
  inflammation of 342
  lizard 189
  magenta red color of 187f
  moist 188
  mushroom like 189
  pale 186
  paralysis 219
  purple color 187
  pushes 241
  raspberry 187
  red color 186
  scrotal 188f
  slate-blue 187
  strawberry 187, 187f
  tremors of 189
  trombone 189
  white 186
Total iron-binding capacity 344
Toxic fumes 30
Trail's sign 31
Transcortical aphasia, mixed 217
Transcortical sensory 217
Transcorticalmotor 217
Transient ischemic attack 213
  types of 213
Transjugular intrahepatic
    portosystemic shunt 25f

Transjugular liver biopsy 182
Transudative effusion 18t, 22
Trapped lung 28
Traube's sign 98
Tremor 333
  classification of 333
Tricuspid opening snap 66
Tricuspid regurgitation 82, 82t, 105, 119t
Tricuspid stenosis 105
Tricuspid valve 105, 196
Tripod sign 10
Trisomy 21 126
Tromner's sign 270f
Tropical splenomegaly syndrome 175b
Tubercular lesion 268
Tubercular meningitis,
    neurological complications
    of 220
Tubercular ulcer 189
Tuberculosis 29, 264, 351
  active and healed 46, 47f
  causes ascites 180
  complications of 46
  pleural effusion, management
    of 27f
Tuberculous mastitis 29
Tuberculous pleural effusion 26
Tubular bronchial breathe sounds 32
Tumor 333
  embolism 242
Turner syndrome 126

## U

Ulcer 188
  on leg 364f
  recurrent 189
  single 189
  traumatic 189
Ulnar nerve 291
  branches and supply 288f
  palsy
    muscles affected in 288
    signs of 288
Uncal herniation 228
Uninhibited bladder 268
Unstable angina 79
Upper extremity 199
Upper limb 162
Upper lobe
  mass lesion of 48
  pulmonary fibrosis 33
Upper motor neuron 206, 282, 330t
  causes 260
  facial
    nerve palsy, bilateral 297, 297t
    palsy 236

involvement
	signs of 330
	symptoms of 330
	weakness 237, 237t
Upper respiratory tract examination 4
Urethritis 366

## V

V sign 322
Vacuolar myelopathy, differential diagnosis for 270
Valley sign 325f
Valsalva maneuver 78f, 273, 301t
	sympathetic activity 78f
Valve
	anatomy 64, 65
	area 63
	disease 131, 132
	leaflets, damage to 77
	lesions 82
Valvular aortic
	sclerosis 95, 96
	stenosis 89
Valvular aortosclerosis 95t
Valvular diseases
	effect of 92t
	surgical management for 106
Valvular heart disease 57, 60

Van der Hoeve's syndrome 345
Vapors 30
Varicose bronchiectasis 44f
Vascular claudication 273, 274, 274t
Vascular complications 46
Vascular disease 353
Vascular malformation 333
Vascular spiders 144t, 171
Vascular supply 213, 214
Vasculitis 30
Vasodilators 93
Venous hum 122, 122t
	characteristics of 154
Venous pooling 34
Venous-to-arterial embolism 242
Ventral pontine syndrome 210f
Ventricular premature beats 58
Ventricular septal defect 83, 116, 119t
	absent murmur in 118
	associations of 116
	causes of 118
	complications of 119
	correction 120t
	moderate 119
	signs of 117
	spontaneous closure of 117
	surgical correction of 120

symptoms of 117
	treatment of 120f
	types of 116, 117f
Ventricular septum, development of 117
Vertebra, adjacent 263f
Vertebral artery bruit 241f
Vertebral bodies 255t
	corresponding 255
Vertebral deformities, types of 272
Vertebral lesion 263
Vessel infarcts, large 232
Vestibulocochlear nerve 197
Vestibulo-ocular reflexes 228
Vincent's angina 79, 188
Virchow node 353
Visual disorder 148f
Visual path, sites of lesion of 230
Visual system, affecting 292
Vital 140
	examination 54
	signs 276
Vitamin $B_{12}$ 295
	deficiency 295
Vocal fremitus 5
	causes of
		decreased 35
		increased 35
Vocal resonance 5
Volume deficiency hypothesis 176

von Sölder phenomenon 328
von Willebrand syndrome 89

## W

Waardenburg syndrome 271
Wallenberg syndrome 207
Warm hands 21
Water hammer 100f
	pulse 100
Weakness 193
	asymmetric proximal 282
	distribution of 193
	progression of 193
Weber's syndrome 206
Wernicke's area 216
Wernicke's encephalopathy 233
Wernicke's sensory 217
Wheeze 3
Whooping cough 189
Wide pulse pressure 121
Wilkins score 70t
William's syndrome 95, 126
Wilson's disease 333
Wing-beating tremor 309
Winterbottom sign 353
Withdrawal seizures, treatment and prevention of 306
Woody dullness 20
Wrist 198